Health Assessment for Professional Nursing
A Developmental Approach

Second Edition

With the assistance of:

Mary K Dempsey-Noreika, R.N., M.S., F.N.P.,C.
Executive Director, Twin Tier Home Health Services, Inc.
Binghamton, New York

Mark A. Goodman, M.D.
Assistant Professor of Orthopedics
University of Pittsburgh
Pittsburgh, Pennsylvania

Jane McGuire, R.N., M.S.N., F.N.P.
Lecturer
State University of New York at Binghamton
Binghamton, New York

Elizabeth A. Phelps, R.N., M.N.
Clinical Specialist in Gerontology
Binghamton, New York

Toni Tripp-Reimer, R.N., Ph.D.
Associate Professor
College of Nursing
University of Iowa
Iowa City, Iowa

Linda Harrison Zoeller, R.N.,C., M.P.H.
Assistant Professor
Department of Public Health Nursing
College of Nursing
University of Illinois at Chicago
Chicago, Illinois

Health Assessment for Professional Nursing
A Developmental Approach

Second Edition

Gloria J. Block, R.N., M.S.N., F.N.P.,C.
Presently in private practice
Endwell Family Physicians
Endwell, New York
Former Assistant Professor
Family Nurse Practitioner Program
State University of New York at Binghamton
Binghamton, New York

JoEllen Wilbur Nolan, R.N.,C., Ph.D.
Assistant Professor
Department of Public Health Nursing
College of Nursing
University of Illinois at Chicago
Chicago, Illinois

 APPLETON-CENTURY-CROFTS/Norwalk, Connecticut

To Jon—with all my love and respect—G. J. B.

*To my family, Paul and Katie, and to the family nurse practitioner/
clinician students I have had the pleasure of knowing.—J. W. N.*

0-8385-3661-1

86 87 88 89 90 / 10 9 8 7 6 5 4 3 2 1

Prentice-Hall of Australia, Pty. Ltd., Sydney
Prentice-Hall Canada, Inc.
Prentice-Hall Hispanoamericana, S.A., Mexico
Prentice-Hall of India Private Limited, New Delhi
Prentice-Hall International (UK) Limited, London
Prentice-Hall of Japan, Inc., Tokyo
Prentice-Hall of Southeast Asia (Pte.) Ltd., Singapore
Whitehall Books Ltd., Wellington, New Zealand
Editora Prentice-Hall do Brasil Ltda., Rio de Janeiro

Library of Congress Cataloging in Publication Data

Block, Gloria J., 1952–
    Health assessment for professional nursing.

    Bibliography: p.
    Includes index.
    1. Physical diagnosis. 2. Nursing. I. Nolan,
JoEllen W., 1946–   II. Title. [DNLM: 1. Nursing
Process.   WY 100 B651h]
    RT48.B56 1986   616.07'54   86–1189
    ISBN 0-8385-3661-1

Design: Jean Sabato-Morley
Cover: M. Chandler Martylewski
PRINTED IN THE UNITED STATES OF AMERICA

Contents

Preface to the Second Edition

A second edition is an exciting opportunity for authors. It provides a chance for evaluation, refinement, and expansion of the work done in the first edition. Much thought and planning went into the changes and additions made for the second edition. The result of an extensive effort is a markedly improved product. The authors were very pleased with the acceptance and success of the first edition. Over the last five years the authors' many students and colleagues spent both time and effort feeding back thoughts about strengths, weaknesses, and ideas for future editions. This information helped the authors plan an organized and comprehensive revision and expansion of the book. A description of these exciting changes follows.

The layout of each chapter remains essentially the same. In each physical assessment chapter an entire new section has been added discussing the developmental changes of that system throughout the lifespan. The developmental focus was a favorite feature of the first edition. For this edition we have expanded that content significantly. For example, when one assesses the eye, it is important to consider the age of the patient while doing this assessment. An infant does not have 20/20 vision during the first year of life. An elderly person might have decreased peripheral vision. Noting these variations makes a great deal of difference in what the nurse might expect to find when she conducts her examination of the eye. A well known gerontological clinical-nurse specialist helped us with the aging content throughout the book. The authors felt that having the knowledge of experts in this field would enhance the content of the book regarding the aging population. The information was especially helpful in each physical assessment chapter.

Another helpful feature within each chapter is the summary outline of a screening examination for the system under consideration. This helps the reader differentiate the examination measures to be utilized with the well patient versus the more extensive examination that is necessary with the ill patient. It also differentiates those examination techniques that are to be used exclusively with children versus those used with adults.

Each chapter has been changed depending on its needs; clarification and expansion took place throughout the text. Charts and tables were added to help the reader synthesize the knowledge being presented. Each chapter was updated with the most recent data. For instance, in Chapter 9, the latest figures for acceptable blood pressures were used, and in Chapter 2, updated Metropolitan Life Insurance figures for men's and women's height and weight have been added.

The artwork for the second edition has been expanded and changed extensively. Many photographs were added to further illustrate the text. Where new techniques were discussed within a chapter, new photographs were included to illustrate these points. Many of the figures drawn for the first edition were redrawn to elaborate detail which the authors felt would make it easier for the students to learn the assessment process. The new artwork and photography add an exciting dimension to the second edition.

The final new addition to this book is Chapter 16—"The Prenatal Patient." Many students and colleagues recommended that a chapter such as this be included. Although the chapter varies somewhat in style from the others, the authors agreed it was information that was needed in a health assessment textbook. The chapter includes discussions on fetal development and maternal changes during pregnancy. An extensive section on these topics was included because the authors felt it would help the beginning student understand why certain history and physical assessments were necessary at various times during the pregnancy. For the student who may have already studied maternal–child nursing, this review of the physiological changes in the mother and baby may be helpful. A section on the psychosocial needs of the mother and father is also included. The authors feel that a nurse should not consider her assessment complete until the parents' feelings about the pregnancy, its progression, and the upcoming changes in their lives have been addressed. The last section of the chapter gives the student some general guidelines about the actual assessment of the prenatal patient. This section includes the appropriate history and physical data needed throughout the pregnancy. Many students in both graduate and undergraduate programs spend time in settings with pregnant patients. This chapter provides valuable information in order to meet the needs of these patients and their families.

Now that this edition is complete, it is the readers' turn to take the next step. While using this textbook, it is the authors hope that our students and colleagues will be as helpful to us once again in evaluating the effectiveness of our book. Many of the changes and improvements made were in response to our readers' suggestions. We feel we have made some very exciting changes in this edition and at the same time are continuing to address the challenges and growth of the nursing profession.

Gloria J. Block
JoEllen Wilbur Nolan

Preface to the First Edition

Nursing and nurses are growing—qualitatively! The role of the professional nurse is changing in all health care settings. Nurses are being called upon to make in-depth nursing assessments. In order to do this, they need tools at their disposal to validate their findings. A sound data base is needed by all nurses upon which to base assessments. The purpose of this book is to provide the professional nurse or the professional nursing student with the knowledge to elicit this important data.

Nurses have special qualities that often direct them into nursing. Generally they are excellent listeners and observers. Their basic education should and does nurture these characteristics. Nursing, however, as a discipline, determines its own scientific data base that has evolved far beyond listening and observing. Professional nurses are functioning more independently and making more autonomous decisions. Taking the patient's blood pressure was once the sole purview of the physician. Over the years the scope of nursing practice has expanded far beyond measuring blood pressures to the monitoring and use of complex sophisticated equipment. The nurse is expected to evaluate the patient's condition and response to increasingly complicated modes of treatment. This evaluation requires a greater knowledge of and responsibility for determining the state of health of the patient. Another word for the phrase "determining the state of health of the patient" is assessment. Assessment is the first phase of the nursing process. The level and depth of nursing assessment is expanding to meet the greater expectations of the nurse. Tools and techniques are being used to make more complex assessments. For example, the stethoscope once used for blood pressures and apical pulses is used now also to separate normal vesicular breath sounds from ronchii or normal heart sounds from murmurs.

The nursing history encompasses the health history. Eliciting the health history and performing a physical examination are today a part of nursing. Together they provide the data for the nursing assessment. It is a goal of this book to provide information for the professional nurse seeking to attain these skills.

It is the belief of the authors that they offer a unique approach to a health assessment text. Much thought went into this book before any writing was begun. The authors have had experience in teaching and practice. All three have taught health assessment to undergraduate and graduate nursing students as well as nurses in continuing education programs. All three practice as family nurse practitioners to maintain their role as providers in the nursing profession. All three were once students learning health assessment themselves. Because of this transition from student to educator and practitioner, the authors feel they have the expertise to present the right amount of knowledge in the most appropriate fashion. This book represents the culmination of their efforts.

A developmental framework with an integrated approach was selected as a design for the book. This has two benefits. First, health assessment can be discussed by each body system and each system can then be developed according to particular concerns and differences of each age group. Secondly, the book's structure can be easily utilized in an integrated curriculum model in a school of nursing. Thus, each system can be presented as it occurs in the sequence of the curriculum design. If the course is taught independently in a nursing curriculum, the framework works well, too.

The developmental framework was chosen by the authors as it offers the most adaptable design for their beliefs about patients and health. The patient is envisioned as a holistic being composed of biopsychosocial needs. The nurse assumes "wholeness" and attempts to make assessments that include biopsychosocial facets. The person then is assessed within their life cycle as a whole person with integrated complex needs. The nurse assesses the relative health of the person. Thus, the patient receives the benefits of health assessment implemented with this philosophy as a guide.

For this book the term "health assessment" was selected for two reasons. Firstly, the authors believe that nurses do more than "illness assessment." The nurse who evaluates her patients holistically looks at where they are situated on a continuum of health. It is as important to emphasize the patient's health as well as his illness. For this reason this book's emphasis is on "normal" health assessment with "abnormal" findings highlighted appropriately to the needs of the student learning this process. The goal of this book is not to make an expert diagnostician out of the reader, but to give her enough knowledge about health assessment to substantiate the actions she takes in her nursing decisions.

Secondly, the term health assessment was selected because it is more comprehensive than physical assessment or physical diagnosis, phrases commonly used in the past to describe this process. Health assessment features a holistic approach. It not only includes the results of the physical examination, but also what the patient tells you about his wellness or illness. In other words, the term health assessment includes the process of history taking and physical examination.

The following statement is often professed to students on the first day of their health assessment course. "If you can learn to elicit a thorough and accurate history, you can be almost certain about what you will discover on the physical examination." The authors believe this statement to be entirely true. With that in mind we have selected to emphasize and reemphasize the history taking process throughout the book.

The first chapter is devoted exclusively to the health history.

This chapter begins by reviewing some basic information about listening, questioning, and providing a supportive environment for the patient while collecting the data. This section not only discusses the principles of history taking, but also provides the student with suggestions for questioning the patient most effectively.

The components of the health history are then developed at length. The features of this chapter which give this book an extensive nursing emphasis are the psychosocial and nutritional sections. As nurses, we believe that developing these areas in the history is essential to evaluating the patient's overall health status. Therefore, within the chapter, the developmental, sexual, and nutritional histories are discussed according to every age and stage throughout the lifespan. Each section includes the necessary content that the student needs to be familiar with to explore specific areas with the patient.

In addition, each section provides examples of questions that can be used to elicit the data. The authors find this especially helpful for students who are struggling with how to ask the patient about his perception of his achievement of developmental tasks or feelings concerning his sexuality. It is not hard to convince students that this information is necessary to obtain, but they do seem to have a great deal of difficulty knowing how to elicit the data. Therefore, the emphasis is on the "how to's" of eliciting the data in these less tangible areas of the health history.

In addition to the chapter devoted to the health history, there are short histories at the beginning of each chapter reviewing the body system being discussed. It is important for the student to understand that each system of the body when being evaluated has more than the physical findings which contribute to the final assessment of the condition of that system. For instance, when a stethoscope is placed on a patient's chest and abnormal breath sounds are heard, and whether the patient has a previous diagnosis of congestive heart failure or has had an elevated temperature for three days, will channel the nurse's thinking about the nature of the problem. It is the combination of the history of the presenting complaint and the physical findings that lead the nurse to her assessment.

Each physical assessment chapter is organized in a similar fashion. There are four major sections: the historical review of the system being discussed, an overview of the necessary anatomy and physiology to assess the organs involved, the methods of physical examination used to evaluate the system and an example of how to record a chief complaint, history of present illness and physical findings of a problem commonly occurring in that system.

The repetitive format of each physical assessment chapter reinforces the necessity of a systematic approach to a physical examination. This is most important for the novice learning the process of health assessment.

Another unique feature of each chapter is the inclusion of transcultural aspects and physical features of various populations in the world. A nursing leader who is doctorally prepared in anthropology and sociology has incorporated this type of information throughout the book. All these very extensive discussions and highlighted areas throughout the book reflect the authors' holistic approach to health assessment with its variations throughout the life cycle.

"Nursing means caring, comforting, counseling, teaching, guiding."* Caring and comforting are a great part of what this book is all about, for to take care of and give comfort to, a nurse must first listen, touch, and observe. Of all those whom the patient sees for health care, the nurse is likely to be the most consistent contact and the most available to evaluate the patient with tender compassionate interest.

Much has been written and continues to be written about the changing role of the professional nurse in the delivery of health care. The entire system is in a state of dynamic change at every level. These changes are especially apparent in legislative enactments, professional education, third-party payment demands, and the redistribution of responsibility among providers of health care. The role of the nurse has already changed a great deal. As the entire system changes, the function of the professional nurse will continue to develop. It is absolutely essential for the nurse to recognize how much the role of the professional nurse has already changed, if she is to be a full participant in the delivery of health care and especially if she is to be a creative contributor shaping still other changes which are bound to come.

The very fact that you, the nurse, have begun to read this book and study this subject, indicates that you acknowledge your awareness that the changes have indeed taken place and that you are making the professional decision to add to your learning and your skills, to the end that you will be doing all in your power to ready yourself for the professional demands of the nurses' role.

This knowledge can be incorporated into any area of nursing practice. Some nurses may find certain portions of the content more appropriate to their specialty. However, the book is written to meet the needs of the nurse in any health care setting. The nurse in a cardiac intensive care unit may become very proficient at listening to heart and breath sounds, but the very fact that she has the knowledge to evaluate psychosocial status or a skin rash reinforces the concept of holistic nursing care.

The nurse practicing in a primary care setting will probably use this information for more generalized assessments as opposed to the nurse who has a highly specialized area of expertise. The authors wrote the book with the intention of meeting the needs of the professional nurse in any clinical setting.

Ideally, the book should be a valuable tool for nurses and nurses-to-be . . . and of equal worth to their teachers. This means that far more is envisioned than a "How To" teaching manual. The book, on the one hand should serve the already present desire of students to acquire new professional skills, without losing sight, on the other hand, of the importance of serving as a stimulus to the generation of ideas by the students themselves. The new nursing role calls for a greater degree of creativity and originality than was historically permitted.

The book, therefore, should be seen as opening doors for nurses in their expanding roles in the developing system of delivery of overall health care. "Expanding" is just the right word. The system is

---

* Mauksch, Ingeborg. "The Future of Nursing." Presentation delivered in Binghamton, New York, May 1979.

expanding. The nurses' roles are expanding. The book, too, should be designed for expansion . . . to keep pace with the dynamism of the nursing profession.

Nurses need to win the right to practice in settings which traditionally have provided little room for such nursing functions. To be successful, the book ought to help individual nurses learn to accept new responsibilities, to be comfortable where reliance is placed on their shoulders in unaccustomed professional areas, and finally, to be pioneers . . . that is, to show leadership in encouraging other professionals to accept them in wider roles.

The intention of this book is to give our nursing colleagues and nursing students the information they will need to be "astute assessors." Lacking this knowledge is like not having frosting on a layer cake. The cake might be adequate without it, but the frosting adds a flavor and richness that completes the taste. This book is for nurses who want to remain nurses!

Gloria J. Block
JoEllen Wilbur Nolan
Mary K Dempsey

Acknowledgments

Books such as this one never get completed without the efforts of many people. We are grateful to our models Jamie Allen, Lauren and Ellen Appel, April Button, Lynn Dunn, the Elinoff family, Johann Fiore, Jeff France, Kara Geller, Jon Harris, Katie Nolan, Dave Samsonik, Maggie Shea, and Chris Wang; our typist, Mary Ann Samsonik; our nursing and physician colleagues for their consultation, Jon Harris, Victor Elinoff, Johann Fiore, and Judy Czerenda; our friend, Barb Salisbury, and everyone at 415; and our families for their endless support and love.

For the new illustrations in this edition, we wish to thank Sue Cottrill, Deirdre Alla McConathy, Robert F. Parshall, Diana Martia Salaty, and William R. Schwarz from the Department of Biocommunication Arts, University of Illinois at Chicago. We would also like to thank Stephen Appel, from Binghamton, New York, for the new photography for the second edition.

A special thanks goes to our Editor, Marion Kalstein-Welch and our Production Editor, Kathy Drasky.

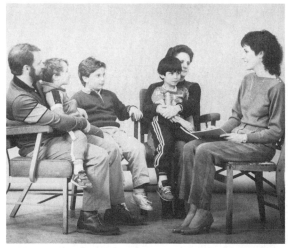

1

The Health History

The information obtained for a complete patient assessment includes a health history, physical findings, and laboratory data. The history is the first and most important part of the data base. It serves as the foundation for the physical and laboratory data by directing the examiner toward the systems that should be examined. If a patient were to give a history of sore throat and rhinorrhea, the nurse would focus on (but not limit herself to) an examination of the ear, nasopharyngeal area, and neck nodes. A detailed neurologic examination would be neither necessary nor appropriate. In addition to its influence on the course of the examination, the history gives meaning to the physical findings. Wheezing heard in the chest of an adult patient can be the result of a variety of causes. Knowledge of a 30-year history of heavy tobacco use might lead to the assessment: "Wheezes as a result of smoking." Without the support of historical data this wheezing would have been an isolated finding and the cause would have been difficult to determine. It is hard to overemphasize the importance of the history. It is fair to say that at least 80 percent of all diagnoses could be accurately made on the basis of history alone.

At this point it is important to distinguish between historical data and data obtained on physical examination and through laboratory tests. The information given by the patient during the health history is subjective data. This is the patient's perception of his state of health. Subjective data includes health enhancing behaviors as well as a patient's description of a sensation or situation which is interfering with his* physical or mental comfort. On the other hand, objective data are evidence of the patient's state of health identified during the physical examination and from laboratory data. This information the examiner sees, feels, or hears with her own senses. Examples of objective data are palpation of an abdominal mass and a 20/20 vision examination. Subjective data are recorded in the history and objective data are recorded in the physical examination.

This chapter will cover the complete health history, while following chapters will present the historical data and physical examination data pertinent to specific systems. Accompanying each chapter will be a discussion of the developmental changes that occur in the system during the life span. A suggested approach to the screening examination of each system and an example of a written history and physical are presented at the end of each chapter. This book will not address specific laboratory techniques, with the exception of Chapter 12, The Female Genitalia.

THE HEALTH HISTORY

Traditionally, the patient's record contains histories from a variety of disciplines. Under the premise that there is a body of knowledge specific to its field only, each professional group feels it necessary to gather its own information. This results in separate histories for nursing, medicine, nutrition, social service, and so forth. The main disadvantage of this system is that much of the data collected is often redundant. The patient is subjected to many interviews consisting of repetitious questions. Because health care providers feel (perhaps with some justification) that information collected by other professionals does not meet their needs, they ignore it. This was often the case with the traditional nursing history, which was somewhat superficial and included such items as personal belongings brought with the patient to the hospital.

Nurses today are accountable for their actions. If a nurse is to arrive at an assessment,

---

* For the purposes of clarity, throughout the book the nurse (or examiner) will be referred to as "she" or "her" and the patient as "he" or "him."

to determine the course of management or to make an appropriate referral, her decisions must be based on a body of professional knowledge combined with factual information about the patient under consideration. These data are then clearly documented.

The history is the primary source of patient information. It is a comprehensive record of the patient's present and past state of health. It reflects the patient as a complete entity both physically and psychosocially. The format to be presented can be used with the well or ill patient at any point in his development. Once the history is recorded, it gives any reader a clear picture of the patient and his problems. The availability of the history for use by all members of the health care team eliminates the need for repetitious interviews. Another professional may ask the patient to elaborate on a particular area, but then should not independently repeat material already collected. Thus time spent with the patient is used more efficiently, enhancing the interdisciplinary approach to health care.

Obtaining the History

The source of information may be the patient, relatives, friends, old records, or any combination of these. Depending on the nature of the visit or severity of a problem, the history may take up to a half hour to an hour to collect and an additional half hour to an hour to record. Ideally, all the information is collected at the time of the first patient encounter and ongoing data are obtained at subsequent visits. Realistically, time is often limited and portions of the history must be obtained during several patient contacts. The examiner should be sure to record in the notes the important facts to be elaborated on at the next meeting.

To ease the nurse's task, a predetermined format should be used to guide the interview. (See Worksheet for Patient History, Appendix A.) This is merely a skeleton outline and not a check list or series of questions; the nurse's questions should be prompted by her knowledge of patient care. The structure keeps the interview efficient, and the nurse is better able to keep the patient on the topic at hand. This is not to say that flexibility is detrimental. If the patient jumps to the end of the outline, but the information is valuable, he should be allowed to discuss what is on his mind at that time. The gaps can be filled in later. (A completed Worksheet for Patient History is shown in Appendix B.)

Taking occasional notes is necessary due to the volume of information obtained. Before beginning the interview, the examiner should inform the patient that she will be writing down some of the things he tells her. It is often reassuring to patients to know that their words are important enough to be recorded. The examiner should try to maintain eye contact while writing and record just enough to later recall the data. It is important to remember that members of many ethnic groups may not wish to engage in direct eye contact. For example, some Appalachians, American Indians, and Orientals consider direct eye contact impolite and avert their eyes during an interview. This behavior should be respected and not misunderstood as disinterest or dishonesty (Tripp-Reimer & Friedl, 1977).

Approach to the History

The nurse's first contact with the patient is usually for the purpose of obtaining a health history. Ideally, this is time when the nurse establishes a trusting relationship that will facilitate the course of the patient's health care.

The patient can quickly detect whether the nurse is objective or judgmental and nonaccepting. There are several ways the nurse can help to make the patient feel comfortable and gain his trust. First, the interview should be conducted in a private environment. If this is impossible, the nurse should make sure that curtains are pulled and should talk only loud enough for the patient to hear.

Second, the nurse should provide a relaxed setting. This is often accomplished by moving the interviewer's chair out from behind a desk, avoiding an authoritarian approach. When interviewing an elderly client it is best to sit in front of the person in order to be more easily heard and understood.

Third, the nurse should make appropriate introductions, acknowledging all persons and their roles. If a young child has come with his parent, the nurse should be sure to recognize the child as well as the adult by name. Initially the nurse should address the person by his first and last name or by title such as Ms., Miss, Mrs. or Mr. It is important to estab-

lish how the patient would like to be addressed. Calling the elderly person by his or her first name may be viewed by the patient as demeaning. The nurse should tell the patient her name in the way she would like to be addressed in the future.

Fourth, the nurse should determine who will be present during the interview. In the case of the young child it is clear that the person accompanying him to the visit will be present during the entire history. This is not always so with adolescents and adults. Once the nurse is alone with the patient she may ask if he would like to have the person who accompanied him to the visit be present during the interview. This question can be very uncomfortable to the patient if asked in front of the accompanying individual. If the adolescent or adult wishes to be accompanied by a family member the nurse should acknowledge both but seek information from the patient first before seeking clarification or additional information from the family member.

Fifth, if possible, the nurse should take most of the health history prior to the physical exam, while the patient is still fully clothed. This gives the patient a sense of security. The nurse should avoid introducing new questions once the physical exam has begun—the patient may become very anxious if he thinks a problem has been found. In most cases it is best to wait to ask these questions until after the examination is completed, although exceptions do occur and this approach may have to be modified. For example, some children are so frightened when they arrive for health care that it is best to take a brief history and quickly proceed to the physical examination. Once this is completed, the child may be sufficiently relaxed for the parent/guardian to give a detailed explanation of the problem.

There are several additional points to be aware of when approaching children, adolescents, and elderly adults for a health history.

CHILDREN

If the child is very young, the parent or guardian will give the information. Infants usually remain quietly in the parent's arms. An active toddler can be occupied with toys at this time. The toys in the Denver Developmental Screening Test kit (see Chapter 15) can be used or the nurse may gather together age appropriate toys to have on hand for such occasions. A school-age child, and occasionally a pre-schooler, is old enough to make a significant contribution to the history. The nurse should include the child in the questioning and allow him to speak without interruption (Fig. 1.1). The child can provide valuable information about himself, which is often very revealing to his parent. Sensitive areas regarding the child's problem are best discussed with the parent in private. Because the school-age child may become concerned about what is transpiring in his absence, the nurse should talk with the parent when the child is occupied with, for example, vision screening or laboratory work.

ADOLESCENTS

Children in early adolescence are beginning to assert their independence. Their parents however still want to be, and should be, involved in their children's care. The question of confidentiality can be awkward for the nurse. She must weigh the effect that talking with the parents will have on the youth's physi-

cal and mental well-being against the benefits of parental involvement. In order to retain trust, the nurse should discuss with the teenager which information will be shared with the parents and which will be kept confidential. If time allows, it is best to talk with the adolescent and parent separately and together. By late adolescence the teenager's parents are less frequently involved and questions of confidence rarely arise.

ELDERLY ADULTS

The elderly patient is sometimes the most difficult patient from whom to obtain a history. Many factors contribute to this. First, their medical history is often complicated with multiple hospitalizations and a long list of prior illnesses. Second, the individual's recall may be vague, adding more confusion to the history. Some elderly persons have impairment for recent memory, but have vivid recall of past events. Third, some older persons may not share vital information. This too may be due to the patient's failure to understand the

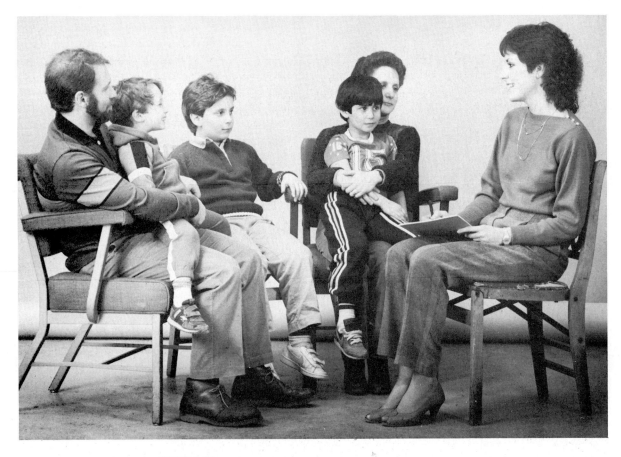

FIGURE 1.1
Interviewing the young family; the children share their feelings.

significance of his symptoms, attributing many to his age, or he may be afraid to have his fears of illness confirmed. Lastly, common physical changes that occur with age can have an impact on the health history interview. For example, the patient may have vision impairment, hearing impairment, or arthritic problems that make it difficult to sit for long periods.

The interview of an elderly patient should be conducted in a well-lighted room without any glare to compensate if the patient has visual deficiencies. When a hearing impairment exists, the nurse should position herself close to the patient's good ear and far enough in front of the patient so he can see her mouth. Also, the room should be without any interfering background noise. All questions asked should be simple and direct. Avoid rewording or repeating the question until the patient has attempted to answer the first time. The need for a complete history at the first encounter must be determined. It may be beneficial to complete the history at a second meeting.

Often the elderly patient feels uncomfortable discussing personal aspects of his life. This may be related to his having been raised in a less open era, and this uneasiness can be magnified if the nurse obtaining his history is young. The nurse should tread slowly into areas that are upsetting, always respecting the patient's privacy. She may need to wait until a firm relationship is established before probing sensitive areas.

Prior to beginning work with the elderly, the nurse should be aware of her own feelings about the aged and the aging process. Today many myths and stereotypes about aging still exist. An example of a myth is that all elderly are senile and forgetful. Estimates made of community elderly in the United Kingdom report that only about 4.1 percent of the population older than 65 years have senile dementia, and 10 to 11 percent have some degree of dementia (Kay, 1972). Another myth is that all elderly are inflexible and unable to change. The ability of the older person to change is dependent on his earlier life experiences, personality, physical health, and social supports. Most people change and remain open to change throughout life. If the nurse ascribes to any of these myths she may structure her interview in such a way that she could miss important pieces of information.

Finally, remember that the patient is your primary source for information. If statements are unclear, indicate this to the patient and ask him for additional information. It may be necessary, however, to obtain information from other sources, such as old medical records, spouses, or children.

The Principles of History Taking

The principles of history taking include listening, questioning, observation, and integration (Prior & Silberstein, 1981).

LISTENING

The interviewer should sit back and listen attentively as the patient tells his story (Fig. 1.2).

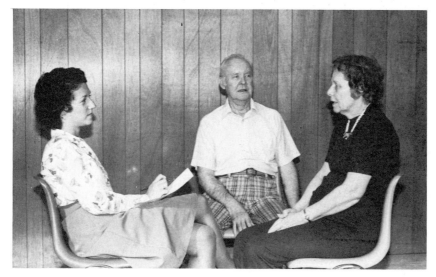

FIGURE 1.2
The art of attentive listening.

A great deal of factual information can be obtained by letting the patient talk without interruption. This period of silence for the interviewer allows time to learn about the patient's personality and emotional status and to assess his background, experience, and general level of intellectual functioning. It is important to evaluate these factors during the initial phases of the interview in order to be able to frame questions appropriately.

QUESTIONING

After the patient has completed his story, the interviewer should ask specific questions to gain additional information. Some pertinent areas of the history may need clarification; other areas may have been omitted entirely. The nurse should resist the tendency to formulate the next question while the patient is still answering an earlier question. Valuable information may be lost by neglecting to give full attention to each response.

An open-ended approach should be used whenever possible—for example, "Tell me about your chest pain." This encourages verbalization, although some interviews can become rambling if too many open-ended questions are used. A more direct approach can refocus and expedite the process. When a patient is having difficulty describing a problem, such as pain, the interviewer might offer descriptive words such as sharp, dull, throbbing, etc. Giving the patient the opportunity to choose among several adjectives provides more information than eliciting a simple yes/no response. The disadvantage in using direct questioning is that too many pointed inquiries tend to overwhelm the patient and put words in his mouth.

The nurse should avoid the use of leading questions, such as, "You don't have a history of emotional illness, do you?" This gives the patient an idea of the answer desired and, in an effort to please the interviewer, the patient often responds accordingly. The nurse's body movements, expression, and paralinguistics all indicate to the patient the expected response. The nurse should strive for a neutral demeanor by eliminating personal idiosyncrasies, such as head nodding, while asking the questions.

Areas that may make the patient uncomfortable should be handled in a factual but not impersonal manner. If the interviewer conveys to the patient that she is comfortable with the information being obtained, the patient will usually respond honestly. Often patients are relieved when asked questions regarding personal matters which they may have been too embarrassed or afraid to introduce. However, the interviewer should not force sensitive issues the patient may not wish to discuss. These issues can be addressed later in the relationship, after trust has been established.

OBSERVATION

The collection of objective data which later become part of the physical exam begins during the history. The patient should be observed during the interview for factors that may relate to his presenting problem. These include the patient's general appearance, demeanor, and stature and his attitudes toward himself, the interviewer, and his problems. Such information gives clues regarding the patient's sense of physical and mental well-being. The elderly, however, may have less facial expression than younger patients. This should not be misinterpreted as a lack of understanding or lack of emotional response. If the patient is accompanied to the interview by someone else, as in the case of a child, or elderly adult, their interactions should be observed. One can occasionally detect an emotional basis to a seemingly physical problem.

INTEGRATION

It is helpful to periodically summarize the data that have been collected so far during the history. This clarifies the information and keeps the interview directly focused. The final summary is an integration of all the information gathered in the health history. If the task has been performed properly and completely, the nurse will have an accurate understanding of the patient and his problem.

Recording the History

The history should not be recorded during the interview. The nurse needs time to digest, sort, and integrate the information so that it can be put into a concise, coherent narrative. The same format used to guide the interview should be used to write it. It should be remembered that the history consists of the information gathered from the patient free of embellishment or reinterpretation by the interviewer. Interpretation should encompass all available information (history, physical, and laboratory data). Obviously, this is only possible at the end of the entire process.

OUTLINE FOR THE HEALTH HISTORY

A. Demographic data
B. Chief complaint/reason for visit
C. History of present state of health
   1. The well patient
      a. Usual state of health
      b. Reason for last examination and interim health
      c. Developmental status
      d. Nutritional status
   2. The ill patient
      a. Usual state of health
      b. Chronologic story
         (1) Sequency and chronology
         (2) Frequency
         (3) Location and radiation
         (4) Character of the complaint
         (5) Intensity or severity
         (6) Setting
         (7) Associated phenomena
         (8) Aggravating or alleviating factors
      c. Relevant family history
      d. Disability assessment
D. Past history
   1. Childhood illnesses
   2. Immunizations
   3. Allergies
   4. Hospitalizations and serious illnesses
   5. Accidents and injuries
   6. Medications
   7. Habits
   8. Prenatal history*
   9. Labor and delivery history*
   10. Neonatal history*
E. Family history
F. Review of systems
   1. General
   2. Skin
   3. Hair
   4. Nails
   5. Head
   6. Eyes
   7. Ears
   8. Nose and sinuses
   9. Mouth
   10. Throat
   11. Neck
   12. Lymph nodes
   13. Breast
   14. Respiratory
   15. Cardiovascular
   16. Gastrointestinal
   17. Genitourinary
   18. Back
   19. Extremities
   20. Neurologic
   21. Hematopoietic
   22. Endocrine
G. Nutritional history
H. Social data
   1. Family relationships and friendships
   2. Ethnic affiliation
   3. Occupational history
   4. Educational history
   5. Economic status
   6. Daily profile
   7. Living circumstances
   8. Pattern of health care
I. Developmental history
J. Sexual history
K. Exercise and activity patterns
L. Stress patterns

Demographic Data

There are some biographic facts that are necessary to the patient's record. This information is standard in all health facilities. The data to be collected for this section include:

1. Name
2. Address
3. Phone number of the patient or neighbor/relative
4. Age
5. Sex
6. Marital status
7. Race
8. Religion
9. Usual source of medical care

---

* Recorded for all children 5 years of age and under and older children with congenital or developmental problems.

Usually most of this data is collected by someone other than the nurse prior to the history. A careful review of this information by the nurse before seeing the patient gives her baseline information from which to start the interview.

Chief Complaint/Reason for Visit

The patient has arrived in the clinic office, signaled with his call bell in the hospital, or phoned the Public Health Department for a definite reason. The chief complaint (CC) is a brief statement of things that are troubling the patient and the duration of time the problem(s) has existed. Generally, it is the answer to the question, "What is troubling you?" or "What brought you to the clinic today?" or "Why did you come to the hospital?" Ideally the CC is the patient's first response to the nurse's question and is written in quotation marks. However, the patient may give a vague answer, such as, "I haven't felt well for the past week." It is important to be precise in exploring the patient's problem. A better CC would be, "I have felt weak and tired for the past week." Health-oriented terminology or disease entities should not be included in the CC. If a patient says his eyes are "yellow," his complaint should be recorded in his own words. It is not correct to record that the patient is complaining of "scleral jaundice." Using the name of a disease, such as "rheumatoid arthritis," tends to bias the subsequent readers of the record prior to adequate exploration of the problem. A better way of stating the CC would be, "Hands swollen and stiff for 10 days."

In the case of a well patient seeking a routine physical, there is no actual CC. Data to be obtained include his reason for the visit and date of his last contact with the health care system. An example is, "Here for a physical examination, last complete exam two years ago." When a child comes to the clinic for an immunization, the CC is written, "Immunization needed. Second DPT two months ago." Brevity is important; elaboration of the CC is dealt with in the "history of the present illness."

The primary purpose of the CC is to focus the nurse's attention on the reason for the patient's visit. For the elderly the CC may represent multiple chronic medical conditions. The symptoms may not fit into a defined pattern in light of the complex nature of chronic disease. It is easy to make assumptions as to the reason the patient is seeking care. For example an elderly person who is being followed for elevated blood pressure may not define his health need as elevated blood pressure, but may be concerned about his constipation. The problem that is bothering the patient may seem trivial when compared to a problem that is more obvious to the health care provider. However, what the patient sees as a problem should be made a priority.

History of the Present State of Health

The History of the Present State of Health (HPH) is the narrative portion of the history. It gives the reader a clear idea of the patient's present state of well-being. When the patient is well and seeking a routine screening examination, the HPH gives a brief overview of the patient's physical and mental health since his last contact with the health care system. When the patient is ill, the HPH provides a sequentially developed elaboration of the reason for his visit.

THE WELL PATIENT
The narrative opens with a brief statement of the patient's usual long-term state of health. This gives the nurse an idea of how the patient evaluates his health. The well child or adult is asked the reason for his last examination or contact with the health care system and how his health has been in the interim. The patient is questioned about his nutritional and developmental status since his last examination. Nutritional and developmental data will be discussed in detail later in this chapter. Each well patient is questioned regarding any present concerns; detail is obtained if he has concerns. When no concerns exist, this is recorded as such.

THE ILL PATIENT
The HPH for the ill patient is divided into four sections: *usual health, chronologic story, relevant family history,* and *disability assessment.* As with the well patient the narrative is opened with a brief statement of the patient's usual long-term state of health. The opening state-

ment may read, "The patient considered himself in good health until yesterday, when. . ."

Chronologic Story. The chronologic story is the detailed section of the HPH. This is where the problem that brought the patient in is written down in the proper sequence of events. A great deal of time and investigative skill is needed to come up with meaningful data. There are general questions that help in the analysis of almost any symptom. These are referred to as the *eight areas of investigation* and should be learned thoroughly and used frequently. The eight areas of investigation are (1) sequence and chronology, (2) frequency, (3) location and radiation, (4) character of the complaint, (5) intensity or severity, (6) setting, (7) associated phenomena, and (8) aggravating or alleviating factors.

Sequence and Chronology. When investigating the sequence and chronology, the nurse should determine when the symptoms first began. She should make it clear to the patient that she wants to know when the mildest symptoms were experienced and how long it took for them to reach a peak and subsequently fade. The timing of symptoms should be identified as being continuous or intermittent. If intermittent, the time between occurrences must be established. Notation is made of the actual time units if possible (e.g., minutes/hours/weeks, etc.). Symptoms in the elderly are more apt to be of long duration making it more difficult to determine the exact onset. The examiner should also ask the patient if the onset of the problem was sudden or gradual. In the case of an episodic problem (such as an asthma attack) it is necessary to learn about the initial and later attacks. Whenever possible, specific dates should be used. Terms such as "two years ago" or "last week" are confusing to other readers of the record.

There are two approaches that can be taken when writing the narrative. The nurse can record the most recent event first and then trace events backwards sequentially or she can start from the beginning, moving chronologically forward. Patients can usually give a clearer picture of the most recent episode of a problem. Regardless of the order used, it is important that the narrative be written according to a logical format.

Frequency. Frequency refers to how often the problem occurs. It is common for patients to be vague on the frequency of a problem. The interviewer should help the patient with direct questions, such as, "Does your headache occur more than once a month or more than once a week?" Another method of helping a patient to be more specific is to ask him to relate certain activities to the problem. This may help him recall the time frame more clearly.

Location and Radiation. The location is where the distress is situated. Patients often use confusing terms when discussing the location of their problem. For example, a patient may say he has a "stomach ache" and really have prostatic pain. It is helpful to have the patient point with one finger to the exact location of his discomfort. Noting the exact location is beneficial when considering differential diagnoses. In the above example the examiner would focus her examination on the genitourinary organs and the epigastric area. When pain is reported, it is important to not only determine the location, but to pursue any radiation and determine whether the pain is on the surface or present in deeper organs of the body.

Character of the Complaint. When exploring the character of the complaint, the interviewer should try to get a description of the quality of the discomfort. She should first try an open question—for example, "Could you tell me about the chest pain?" If this does not elicit the data needed, a "laundry list" type of questioning might be used, in which the patient is given a number of alternate adjectives or descriptive phrases to use. Some examples are: burning, sharp, dull, aching, gnawing, throbbing, shooting, viselike, and constricting. If the symptom is other than pain, such as vomiting, sputum, or discharge, the quality would be described in terms of color and odor.

Character also refers to quantity and consistency of symptoms other than pain. Quantity is the best approximation of size, amount, and extent. The size of a lesion or mass is determined in centimeters or by comparing it to such common items as a nickel, a pea, or a walnut. Discharge is best measured in terms of teaspoons, tablespoons, and cups. If this is not possible, it can be estimated in terms of the number of pads or dressings saturated in a given period of time. Consistency is a description of composition and texture. For example, stool can be described as being soft, firm, or watery.

Intensity or Severity. This refers to the degree of disability caused by the problem. A helpful way to find out about the degree of discomfort is to ask the patient if the pain interferes with his daily activities. The elderly have a decreased sensitivity to pain which makes this a less reliable indicator of the severity of the problem compared with the younger patient.

Setting. Setting most commonly refers to the activity the patient was involved in at the time his problem occurred. A pattern should quickly emerge. It may also be discovered that a problem is related to a season of the year or to a particularly stressful event. Questions like "Where were you or what were you doing when the problem occurred?" will be helpful in eliciting this information.

Associated Phenomena. Associated phenomena are symptoms that occur along with the chief complaint. These symptoms (or their absence) are additional aides in the assessment. With clinical experience and knowledge the nurse soon learns which systems of the body may be contributing to the CC. The nurse must inquire about each system involved in the complaint, looking for related symptoms. For example, if the patient is complaining of chest pain, the cardiac, respiratory, and gastrointestinal systems must be thoroughly reviewed. All positive and negative responses should be recorded. Those symptoms that do not occur with the CC but could be related to it are referred to as *pertinent negatives.* For instance, if a nurse is interviewing a patient who has a CC of vomiting it is important to find out if there has been a fever accompanying the vomiting to rule out systemic illness. If not, recording "no fever associated with vomiting" is known as a pertinent negative. If the nurse fails to record a pertinent negative response, subsequent readers will not be able to rule out that symptom as being related to the chief complaint. Pertinent negatives are recorded after the positive responses.

Aggravating or Alleviating Factors. Most patients are aware of the factors that aggravate their problems. Some of the factors that may con-

tribute to a problem are emotional stress, fatigue, physical exertion, pregnancy, and use of certain drugs. Alleviating factors are those treatments the patient initiates or which have been prescribed to ease his distress. The success or failure of such treatments should be recorded. It may be discovered that the treatment utilized by the patient is harmful. The beginnings of a patient teaching plan are often formulated on the basis of this information.

Relevant Family History. The third section of the HPH concerns relevant family history. The patient is questioned about related problems of family members. For example, if the patient is having chest pain he is asked if there is any family history of heart disease. When a contagious illness is being considered, it is important to ask if the patient recently has been around anyone with similar symptoms. If there is a positive history the specific family member or acquaintance and his problem are recorded.

Disability Assessment. The last section of the HPH is the disability assessment. This is often a sensitive area because it explores the patient's feelings concerning the disruption of, or interference with daily life from his problem. The problem may result in strained family resources and relationships. For example, if the head of the household is ill, he may be unable to work. A child may be unable to attend school, resulting in his falling behind in his studies. The elderly may accept problems as part of the aging process, and try to ignore the severity of the disruption or interference with daily life. With a long-term problem, relationships can become strained when all family energies are focused on the ill member. The disability assessment is important to the nurse in that it provides information regarding the patient's perspective of the severity of the problem.

Past History

The past history provides background for understanding the patient as a whole and his present illness. It is also a storehouse of information that may be relevant to management of the present illness. For example, if a patient comes to the clinic with right-lower quadrant pain and he has a past surgical history of an appendectomy, the possibility of appendicitis is ruled out.

Included in the past history are (1) childhood illnesses, (2) immunizations, (3) allergies, (4) hospitalizations and serious illnesses, (5) accidents and injuries, (6) medications, and (7) habits.

CHILDHOOD ILLNESSES

The patient is asked if he has ever had chicken pox, mumps, rubella, rubeola, streptococcal infections, or scarlet fever. All patients are asked if they remember having had rheumatic fever. Most people cannot recall the dates of childhood illnesses. If they can, this is helpful information and should be recorded. If not, the approximate age at which they had the diseases should be recorded. The adult woman of childbearing age is asked when she had rubella. If there is a history of other significant childhood illness, then the dates, symptoms and signs, course of illness, treatment, complications, and follow-up should be recorded.

IMMUNIZATIONS

The parent should be asked for the dates the child received the following immunizations: initial DPT series and boosters; measles, mumps, rubella (MMR); and oral polio vaccine (OPV). The nurse should inquire about the occurrence of side effects. Also important are the dates and results of screening tests, such as the tuberculin skin test, the sickle cell test, and the G-6-PD (glucose-6-phosphate dehydrogenase deficiency). It is not necessary to obtain a complete immunization history from an adult, but the nurse should make sure that the necessary immunizations have been given and should note the date of the patient's last tetanus shot.

ALLERGIES

All patients should be asked about the presence of allergies to drugs (specifically penicillin), animals, insects, foods, and environmental agents or irritants. It is not sufficient to record just the name of the offending allergen. The nurse should investigate exactly what type of reaction occurs and the treatment implemented. All types of untoward reactions to foods should also be discussed at this time. It is important to identify the offending food as well as the nature of the response, for this may be important in other areas of physical assessment. Thus, a true food allergy may present as an urticarial reaction to egg consumption. This response has different assessment implications than a response of hemolytic crisis when a person with Mediterranean G-6-PD deficiency consumes fava beans; or a response of bloating, flatulence, diarrhea, and cramping when a person with lactase deficiency consumes a threshold quantity of milk.

HOSPITALIZATIONS AND SERIOUS ILLNESSES

When asking about hospitalizations, the nurse should obtain exact information on the dates of hospitalization; the location or name of the hospital and the name of the attending physician; and the reason for the hospitalization, surgery performed, complications, and course of recovery. If the elderly patient has had many hospitalizations or his memory is vague, you may want to obtain hospital summaries to determine details of hospitalizations. Obstetrical hospitalizations may be recorded here or in the review of systems under genitourinary. The patient should be asked about serious past illnesses (which may not have required hospital admission), including dates, duration, severity, degree of recovery, and any sequelae. Some of the illnesses included in this category are high blood pressure, diabetes, pneumonia, pleurisy, tuberculosis, malaria, hepatitis, infectious mononucleosis, unexplained high fevers, and frequent colds and sore throats.

ACCIDENTS AND INJURIES

The patient is asked about accidents, harmful ingestions, and injuries that have occurred, regardless of whether or not he was hospitalized. The interviewer should determine how the accident happened, where it happened, the type of injury, the treatment received, and sequela. The interviewer should be alert to a pattern of injury. Falls in the aged can be a particularly difficult problem. In 1978, 70.3 percent of all fatal accidental falls occurred in persons aged 64 years or older (Burnside, 1981). The nurse will want to be alert to changes that can be made in the home environment to prevent further falls. The young child or the frail elderly living with others may be the object of abuse. Repeated accidents and injuries are frequently the major clues.

MEDICATIONS

The patient is asked the names of prescribed medications he is taking currently or took for an extended period of time in the past. The nurse should also inquire about the use of over-the-counter medications. Patients may neglect to mention that they use vitamins, aspirin, nasal sprays, and laxatives that are obtained without a prescription. Because many patients, particularly those retaining strong ethnic ties, will prepare folk treatments themselves, patients should also be asked if they are using any home remedies or tonics. If they respond affirmatively, the method of preparation and administration as well as the frequency of use should be elicited. Many women do not consider the birth control pill a medication. A specific question about this is necessary. Although the patient may not be taking the pill currently, past use, side effects, and the reason for stopping use constitute important information and should be recorded (this may also be recorded in the review of systems). The dosage, routes of administration, frequency of administration, and reason for use should be noted for all medications.

HABITS

The nurse should inquire about the use of illicit or recreational drugs; caffeinated soft drinks, coffee and tea; alcohol; and tobacco. When asking about illicit or recreational drugs, she should be sure to include drugs that were used extensively in the past. She should also ask about the frequency and duration of use and the good and bad effects.

Inquiry should be made into the amount of caffeinated beverages the patient drinks per day. It is interesting to ask about the use of sugar and cream in coffee and tea. This may account for a number of extra calories.

When asking about the patient's drinking habits, the interviewer should include types of alcohol, amount of alcohol consumed, pattern of drinking (morning or evening), drinking binges, and past treatment for alcoholism. It is sometimes difficult to assess the patient's consumption of alcohol. The nurse should obtain the exact number of bottles of beer or glasses of wine the patient drinks in a specified period of time. This lets the nurse, rather than the patient, decide whether the patient's drinking is occasional or not. Also obtain any past history of alcohol consumption. Do not as-

sume the elderly patient no longer drinks. This can be a sensitive area for both the nurse and the patient if a problem exists. Therefore, open-ended questions may be advisable, since they are less pointed and threatening.

In the case of cigarette use, the nurse should ask about the number of packs smoked per day, the type of cigarette, and the number of years the patient has been smoking. It is important to note the number of years the patient has been smoking rather than just his daily rate of consumption. A past history of smoking should also be obtained. This includes the number of years he smoked, the number of cigarettes, and the number of years since he stopped. Cigar and pipe smoking warrant obtaining the same information.

Habits specific to the child 5 years of age and younger include the presence of excessive bedwetting, masturbation, thumbsucking, nailbiting, temper tantrums, use of a favorite blanket or toy. Additional information is obtained regarding the child's sleeping patterns including hours, disturbances, dreaming, and nightmares.

ADDITIONAL PAST HISTORY

The prenatal, labor and delivery, and neonatal histories are obtained on all children 5 years of age and younger and all older children who have a congenital or developmental problem.

Prenatal History. The gravity, parity, and number of abortions a mother has had may be important to the child's health. The mother should be asked when she first sought prenatal care for this child, how she felt physically and emotionally during pregnancy, the couple's feelings and acceptance of the pregnancy, and whether or not the baby was planned. All of these data may reveal very helpful information about the family's dynamics and health.

The nurse should explore for the presence of difficulties during the prenatal period. Some possible problems are diabetes, hypertension, excessive weight gain, poor nutrition, infections, rubella, vaginal bleeding, convulsions, and excessive stress. The use of alcohol, medications (amount and types), and tobacco during pregnancy should be recorded.

Labor and Delivery History. Difficulties during labor and delivery may indicate potential problems during childhood. The nurse should ask about the length and difficulty of labor, type of delivery, the presence of significant other, complications during the delivery, gestation, and birth weight. She should also inquire about problems specific to the child at the time of delivery. These include difficulty in breathing, seizures, jaundice, or low birthweight.

Neonatal History. A good general question for establishing an idea of the newborn's health is, "Did your baby go home with you?" or "When was the baby discharged from the nursery?" If the baby did leave the hospital with his parents, the nurse should inquire about the baby's first month of life. Helpful questions include: "Were there any problems? Was the baby unusually fussy? How did the parents feel they adjusted to this new family member? What type of feeding was the baby on—breast or bottle? Was there any difficulty with feeding? Can the parents remember the frequency and give a description of bowel movements? How many times a day did the baby void? What were the baby's sleeping patterns?

If the baby remained in the hospital or was in a special nursery, the parents will probably recall special incubators or lights used. A detailed description of the prolonged hospitalization is necessary, if that was the case.

The mother is asked specifically if the child had any of the following problems in the postnatal period: cyanosis, jaundice, fever, congenital abnormalities, rashes, weight loss, or difficulty sucking.

Family History

The purpose of the family history is to identify genetic problems, communicable diseases, environmental problems, and interpersonal data. This information enhances understanding of the environment in which the patient and his family live. Specific inquiry should be made regarding paternal and maternal grandparents, parents, siblings, spouse, and children. Their ages, general state of health, and health problems, if any should be recorded. If any family members are deceased, the nurse should record the age at death and the cause. The patient should be asked if any other family members (aunts, uncles, or cousins) have any of the following diseases: cancer, tuberculosis, heart disease, hypertension, epi-

lepsy, allergy, mental retardation, nervous or mental disease, and endocrine (diabetes) or other metabolic disorders. If any family member has a positive history of disease, minimal additional information to be obtained includes age of onset and treatment.

Family history data may be recorded in the form of a list, but the use of a family tree or genogram is more practical. Figure 1.3 is an example of a blank family tree and Figure 1.4 is a legend of a brief coded classification of diseases, health problems, social events, and family interactions (Jolly, et al., 1980). A family tree clearly indicates all family relationships including deaths, divorces, subsequent marriages, etc. Figure 1.5 is an illustration of a completed genogram.

The family history of the elderly patient is less important as a diagnostic tool than with a young patient. It does, however, represent the patient's experience with disease. In the case of an adopted patient who is unaware of his blood relatives, it is nevertheless beneficial to get a history of his adoptive family. The nurse notes on the record that the patient is adopted and has no access to his biological family's history.

Review of Systems

The review of systems (ROS) is a review of all complaints by body system, moving from head to foot. It is an evaluation of the past and present status of each system. The purpose of the review of systems is to act as a double check to prevent omission of data relevant to the present illness and to uncover other problems that might have been missed.

The review of systems is a list of symptoms that can be asked fairly quickly in a checklist manner. However, it is important to allow enough time for the patient to consider each symptom and to reply. The list of symptoms is fairly long and difficult to remember. It is therefore recommended that the nurse keep them on a reference card for easy access. Once she becomes practiced with the list, she will have it memorized. It is essential to record all negative as well as positive answers. If just the positives are written down the reader has no way to determine what other questions were asked. If there is a positive response, it should be explored via the eight areas of inves-

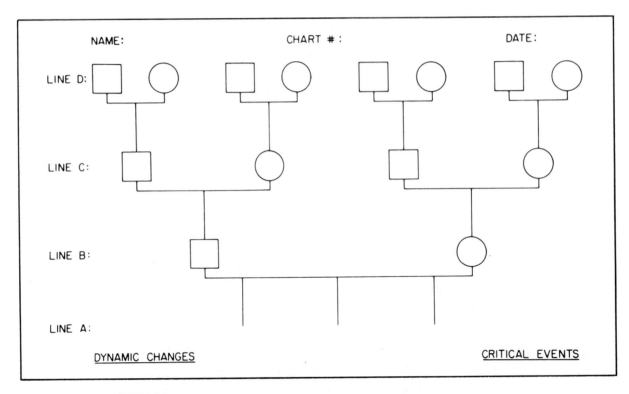

FIGURE 1.3
The genogram. (Reprinted from Jolly, W., et al. The Journal of Family Practice, 10(2), 1980, p. 252, with permission.)

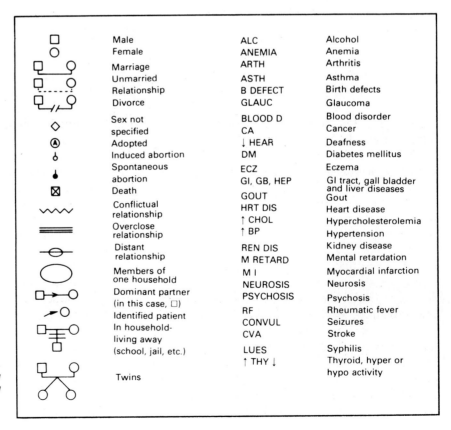

Male	ALC	Alcohol
Female	ANEMIA	Anemia
Marriage	ARTH	Arthritis
Unmarried	ASTH	Asthma
Relationship	B DEFECT	Birth defects
Divorce	GLAUC	Glaucoma
Sex not specified	BLOOD D	Blood disorder
	CA	Cancer
Adopted	↓ HEAR	Deafness
Induced abortion	DM	Diabetes mellitus
Spontaneous abortion	ECZ	Eczema
	GI, GB, HEP	GI tract, gall bladder and liver diseases
Death	GOUT	Gout
Conflictual relationship	HRT DIS	Heart disease
Overclose relationship	↑ CHOL	Hypercholesterolemia
	↑ BP	Hypertension
Distant relationship	REN DIS	Kidney disease
	M RETARD	Mental retardation
Members of one household	M I	Myocardial infarction
Dominant partner (in this case, □)	NEUROSIS	Neurosis
	PSYCHOSIS	Psychosis
Identified patient	RF	Rheumatic fever
In household- living away (school, jail, etc.)	CONVUL	Seizures
	CVA	Stroke
	LUES	Syphilis
Twins	↑ THY ↓	Thyroid, hyper or hypo activity

FIGURE 1.4
Genogram symbols. (Reprinted from Jolly, W., et al. The Journal of Family Practice, 10(2), 1980, p. 254, with permission.)

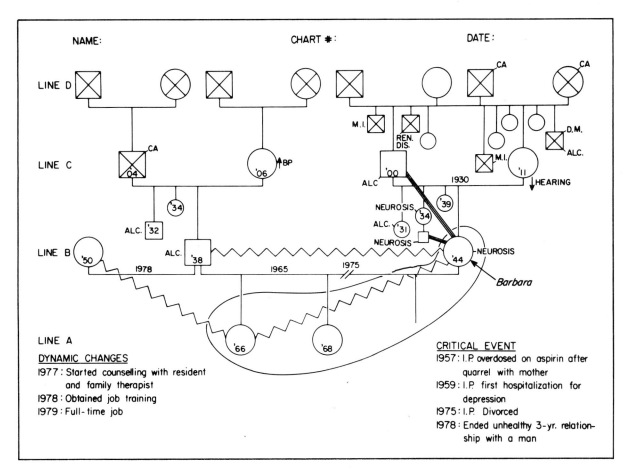

FIGURE 1.5
Example of a completed genogram. (Reprinted from Jolly, W., et al. The Journal of Family Practice, 10(2), 1980, p. 254, with permission.)

tigation utilized in the "history of present illness." When a response relates to the present illness it should be recorded under "present illness" and the following statement should be made in the ROS: "See HPH."

Nurses first learning the art of history taking often confuse the review of systems with a physical exam. This is evident when they record the history. The nurse will mistakenly write physical findings in the review of systems. It must be remembered that the review of systems contains subjective data given by the patient.

Following is a list of symptoms or problems that relate to each system. Some of the terminology may not be familiar to all patients. It is often necessary to change the wording according to the patient's age and level of understanding.

- **General:** Height, unusual/unexpected shift in weight, fatigue, chills, fever, weakness, night sweats.
- **Skin:** Scaling, change in pigmentation, tendency toward bruising, lesions, birth marks, changes in moles, pruritis, rashes, dryness.
- **Hair:** Amount, thickness, color, texture, alopecia, chemical treatments.
- **Nails:** Color changes, biting, clubbing, splitting, change in shape, lesions under the nail.
- **Head:** Problems with headache(s), falls resulting in unconsciousness or injury, dizziness, syncope.
- **Eyes:** *Adult and Child:* Difficulty seeing, glasses (what for?), excessive tearing, pain, photophobia, diploplia, color blindness, cataracts, glaucoma, discharge, his-

tory of infections, date of last eye examination. *Child:* Problems with eye coordination.

- **Ears:** Discharge, tinnitus, history of infections, vertigo, pain, prosthetic devices, hearing ability.
- **Nose and Sinuses:** Rhinorrhea, epistaxis, sinus problems, frequent colds, obstruction, loss of smell.
- **Mouth:** *Adult and Child:* Sore or bleeding gums; lesion on lips, tongue, or mucosa; excessive salivation; date of last dental exam; poor speech pattern; hygiene practices; prosthetic devices (dentures, braces, etc.); history of cold sores. *Child:* Age of eruption of deciduous and permanent teeth; thumbsucking.
- **Throat:** Soreness, hoarseness, frequent streptococcal or viral sore throats, difficulty swallowing, change in taste.
- **Neck:** Swelling, stiffness, limitation of motion, thyroid disease, enlarged nodes.
- **Lymph Nodes:** Any swelling in the nodes of the neck, axilla, groin or epitrochlear areas.
- **Breasts:** *Child and Adolescent:* Pattern of development. *Adult Female:* Discharge from nipples, masses, lesions, pain, pattern of self-examination of breasts, history of breast masses (dates and treatment), date of last mammogram and results. *Male:* discharge from nipples, masses, lesions, pain, enlargement.
- **Respiratory:** Chest pain with breathing; cough; shortness of breath; night sweats; wheezing; frequent upper respiratory infections; history of emphysema, pneumonia, asthma, tuberculosis, bronchitis, or hemoptysis; date of last chest x-ray and results, if known; smoking habits; date and results of last tuberculin skin test.
- **Cardiovascular:** *Child:* Fatigue, cyanosis, congenital heart disease, tiring with feeding, heart murmur. *Adult:* Orthopnea, paroxysmal nocturnal dyspnea, edema, varicosities, chest pain, palpitations, claudication, history of heart murmur, hypertension, rheumatic fever, heart failure, heart attack (questions regarding rheumatic fever and smoking habits may appear in more than one place; answers only need to be recorded once).
- **Gastrointestinal:** *Adult and Child:* Appetite, bowel patterns, changes in stools, diarrhea, constipation, abdominal pain, excessive flatulence, hemorrhoids, rectal bleeding, jaundice, dysphagia, tarry stools, anal itching, past history of peptic or other ulcer, gallbladder disease or "attacks" and hepatitis. *Child:* Encopresis.
- **Genitourinary:** *General:* Frequency, dribbling, pain, incontinence, pyuria, nocturia, urgency, color change of urine, hesitancy, hematuria, history of venereal disease (type of infection and treatment), history of urinary tract infection (type of infection and treatment). *Toddler:* Toilet training. *School Age:* Bedwetting. *Adolescent and Adult Female:* Menstrual history including menarche, length of cycles, duration of menses, regularity, amount, dysmenorrhea, premenstrual symptoms (breast tenderness, moodiness), menorrhagia, metrorrhagia, intermenstrual spotting, date of last menstrual period, and date of last Pap smear. Genital history including vaginal discharge, vaginal itching, lesions, dyspareunia, odor, and past history of vaginal infections (type and treatment). Birth control history including type, duration, and satisfaction. An obstetrical history is taken for all women, including those who are postmenopausal. The dates of birth, types of deliveries, weights of babies, lengths of gestation, and complications or illnesses during prenatal and postpartum periods are obtained. This is an appropriate point to proceed with an age appropriate sexual history (see pages 25, 30–35). *Adolescent Male:* Nocturnal emissions. *Adolescent and Adult Male:* Lesions, impotence, prostate problems (symptoms and treatment), penile discharge, swelling of testicles, difficulty starting or stopping stream, and pattern of testicular self-examination. This is an appropriate point to proceed with an age appropriate sexual history (see pages 25, 30–35).
- **Back:** Pain, stiffness, limited movement, history of injury or disease.
- **Extremities:** Pain, swelling, redness, stiffness, or deformities of joints; limitation of movement; crepitation, varicose veins, gout, edema; history of fractures, injuries, or disease.
- **Neurologic:** Seizures, tremors, difficulty with balance, speech disorders, weakness,

paralysis, limps, paresthesias, sleep disturbances, fainting, loss of memory, disorientation, mood swings, anxiety, depression, phobias.
- **Hematopoietic:** History of anemia (type and treatment), sickle-cell trait, spontaneous bleeding, blood dyscrasia, transfusions (reason for and reaction to).
- **Endocrine:** Change in glove or shoe size, hirsutism, excessive sweating, polyuria, polydypsia, polyphasia, history of goiter, heat or cold intolerance.

Nutritional History

The nutritional history is a vital part of the total picture of a person's health. The cliche, "A person is what he eats," is somewhat extreme, but does have some accuracy.

Our society tends to have problems with nutrition. As a whole we overeat; we eat the wrong types of foods; we cook in excess fat; we cover foods with extra calories and nonnutritional sauces; and we eat most of our calories at the wrong time of the day.

However, there is hope! More healthful nutritional practices are presently a trend. This is demonstrated by the fact that during the past 10 years there has been a decrease in coronary heart disease. This is thought to be due in part to the public's modification of fat intake in their diet. If we, as health care providers, reinforce the importance of good nutrition while it is in its "trend" state, maybe "the balanced diet" will become a way of life. Even the fast food restaurants, which have become so much a part of our lifestyle, are stressing items that are nutritionally beneficial. The push in this direction is strong, so let's not lose it!

Good nutrition is essential from birth to death. For this reason it is important to consider the nutritional history in a developmental framework. If specific questions are directed to the nutritional requirements of a particular age group, more accurate information will be obtained. Before approaching the nutritional history developmentally, there are certain general areas to explore.

Eliciting a 24-hour diet history is a good way to gain some insight into a person's diet. The patient should be questioned about what he ate yesterday or the day before including all meals, snacks and beverages. It is not meaningful to merely ask the patient what he usually eats. Most people have some idea of a balanced diet and consciously or unconsciously recite this back to the nurse. Encouraging the patient to reflect on specific foods he ate in the last 24 hours is often revealing not only to the nurse, but to the patient himself. It is also helpful to ask the patient if *he thinks* he eats a nutritionally balanced diet. Does he see himself as overweight or underweight, and how much? Have there been any recent weight gains or losses? This information provides the nurse with the *patient's perspective* of his nutritional status. Most people are aware of the quality of their diets. However, the patient should give his view and the nurse should not judge.

Other important general questions to ask are: Who does the cooking at home? What kind of facilities are available? Who does the grocery shopping? Are you concerned about obtaining groceries? Do you eat out? How many times per week? What kinds of restaurants (i.e., fast foods, what types)? Do you have any financial concerns in terms of money spent on food? Are you or any family members on special diets? How does this affect the family's eating practices? And finally, it is advantageous to find out if there are any unusual weight problems in the family or any family history of obesity.

With ethnically distinct patients, food patterns are a particularly crucial area for assessment. An individual's culture defines what may be considered food. Within this range of culturally approved items, an individual diet depends on a host of economic, religious, psychologic, and personal preference factors. Because food traditions are among the last traditional ethnic customs to change, and because of the ethnic diversity in American society, the patient's "foodways" may vary dramatically from those of the examiner. It is essential for the nurse to respect the food habits and preferences of all patients. It is important to investigate this area with culturally distinct patients, asking about methods of food preparation, meal ingredients, timing and frequency of meals, and foods considered harmful or beneficial to health.

Methods of *food preparation* merit special attention in the diet history. While some methods may remove nutrients (as in overcooking vegetables), other methods may increase available nutrients (soaking corn for tortillas in lime water adds calcium to the diet).

The *ingredients* used in cooking constitute another crucial area for diet assessment. Indochinese patients should be asked questions regarding the use of soy or MSG (monosodium glutamate) in addition to salt. Specific ingredients of ethnic foods should be elicited if the foods are not familiar to the examiner. For example, most nurses are familiar with lasagna, but not with pastitsio, a comparable Greek dish.

In addition to learning what is eaten and how it is prepared, it is important to determine the *timing and frequency of meals.* The examiner cannot assume that all persons eat three meals a day, with the largest meal in the evening. An often missed area of assessment concerns the timing of medications and treatments. Patients are often told to take a medication before or after meals, assuming a breakfast–lunch–dinner pattern. Variations in mealtime patterns should be noted in the record.

In obtaining a diet history, the nurse should also try to determine what the patient believes about *food and its relationship to health.* In many ethnic groups, infants and women during pregnancy and after delivery are placed on special diets, with some foods considered health-promoting and others considered dangerous. This is also true of menstruating women who are warned to avoid some foods and eat others during menstruation. Some of these beliefs are based on theory and others are primarily myths. Many people, including the majority of those in Asian and Spanish-speaking groups, classify foods as *hot* or *cold* on the basis of inherent characteristics of the food, and not on their actual temperature. In this hot/cold system, foods are balanced for optimum health. In addition, if a person has a "cold" illness or condition, such as colic or earache, he should consume balancing or "hot" foods.

Assessing compliance with a prescribed therapeutic diet may pose difficulties for nurses unfamiliar with ethnic foods. To augment the examiner's skills, dietary exchange lists are available for some major ethnic groups (Bierman, 1974; Whitaker, 1976).

In addition to exploring these topical areas, Branch and Paxton (1976) suggest asking the following specific questions when assessing the diet of ethnic people of color. However, they are important questions to ask of all individuals.

1. What times during the day do you usually eat?
2. Are there any circumstances that make you want to eat?
3. What takes your appetite away?
4. What foods do you like most?
5. What foods do you like least?
6. What foods are neutral?
7. What seasonings do you use regularly in preparing your foods?

After this information is obtained the nurse can further discuss the nutritional practices of the patient by considering his age. To make the *elicitation* of this easier, Chart 1.1 is available for reference. This chart is sectioned into various age groups. The questions included in the chart will help the nurse to gather a complete nutritional history. When the patient is in for a well visit this information is recorded in the HPH.

Social Data

Social data include family relationships and friendships, ethnic affiliations, occupational history, educational history, economic status, daily profile, living circumstances, and patterns of health care. The nurse has traditionally given careful consideration to this area. However, when a nurse first becomes involved in taking the in-depth health history she sometimes neglects this area and concentrates on sections that are new to her. She must be reminded that she is to synthesize both the physical and social aspects of the patient history to make a meaningful assessment.

FAMILY RELATIONSHIPS AND FRIENDSHIPS

This can be a sensitive area and must be approached with care. Questions are directed toward assessing the quality and dynamics of the patient's significant relationships. The patient is asked how he gets along with family members and how he feels the other family members relate to him. He is asked such questions as, "Who do you feel close to in your

CHART 1.1
DEVELOPMENTAL APPROACH TO THE NUTRITIONAL HISTORY

Neonate (first 4 weeks)

Breast

1. How often?
2. How long on each breast?
3. Relief bottles: What brand of formula? Type of nipple and bottle? How often?
4. Mother's caloric intake, fluid intake, drug usage, foods that bother her or infant? Is mother experiencing any difficulties (i.e., cracked nipples, engorgement)?
5. Is the feeding relationship pleasurable? Any problems? Concerns? How does father feel about breast feeding?
6. How long does mother plan to breast feed?
7. Does the child drink any water? How much?
8. Is the water supply fluoridated? How much?
9. Supplements (i.e., food, vitamins, vitamins with iron)?

Bottle-fed

1. How often?
2. How much? Ounces per bottle, bottles per day?
3. What brand of formula? Does the formula contain iron?
4. What type of formula (powder, concentrate, ready to feed)?
5. What dilution? How is the formula prepared?
6. Type of nipple and bottle?
7. Is the water supply fluoridated? How much?
8. Who feeds the baby?
9. Is the feeding relationship pleasurable? Problems?
10. Supplement (i.e., foods)?
11. Does the infant take a bottle to bed at night?

Infancy (1 month–12 months)

Milk intake

1. Is the child weaned from the breast? (If no, repeat questions for breast fed above and if yes, repeat questions for bottle fed above.) Age weaned?
2. Questions/concerns regarding breast weaning?
3. Has the infant started cow's milk? When? Type (whole, 2%, skim)? Questions/concerns regarding introduction of cow's milk?
4. Does the infant hold his own bottle?
5. Has the infant started to drink from a cup? When?

Intake of Solids and Other Supplements

1. When started?
   a. Cereal? How much? What type?
   b. Vegetables? How much? What type?
   c. Fruits? How much? What type?
   d. Juice? How much? What type?
   e. Meats? How much? What type?
   f. Eggs? How much? What type?
2. How are foods prepared? At home? Bought? Brand?
3. How far apart are new foods introduced?
4. What is a typical 24-hour diet?
5. Have any allergies developed? With which foods? How manifested?
6. Likes and dislikes?
7. H_2O intake?
8. Fluoride in water?
9. Vitamins? Iron?
10. Who feeds the infant?
11. Does the infant feed himself with his fingers? What foods?

Toddler (1 year–3 years)

1. Typical 24-hour diet (include amounts of food, fluid, and H_2O)?[a]
2. Milk intake (type, how much, cup used, etc.).
3. Who does the child eat with?
4. Does he feed himself?
5. Snacks? What types? How often?
6. Foods as rewards? Punishments?
7. Allergies? Which foods? How manifested?
8. Likes and dislikes?
9. Vitamins?
10. Parental concerns?

Preschool (3–5 years)

1. Independence in eating?
2. Willingness to try new foods?
3. See 1, 2, 3, 5–10 under *Toddler.*

School Age (6–12 years)

1. Does child eat breakfast before school? What?
2. Does child eat school lunch? What does he eat? Does he take his own lunch? What does he take?
3. Attitude towards food?
4. See 1, 2, 3, 5–10 under *Toddler.*

(continued)

CHART 1.1—*Continued*

Adolescent and Adult

1. Typical 24-hour diet?
2. Typical daily activities? Exercise?
3. Does patient eat at home? How often? With whom?
4. Does patient eat out? How often? With whom? What types of food?
5. Snacks? What types? How often?
6. Fluids (types, amounts, H_2O)?
7. Likes and dislikes?
8. Allergies to foods? Which foods? How manifested?
9. Vitamins? Types? Amounts? How long taken?
10. Recent weight gain or loss?
11. Salt intake? How much (including that in canned foods, added salt to foods)?
12. Alcohol intake? What type? How often? How much?
13. Does patient feel knowledgeable about nutrition?

Older Adult

1. Typical 24-hour diet or 3-day intake?
2. Interest in food?
3. Who cooks? How often?
4. Who shops? How often? Does patient eat out? How often?
5. Are frozen or canned foods used extensively?
6. How does food taste?[b]
7. Salt intake? How much (including that in canned foods, added salt to foods)?
8. Vitamins? What type? How much? How often? For how long?
9. Recent weight gain or loss?
10. Dentures? Condition and fit? Difficulty chewing?
11. Own teeth? Condition? Difficulty chewing?
12. Fluids (types, amounts, H_2O)?
13. Snacks? What types? How often? Type and frequency of between meal snacking?
14. Alcohol intake? What type? How often? How much?
15. Likes and dislikes?
16. Economic aspects? Amount of money available for food on a weekly basis?

[a] Sometimes a weekly diet history will give a better idea of the balance in the diet.
[b] Smoking may influence taste.

family?" The nurse should determine whether anyone in the family is sick or has problems with behavior, school, work, drugs, or alcohol. If any of these problems are present, the nurse should ask how the patient feels they affect the rest of the family. The nurse should also ask if there are extended family members nearby to offer support in times of stress. Nearby extended family members may be particularly important to the elderly person because they can often provide much support as physical disabilities increase. It is important to determine how the patient feels about these relationships.

In our mobile society today there are many different types of relationships and "family" arrangements. For instance, the college student's "family" may be his roommates. A young man in the service may have a similar living arrangement and support system. Other families include single parents, unmarried couples, homosexual couples, etc. As people age, the importance of lasting relationships as a means of psychological support increases. It is important, therefore, to know whom the elderly patient identifies as a close friend. The presence of these significant relationships should be explored.

The married patient should be questioned about the length of his marriage, previous marriages, duration of past marriages, how he feels about his relationship with his spouse, and the number of children from previous marriages. The recently widowed patient should be questioned about his emotional and physical adjustment to the loss. The widowed are more apt to seek medical care during the first year of bereavement. The stress of the change may lead to changes in health status to which the nurse should respond.

1. THE HEALTH HISTORY / **23**

ETHNIC AFFILIATION

Cultural diversity accounts in large part for variations in family relationships, food preferences, religion, communication, and value patterns, as well as in health beliefs and behaviors. Ethnic affiliation differs from race, although both are important in health assessment. Ethnic identity concerns the cultural and social characteristics of a group of people. Racial identity has to do with biophysiologic differences among populations. Although there are certainly more biologic differences *within* a population than *among* populations, race is an important assessment variable because it indicates particular areas of attention. For example, persons of Mediterranean ancestry are routinely screened for glucose-6-phosphate dehydrogenase deficiency, blacks are commonly checked for sickle-cell anemia and hypertension, and Caucasians are the only group having a high rate of multiple sclerosis.

Ethnic affiliation may be determined by direct questioning as well as indirect assessment of such variables as language, manner of dress, and food preferences. While it is essential not to stereotype individuals, ethnic affiliation can serve as a clue in assisting the nurse in understanding client customs or beliefs. Sensitivity to ethnic differences is an important element in the delivery of quality health care. This variable should not be ignored because of a misguided notion that all people are the same. It is helpful to ask the patient if he is aware of any ethnic or religious customs that might affect his response to illness, wellness, or therapy that may be prescribed.

OCCUPATIONAL HISTORY

The occupational history is geared toward identifying workplace hazards, job satisfaction, and sources of work-related psychological stress. The history should include a chronological listing of all jobs the patient has held, including the type of work, job title, location, and duration of employment. The interviewer should obtain a thorough description of the physical work environment, including the size of the work area, ventilation, noise levels, room temperature, safety measures, cleanliness, and exposure to chemical substances (Ginnetti & Greig, 1981). Names of all chemical substances should be obtained with special note taken of those known to be carci-

nogenic (i.e., asbestos, arsenic, benzene, mustard gas, soots, tars, and oils) (Newell, 1983). In addition, the patient should be screened for job related stress. This stress includes deadline pressures, relationships with his employer and peers, boredom, and effects of the work situation on other family members. Many people are satisfied and fulfilled with their jobs or careers and this should be recorded, too.

The patient should be asked if he has ever been required to change jobs because of illness and how he feels about that. The nurse should not neglect to obtain a job history for housewives. Note exposure to chemical substances such as cleaning fluids. Explore her satisfaction with her role and determine how she copes with pressure. She should be asked if she is able to find relief time from her responsibilities (i.e., the use of babysitters and help from other family members). If a woman has no work experience outside the home she may be at risk for adjustment problems when the children leave home or she loses her spouse.

Many elderly patients have retired from life-long occupations. It is important for the nurse to know what kind of work the patient did, for how long, and when he retired. There are important implications in this information. If the patient recently retired there may be symptoms of an underlying depression due to a sense of loss or economic worries. Another concern is long-term exposure to a chemical agent that may result in disease later in life.

EDUCATIONAL HISTORY

When interviewing a child the nurse should ask his grade level and the type of school he attends. It is important to ask the child if he likes or dislikes school. The parent and child are asked about school progress. Special aptitudes and any problem with school behavior are identified.

The interviewer asks the parent of a grade school child how the student learns in relation to children of the same age and in relation to members of the same family. The parent is asked if the child has ever had to repeat a grade or has ever been told he has a learning disability. The nurse asks the child if he likes to learn. Inquiry is also made as to how the child relates to his teachers and peers at school.

The nurse should determine whether the high school student is satisfied with his academic performance and what he plans to do after high school. The student should be asked how he relates to his teachers and peers at school, too.

The nurse should record the highest level of education attained by adult patients and determine whether the patient feels this education is adequate. Inquiry is also made about past difficulties with learning in school. These difficulties can influence plans for patient education. More adults are returning to school to begin a career or to make a career change. The nurse should explore with the adult learner how he and his family are adjusting to this change.

ECONOMIC STATUS

Inquiry into the family's economic status is another sensitive area. The nurse should determine whether the patient feels the family income is sufficient to meet the family's basic needs. The patient should be asked how he is paying for his medical care. This includes the type of medical and hospitalization coverage he holds. Exploring the medical coverage of an elderly patient is especially important. This population is often too proud to admit hardship and patients may not purchase drugs or other services if they cannot afford to. If illness exists the nurse should ask how it has affected a patient's savings.

DAILY PROFILE

The patient is asked to describe the events of a usual day starting with the time he arises and ending with bed time. Special attention is paid to sleeping, eating and exercise patterns.

LIVING CIRCUMSTANCES

In this section the adequacy of the home and surrounding community is assessed. This can be done by questioning the patient and his family. However, the information is best obtained by making a home visit. The nurse should ask about the type of home (i.e., apartment, single family) and whether it meets the present needs of the family. Do family members have enough privacy? The nurse should determine whether the location provides easy access to shopping, schools, churches and parks. In rural locations, transportation may be a problem. The nurse should assess the safety of the neighborhood and home. In large metropolitan areas, elderly persons frequently remain in communities which have changed into high crime areas. Ask the patient if he has a fear of crime in his neighborhood. The nurse should also question whether the home is near any industrial sites that may present an environmental hazard.

The safety of the home should be explored in detail if there are children or elderly people living there. For young children it is important to discuss placement of poisonous substances (such as cleaning solutions), home repair equipment, medications, and house plants. Child proof safety locks should be in place on all drawers and cupboards containing dangerous materials. The parent should be asked if there is any peeling paint in the home because it would put the young child at risk for lead poisoning. Toys belonging to older children that are unsuitable for infants and toddlers must be stored out of reach. It is necessary to cover electric sockets when there are toddlers in the home. Additional safety information includes the use of car seats for children under four years of age and the use of safety belts for older children and adults; compliance with water, bike and sports safety.

Accidents in the home are also common for the elderly. Are there loose rugs or mats around? Are there stair railings? Are the stairs getting harder to maneuver without help? Is there a bathroom on the first floor? Does the toilet have a raised seat or handlebars? Is there a shower stall or is the bath tub equipped with safety rails and a mat? Is there adequate light to find the bathroom at night? If the individual uses a cane, walker or wheel chair, determine if he has sufficient space to move within his home. All this information may prove crucial in preventing an accident and is the basis for good preventive teaching.

PATTERNS OF HEALTH CARE

Interesting information is obtained by inquiring about the patient's pattern of health care. In an age of specialization, many patients refer themselves to specialists. The patient may have a variety of health care providers meeting specific needs. However, there may be no one who is treating the individual holistically. This can also result in duplication of services. The patient should be asked about the resources he uses for regular ambulatory care and emergency care. The nurse should record all other health resources that are currently used and that were utilized in the past, including periodic visits to dentists, eye doctors, etc. If folk practitioners, such as herbalists and curanderas are also treating the patient, the nurse should obtain information concerning the nature of and reasons for treatment.

Inquiry should be made into the sources of health care received by other members of the family. The children may see a pediatrician, the mother a gynecologist, and the father may have no health care provider.

The patient's general attitude toward the health care system should be obtained. The patient should be asked if he feels the care he is receiving is adequate. Any bad experiences with health care providers, either personal or involving family members or friends, should be recorded, compliance with past health care recommendations should be obtained. The nurse should explore factors that may have interfered with the family's ability to procure medical care when needed (i.e., no transportation, little money, no babysitter).

Developmental History

The developmental history is elicited to collect information regarding a person's accomplishment of developmental tasks within a particular stage of the life cycle. Erikson's (1963) developmental framework is a universally accepted method of assessing a person's stage of development.

Chart 1.2 is constructed to help the health care provider gather data to evaluate whether or not a person has accomplished the tasks within each stage. This chart provides *examples* of questions used to elicit the appropriate material.

Some of the developmental information will be collected in other areas of the health history (i.e., neurologic history, sexual history). There is no need to repeat this information in two places. It is important, though, to record all pertinent data regarding the accomplishment of the developmental tasks somewhere within the total health history. When

the nurse sees the patient for a well visit this information is recorded in the HPH.

Sexual History

The discussion of the sexual history is based on the premise that man is a holistic being and his sexuality is part of that holism. If we as nurses believe that statement, then the sexual history is as important as any other component of the total health history. Worthy of consideration, too, is the fact that many physical ailments are a result of or are incorporated with psychosocial stresses. This relationship is reciprocal—stresses can precipitate a sexual dysfunction or, similarly, a sexual dysfunction can produce biopsychosocial responses.

Until recently, elicitation of the sexual history as an integral part of the health history was given little attention. There is one recurrent reason why nurses and other health providers deemphasized their role in this process—namely their own discomfort. These feelings inhibit them in broaching the subject with a client. Four key factors can contribute to this discomfort: (1) lack of acceptance of self as a sexual being, (2) lack of acceptance of other definitions of sexuality, (3) a lack of knowledge about human sexuality, and (4) a lack of self-confidence as a professional in this area.

Regardless of how a person defines his sexuality, it is of the utmost importance that he be comfortable with this aspect of his life. To be comfortable does not necessarily mean that this person is sexually active (engaging in intercourse). It does mean that he is comfortable with however he chooses to define his sexuality.

Accepting another person's sexual beliefs can be very difficult. If a person tells the nurse that he is a homosexual or bisexual and that poses a conflict for her in terms of her own values, then she must recognize these feelings and attempt to elicit information without imposing her values. Her responsibility as a health care provider is to offer the patient the highest quality of care that she is capable of giving. In this instance that may mean that she identifies and accepts her feelings and refers this patient to someone who is comfortable dealing with people who define their sexuality in that way. That is a mature and honest

CHART 1.2
THE DEVELOPMENTAL HISTORY

Developmental Tasks	Examples of Questions to Elicit Data

Age: Birth–12 Months
Developmental Stage: Infancy
Developmental Crisis: Trust vs. Mistrust

1. Adjusts physiologically to his physical environment after birth.

(Address questions to parents.) Did you take your baby home with you when you went home from the hospital? Were there any problems after birth? Do you remember the Apgar score? How is the baby sleeping? How is he eating? Does he seem fussy? Does anything in particular bother him?

2. Totally depends on others, but establishes a separateness.

How is your baby special? What seem to be his own unique habits and responses? How does he let you know when he needs you?

3. Becomes a social being, can differentiate between people and objects and strange and familiar.

How does your baby know and respond to you? Your faces? Your voices? Some of your habits? Does he smile? After 6 months: Does he recognize his own environment (i.e., room, toys)? Does he seem to be afraid of strangers?

4. Develops need for affection and returns affection to others.

How does your baby respond to hugging and kissing? Does he seem to "love" back (i.e., hugging, kissing, reaching out to be picked up)?

5. Begins to interpret expectations of others.

How can you tell when he detects displeasure? How does he respond to "no"?

6. Makes strides developmentally.

(See Denver Developmental section in Chapter 15 for questions appropriate to age.)

7. Explores world around him.

Depending on age: Does he follow objects with his eyes? Does he reach out for things? Does he try to move to what is intriguing him?

8. Develops a communication system.

How does he let you know when he wants something? Is he happy? Is he sad?

Age: 13 Months–3 Years
Developmental Stage: Toddler
Developmental Crisis: Autonomy vs. Shame and Doubt

1. Begins to adjust to daily routines.

What does the toddler do all day? What are his activities? His resting patterns? Does he sleep through the night? Does he have a planned bedtime and bath time? Are parents consistent with maintaining structure in the schedule?

2. Develops good nutritional practices.

What times does he eat? Snack? Does he eat table food? What? What utensils does he use? Who does he sit with at mealtimes? (See nutritional history for further detail.)

3. Begins to demonstrate the basics of toilet training.

Earlier stages: Does he indicate when his diapers are dirty? How does he tell you that he has to "go potty"? Does he have a bowel movement when placed on the toilet? Later stages: Does he begin to indicate signs of nighttime control?

4. Develops physical skills appropriate to his age and stages.

What gross-motor, fine-motor, language, and personal-social skills does he demonstrate? (See Denver Developmental section in Chapter 15 for further detail.)

5. Begins to participate as a family member.

What does he enjoy doing with the family? How does he get along with members? Who is he close to? How does he demonstrate affection? How does he play with his brothers and sisters? How does he want to help mommy and daddy?

6. Begins to communicate with people outside his immediate family circle.

How does he play with other children, other adults? How does he communicate with people other than his family?

7. Shows signs of autonomous behavior.

How does he express his needs, wants, likes, and dislikes? What does he do for himself?

Age: 3–5 Years
Developmental Stage: Preschool
Developmental Crisis: Initiative vs. Guilt

1. Adjusts to daily routines of good nutritional habits, physical activity, and appropriate amounts of rest.

What does the preschooler do all day? What are his activities? Eating practices? Who does he sit with at mealtimes? What time does he eat? Snack? Rest? When does he nap? For how long? How many hours of sleep does he get at night?

CHART 1.2—Continued

Developmental Tasks	Examples of Questions to Elicit Data
2. Develops physical skills appropriate to his age and stage.	What gross-motor, fine-motor, language, and personal-social skills is he capable of? (See Denver Developmental section in Chapter 15 for further detail.)
3. Participates actively as a family member.	What does he enjoy doing with the family? How does he get along with members? How does he show affection? Who is he close to in the family? What responsibilities does he assume as a family member (household chores, picking up toys)? What are the feelings between siblings?
4. Becomes toilet-trained	Is he bowel and bladder trained? Since when? Any enuresis or encopresis? Day or night? What problems did he have?
5. Tries to monitor impulsive actions and reactions.	Does he laugh and cry at seemingly appropriate times?[a] What does "no" mean to him (7)?[a] How does he show anger? How do parents deal with anger or temper tantrums?
6. Responds to expectations of others.	How is discipline handled? Is praise given, too? How does he respond to praise, direction, discipline?
7. Develops appropriate emotional expression for various experiences.	Does he seem like a happy child? Is he unusually afraid (5)?[a] What does he do to show happiness, sadness, affection?
8. Learns to communicate effectively with more and more people.	Does he talk? What does he say or talk about? How are his sentences formed—two words, three words, complete? (See Denver Developmental section in Chapter 15—language skills.) Does he listen to you as well as others? How is his attention span? Does his social circle go beyond the immediate family? How does he act around strangers?
9. Begins to handle potentially dangerous situations.	What does he do if he is confronted by a barking dog? What does he understand about poisons, electrical outlets, hot stoves, etc.? What safety signals does he understand?
10. Is developing autonomy.	What things does he want to do for himself (i.e., dress, bathe)? How does he differentiate between and explore the concepts of boy and girl? What typical "little boy" ("little girl") things does he do?
11. Begins to understand life's meaning ethically, religiously and philosophically?	What seems to be important to him? What does he understand about religion, the church, or God (if this is a family value)?

Age: Juvenile Period, 6–9 Years
    Preadolescence, 10–12 Years (Onset of Puberty)
Developmental Stage: School Age
Developmental Crisis: Industry vs. Inferiority

1. Becomes an active and cooperative family member, at the same time decreasing dependency on family for total love and support.	(These questions are directed to the child.) What do you do to be helpful as a family member (i.e., chores)? What does the family do together? Do you have friends outside the family? Who is your best friend?
2. Develops physical characteristics and skills to join in activities in school and with peers.	What kinds of things do you like to do with your friends (i.e., games, hiking, riding)? Do you like sports, running games, etc.?
3. Begins to show active problem solving, especially relating to activities of daily living (ADL) and role for this age.	What do you do when you have a problem with a friend? If you come home from school and no one is home yet, what do you do? What happens when you disagree with your brother or sister?
4. Begins "realistic" communication with parents, siblings, teachers, etc.	What do you and your family talk over together? When you plan a family project, does everyone talk it over? When you have a problem, who do you talk to? When you don't agree with your parents (i.e., at bedtime, going somewhere with a friend), what usually happens?
5. Begins to understand the definition of friend and to learn about give and take with family and peers.	How do you feel about sharing (1, 2, 4)?[a]
6. Begins to learn how to handle money in both saving and spending aspects.	What do you do with your own money? How do you get it? What chores do you do around the house? Do you get an allowance? How do you save money?
7. Handles strong and impulsive feelings.	When you are very happy, how do you show it? When you get very mad, how do you show it? When you are sad, what do you do?

(continued)

CHART 1.2—*Continued*

Developmental Tasks	Examples of Questions to Elicit Data
8. Acknowledges body changes and understands some concepts of masculinity and femininity.	What do you notice that is different about your body? How do you feel about that (see sexual history, page 31)?
9. Relates to aspects of society beyond self—religious (if it is a family or personal value) and community participation.	What kinds of groups or clubs do you belong to? (Girl Scouts, Boy Scouts) What activities does the group participate in? Community programs? Charity projects? How do you feel about going to church? Sunday school? What about religion is special to you?
10. Thinks of self as healthy and engages in healthy activity.	Do you like yourself (1, 2, 4, 8, 9)?[a] Do you feel healthy? How could you be more healthy?

Age: Early, 12–14 Years (Female)
14–16 Years (Male)
Middle, 15–18 Years (Female)
16–20 Years (Male)
Late, 20–25 Years
Developmental Stage: Adolescence
Developmental Crisis: Identity Formation vs. Identity Diffusion

1. Acknowledgement and acceptance of physical changes in body and body image.	(These questions are directed to the adolescent.) How do you see your body changing? How do you feel about it?
2. Attains male or female role.	In today's world, what do you think it means to be a man (woman) (1)?[a] How do you see yourself as a man (woman)?
3. Understands body function and utilization.	What do you understand about reproduction, lovemaking, birth control, etc.? Where did you get this knowledge? What further questions do you have (1)?[a] (See sexual history, page 31—adolescent.) If you have decided to be sexually active, what are your beliefs about and practice of birth control?
4. Has peer relationships of both sexes.	Do you have friends that you enjoy? Male and female? What kinds of activities do you and your friends participate in? Do you have a best friend?
5. Seeks more of a peer relationship with parents, changing from dependence to supportive.	How would you describe your relationship with your parents? What kinds of issues do you agree about? Disagree about? Do you feel they listen to your reasoning? How do you help them to understand you?
6. Begins to make decisions regarding future career, etc. (occupation).	What kind of work would you like to do? Do you have a job now? What will you do when you finish high school? Do you "wish-dream"? What about?
7. Develops a relationship on a deep personal level with future commitment in mind (although this is not the central focus of this task at this age).	Do you date? Do you have a boyfriend (girlfriend)? If so, what kinds of things do you enjoy talking over and doing together? What issues do you disagree about? How do you resolve the discussion when you disagree?
8. Considers role as citizen and contributions that can be made to community life.	What projects do you get involved in that benefit others? Do you belong to a club of any sort? What kind?
9. Develops a set of values, ideals, and ethical standards that contributes to a philosophy of life.	What in life is important to you? What are your personal goals? How do religion and/or spiritual beliefs fit into your life?
10. Promotes good health.	What do you do to be happy and healthy? What sports do you engage in? What do you do if you get sick or need information regarding your health?

Age: 25–45 Years
Developmental Stage: Young Adult
Developmental Crisis: Intimacy vs. Self-isolation

1. Stabilizes self-image.	How do you feel about yourself as a person? How do you feel about the direction your life is taking?
2. Establishes personhood away from parent's home and financial support.	Where do you live? Do you live alone? Are you satisfied with where and with whom you live?
3. Selects a job or career which supports a strong self-image, financial independence, and satisfaction.	What career choice have you made? How did you choose your occupation? Are you satisfied with that decision? What direction is your career taking? Does your income meet your basic needs?
4. Is having (or has had) an intimate relationship which is more than infatuation or just for the purpose of self-gratification.	Are you involved in an intimate relationship (have you been at some point)? How does (did) this relationship

CHART 1.2—Continued

Developmental Tasks	Examples of Questions to Elicit Data
	enrich your life? What do (did) you find particularly satisfying in this relationship? Do you wish to have an intimate relationship in the future?
5. Makes and maintains a home.	How does your home meet your needs (i.e., comfort, life space) (2)?[a]
6. Has a meaningful social life.	Do you have friends that you enjoy? What activities do you participate in together? How do you seek out an interesting life outside your work?
7. Determines desires for having a family.	Do you see yourself becoming a parent? How do you think parenthood will fit into your life and personal goals?
8. Participates in social, civic, and community roles.	Are you involved in any community activities (i.e., PTA, school board, community organizations)? How do you contribute to this (these) group(s)?
9. Maintains an optimal level of wellness.	What is your daily diet? What physical exercise do you do? How do you relax? How much rest do you need? Do you get it? From whom do you obtain your health care?
10. Formulates philosophy of life. Continues to develop values and ethical standards that contribute to this philosophy.	What gives your life meaning? What in life is important to you? What are your personal goals in life? How do religion and/or spiritual beliefs fit into your life?

Age: 45–65 Years
Developmental Stage: Middle Age
Developmental Crisis: Generativity vs. Self-absorption and Stagnation

Developmental Tasks	Examples of Questions to Elicit Data
1. Acknowledges and accepts the physical and emotional changes of the middle years.	What physical changes do you see happening to you? What emotional changes are you aware of? How do you feel about these changes?
2. Works on marriage (or significant relationship) and its growth by developing new joint activities and goals with spouse as well as building on existing love and friendship (including sexual relationship). If need be, they together reassess feelings and commitment and build on that or restructure the relationship in a way appropriate to both members.	How do you feel about your marriage (or significant relationship)? How do you spend your time together? How do you feel about the communication in the relationship? What do you like best and least about being married? How do you see your spouse: as a friend, lover?
3. Fosters independence of grown children.	Are your children still home? Where do they live? How do you feel about your relationship with them? How do they fit into your lives? How do you encourage independence in your children?
4. Finds satisfaction and accepts new responsibilities in work. May be peak time in career.	How do you feel about your work? What do you see yourself doing in later years? How do you feel about retirement?
5. Considers plans for retirement.	How will you keep busy after you retire (4)?[a] How will you maintain economic stability during these years?
6. Creates a comfortable living environment.	Do you feel that your home offers a safe and comfortable environment? How do you maintain your home to your satisfaction?
7. Assists aging parent(s) in finding satisfactory living accommodations and lifestyle for their later years.	Where are your parents living? Are they healthy and independent? How do you see yourself helping them in the future?
8. Maintains and/or enhances civil and social responsibilities.	How do you contribute to your community and/or charity organizations?
9. Develops friendships with new and old friends of both sexes and assorted ages.	Do you have a social life that you enjoy? What activities do you and friends participate in together? Do you find rewards in friendships with people of all ages, and both sexes?
10. Spends leisure time satisfactorily.	What do you do to relax? What do you do in your free time (9)?[a]
11. Practices preventative health care and maintains stability with existing chronic disease, if possible.	What is your daily diet? In what physical exercise do you participate? How much rest do you require (10)?[a] Do you get it? From whom and for what do you obtain health care? Are you satisfied with this (these) resource(s)?
12. Continues to build on existing philosophy of life, if pleased with it, or changes as needed.	What gives your life meaning? What in life was, is, and will be important to you? How do religion and/or spiritual beliefs fit into your life? What are your future goals and plans?

(continued)

CHART 1.2—*Continued*

Developmental Tasks	Examples of Questions to Elicit Data
Age: 65 and over (Questionable; May be 70 and over) **Developmental Stage: Later Maturity** **Developmental Crisis: Ego Integrity vs. Despair**	
1. Makes decisions concerning how and where to live for the rest of his life.	Where do you live? Does your family live nearby? How and where would you choose to live for the rest of your life?
2. Provides self with safe and pleasant living environment within economic means.	Where and how do you see yourself situated if illness or a loss of independence becomes a problem (1)?[a] Whom do you call in an emergency? Do you think your home is safe (i.e., throw rugs, stairs)?
3. Continues close, warm, loving relationship with spouse and helps her (him) to adjust to life in these years.	Do you enjoy the companionship of your spouse? What sort of things do you do together?
4. Adapts to retirement by developing both old and new interests and activities.	How do you spend your day? Do you feel satisfied with your daily activities? Do you feel the need to be productive, if so, are you? Are you active in any clubs, groups, etc.?
5. Acclimates himself to retirement income and augments this if desirable and possible.	Does your income meet your needs? In what areas is most of your income spent?
6. Promotes for himself and spouse the highest level of wellness possible. Seeks care and complies with and practices prevention wherever possible.	How do you feel physically and emotionally? What type of diet do you follow? What exercise do you get? How do you see your body changing? How do you feel about its changes? For what and from whom do you seek health care? Do you have Medicare? What other agencies do you use? Do you go for follow-up visits at recommended times (2)?[a]
7. Maintains close relationships with children, grandchildren, and other relatives and friends.	How often do you correspond and visit with your family? Do they live nearby? How often are you able to visit and communicate with friends and relatives?
8. Maintains old interests and develops new ones with both activities and people.	How often are you able to communicate with friends? How have your friendships developed new meaning over the years? Do you have new friends?
9. Copes with and accepts illness or death of spouse, aging relatives, and friends.	(Questions will vary according to the recency of deaths. For the most part, open-ended questions like "How are you feeling since your wife [husband] died?" will open communication.)
10. Continues to uphold his philosophy of life and feeling of self-worth.	How do you see that your life has meaning, to you and to others? How do religion and/or spiritual beliefs fit into your life?
11. Develops his philosophy of life so that death is accepted as a part of life. Accepts prospect of own death, secure in knowledge that his life has made a contribution to mankind.	Have you thought about death? How do you feel about dying? Do you feel you have your affairs in order to your satisfaction (i.e., wills, finances)? Do you feel you have made a contribution to others in your life? How do you feel you will be remembered?

[a] Questions may fit in with other categories. Numbers in parentheses refer to the developmental task and its corresponding questions.

way of dealing with such feelings. The nurse should not consider herself inadequate because she refers the patient to another provider.

A knowledge base about the physiologic, cultural, and developmental aspects of human sexuality is essential if the nurse expects to be effective. It is not enough for the nurse to be able to answer questions that a patient may have. The nurse as a teacher and counselor must assess the patient's developmental level, health or illness status, and his unique characteristics as a human being. She is then in a position to provide anticipatory guidance as he needs it.

If a nurse accepts her own sexuality and the sexuality of others and has a strong knowledge base on the subject, then her level of self-confidence in this role will improve markedly. If she can convey an attitude of self-assuredness and trust, the patient will most likely respond to her with frankness and honesty.

The primary goal of taking a sexual history is for the nurse to gain knowledge about the patient's feelings or concerns about his sexuality so that teaching, counseling, and support may be given to the patient when necessary. A most important fact to remember is that there is no one way to elicit a sexual history. Every nurse must find a method that is comfortable for her and her patients. It is expected that the nurse will develop her own style as she gains confidence in the art of taking a sexual history. Knowing the patient's developmental stage is helpful in deciding upon an approach to use in eliciting appropriate and pertinent information. The questions asked of a school-age child will obviously differ from those asked of an older person. Therefore, the best way for the nurse to develop an approach is by starting with an assessment of the developmental stage. Following are a few suggestions to help in taking a sexual history.

INFANCY THROUGH PRESCHOOL

The sexual history of the very young child focuses primarily on parental concerns and approaches they are taking in educating their child and instilling their own values about sex. Some of the following questions may help to open the discussion.

1. Do you have any questions or concerns about the development of your child's genitalia?
2. Do you have any questions or concerns as how to proceed, now and in the future, with sex education for your child?
3. Has your child begun to notice that other people are not identical to him? (commonly occurs between the ages of 3 and 5)
4. Are there rules for bathroom and bedroom privacy in your home? Is there family agreement on this issue?
5. What terms do you use with the child for his anatomy?
6. Has he begun to ask questions about procreation? How do you feel about this?
7. Do you have any concerns regarding sexual abuse? Are you knowledgeable about teaching your child to protect himself from sexual abuse?

SCHOOL AGE

The child in these years is very curious and asks a lot of questions. The "rule of thumb" is to be honest and straightforward when responding. The nurse should *not* make assumptions about what the child does or does not know. In addition, it is important to consider the parents' feelings about what and where their child learns about the "facts of life." It should be remembered, too, that when a child asks a sex-related question, one should clarify what the child wants to know. The following questions are *examples* of how a nurse might elicit a sexual history from the school-age child.

1. What do you know about having babies?
   a. From whom and where did you learn this information (school, friends, etc.)?
   b. When you have questions about having babies, etc., whom do you ask?
2. What do you notice about your body changing? How does that make you feel?
3. What do you know about having "periods?"
4. What other questions do you have?

This information will provide a beginning data base regarding the child's perceptions and knowledge about pregnancy and puberty. The nurse can then decide whether the child is adequately informed. If he is not, she must make some decisions about what to say to the parents. This can be a sensitive area, especially if the parents do not feel secure discussing sex with their children. In any case, the nurse must see that the child has access to appropriate information, so that any major physical changes in the child do not frighten or repulse him.

ADOLESCENCE

The physical and emotional changes that a teenager undergoes affect his sexual identity. Each adolescent responds differently to these changes. Some will be more embarrassed than others. Some will try to deny the existence of these changes. Others will explore all facets of their development. A teenager's attitudes and acceptance of these changes may reflect how he feels about himself as a person. The accomplishment of the developmental tasks will depend in great measure on the adult support and guidance available to him during this period. Peer relationships will also influence risk-taking and testing. The nurse should be prepared to listen objectively and offer support and factual information. Directness is very important, as is mutual understanding of the terms used in the dialogue. Privacy and confidentiality are fundamental to the trust that develops in this relationship.

Prior assessment of the youth's level of maturity and development is helpful in identifying appropriate questions to ask. Once assured that the patient can answer the questions appropriate for school-age children, the nurse may gather information more directly by asking the questions for adolescents.

The teenager may have already had a sexual experience. It may have been heterosexual, bisexual, or homosexual. The nurse should be prepared to respond as she would to any other information the patient reveals. However, without making any assumptions, the nurse must find out whether the adolescent is sexually active or not. Once she determines this, she can guide the conversation accordingly.

Some nurses have found that an appropriate time to approach the sexual history of the adolescent is after the completion of the physical examination. Both young males and young females need reassurance that they are developing normally. The nurse can share with the adolescent male that his testicles are fine and his penis is growing as it should for his age. She can then say that it is not uncommon for boys his age to have wet dreams and that he is at the age when he is capable of fathering a child. The young girl can be reassured that her breasts and genitalia are developing normally, and since she is now menstruating, she can become pregnant. More intimate questions can flow from this point.

There are several methods of approaching the question, "Are you sexually active?" Sometimes a general statement to open the dialogue is helpful. An example is, "Some teenagers have decided to be sexually active. How do you feel about that?" (Be sure to use terminology familiar to the patient.) From the patient's response there will probably be some cues that the nurse can pick up and use for further exploration by saying, "How does that fit into your life?" The nurse should keep in mind that "being sexually active" can have varied meanings. The activity may include vaginal–penile, oral–genital, or rectal intercourse, as well as other variations. It may not be necessary to identify the patient's specific preferences or practices; this is left to the judgment of the individual practitioner. The primary concern with the adolescent is that he or she has an understanding of conception. If it is determined that the patient is sexually active, then birth control and satisfaction with any relationship should be discussed. The following questions are *examples* that may be helpful to the nurse:

1. Birth control
   a. Do you use birth control measures?
   b. What birth control method(s) are you using?
   c. What do you like or dislike about it (them)?
   d. What other methods are you familiar with? What do you know about (them)?
   e. What other method(s) have you used in the past?
      (1) What did you like or dislike about it (them)?
      (2) What problems did you have with it (them)?
   f. Are there other methods you would like to consider?
      (1) What do you know about the method?
      (2) Why do you feel that method would be good for you?
   g. If pregnancy were to occur, how would you feel? How does this affect your sexual pleasure or relationship?
2. Satisfaction with the sexual relationship
   a. How do you feel about your sexual relationship? Do you talk over your feelings, pleasures, and displeasures with your partner(s)?
   b. For women
      (1) Do you have pain with intercourse? Dryness?
         (a) At what point during intercourse does this occur? With entry? With deep thrusting?
         (b) Do some positions cause the symptom(s) more than others? Which position(s)?
      (2) Do you have orgasms?
         (a) Do you notice that they occur more easily when you are relaxed, rested, and feeling good about yourself and the relationship?
         (b) Do you notice that they occur more easily if you have more

time, privacy, and/or fore-
play?"
(3) Is the frequency with which you
have intercourse satisfactory to
you?
(4) Many people find masturbation to
be a satisfying sexual outlet. How
is this for you?
  c. For men
(1) Do you have any problems with
having or maintaining an erection? If yes:
  (a) How often?
  (b) Do you notice that fatigue,
stress, and how you are feeling about yourself and the relationship affect this?
(2) Do you have problems with ejaculation?
  (a) What happens?
  (b) How often?
  (c) Do you notice that fatigue,
stress, and how you are feeling about yourself and the relationship affect this?
(3) Is the frequency with which you
have intercourse satisfactory to
you?
(4) Many people find masturbation to
be a satisfying sexual outlet. How
is this for you?

If the teenager is not sexually active, it
is important to determine whether he antici-
pates becoming active in the near future. The
nurse should discuss the patient's feelings
about not being sexually active. There may
be some peer pressure either to alter or maintain his present state. How does the patient
handle that pressure? This is a good time in
the interview for the nurse to provide anticipatory guidance regarding responsibility for
birth control, including information about
various methods and about facilities that provide birth control services. The nurse's confidentiality as well as availability as a resource
person must be emphasized to the patient.

YOUNG ADULT

For all adults, the sexual history usually flows
easily from the genitourinary history in the
review of systems. Asking a woman about her

menstrual pattern, facilitates the discussion
of her sexuality. For the male, the dialogue
can continue from questions pertaining to urinary symptoms, etc.

For the single young adult the same approaches that are used with the unmarried adolescent may be employed to elicit the sexual
history. A general comment can be used to
open communication, such as "Many single
people decide that being sexually active fits
into their lifestyle. How do you feel about
that?" As with the teenager, it is necessary to
establish whether or not the patient is sexually
active and what his feelings are about his
choice. If the patient is engaging in intercourse, the same questions that are used with
the sexually-active teenager may be used. If
the patient is not active, the basic approach
used with the nonactive adolescent may be
helpful to the nurse.

When the patient is married, discussing
how he feels about his relationship with his
wife may flow easily into his sharing how he
feels about their sexual relationship. Care
should be taken not to make any assumptions
regarding marital fidelity or the lack of that
commitment. Open-ended questions such as,
"How would you describe your sex life?" or
"How are things for you sexually?" will prevent falling into an embarrassing trap.

When children are born into a marriage,
a couple's energy dissipates in new directions.
This is a common time for sexual tension to
occur. The patient should have an opportunity
to express his/her feelings about the changes
that occur in a growing family. Again a general statement might open communication,
such as, "Many couples notice that when they
have children their own relationship changes
significantly. What have you noticed that's different in your relationship since the birth of
your child(ren)?" After the patient has shared
his/her feelings about this, the nurse should
further explore the patient's overall satisfaction with his sexual life. (See questions regarding satisfaction in sexual relationships under
"Adolescence."

The desire to have children can affect the
purposes of lovemaking. If there is a difficulty
with conception, lovemaking can become
task-oriented. Here again, the nurse should
give the patient an opportunity to identify this
aspect of the relationship and share his feelings about it. As the quality of the sexual rela-

tionship is discussed the presence of this task orientation often becomes clear.

In this developmental stage, career goals or job related stresses are often a major focus of the patient's life. Many times, working towards achieving these goals or resolving the stresses takes a great deal of physical and emotional energy. The result of these efforts and the time commitment involved may cause unusual fatigue and strain, thus affecting the patient's libido and sexual abilities. Unusual financial concern may also have the same effect. It is important to explore this with the patient. A general statement such as the following may facilitate conversation: "Some people notice that when they are under severe job or financial pressure there is a change in their sexual abilities or desires. Have you noticed this happening to you?" If yes, "What have you noticed that is different? How do you feel about that?" These kinds of life stresses are not necessarily unique to any particular developmental stage and should be considered whenever the possibilities exist.

MIDDLE AGE

Whether a person is single, married, widowed, or divorced, general inquiry about how he feels about his sexuality is appropriate. However, in this age group there are some key areas that might affect the patient's feelings, desires, and self-image.

For the female, the most obvious physiologic change that is likely to occur is menopause. This can have a positive or negative effect or even no effect at all. For some women, freedom from fear of becoming pregnant makes menopause a great relief. For others, no longer having the ability to become pregnant may seem like a loss. Before making any assumptions, the nurse should explore how the patient feels about the changes taking place in her body (a discussion of what she notices happening will probably precede this in the menstrual history). Once her feelings have been discussed and the fact that she remains sexually active has been established, it is important to share with her that some women notice dryness or pain with intercourse after menopause because of physiologic changes in the vagina. Such symptoms are a common problem and can often be treated effectively with lubricating creams, if

the physiologic change is the primary reason for the problem. The nurse should find out whether or not there are situational or self-image crises. If there are emotional stresses superimposed on the physiologic changes, then these feelings should be explored as well.

Physiologically, the male at this stage has changes, too. Attainment of an erection takes longer, sustainment time decreases, and ejaculatory force lessens (Masters & Johnson, 1966). These changes are likely to happen gradually throughout the aging process. The nurse should explore with the patient his fears and feelings about these occurrences.

The nurse should be alert to common life stresses during these years. The patient may be at the height of his career, or he may be trying to keep his job safe from the "younger fellow in the department." There may be a problem with physical illness that keeps him from doing his job. He may have major expenses in terms of educating his children or helping his retired parents financially. In any event, the impact of these types of stresses can affect his sexual desires and abilities. The nurse must be able to elicit information to help the patient identify the presence of these problems. She can then follow with a discussion of how he feels about his sexual life. (It is important not to make assumptions or inferences about the existence of one or more than one partner.)

After exploring these areas with the patient it is important to discuss his feelings about the quality of the existing relationship(s). Such questions as the following are helpful in eliciting information on these feelings: How would you rate your marriage sexually? How do you think your wife would rate it? What would you do to make it better? What could your wife do to make it better? These questions can be asked of any patient who has a significant relationship. Anticipatory guidance regarding normal developmental struggles may help the patient avoid long-term concerns which can cause sexual problems.

LATE MATURITY

Emotional well-being and personal security are promoted when a person is involved in a close relationship. This is particularly important for the elderly. At this stage of development the major deterents to continuing sexual activity are societal conventions, lack of a partner, and illness (Gioiella & Bevil, 1985). Unfortunately, society has viewed sexual activity as being for the young and not the aging individual. Some elderly persons use this societal convention as an excuse for discontinuing sexual activity. Therefore, the nurse is concerned not only with present, but past relationships. What is particularly sad are those persons who have enjoyed the closeness of sex and would like to continue, but lack an available partner. At this stage of life, chronic illness often exists and can abruptly interrupt a person's sexual life. With this information in mind the nurse directs her sexual history of the older adult accordingly.

A general statement to open the dialogue is: "Many older people enjoy a close physical relationship with a loved one. How do you feel about that?" Then a question regarding how the patient feels about his present and past sexual function should be asked. It is especially important to ask the individual if he has any discomforts or problems with sexual activity. The same questions discussed earlier regarding sexual satisfaction should be asked of those individuals who have a partner. The nurse should explore the feelings of the elderly person who is alone and help identify alternative outlets.

Sensitivity on the nurse's part is important, too. Some patients may prefer not to share this information or may need a long-established relationship before they can do so. The nurse must decipher the patient's verbal and nonverbal cues. She must try to ascertain what the patient is really trying to tell her. In addition, the nurse must be aware of traditions and long-standing cultural beliefs and stereotypes especially related to aging and sexual behavior. This will add to her ability to provide anticipatory guidance in these situations because her knowledge base will be broader.

Exercise and Activity Patterns

This category of information has four purposes. First, it provides the nurse with knowledge regarding the patient's perception of his approach to maintaining an optimal level of wellness, both physical and emotional. Sec-

ond, the patient has an opportunity to share with the nurse his own ideas (or lack thereof) of what he does to maintain his health. Third, these data give the nurse an idea of the patient's leisure activities which contribute to his health. Fourth, it alerts a patient to the fact that he has responsibilities for his health.

Eliciting information regarding the patient's hobbies (cooking, stamp collecting, etc.), recreational interests (fishing, camping, etc.), and physical activity (jogging, swimming, etc.) will give the nurse further insight into the patient's lifestyle. The following questions are helpful in assessing the exercise and activity patterns of the young child:

1. What are the child's favorite toys?
2. What are the child's favorite play activities?
3. How much time does the child spend watching television?
4. What types of television programs does he enjoy?

Additional questions to be asked of the school-age child and adolescent include:

1. Do you participate in any group sports? What type?
2. Do you participate in any individual sports? What type? How often?
3. Do you have any hobbies? What are they?

Questions to be asked of the adult include:

1. Do you have an exercise program? What is it?
2. How many times per week do you exercise? How much time do you spend per session?
3. How would you describe the level of exertion you reach during exercise?
4. Do you find barriers to exercising on a regular basis? What are they?
5. What do you enjoy doing during your leisure time?
6. How active are you compared to others in your age group?

Stress Patterns

The nurse has two objectives: to identify stress in the patient's life that may lead to illness; and to determine the patient's ability to pre-

CHART 1.3
LIFE-CHANGE INDEX

Please check those life changes that you have experienced personally during the past *two years.*

Life Event	Scale of Impact Units	
Death of Spouse	100	_____
Divorce	73	_____
Marital separation	65	_____
Jail term	63	_____
Death of close family member	63	_____
Personal injury or illness	53	_____
Marriage	50	_____
Fired at work	47	_____
Marital reconciliation	45	_____
Retirement	45	_____
Change in health of family member	44	_____
Pregnancy	40	_____
Sex difficulties	39	_____
Gain of new family member	39	_____
Business readjustment	39	_____
Change in financial state	38	_____
Death of close friend	37	_____
Change to different line of work	36	_____
Change in number of arguments with spouse	35	_____
Mortgage over $20,000	31	_____
Foreclosure of mortgage or loan	30	_____
Change in responsibilities at work	29	_____
Son or daughter leaving home	29	_____
Trouble with in-laws	29	_____
Outstanding personal achievement	28	_____
Spouse begins or stops work	26	_____
Begin or end school	26	_____
Change in living conditions	25	_____
Revision of personal habits	24	_____
Trouble with boss	23	_____
Change in work hours or conditions	20	_____
Change in residence	20	_____
Change in schools	20	_____
Change in recreation	19	_____
Change in church activities	19	_____
Change in social activities	18	_____
Mortgage or loan less than $20,000	17	_____
Change in sleeping habits	16	_____
Change in number of family get-togethers	15	_____
Change in eating habits	15	_____
Vacation	13	_____
Christmas (if approaching)	12	_____
Minor violations of the law	11	_____
Total		_____

(Reprinted from Holmes, T., & Rahe, E. Journal of Psychosomatic Research, 1967, 11, 214. Copyright © 1967, Pergamon Press, Ltd., with permission.)

CHART 1.4
SCORING THE LIFE-CHANGE INDEX

Score Range	Interpretation
0–150	No significant problems, low or tolerable life change
150–199	Mild life change (approximately 33% chance of illness)
200–299	Moderate life change (approximately 50% chance of illness)
300 or over	Major life change (approximately 80% chance of illness)

(Reprinted from Holmes, T., & Rahe, E. Journal of Psychosomatic Research, 1967, 11, 213. Copyright © 1967 Pergamon Press, Ltd., with permission.)

vent or cope with stress. Holmes and Rahe (1967) developed a tool to measure life change in adults as a predictor of the probability of becoming ill. Chances of becoming ill increase with the number of life changes a person expe-

riences in a 2-year period. The Life-Change Index can be self-administered or done in the form of an interview (Chart 1.3). The scoring procedure for the index is given in Chart 1.4. Coddington modified the index for children (1972) utilizing the methods developed by Holmes and Rahe (Charts 1.5 to 1.8). The amount of change the child has undergone during a year is determined by adding the scale of impact units. This provides a measure of the environmental factors effecting the child.

Following an assessment of stress factors the nurse should explore how the individual prevents or copes with stress. Questions to ask include:

1. What situations cause stress?
2. How do you react to a stressful situation?

CHART 1.5
LIFE-CHANGE INDEX FOR THE PRESCHOOL AGE GROUP

Please check those life changes that your child has experienced in the past year.

Life Event	Scale of Impact Units	
Death of a parent	89	_____
Divorce of parents	78	_____
Marital separation of parents	74	_____
Jail sentence of parent for 1 year or more	67	_____
Marriage of parent to stepparent	62	_____
Serious illness requiring hospitalization of child	59	_____
Death of a brother or sister	59	_____
Acquiring a visible deformity	52	_____
Serious illness requiring hospitalization of parent	51	_____
Birth of a brother or sister	50	_____
Mother beginning to work	47	_____
Increase in number of arguments between parents	44	_____
Beginning nursery school	42	_____
Addition of third adult to family (i.e., grandparent, etc.)	39	_____
Brother or sister leaving home	39	_____
Having a visible congenital deformity	39	_____
Increase in number of arguments with parents	39	_____
Change in child's acceptance by peers	38	_____
Death of a close friend	38	_____
Serious illness requiring hospitalization of brother or sister	37	_____
Change in father's occupation requiring increased absence from home	36	_____
Jail sentence of parent for 30 days or less	34	_____
Discovery of being an adopted child	33	_____
Change to a new nursery school	33	_____
Death of a grandparent	30	_____
Outstanding personal achievement	23	_____
Loss of job by a parent	23	_____
Decrease in number of arguments with parents	22	_____
Decrease in number of arguments between parents	21	_____
Change in parents' financial status	21	_____

(From Coddington, R. Journal of Psychosomatic Research, 16, 13, 1972, with permission.)

CHART 1.6
LIFE-CHANGE INDEX FOR THE ELEMENTARY SCHOOL AGE GROUP

Please check those life changes that your child has experienced in the past year.

Life Event	Scale of Impact Units	
Death of a parent	91	_____
Divorce of parents	84	_____
Marital separation of parents	78	_____
Acquiring a visible deformity	69	_____
Death of a brother or sister	68	_____
Jail sentence of parent for 1 year or more	67	_____
Marriage of parent to stepparent	65	_____
Serious illness requiring hospitalization of child	62	_____
Becoming involved with drugs or alcohol	61	_____
Having a visible congenital deformity	60	_____
Failure of a grade in school	57	_____
Serious illness requiring hospitalization of parent	55	_____
Death of a close friend	53	_____
Discovery of being an adopted child	52	_____
Increase in number of arguments between parents	51	_____
Change in child's acceptance by peers	51	_____
Birth of a brother or sister	50	_____
Increase in number of arguments with parents	47	_____
Move to a new school district	46	_____
Beginning school	46	_____
Suspension from school	46	_____
Change in father's occupation requiring increased absence from home	45	_____
Mother beginning to work	44	_____
Jail sentence of parent for 30 days or less	44	_____
Serious illness requiring hospitalization of brother or sister	41	_____
Addition of third adult to family (i.e. grandmother, etc.)	41	_____
Outstanding personal achievement	39	_____
Loss of job by a parent	38	_____
Death of a grandparent	38	_____
Brother or sister leaving home	36	_____
Pregnancy in unwed teenage sister	36	_____
Change in parents' financial status	29	_____
Beginning another school year	27	_____
Decrease in number of arguments with parents	27	_____
Decrease in number of arguments between parents	25	_____
Becoming a full fledged member of a church	25	_____
Total		_____

(*From Coddington, R. Journal of Psychosomatic Research, 16, 14, 1972, with permission.*)

CHART 1.7
LIFE-CHANGE INDEX FOR THE JUNIOR HIGH SCHOOL AGE GROUP

Please check those life changes that you have experienced personally during the past year.

Life Event	Scale of Impact Units	
Unwed pregnancy of self	95	_____
Death of a parent	94	_____
Divorce of parents	84	_____
Acquiring a visible deformity	83	_____
Marital separation of parents	77	_____
Jail sentence of parent for 1 year or more	76	_____
Fathering an unwed pregnancy	76	_____
Death of a brother or sister	71	_____
Having a visible congenital deformity	70	_____
Discovery of being an adopted child	70	_____
Becoming involved with drugs or alcohol	70	_____
Change in your acceptance by peers	68	_____
Death of a close friend	65	_____
Marriage of parent to stepparent	63	_____
Failure of a grade in school	62	_____
Pregnancy in unwed teenage sister	60	_____
Serious illness requiring hospitalization of self	59	_____
Beginning to date	55	_____
Suspension from school	54	_____
Serious illness requiring hospitalization of parent	54	_____
Move to a new school district	52	_____
Jail sentence of parent for 30 days or less	50	_____
Birth of a brother or sister	50	_____
Not making an extracurricular activity you wanted	49	_____
Loss of job by a parent	48	_____
Increase in number of arguments between parents	48	_____
Breaking up with a boyfriend or girlfriend	47	_____
Increase in number of arguments with parents	46	_____
Beginning Junior High School	45	_____
Outstanding personal achievement	45	_____
Serious illness requiring hospitalization of brother or sister	44	_____
Change in father's occupation requiring increased absence from home	42	_____
Change in parents' financial status	40	_____
Mother beginning to work	36	_____
Death of a grandparent	35	_____
Addition of third adult to family (i.e. grandparent, etc.)	34	_____
Brother or sister leaving home	33	_____
Decrease in number of arguments between parents	29	_____
Decrease in number of arguments with parents	29	_____
Becoming a full fledged member of a church	28	_____
Total		_____

(From Coddington, R. Journal of Psychosomatic Research, 16, 15, 1972, with permission.)

CHART 1.8
LIFE-CHANGE INDEX FOR THE SENIOR HIGH SCHOOL AGE GROUP

Please check those life changes that you have experienced personally during the past year.

Life Event	Scale of Impact Units	
Getting married	101	_____
Unwed pregnancy of self	92	_____
Death of a parent	87	_____
Acquiring a visible deformity	81	_____
Divorce of parents	77	_____
Fathering an unwed pregnancy	77	_____
Becoming involved with drugs or alcohol	76	_____
Jail sentence of parent for 1 year or more	75	_____
Marital separation of parents	69	_____
Death of a brother or sister	68	_____
Change in your acceptance by peers	67	_____
Pregnancy in unwed teenage sister	64	_____
Discovery of being an adopted child	64	_____
Marriage of parent to stepparent	63	_____
Death of a close friend	63	_____
Having a visible congenital deformity	62	_____
Serious illness requiring hospitalization of self	58	_____
Failure of a grade in school	56	_____
Move to a new school district	56	_____
Not making an extracurricular activity you wanted	55	_____
Serious illness requiring hospitalization of parent	55	_____
Jail sentence of parent for 30 days or less	53	_____
Breaking up with a boyfriend or girlfriend	53	_____
Beginning to date	51	_____
Suspension from school	50	_____
Birth of a brother or sister	50	_____
Increase in number of arguments with parents	47	_____
Increase in number of arguments between parents	46	_____
Loss of job by a parent	46	_____
Outstanding personal achievement	46	_____
Change in parents' financial status	45	_____
Being accepted at a college of your choice	43	_____
Beginning senior high school	42	_____
Serious illness requiring hospitalization of brother or sister	41	_____
Change in father's occupation requiring increased absence from home	38	_____
Brother or sister leaving home	37	_____
Death of a grandparent	36	_____
Addition of third adult to family (i.e., grandparent, etc.)	34	_____
Becoming a full fledged member of a church	31	_____
Decrease in number of arguments between parents	27	_____
Decrease in number of arguments with parents	26	_____
Mother beginning to work	26	_____
Total		_____

(From Coddington, R. Journal of Psychosomatic Research, 16, 15, 1972, with permission.)

3. Have you identified any means of preventing or alleviating stress? How?
4. Does stress interfere with the way you interact with others at home, school, work? How?
5. Do you have someone close to you who is of comfort to you at times of stress?

For the child, questions are directed more toward displays of anger and how he handles his anger.

SUMMARY

The reader has probably noted that there are areas of overlap in health history. To some extent this is built in to ensure accuracy. Questions may go unanswered because they are unclear or forgotten. A similar question asked again may jog the patient's memory or be understood this time. Some repetition serves as a check on the reliability of the information the patient provides and is a check on his consistency. Where to record the data is sometimes clear, but is often left up to the interviewer's judgment. For example, the patient may have forgotten to mention a past surgical experience when asked about his hospitalizations, but mention it in the review of systems. This surgery should be recorded under the section on past history and a notation to see past history would be made in the review of systems. It is not necessary to record data more than once. The recorder need only refer to where the information occurs in the history. Taking and recording a health history is a highly complex skill that requires knowledge, experience and frequent self-appraisal. See Appendix A for the blank worksheet for recording the patient history. (See also Appendix B for the completed worksheet.)

EXAMPLE OF A HEALTH HISTORY ON AN INFANT

NAME K. J.

ADDRESS

AGE 1 month   SEX F   Marital Status S

RACE Caucasian RELIGION Protestant

OCCUPATION Not applicable

USUAL SOURCE OF MEDICAL CARE HMO

SOURCE AND RELIABILITY OF INFORMATION Mother, who appears

articulate and reliable

CHIEF COMPLAINT/REASON FOR VISIT:

"She's due for her 4-week-check-up, but I think she looks thin."

HISTORY OF PRESENT STATE OF HEALTH:

Mother says the baby has been "healthy" and "doing well" since birth.

The baby came home from the hospital with her mother 2 days postpartum. She was born after an uncomplicated spontaneous vaginal delivery (see Labor and Delivery History). She cried immediately. Her weight was 8 lbs. 6 oz.; length 21″. She had a stool shortly after birth and the mother thinks she urinated at the time.

Mother states baby could not suck breast for the first 24 hours. Sterile water and 1 supplemental bottle given. Second day, baby was able to nurse 5 minutes on each breast with use of nipple shield. Continued like this for 3 more days. Mother "frustrated and ready to give up." Mother then developed "clogged nipples and ducts." The next few days baby "struggled with grasping the breast, but eventually was able to nurse 10 minutes on each breast." Until 2 weeks ago, nursed 6 times/day. Mother now gives pacifier after baby nurses 20 minutes (10 minutes/side), to "satisfy sucking." Takes fluoride drops and Vit. D. Burps easily after 5 minutes of feeding and then at end of feeding.

The last 2 weeks things much improved. Continues to nurse 4 to 5 times per day. Both mother and baby "satisfied." Baby does not like H_2O. She urinates "6 to 9 times per day." Has "squirty, soup-like" yellow stool every day or every other day. Moderate to large amount ("fills diaper"). The cord came off 2 weeks ago—no bleeding or discharge.

Sleeps for 4 to 6 hour periods. Does not cry often if not hungry or wet. Mother states her husband is "very supportive and helpful. He's thrilled to death with the baby. He knows the first few weeks are a big adjustment and tries to remind me of that."

In general, mother feels things are going "as smoothly as possible now." She's concerned about the baby being "too thin because of our problem in the beginning, and she just looks small to me."

PAST HISTORY

Childhood Illnesses: None yet.

Immunizations: None yet.

Allergies: None known to foods, clothes, soaps.

Hospitalizations and Serious Illnesses: None yet.

Accidents and Injuries: None yet.

Medications: None since birth.

Habits: Not applicable.

Prenatal History: Mother had no health problems during pregnancy. Considered herself in "excellent health." We were anxious to become parents and the timing could not have been better." Mother tried to eat balanced diet with right amount of vegetables, meat, fruit. Mother took no alcohol or medication during pregnancy. Gained 25 lbs. Had "low blood count." M.D. prescribed FeSO₄ tablets t.i.d. No toxemia, diabetes, heart disease, or depression during pregnancy. Felt life at "4 months." Baby carried to term. Duration of pregnancy: 40 weeks.

Labor and Delivery History: Modified LeBoyer birth. Father present throughout. Mother feels labor was "easy." Ten hour duration. Delivered vaginally. No forceps. Pudendal block used. "Very effective." Baby cried instantly. Weighed 8 lb. 6 oz. Then given to father so he could hold and give bath. After bath, mother, dad, and baby spent 2 hours together in recovery room. "Apgar 9."

Neonatal History: (See HPH.) No respiratory distress, jaundice, seizures, paralysis, congenital anomalies, or blood group incompatibility.

FAMILY HISTORY:

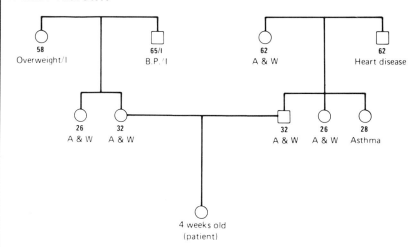

O = female; □ = male; no family history of cancer, epilepsy, stroke, tuberculosis, diabetes, mental illness, mental retardation, or kidney disease.

REVIEW OF SYSTEMS:

General: "Pink and healthy." (See HPH.)

Skin and Mucous Membranes: No rashes, no diaper irritation, moles, birthmarks. "Black and blue" bruise on frontal area of scalp from birth—disappeared at 2 weeks.

Hair: "Light peach fuzz on head."

Nails: Seem to grow fast. Must trim 2 ×/wk.

Head: No lump, lesions. "Soft spot" in top of head; it seems to "pulsate" sometimes. Baby has no hair yet, "fuzzy light hair" covers scalp.

Eyes: No discharge, redness. Can cry real tears. Looks at mobile in crib. Squints in bright light.

Ears: No discharge, redness, lesions. Seems to listen to music box in mobile. Responds with a startle to loud noises.

Nose and Sinuses: No discharge, no bleeding.

Mouth: No drooling, lesions, teeth. Can purse lips to suck.

Throat: "Floppy." No masses or stiffness.

Nodes: No masses noted in cervical, axillary, epitrochlear, or inguinal areas.

Breast: Had "small breast buds" when born. Resolved at 2 weeks. No discharge then. No masses, discharge now.

Respiratory: No cough, breathing difficulties, wheezing, or history of respiratory illness.

Cardiovascular: "Can feel her heart beating when I hold her against me." No cyanosis, peripheral edema, or varicosities.

Gastrointestinal: "Nurses well." Burps 2 to 3 times during feedings. No apparent colic or abdominal cramping. No constipation, diarrhea. (See HPH.)

Genitourinary: Voids yellow, not strong-smelling liquid 6 to 8 times per day. No vaginal discharge.

Menstrual History: Not applicable.

Back: No noticeable curvature of spine. Able to lift head from bed when lying on abdomen. Cannot hold head up without support.

Extremities: Fingers and toes symmetrical bilatcrally. Legs "long and thin." Feet and hands warm to touch. No apparent redness, edema, stiffness, or deformity.

Neurologic: No seizures, paralysis, tics, tremors, projectile vomiting; no difficulty sucking. Cries when hungry or wet. (See Developmental.)

Hematopoietic: No known anemia, need for "purple light" after birth. No bleeding or bruising tendencies. Mom and dad's blood type both A positive.

Endocrine: No apparent heat or cold intolerances. No hair on body.

NUTRITIONAL HISTORY:

Breast feeding. (See HPH.)

SOCIAL DATA:

Family Relationships and Friendships: "We hope she is as pleased with us as we are with her." Grandparents on both sides live nearby and visit often. They like to babysit. No siblings.

Ethnic Affiliation: Mother denies any ethnic or religious customs that might affect her response to health and illness.

Occupational History: Not applicable.

Educational History: Not applicable.

Economic Status: Parents both work. Income meets needs. No extras right now. Mother plans to return to part-time in 3 months. Working on babysitting arrangements.

Daily Profile: See HPH.

Living Circumstances: Family lives in 3-bedroom ranch house in suburb. All conveniences: gas heat, city water, air conditioning, etc. Baby has own room. In cradle at present. Will move to her crib when she gets bigger.

Pattern of Health Care: Family practice M.D. and nurse practitioner team. Parents very satisfied with availability, teaching, and care by the team.

DEVELOPMENTAL HISTORY:

Mother notices that when she strokes baby's cheek she begins to suck; there is no difficulty sucking; when finger is inserted in baby's hand, she grasps finger; if loud noise, baby is startled; when she is held in a standing position and her feet touch a flat surface she "tries to step"; she lifts her head up when lying on abdomen, but cannot hold it straight yet (for vision and hearing see Review of Systems)

SEXUAL HISTORY:

No present concerns.

EXERCISE AND ACTIVITY PATTERNS:

See HPH.

STRESS PATTERNS:

Not applicable.

EXAMPLE OF A HEALTH HISTORY ON A YOUNG ADULT

NAME L. R.

ADDRESS Harvey University, Boston, MA

AGE 21   *SEX* F   *MARITAL STATUS* S

RACE Caucasian *RELIGION* Baptist

OCCUPATION Student; part-time nurse's aid (home care of elderly)

USUAL SOURCE OF MEDICAL CARE Family physician

SOURCE AND RELIABILITY OF INFORMATION Patient, who appears reliable.

CHIEF COMPLAINT/REASON FOR VISIT:

"I need a physical. I haven't had a good one in 3 years."

HISTORY OF PRESENT STATE OF HEALTH:

This 21-year-old female considers herself to be in "excellent" health. States she has never been seriously ill or hospitalized and has never had surgery. Patient states she was diagnosed with "anemia" by a blood test at her "doctor's office" in 1980. She was treated with $FeSO_4$ gr. V. q.d. × 1 month. Rechecked at that time. Blood test revealed "anemia gone." No further treatment. In the summer of 1984 began to feel weak and tired. Went to M.D. He did a "CBC" and it showed that she "was mildly anemic." He gave the same "iron pills" to take 3 times a day for 1 month. "I haven't been back since I stopped the pills, I feel so much better."

Patient feels she has no major concerns or stresses at the moment. She is graduating from nursing school this spring and is anxious to "go to work" for a few years. She states she "likes herself as a person," although there are times when "we don't feel as good about ourselves as other times." She feels that her friends and family respect her, as she does them. She exercises daily (since 3 months ago jogs 1 mile) and tries to eat a balanced diet with "extra red meat and leafy vegetables."

PAST HISTORY:

Childhood Illnesses: Mumps, German measles (rubella), rubeola, chicken pox under 10 years of age. No strep throats or scarlet fever. (See Chest and Respiratory section.)

Immunizations: Had usual immunizations—doesn't remember which ones or when. Had tetanus booster this past summer (1980).

Allergies: No allergies to foods, medications, or environmental factors.

Hospitalizations and Serious Illnesses: None.

Accidents and Injuries: None.

Medications: ASA gr. × approx. 1 time per month for headache; Mycolog cream; Nystatin cream q.h.s. (see Skin section).

Habits: Does not smoke cigarettes or "grass." Drinks 1 or 2 glasses of wine on weekends; 1 or 2 cups of coffee or tea per day. No soda.

FAMILY HISTORY:

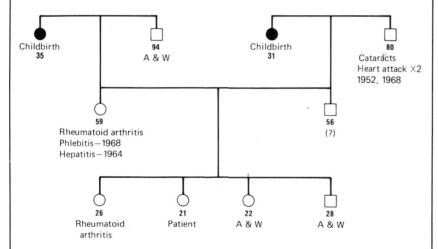

O = female; □ = male; ●, ■ = deceased; denies family history of cancer, diabetes, tuberculosis, epilepsy, mental retardation, mental illness, kidney disease, or asthma.

REVIEW OF SYSTEMS:

General: Height 5′4″. Usual minimum–maximum weight 120–125 lbs. No recent weight gains or losses. Denies fatigue, malaise, or weakness.

Skin: Winter 1981 had "rash" consisting of "little dry, flat, brown spots" covering area from axilla to waist in midaxillary lines (R and L). Went to M.D. because of itching. Doesn't remember diagnosis. Prescribed Mycolog cream during day, Nystatin at night. Continued with medications for 3 months until rash subsided completely. Last month noticed same type rash about 6" to 8" underneath axilla, at midaxillary line. Did not visit M.D. Started using Mycolog and Nystatin again. No associated pruritis or scaling of this area. Rash improved slowly. No further rashes, spreading, or itching. No lesions, color changes, tendency toward bruising.

Hair: No alopecia or brittleness. Washes daily, no use of dyes or other chemicals.

Nails: No splitting, peeling, cracking, biting, or markings on or under nails.

Head: No pain, dizziness, vertigo, or history of injury or loss of consciousness. Never has headaches.

Eyes: Wears corrective lenses for distance vision. Last eye exam 1 year ago. No recent change in visual acuity. Denies pain, infection, watering or itching eyes, diplopia, glaucoma, cataracts, blurred vision, or difficulty with night vision.

Ears: Denies hearing loss, discharge, pain, irritation, or tinnitus. Impacted cerumen in both ears during Jr. High School. Visited physician, irrigation without further occurrence of this condition. Occasional ear infections as a child. Does not remember treatment or outcome.

Nose and Sinuses: No sinus pain, congestion, postnasal drip, impairment in olfaction, discharge, sinus infection, sneezing. Infrequent cold, 1 ×/year, lasting a few days. No meds for cold.

Mouth: No problems with teeth. Sees dentist yearly. Few cavities. None in years. No bleeding or swelling of gums, lips, mouth, or tongue. Rare sore throat, 1 ×/year. No meds. Brushes teeth twice daily. No history of cold sores.

Throat: Denies hoarseness or frequent sore throats.

Neck: Denies pain, stiffness, limitation of motion, swelling, or history of goiter.

Nodes: No node enlargement or tenderness in cervical, axillary, or epitrochlear areas.

Breast: No masses, pain, tenderness, or discharge. Does self breast exam every month 7 days after menses in lying down position. Learned about it in nursing magazine and nursing class.

Respiratory: No history of chest pain with breathing, cough, dyspnea, asthma, or hemoptysis. Pneumonia age 4— visited physician.

No hospitalization. Doesn't remember meds. During early childhood years, yearly occurrence of bronchitis. Seen by physician each time. No hospitalizations. No recurrence since 11 years old. No TB, asthma, emphysema. Denies orthopnea and night sweats. Tinné test done summer 1984 for employment—negative. Does not recall ever having a chest x-ray.

Cardiovascular: No precordial pain, palpitations, cyanosis, edema, or varicose veins. Denies Hx [history] of heart murmur, heart disease, high blood pressure, or rheumatic fever. Rheumatic fever in family—sister. No complications. (See Family History.)

Gastrointestinal: No abdominal pain or disease. Appetite "too good, sometimes." Belching after eating for a few hours. "Think it is a nervous habit." No food intolerances or M.D. care for this. No associated pain. No dysphagia, nausea, vomiting, diarrhea, constipation, hemorrhoids, hematemesis, jaundice. Bowel movement q.d. or q.o.d.—moderate amount firm, brown stool.

Genitourinary: Denies history of bladder or kidney infection, hematuria, urgency, stones, frequency, dysuria, nocturia, incontinence, polyuria, or venereal disease.

Menstrual History: Menarche 12 years. First 1½ years of menstrual cycle 19 to 21 days. Since has had 26 to 28 day cycle. Duration 4 to 5 days. First 2 days uses tampons × 7; days 3 to 5, decreased flow, uses 3 to 4 (tampons). No cramping, slight bloating, mood change (irritable first couple days), and breast tenderness. Denies dysmenorrhea, menorrhagia, infection, or pruritis. No history of pelvic exam with Pap—has had no problems, "never got around to go for an exam."

Back: No past problems. Denies pain, stiffness, limitation of ROM, postural problems.

Extremities: No history of disease. No coldness, deformities, discoloration, varicosities, crepitation, pain, history of phlebitis. Denies muscle weakness, pain. No joint swelling, stiffness, redness, limited ROM, or history of fracture. No history of arthritis.

Neurologic: One episode of fainting in 1980. "Blacked out" for 10 to 15 seconds. Got up in the night to go to the bathroom and "passed out." Went to M.D. No diagnosis offered or studies done. No repeat incident. Denies loss of consciousness, change in sleep patterns, weakness, tic, tremor, numbness, tingling, speech disorder, paralysis, anxiety, phobias, mood change, difficulty with balance, seizures, aphasia, change in memory, disorientation, hallucination, or severe depression. Denies pain and paresthesia.

Hematopoietic: See HPH. No bleeding tendencies, transfusions, blood diseases. Does not know blood group or type.

Endocrine: No change in eating patterns; no unusual growth patterns, thyroid problems, heat or cold intolerance, polyuria, polydypsia, polyphagia. No change in glove or shoe size or hirsutism.

NUTRITIONAL HISTORY:

Tries to include basic four food groups daily. Likes most foods except for an occasional vegetable. Eats out with friends at fast food places 2 or 3 times per week.

A.M.: Eats breakfast q.o.d. or so (does not always have time). Grapefruit; cereal with milk, no sugar; coffee with cream

Lunch: Sandwich (2 slices bread with 2 slices lunch meat); 1 piece fruit; 1 glass of 2% milk

Dinner: 1 portion meat or fish (2 slices); 1 vegetable (1 cup frozen); 1 dish of salad with dressing (2 tbsp.); 1 glass milk (8 oz.)

Snacks: Popcorn, chips approximately q.o.d.

Beverages: Drinks "lots of water" daily.

SOCIAL DATA:

Family Relationships and Friendships: Feels positive about relationship with mother and brother and sisters. Feels they relate well, talk over problems, are close to one another. Enjoys being with family. Father and mother divorced for 18 years. Doesn't remember father. "He doesn't come around or keep in touch. I'm not angry anymore, but I'd like to know him." Presently lives with four housemates. "We're all good friends." Rarely disagree. "I'll really miss them next year."

Ethnic Affiliation: Denies any ethnic or religious customs that might affect her response to health and illness.

Occupational History: Attends baccalaureate nursing program full-time. Work-study in office on campus 10 hrs./wk. Takes care of elderly woman 6 hrs./day on weekends. Feels satisfied with job and school. Wishes she had more leisure time.

Educational History: Senior undergraduate nursing student.

Economic Status: Income satisfactory. Putting herself through school. Receives adequate financial aid. Just has to pay rent, food, and personal articles. "Everything is O.K. with the finances."

Daily Profile: Up at 8 A.M., breakfast, classes 9 A.M. to 3 P.M., lunch at 12 noon, jogs after classes, supper at 6 P.M., studies or watches TV until 11 P.M. bedtime.

Living Circumstances: Lives with four others in apartment. Own bedroom, two bathrooms, large living room, and kitchen with appliances.

Pattern of Health Care: No routine health maintenance, except for dentist and eye doctor. Only sees physician when ill. Doesn't want to spend money to see physician when well.

DEVELOPMENTAL HISTORY:

Patient considers herself an adult, having "moved out of the adolescent stage." States she knows the direction she would like her life to take. She plans to work in nursing for a while and eventually return to school to get a Master's in her area of specialty, which is undetermined at this time. She hopes to marry and have a family, although she has not met anyone yet who "fits the bill." The things in life that are most important to her are her friends, family, and work.

SEXUAL HISTORY:

No sexual intercourse up to present time. "I want the relationship to be special." Not necessarily "saving myself for marriage; just haven't met the right man." Desires a mutually loving relationship in which intercourse would be enjoyable. Knows about birth control methods. Does a lot of reading on the subject. "I'd like to try a diaphragm when the time comes."

EXERCISE AND ACTIVITY PATTERNS:

Enjoys music, going out with friends to movies and parties. Also enjoys walking in forests and reading novels. She feels "good health comes from good food, rest, and a sensible approach to life."

STRESS PATTERNS:

Has experienced no recent stressful events. She does relaxation exercises when she feels stressed.

EXAMPLE OF A HEALTH HISTORY ON AN OLDER ADULT

NAME N. M.

ADDRESS

AGE 71   *SEX* M   *MARITAL STATUS* M

RACE Caucasian   *RELIGION* Catholic

OCCUPATION Full-time engineer.

USUAL SOURCE OF MEDICAL CARE General practitioner, ophthalmologist.

SOURCE AND RELIABILITY OF INFORMATION Patient, who appears

both articulate and reliable.

CHIEF COMPLAINT/REASON FOR VISIT:

"Chronic shortness of breath since childhood which has become gradually worse over the past year."

HISTORY OF PRESENT STATE OF HEALTH:

This 71-year-old man has considered himself to be in good health. He does not feel dyspneic at the moment. As a child, he noticed he would become dyspneic following running sooner than his peers. During grade school and high school he had frequent absences due to bronchitis and asthma for which he was treated at home. During college he was well, but became short of breath with exertion, such as running or pushing a car. In (approximately) 1964, he had a lung capacity test done in Rochester, Minnesota, and was told he had 50 percent lung capacity. In 1976, the test was repeated and again he was told he had 50 percent lung capacity due to emphysema. There is no pain with inspiration, no coughing, no wheezing, no night sweats. Shortness of breath is only associated with exertion, such as lifting a moderately heavy box, walking fast, or playing golf on a hot day. He notices that less exertion causes shortness of breath than was required 1 year ago. When shortness of breath occurs, he ceases activity and it improves in 3 or 4-minutes. His work involves no real physical activity. He has an attack of "asthma" with wheezing 2 or 3 times a year. He uses "a squirt or 2" of Primatene Mist, which relieves symptoms. The asthma can be brought on by humid weather, cold weather, vapors from fried cooking, horses, cats, or excess dust. He does not consider his life stressful at present and also does not feel that anxiety ever precipitated an episode. He has never been formally tested for allergies. No interference with sleep.

For 20 years he smoked 2 to 2½ packs of cigarettes a day without inhaling. He stopped in 1960. He then smoked 2 cigars a day and stopped in 1976. He noticed no change in shortness of breath after he ceased smoking. He drinks 1 beer a day. Other than 2 uncomplicated surgical procedures (see section on Hospitalizations and Serious Illnesses), he has never been ill. His father had asthma and one of his sons has a history of asthma. He does not consider this disease life-threatening, just a "nuisance" which interferes with his golf game on occasion. Last chest x-ray 1980. Does not recall any "unusual comments from the doctor regarding the findings."

PAST HISTORY:

Childhood Illnesses: Chickenpox—under 10 years; "hard" measles—under 10 years; no history of German measles, mumps, strep throat, or scarlet fever. Bronchitis at least twice a year during grade school and high school.

Immunizations: Last remembers being immunized before college. Last tetanus shot 12/70.

Allergies: None known to medications (see HPH).

Hospitalizations and Serious Illnesses: 1950 hernia repair, no complications, Peoria, Illinois. 1952 bilateral vein ligation, no complications, Peoria, Illinois. In February, 1980, bronchoscopy at Wesley Hospital by Dr. Buckingham. At routine physical in January, 1984, "whistling" was heard on right frontal chest. It persisted following one month of cough medicine. "Laminar" chest x-rays were negative. Bronchoscopy negative.

Accidents and Injuries: None.

Medications: Primatene Mist 2 to 3 times per year.

Habits: Not smoking presently, beer (1 × day), no other drug usage; 2 cups decaffeinated coffee per day; does not drink soda.

FAMILY HISTORY:

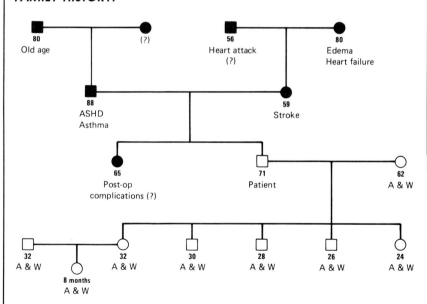

O = female; □ = male; ●, ■ = deceased; no family history of cancer, diabetes, tuberculosis, epilepsy, mental illness, mental retardation, or kidney disease.

REVIEW OF SYSTEMS:

General: Height 6′, Weight 180 lbs. considers himself a "good weight." No recent gains or losses. Denies fatigue or weakness. Feels good, generally.

Skin: Scattered multiple white flat elevations on chest and back present for 10 years. February, 1980 had some removed—none malignant. Have reappeared in greater number. Mild itching of skin on legs in the winter; treated with hand lotion. No rashes, lesions, tendency to bruising.

Hair: Gray, balding on frontal aspect, no dandruff.

Nails: No splitting, cracking, biting, changes in shape, or markings under or on the nails.

Head: No headache, dizziness, or trauma. Occasional pain in anterior to right auricular area, enough to wake him at night. A sharp pain relieved after hot water bottle applied for ½ hour. Occurs approximately once a month for 3–4 years. Not associated with activity or weather. No treatment sought.

Eyes: Glasses for reading for 15 years. Sees ophthalmologist yearly for tonometry test. Was told his pressure is normally high. No diploplia, pain, history of infections, spots, photophobia, excessive lacrimination. No problems with night vision.

Ears: For past year, humming in both ears when he wakes mornings. Goes away when he gets up. Has not sought health care. No discharge, vertigo, earaches, or history of infections.

Nose and Sinuses: Mild epistaxis with colds when he blows his nose. No sinus pain, obstruction, discharge, post nasal drip, frequent colds, trauma, sneezing, or loss of smell.

Mouth: No problems with teeth. Has all his own teeth. No recent extractions, no soreness or bleeding of lips, gums, mouth, or tongue. Brushes teeth twice daily.

Throat: Few sore throats, no disturbance of taste, no hoarseness.

Neck: No pain or limitation of motion, swelling, or history of goiter.

Nodes: No tenderness of cervical, axillary, or epitrochlear areas. Mild swelling in inguinal area first noticed by M.D. in 1969. No change—remains swollen. Was told it is like a varicose vein. No discomfort.

Breast: No pain, lumps, discharge.

Respiratory: See HPH.

Cardiovascular: No palpitation; dyspnea with exertion. Edema of both ankles 1978 to 1979, at end of day. He began wearing socks with loose tops and edema has not been present since 1980. No chest pain, orthopnea, paroxysmal nocturnal dyspnea, cyanosis, history of heart disease, murmur, rheumatic fever, palpitations, ↑ B.P., leg cramps, or varicose veins at present. (See Hospitalizations and Serious Illnesses section.)

Gastrointestinal: No history of abdominal pain or disease; no disturbance in appetite; no indigestion or food intolerances; no nausea, vomiting, belching, flatulence, or jaundice; no change in bowel habits; has one formed brown stool daily. No diarrhea, constipation, use of laxatives, or hemorrhoids.

Genitourinary: No frequency, nocturia, polyuria, hesitancy, hematuria, or kidney stones; no history of UTI or V.D.

Back: No back stiffness, limitation of motion, or injury.

Extremities: No pain, swelling, redness, deformities of joints, crepitation, gout, limitation of movement, or history of fracture, injuries, or disease.

Neurologic: No speech disorder or change in sleep pattern; no tremors or weakness; no convulsions, loss of consciousness, strokes, mental illness, numbness, limps, paralysis, disorientation, mood swings, anxiety, depression, or phobias.

Hematopoietic: In 1957, was told he was anemic, asked to have test rerun as he did not believe diagnosis and then refused test. Took medication (iron) for 1 year. No tiredness. No bleeding tendencies or other blood diseases or transfusions.

Endocrine: No change in eating patterns. No unusual growth problems, thyroid problems, heat or cold intolerance, polyuria, polydypsia, polyphagia. No change in glove or shoe size or hirsutism.

NUTRITIONAL HISTORY:

Wife does all cooking and shopping. Tries to include "meat and vegetables" in diet daily. Dines out one time per month with wife and friends. Enjoys "all" foods, especially desserts. Two meals per day. Lunch—sandwich, fruit; dinner—meat, vegetables, potato, salad, dessert, and a glass of milk; 1 glass of beer in the evening.

Diet Yesterday: A.M.—1 cup of coffee; lunch—ham sandwich (2 pieces of white bread with mayonnaise and 3 slices of ham), 1 apple; snack—1 cup of coffee; dinner—2 slices pot roast with gravy, 1 cup (or so) peas, 1 baked potato, 1 lettuce salad with dressing, 1 piece of apple pie with ice cream, 1 glass of milk; P.M. snack—1 glass of beer.

SOCIAL DATA:

Family Relationships and Friendships: Client feels "positive" about relationship with his family. He and his wife like one another both as people and as spouses: "There are 35 years of affection in our marriage." They talk over problems together and share decisions. His children are grown and he feels close to them. His first granddaughter was born 3 months ago and this gives him "a great thrill."

Ethnic Affiliation: Denies any ethnic or religious customs that might affect his response to health and illness.

Occupational History: Worked for 40 years at L&R Railroad as a chief bridge engineer. Retired in February, 1980 at 65 years of age. Started work full-time at consulting engineering firm the next week. Hopes to work until 75 years old and longer if his health remains good.

Educational History: Obtained B.S. and M.S. in Engineering at Fulton University.

Economic Status: Very happy that he found good employment following retirement. He is involved with different areas in his field which he has found challenging. Receiving retirement benefits. Feels economically secure at present. Helping children through graduate school as best he can.

Daily Profile: Up at 6 A.M., breakfast, 7:30 drives to work, works 8 A.M. to 4:30 P.M., 5 P.M. home, reads the paper, 6 P.M. supper, watches some TV, to bed by 8:30 P.M.

Living Circumstances: Lives in two-bedroom home in a suburb of upstate New York. Has lived in this house for 23 years. He lives there with his wife. This home has gas heat, running water, etc. It is well insulated. There are no loose rugs, mats, etc. The house is easy to manage and he and his wife hope to live there until "our health gives out."

Pattern of Health Care: Sees his M.D. as needed and "every couple of years for a physical." Has eyes checked yearly and also goes to the dentist annually. Doesn't have much faith in physicians. When he questions diagnosis or treatment, responses make him question their reliability. Has a complete record of all medical reports, bills, etc., since the early 1960s.

DEVELOPMENTAL HISTORY:

Client and his wife feel financially secure for the future. They have arrangements with their children for their future residence, health needs, and other relevant concerns. He has strong religious beliefs which "give me courage when thinking of dying." Some of his children live nearby and they visit often. He is proud of his children and their accomplishments. He sees his life's goals as being fulfilled and still "learns new things about himself" every day.

SEXUAL HISTORY:

Believes strongly in marital fidelity and feels he and his wife share very positive feelings about the sexual portion of their marriage.

EXERCISE AND ACTIVITY PATTERNS:

Patient enjoys taking walks with his wife in the neighborhood when the weather permits. He relaxes by reading books in his field. Another favorite pastime is visiting with his family and granddaughter. He feels rest is essential to his "well-being" and retires by 8:30 P.M. every night.

STRESS PATTERNS:

No recent stressful events. He finds that turning to his religion in times of stress is very comforting.

REFERENCES

Bierman, J. (1974). The Diabetes Question and Answer Book. Los Angeles: Sherbourne.

Branch, M., & Paxton, P. (1976). Providing Safe Nursing Care for Ethnic People of Color. New York: Appleton-Century-Crofts.

Burnside, I. (1981). Nursing and the Aged (2nd ed.). New York: McGraw-Hill.

Coddington, R. (1972). The significance of life events as etiologic factors in the diseases of children. Journal of Psychosomatic Research, 16, 7–18.

Erikson, E. H. (1963). Childhood and Society (2nd ed.). New York: W. W. Norton & Co., Inc.

Ginnetti, J., & Greig, A. (1981). The occupational health history. Nurse Practitioner, 6(6), 12–13.

Gioiella, E., & Bevil, C. (1985). Nursing Care of the Aging Client. Norwalk, Conn.: Appleton-Century-Crofts.

Holmes, T., & Rahe, R. (1967). The social readjustment rating scale. Journal of Psychosomatic Research, 11, 213–18.

Jolly, W., Froom, J., & Rosen, M. (1980). The genogram. The Journal of Family Practice, 10(2), 251–55.

Kay, O. (1972). Epidemiological aspects of organic brain disease in the aged. In C. M. Gaitz (Ed.), Aging and the Brain. New York: Plenum.

Masters, W., & Johnson, V. (1966). Human Sexual Response. Boston: Little, Brown.

Newell, G. (1983). Cancer Prevention in Clinical Medicine. New York: Raven Press.

Prior, J., & Silberstein, J. (1981). Physical Diagnosis: The History and Examination of the Patient (5th ed.). St. Louis: C. V. Mosby.

Tripp-Reimer, T., & Friedl, M. (1977). Appalachians: A neglected minority. Nursing Clinics of North America, 12, 41–54.

Whitaker, J. (1976). Guidelines for primary health care in rural Alaska. Washington, D.C.: DHEW (No. 017–026–00049–6).

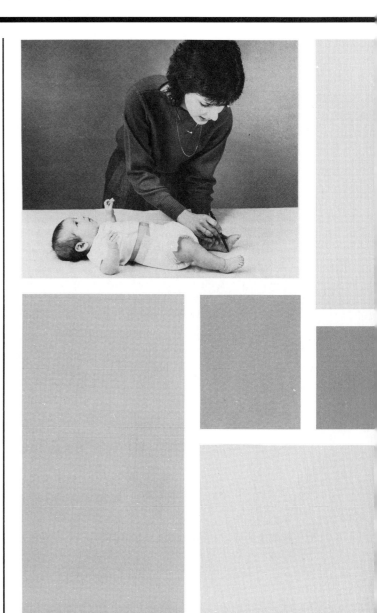

2
The Physical Examination: An Introduction

Ideally, the trusting relationship and rapport between the nurse and the patient have been established during the elicitation of the history. The existence of this kind of relationship will decrease the stress the patient may have in anticipation of what is about to be done *to him*. An additional way to facilitate the physical examination is for the nurse to be meticulous about explaining to the patient what will be done and the reason a particular test is performed. For most people a physical exam is not painful, unless there is something wrong. In many instances, only the area or system involved in an ailment will cause pain during the exam. A patient will be much more relaxed and cooperative if he is assured that he will be told when to expect any discomfort and is given a description of what to expect.

Achieving this trust with children is sometimes more difficult. However, *honesty* is essential. In the long run, the child will benefit from straightforwardness. Some children may have terrible fears and cry from the beginning of the history to the end of the physical. If a child is so terrified that he has to be restrained in order to be examined, evaluating the necessity of the examination is appropriate. In general, most children, if reassured that it is alright to cry when something hurts, and that they will be told in advance, begin to separate the unpleasantness from the more reasonable portions of the exam and cooperate beautifully. It should be remembered, too, that much of this can be made into a game.

Working in an organized and systematic fashion and having all the equipment that will be needed ready and available is another method of making any physical examination as efficient as possible. The more systematic and organized the provider is, the more cooperative and relaxed the patient will be. The patient's participation is essential at various times throughout the exam. He will be asked to sit up, lie down, and stand. If the patient is not asked to do each of these several times, he will be less fatigued. As many of the "sit up" assessments as possible should be done before the "stand up" tests are started. Equally important to remember is the fact that the readiness of the equipment will contribute to the expediency of the exam. Time will be saved and organization will be maintained if the nurse does not have to hunt for equipment either inside or outside the examination room.

Once a thorough history has been elicited, the nurse will have a reasonably good idea about what areas of the patient she will need to examine. The patient should be asked to remove the necessary clothing pertaining to the exam. Most likely a hospitalized patient (in an acute care setting) will be undressed. In the outpatient setting, if a complete physical exam is to be done (from the scalp to the toes), the patient should be completely undressed. For a chief complaint that only involves certain systems, the patient may only have to get partially disrobed (ideally, the patient is able to remain clothed during the elicitation of the history. This does not always work out because of the way a facility may be organized, but it certainly helps preserve the patient's dignity). Whether a complete or partial physical exam is to be done, proper covering should be provided. A gown and sheet (to drape over the patient's lap) should be made available to the patient. Some people, both children and adults, may feel more comfortable leaving their underwear on until the genitalia are examined. This is up to the nurse and the patient. However, it should be remembered that preserving the patient's dignity is an important part of the nurse–patient relationship, and a small consideration like this may contribute significantly to the patient's trust and relaxation.

There are two approaches to doing the physical exam. The approach selected will depend on the reason for the exam. If a patient is in need of, or requests a complete physical exam, then all of the body from the scalp to the toes is examined. On the other hand, if a patient has a specific complaint, then only the involved and related areas are examined.

Two other aspects to consider before starting the exam are the room temperature and the lighting. The temperature should be high enough so that the patient is not chilled during the exam. The light available should be sufficient to see clearly for overall as well as for close inspection.

A last thought to keep in mind relates to the patient's own needs. Every person is unique and has individual concerns. As nurses, we identify as one of our strengths the ability to incorporate those individual concerns into our nursing practice.

THE FOUR TECHNIQUES OF PHYSICAL EXAMINATION

There are four techniques in physical examination: *inspection, palpation, percussion,* and *auscultation.* Unless otherwise specified, they are implemented in this order. Occasionally, the sense of smell is used. This technique is used to help describe the character of things like mouth odors and discharges. Precisely where this is used will be discussed within pertinent chapters.

Inspection

Inspection is the observation portion of the exam. It is probably the most revealing technique, yet the most hastily completed. There is no fancy equipment for this. The quality of the inspection depends on the observer's astuteness as well as the willingness to invest the time to do a thorough job. General inspection begins as the patient walks into the room and continues throughout the entire history taking process.

When a person is looked at as a "whole" (as opposed to looking at a particular portion of his body), notations should be made regarding posture, gait, stance, anomalies, motor activity, affect, and mood (specifications of each are discussed in related chapters). Inspection of specific areas, such as of the abdomen, are done during the physical examination of that system. Information to be obtained includes color, edema, discharge, texture of the surface, and so forth.

The most frequent mistake made during

inspection is rushing through it. This is primarily true because it is hard to take time just to stop and look at a patient without reaching for a piece of equipment or laying on hands. Needless to say, good lighting and exposure of the area(s) which is being inspected are a must.

Palpation

Palpation means to feel (Fig. 2.1). One can feel heat, cold, vibrations, moisture, or masses. Palpation is also used to elicit tenderness. Superficial or light palpation detects palpable findings on the skin surface or the area immediately below. Deep palpation is used to confirm superficial findings, feel deep organs, and elicit deep pain. Some systems do not require palpation. How specific organs are palpated is discussed in individual chapters.

Percussion

Percussion is used to detect air, fluid, or a solid mass in an underlying area. This method of exam involves a "tapping" gesture on the skin (usually the abdomen, thorax, or sinuses) which sets the underlying organs or substance into motion. The result of this tapping creates a sound and a vibratory sensation known as a *percussion note.* These notes can be elicited from areas up to 7 centimeters below the percussed surface.

There are two kinds of percussion: the *indirect* (or mediate) method and the *direct* (or immediate) method. In indirect (mediate) percussion, an object lies between the examiner's percussion finger and the patient's skin, usually the second finger of the examiner's hand (Fig. 2.2). This is the most frequently used method. In the direct (immediate) method, the percussed area is struck directly with the tip

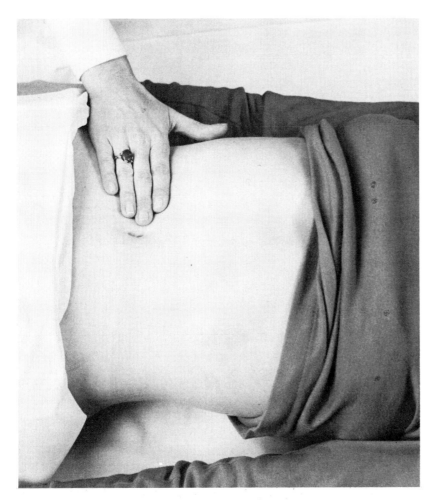

FIGURE 2.1
Palpating the patient's abdomen.

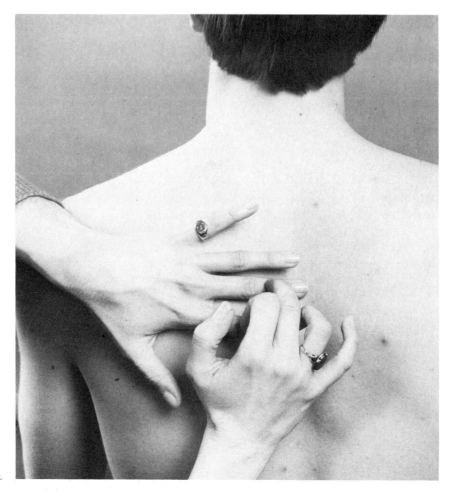

FIGURE 2.2
Indirect or mediate percussion.

of the examiner's finger. Usually the tip of the second finger or the tips of the second, third and fourth fingers are used (Fig. 2.3).

There is a cardinal rule to remember about either method of percussion. Effective technique depends on loose wrist motion.

The procedure for indirect percussion is as follows:

1. The right-handed examiner lays the second finger of her left hand over the area being percussed (positions are reversed for the left-handed examiner). The first and third fingers are elevated so that they are not touching the skin. (Fig. 2.2). The second finger of the left hand is known as the *pleximeter*.
2. With the other hand, the examiner extends and flexes her wrist rhythmically, using the middle finger as the "hammer" or "plexor" tapping the finger already placed on the patient.
3. This motion is repeated two or three times over each area.
4. Each percussion sound is compared to the sound elicited from the same location on the opposite side.

Since this is a gross assessment, any asymmetry of sounds warrants further investigation. Two points to remember are: short nails are a must and percussion over bone will cause great inaccuracy.

There are five percussion notes that can be elicited. These notes vary in quality according to the density of the underlying structures. Each sound has its own intensity, pitch, and duration. The five notes are: *flat, dull, resonant, hyper-resonant,* and *tympanic.* The sounds from percussion can be classified into

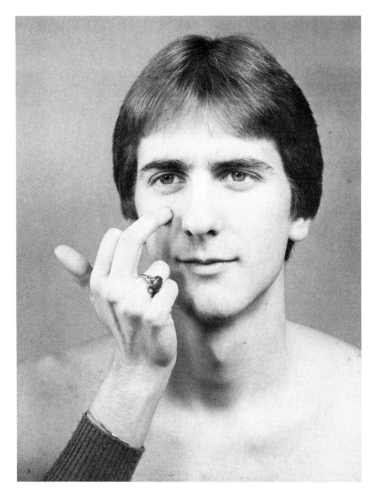

FIGURE 2.3
Direct or immediate percussion.

one of these five notes. (A description of each note is included in Chapter 8, Chart 8.4, page 202.)

Auscultation

To auscultate means to hear. For the purpose of physical examination the terms listening and auscultating are separated. There is little that can be auscultated without a stethoscope. Voices and sounds in the air are listened to. Heart sounds, bowel sounds, and bruits are auscultated.

EQUIPMENT

The discussion thus far indicates the need for

a patient who is appropriately undressed and a room that provides good lighting, warmth, and privacy. In addition to the eyes, nose, and hands of the examiner, other special equipment will be needed (Fig. 2.4):

1. A diagnostic set which includes an otoscope, ophthalmoscope, and various-sized speculum tips
2. A Snellen eye chart (depending on the patient's capability), the illiterate "E" chart, the picture chart, and the alphabet chart (see Figs. 5.5 and 5.6, page 125)
3. A penlight
4. A nasal speculum
5. Tongue blades
6. A tuning fork (500–1000 cycles/second)
7. A wrist watch with a second hand
8. A stethoscope with a diaphragm and bell
9. A sphygmomanometer

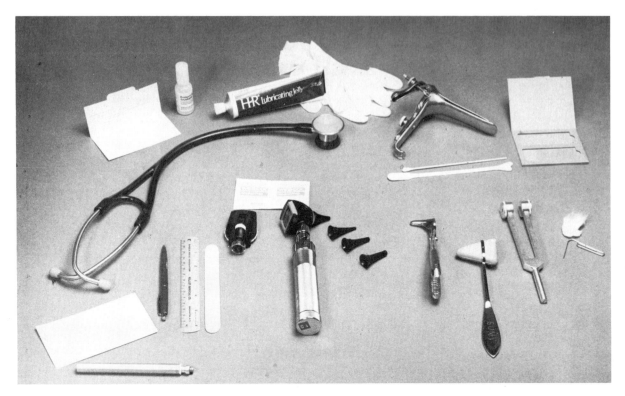

FIGURE 2.4
Equipment needed for a complete physical examination.

10. A reflex hammer
11. A safety pin or a paper clip
12. Cotton
13. A cloth tape measure with centimeter calibrations and ruler
14. A scale with a device that measures height
15. Alcohol swabs
16. Gloves (sterile and unsterile)
17. Lubricant
18. Vaginal speculums
19. Hemocult test slides
20. A microscope and slides

THE GENERAL REVIEW

Before eliciting the review of each specific system in the history or performing the physical (objective) exam, some *general information* is collected.

In the history portion, this category, called *general,* begins the "review of systems" (see p. 17). The information obtained includes the patient's perception of his height and weight, any recent weight gains or losses, and any problem with fatigue or weakness.

As concerns the physical exam, this section includes the measured height and weight, a notation on general appearance, any obvious signs of distress, and the vital signs.

The General Subjective Review

It is important to ask the patient what he weighs and how tall he is. This gives the nurse an idea of how the patient perceives his height and weight. If the information the patient gives differs greatly from the measurements obtained, this is a clue to a possible problem in how the patient views himself. It is helpful when recording the patient's stated weight in the *subjective* review of systems to put quotation marks around the figure, so that it is not confused with the *objective* measurement.

This question provides a good opening to

ask about any recent weight gains or losses. If a positive response is given, further data are needed. The patient should be asked how much weight was lost or gained and over what period of time this occurred. He should be questioned further as to whether this type of weight change has ever occurred before, when it took place, and what the patient's physical condition and stresses were at the time. The nurse should ask him if the change was a desired one and whether it is still desired. Any changes in the patient's life may precipitate this pattern, and he may be very aware of this tendency. This should be confirmed, if possible. Further elaboration can be included in the nutritional review.

The last area to discuss in this portion of the history is any notice of fatigue or weakness. Again, a positive answer always requires an elaboration of the circumstances and events. This area is often particularly difficult to discuss because it is hard to get the patient to be specific. However, a good way to begin is by asking the patient what he means by "fatigue" or "weakness." To some, fatigue may be the result of lack of sleep. To others, all the sleep in the world does not alleviate the feeling of fatigue. After a detailed history of a patient's sleep pattern has been discussed, a look at the psychosocial stresses he is under at the time may prove helpful.

If weakness is a concern, there are many possibilities. Once the patient has tried to define exactly what he means by this sensation, taking him through the *eight areas of investigation* may offer some clues to the source of the problem. With a complaint like this, a complete health history should be elicited to help pinpoint the cause.

The General Objective Review

HEIGHT AND WEIGHT

An accurate recording of the height and weight can be made on a scale that can measure both. The type of scale used will depend on the age and condition of the patient. Infants are weighed on an infant scale on which the child lies or sits. Infants should be undressed, preferably without a diaper. If a diaper is kept on it, it should be weighed separately and this weight of the diaper should be subtracted from the baby's weight with the diaper on.

(A wet diaper will distort accuracy even further.) There are several different types of scales. Balance scales are preferred to spring scales because they are more accurate. At the time a child can stand by himself on an adult balance scale, he may be weighed and measured on it. Infants who are excessively squirmy or uncooperative can be weighed with an adult. Then the adult is weighed and that weight is subtracted from the weight of the adult and child's total weight. An infant should be weighed 6 to 7 times during the first 12 months of his life at routine physicals and other visits that may occur due to illness. Adults can be weighed on a regular balance scale and should also be weighed annually and at each visit. The patient should have on street clothes or only the clothing necessary so as not to "expose" him. No shoes should be worn. Every scale weighs differently, so if accuracy is essential, then an effort should be made to use the same scale each time.

The average weight of a full term infant is 7½ pounds (3.4 kg.). Babies should double their weight by 5 months and triple it by 1 year of age (Smith, et al., 1982). The average length of a full term infant is 50 centimeters or about 20 inches. Length should increase by 50 percent by 12 months, double by 4 years and triple by 12 years for girls and 13 years for boys (Smith, et al., 1982), (Figs. 2.5A–D).

Accurate measurement of height is important as well. An infant can be measured by placing him on a long sheet of paper and marking the point where the crown of the head and the bottom of the heel fall on the paper (Fig. 2.6). The distance between these two points is measured (Fig. 2.7). As with the weight, as soon as the child can stand cooperatively against the scale to be measured, or up against the wall, these methods can be used. A child should be measured as often as he is weighed through the first year of life and annually from then on if there are no problems with his growth and development. An adult should be measured annually.

It is worth noting that a recent survey of several well-child clinics revealed that heights and weights were measured inaccurately up to 90 percent of the time in children below 2 years of age and 75 percent of the time in children above 2 years of age. Children under 2 were measured shorter and children over 2 were measured taller. Errors were due to

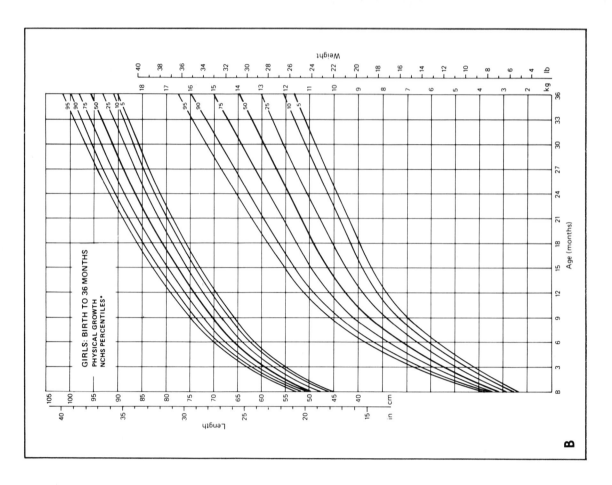

GIRLS: BIRTH TO 36 MONTHS
PHYSICAL GROWTH
NCHS PERCENTILES*

B

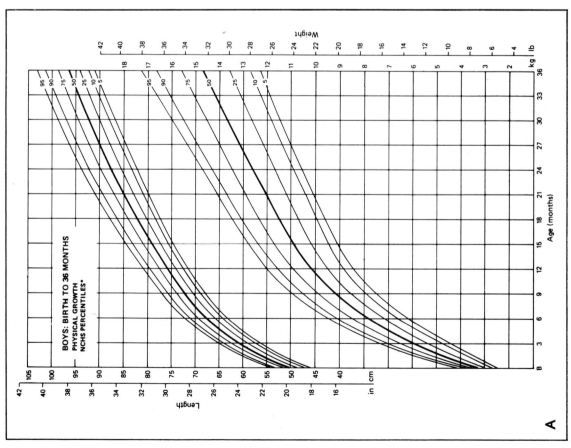

BOYS: BIRTH TO 36 MONTHS
PHYSICAL GROWTH
NCHS PERCENTILES*

A

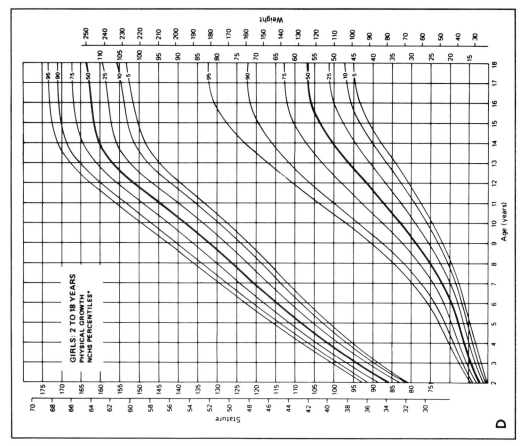

GIRLS: 2 TO 18 YEARS
PHYSICAL GROWTH
NCHS PERCENTILES*

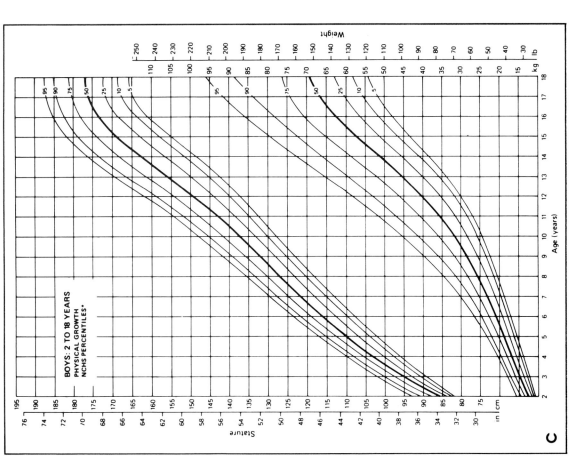

BOYS: 2 TO 18 YEARS
PHYSICAL GROWTH
NCHS PERCENTILES*

FIGURE 2.5A–D
Standardized height and weight charts for children. (Reprinted with permission from Ross Laboratories, Columbus, Ohio. © 1976. Adapted from National Center for Health Statistics: NCHS Growth Charts, 1976. Monthly Vital Statistics Report. Vol. 25, No. 3, Supp. (HRA) 76–1120. Health Resources Administration, Rockville, Md., June, 1976. Data from The Fels Research Institute.)

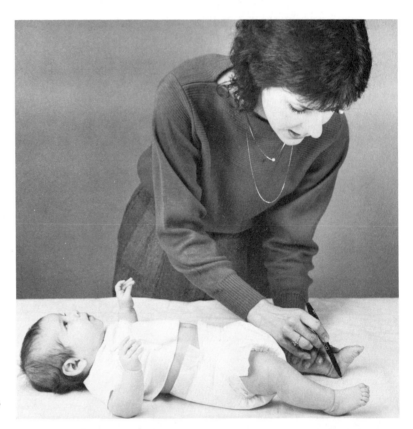

FIGURE 2.6
Marking the point where the heel of
the foot falls on the paper to measure
an infant's height.

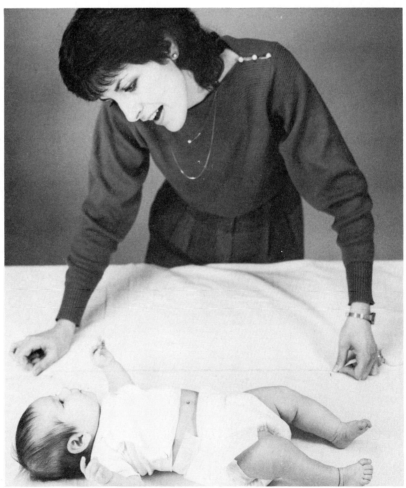

FIGURE 2.7
Measuring an infant's height.

CHART 2.1
DESIRABLE BODY WEIGHTS: MEN[a]

Height		Small Frame	Medium Frame	Large Frame
Feet	Inches			
5	2	128–134	131–141	138–150
5	3	130–136	133–143	140–153
5	4	132–138	135–145	142–156
5	5	134–140	137–148	144–160
5	6	136–142	139–151	146–164
5	7	138–145	142–154	149–168
5	8	140–148	145–157	152–172
5	9	142–151	148–160	155–176
5	10	144–154	151–163	158–180
5	11	146–157	154–166	161–184
6	0	149–160	157–170	164–188
6	1	152–164	160–174	168–192
6	2	155–168	164–178	172–197
6	3	158–172	167–182	176–202
6	4	162–176	171–187	181–207

[a]Weights at ages 25–59 based on lowest mortality. Weight in pounds according to frame (in indoor clothing weighing 5 lbs. for men; shoes with 1″ heels).
(*Courtesy of Metropolitan Life Insurance Company Statistical Bureau, 1983.*)

CHART 2.2
DESIRABLE BODY WEIGHTS: WOMEN[a]

Height		Small Frame	Medium Frame	Large Frame
Feet	Inches			
4	10	102–111	109–121	118–131
4	11	103–113	111–123	120–134
5	0	104–115	113–126	122–137
5	1	106–118	115–129	125–140
5	2	108–121	118–132	128–143
5	3	111–124	121–135	131–147
5	4	114–127	124–138	134–151
5	5	117–130	127–141	137–155
5	6	120–133	130–144	140–159
5	7	123–136	133–147	143–163
5	8	126–139	136–150	146–167
5	9	129–142	139–153	149–170
5	10	132–145	142–156	152–173
5	11	135–148	145–159	155–176
6	0	138–151	148–162	158–179

[a]Weights at ages 25–59 based on lowest mortality. Weight in pounds according to frame (in indoor clothing weighing 3 lbs. for women; shoes with 1″ heels).
(*Courtesy of Metropolitan Life Insurance Company Statistical Bureau, 1983.*)

faulty equipment and technique (McMillan, et al., 1984).

From infancy through early adolescence, the child's height and weight are plotted on standardized growth and development charts. It is important to note that most standardized growth charts are based on Caucasian standards (Figs. 2.5A–D, Charts 2.1, 2.2). Although standardized growth charts for culturally diverse patients have not yet been produced, recent research allows us to make some very gross generalizations. The International Biological Programme has determined that children of predominantly African descent tend to be taller and heavier at all ages than children of European descent, even at somewhat lower economic levels. Individuals of Asiatic descent tend to be less tall at all ages than individuals of European or African descent. Body shape and proportions also differ according to population group. A number of investigators have concurred with Barr and colleagues in stating that "race-specific standards are required before growth achievements in infants and children can be properly evaluated." (Barr, et al., 1972; Eveleth & Tanner, 1976; Robson, et al., 1975). Figures 2.8A–F give examples of differences between population groups of children found in two studies. (Barr, et al., 1972; Eveleth & Tanner, 1976).

APPEARANCE
Note signs of physical age, size, stature, gait, obvious motor dysfunction, deformities, affect, speech, mood, alertness, hygiene, and dress (appropriate to weather).

SIGNS OF DISTRESS
Note any signs of pain, anxiety, depression, or inappropriateness.

VITAL SIGNS
The following should be measured and recorded.

Temperature. Until a child is old enough to hold his lips closed around a thermometer (usually at about 5 to 6 years of age), a rectal temperature is indicated. If a parent is nearby, the child's stress may be decreased if the parent is permitted to take the temperature. In addition, this gives the nurse an opportunity to observe the parent, and if any teaching is necessary, it can be done at that time. Any illness that prevents any patient from closing his lips around the thermometer also requires taking a rectal or axillary temperature. A rec-

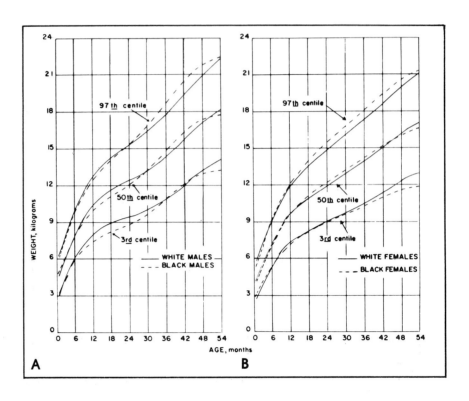

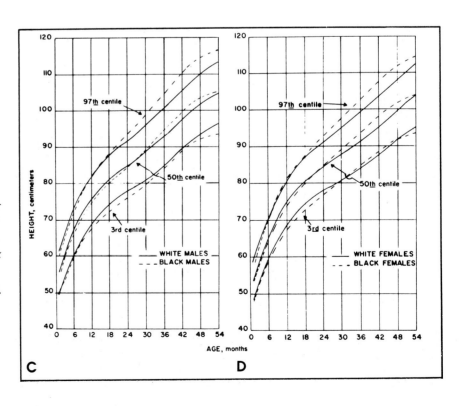

FIGURE 2.8
A. Selected centile estimates for weight by age for young white and black boys. **B.** Selected centile estimates for weight by ages for young white and black girls. **C.** Selected centile estimates for height by age for young white and black boys. **D.** Selected centile estimates for height by age for young white and black girls. (From Robson, J. K., et al., Pediatrics 56(6): 1017–18, 1975, © American Academy of Pediatrics, 1975, with permission.) (Cont'd.)

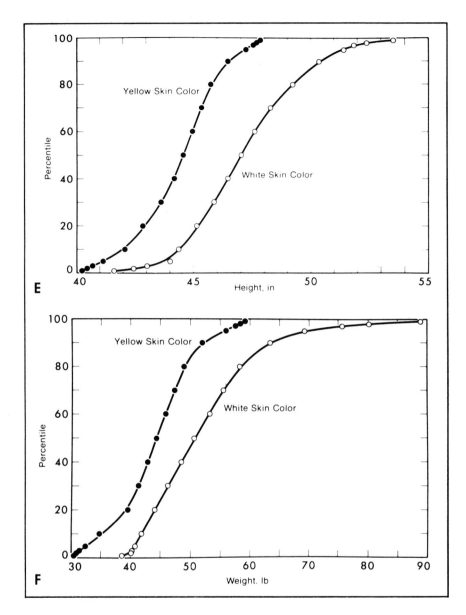

FIGURE 2.8 (*Cont'd.*) **E.** *Percentiles of height compared in 6 year-old boys white and yellow skin color.* **F.** *Percentiles of weight compared in 6 year-old boys of white and yellow skin color.* (*From Barr, G. D., et al.* American Journal of Diseases of Children, *124, 871, 1972, © American Medical Association, 1972, with permission.*)

tal recording provides far more accuracy than an axillary measurement. Some geriatric patients may have difficulty with oral thermometers, too. Again, if accuracy is necessary, a rectal temperature is indicated.

The average body temperature is 98.6°F (37°C). Young children tend to run temperatures higher than normal. There are various ranges of acceptable normal temperatures. Some individuals have a normal temperature of 97°F, others 99°F (Chart 2.3). The important consideration is that whatever is average for that person when he is well should be con-

sidered his normal body temperature. Remember that rectal temperatures may run as much as a whole degree higher than oral temperatures.

Pulse. A pulse can provide valuable information about the patient's health status. An abnormal pulse can be an objective sign of a dysfunctional body system. A rapid pulse, for instance, which is often a sign of cardiac disease, can also be a significant finding in hyperthyroidism.

CHART 2.3
AVERAGE BODY TEMPERATURES IN WELL CHILDREN
UNDER BASAL CONDITIONS

Age	Temperature and Standard Deviation	
	F	C
3 months	99.4 (0.8)	37.4 (0.4)
6 months	99.5 (0.6)	37.5 (0.3)
1 year	99.7 (0.5)	37.6 (0.2)
3 years	99.0 (0.5)	37.2 (0.2)
5 years	98.6 (0.5)	37.0 (0.2)
7 years	98.3 (0.5)	36.8 (0.2)
9 years	98.1 (0.5)	36.7 (0.2)
11 years	98.0 (0.5)	36.7 (0.2)
13 years	97.8 (0.5)	36.5 (0.2)

(Adapted from Lowrey, G. H.: Growth and Development of Children, 7th ed. Chicago: Yearbook, 1978, with permission.)

CHART 2.4
AVERAGE PULSE RATES AT REST

Age	Lower Limits of Normal		Average		Upper Limits of Normal	
Newborn	70/minutes		125/minutes		190/minutes	
1–11 months	80		120		160	
2 years	80		110		130	
4 years	80		100		120	
6 years	75		100		115	
8 years	70		90		110	
10 years	70		90		110	
	Girls	Boys	Girls	Boys	Girls	Boys
12 years	70	65	90	85	110	105
14 years	65	60	85	80	105	100
16 years	60	55	80	75	100	95
18 years	55	50	75	70	95	90

(From Behrman, R. and Vaughn III, V. Nelson Textbook of Pediatrics (12th ed.). Philadelphia: Saunders, 1983, with permission.)

On screening exams for adults, almost all pulses in the body are palpated bilaterally for strength, rhythm, quality or amplitude, contour, and symmetry. The rate is also counted (either apically or radially). Average pulse rates vary among individuals with age. Various rates through the lifespan can be seen in Chart 2.4. A further discussion of pulses can be found in Chapter 9, Chart 9.2, page 235.

Respiration. Respirations are counted and recorded. A discussion of abnormalities and acceptable rates can be found in Chapter 8, page 197.

Blood Pressure. Adults can have their blood pressure taken in various settings: doctors' offices, clinics, dentists' offices, hospitals, shopping malls, etc. Because elevated blood pressure is such a common problem, health facilities have begun checking blood pressure on children, too. All adults should have their blood pressure checked routinely. Children over 3 years (who are healthy) should also be checked annually. Further discussion of technique and acceptable normal ranges can be found in Chapter 9.

APPROACH TO THE PHYSICAL EXAMINATION

The following chapters of this text deal with the assessment of individual systems. For all practical purposes, in adults it is always best to "start at the top and work down." The assessment of some systems will be integrated with others. For instance, the cranial nerves (described in Chapter 15) are usually evaluated while examining the head, ears, eyes, nose, throat, and neck. Every nurse must develop her own system. The most important aspects are thoroughness, organization, and consideration of the patient's needs and abilities.

As the nurse begins to learn the techniques of physical examination, it may be helpful to list these techniques down on cards in the order in which they are performed. Once all the systems are completed, the nurse can take the cards and reorganize the exam using an integrated approach. One important reason for this plan is to organize the examination in a way that limits the number of times the patient changes positions. Also, the nurse should rarely have to change her own position. The right-handed examiner should be able to perform most of the exam from the patient's right side, and the left-handed examiner from the patient's left side. Once the nurse has studied her cards and performed the examination a number of times, the system she has worked out for herself will become automatic. One exception is with the examination of infants and toddlers. When examining a young child, the nurse must be flexible and often examine certain systems when the opportunity arises. For instance, it is easier to listen to the lungs and heart when the child is quiet. Therefore, those systems are often done early in the exam. Usually the ears and mouth are done last because the child often finds this uncomfortable and frequently cries. Each child is different, however, and the nurse must use her judgment in deciding the best way to approach the exam.

REFERENCES

Barr, G., Allen, C., & Shinefeld, H. (1972). Height and weight of 7500 children of three skin colors. American Journal of Disease in Children, 124, 866–72.

Eveleth, P., & Tanner, J. (1976). Worldwide Variation in Human Growth. New York: Cambridge University Press.

McMillan, J., Oski, F., Stockman, D., & Nieburg, P. (1984). The Best of the Whole Pediatrician Catalogue (Vols. 1–3). Philadelphia: Saunders.

Robson, J., Larkin, F., Bursick, J., & Perri, K. (1975). Growth standards for infants and children: A cross-sectional study. Pediatrics, 56, 1017–18.

Smith, M., Goodman, J., Ramsey, N., & Pasternak, S. (1982). Child and Family: Concepts of Nursing Practice. New York: McGraw Hill.

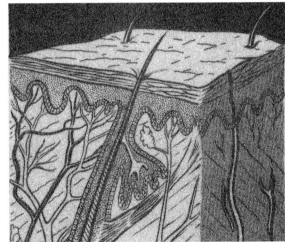

3

The Skin

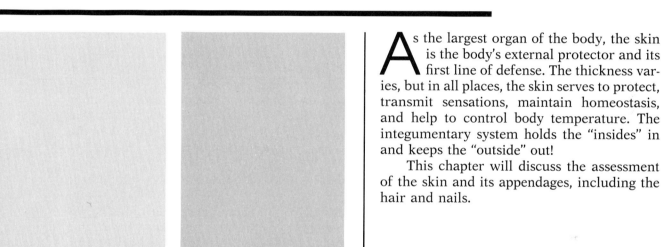

As the largest organ of the body, the skin is the body's external protector and its first line of defense. The thickness varies, but in all places, the skin serves to protect, transmit sensations, maintain homeostasis, and help to control body temperature. The integumentary system holds the "insides" in and keeps the "outside" out!

This chapter will discuss the assessment of the skin and its appendages, including the hair and nails.

DEVELOPMENTAL CHANGES OF THE SKIN, HAIR, AND NAILS THROUGHOUT THE LIFESPAN

Throughout the lifespan, the skin undergoes many changes. This is also true for the hair. Although the nails may change somewhat throughout one's life, the changes are not nearly as striking as those of the skin and hair. From the neonatal period to the elderly years, the changes within the skin, hair, and nails not only help to classify illness, but can also signify very specific life changes.

The skin of a newborn is unique and provides a great deal of information about the infant. When the baby is born, he is likely to be covered with a white, cheesy, odorless covering called *vernix caseosa*. This covering is usually wiped off, but if not, will absorb into the skin in 24 hours. Assessing the amount of vernix helps to determine gestational age. A premature infant will be covered heavily;

the postmature newborn will have very little vernix.

The color of a newborn's skin is significantly red and almost transparent. This erythematous color fades in the first 24 hours of life, then the skin takes on pinker color. Neonates often have red blotchy areas, most noticeable on the trunk. The classic texture is soft and smooth. Their hands and feet may appear somewhat cyanotic. This is called *acrocyanosis* and is caused by vasomotor instability, capillary stasis and the high hemoglobin of the newborn (Jensen, et al., 1981).

The skin of a newborn will shed in certain places. This process, called *desquamation*, will occur several days after birth for the term infant. Desquamation is considered to be an absolutely normal process, but tends to provoke concern from the parents.

Another covering on the neonate's body is called *lanugo*. Lanugo is a fine downy hair that may cover the baby, but is most prevalent on the shoulders, forehead, back, buttocks, and pinnas of the ears. A baby born prematurely will have excessive lanugo, especially over the back. A postmature infant will have little or no lanugo. During the first few months of life, the baby loses this hair, and possibly the hair on his head. If this head hair is lost, it is replaced by permanent hair. The hair of an infant is usually fine and thin. Some babies, especially those who will be blond, often do not get much hair during the first year of life.

Birthmarks in infancy can be very frightening to parents. When parents first see their child, they immediately look for any obvious abnormalities. Accurate information regarding any unusual features of their child must

be provided. Most birthmarks will fade within the first two years of life. The nurse should be able to distinguish between the permanent and temporary birthmarks (Chart 3.1 and 3.7). Some birthmarks are vascular in origin and some stem from abnormal pigmentation. A typical pigment-related birthmark is a *mongolian spot* (Chart 3.1). This blue-black mark varies in size and usually occurs on the lower back or buttocks. This is a common finding in black children. Mongolian spots usually fade by two years of age. *Capillary hemangiomas* (also known as stork bites) and *strawberry hemangiomas* are likely to fade (Chart 3.7). *Port wine stains* and *cavernous hemangiomas* (Chart 3.7) are usually permanent. A port wine stain may also be associated with retardation or other neurologic disease.

The toddler or school-age child may encounter certain infectious diseases (Figs. 3.1, 3.2) such as chicken pox or roseola, accompanied by a skin rash (Chart 3.2). Other than with infectious diseases, the skin does not change much until pubescence.

There are few notable changes in a child's hair as he ages. The hair color may change in children as they get older, but the texture and curl will not change dramatically. Permanent hair may normally be black, brown, red, yellow, or various shades of these colors. Hair fibers are formed into straight, wavy, helical, or spiral filaments, depending on the structure of the protein molecules that make up the hair. This variation in hair fibers makes hair texture range from straight to kinky or wooly.

The skin of the adolescent has most of the qualities of adult skin. The major skin condition that is prevalent in adolescence is acne

CHART 3.1
EXAMPLES OF COMMON SKIN CONDITIONS OF INFANCY

Name	Age	Etiology	Appearance	Resolution
Erythema toxicum neonatorum	First 3 days of life	Unknown	Pinpoint red macular areas; some lesions have pustular centers	Resolves spontaneously within one week
Physiologic jaundice	3rd–4th day of life	↑ number of RBC hemolyzing after birth	Yellowing of skin and mucous membranes, sclera	Fades gradually within first 4 weeks of life
Milia	Neonate–infancy	Collected area of epithelial cysts resulting in plugging of sebaceous glands	Tiny white, raised spots on cheeks, forehead, chin & nose	Resolves spontaneously over several weeks
Mongolian spot	Appears at birth	Clusters of melanocytes in dermis	Blue, black, flat markings usually on buttocks or lower back	Usually fades by 2 years of age

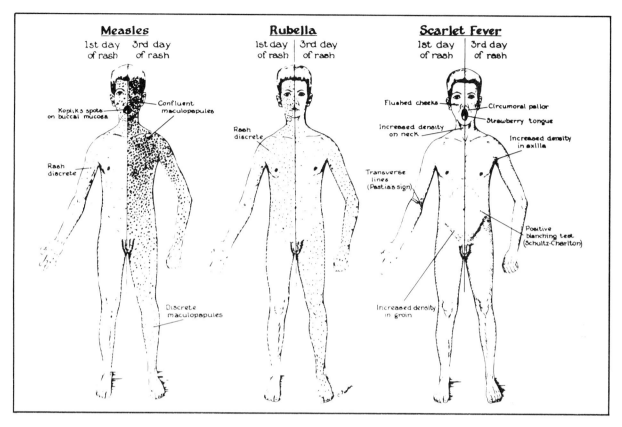

FIGURE 3.1
Signs of communicable diseases. (From McMillan, J., et al. The Whole Pediatrician Catalogue (Vol. 2). Philadelphia: Saunders, 1979, with permission.)

(Chart 3.3). Acne may begin around puberty, or it may not occur until adulthood. The lesions are likely to be on the face, chest, and upper back, where many sebaceous glands are located. Acne is classified by degree and type of lesion.

Grade I acne involves comedones (blackheads). Grade II acne has more pustular lesions in its distribution, in addition to the comedones. Grade III acne includes large painful cysts, plus pustules, and blackheads. Grade IV acne involves widespread cysts and often resulting scars. The latter two stages are hard to treat and can be disfiguring. An adolescent's self concept is often tied up in his appearance and any degree of acne can be of great concern. There have been some significant advances in the treatment of acne over the years. Grades I and II are relatively easy to treat with good results, and researchers are making progress in the treatment of Grades III and IV.

Body hair emerges as puberty begins. In both sexes, axillary and pubic hair are hallmarks of puberty. Hair growth on extremities also appears around this time and continues through the adolescent years. The hair on the legs darkens and thickens. Leg hair on men is more pervasive than on women.

Facial hair also appears on the young adolescent male. The age of facial hair growth differs with each individual. Shaving is often seen as a milestone in a young male's adolescent development.

As a person ages, there are multiple reasons for changes in the integument. A woman who has been pregnant and carried a child to term, might have stretch marks (striae) on her abdomen and breasts for the rest of her life. For some women these fade, but not always. Another individual might notice that the number of skin lesions such as moles or nevi might increase with age.

There are appropriate age-related changes that take place in the adult years. When an individual reaches middle age, he may notice

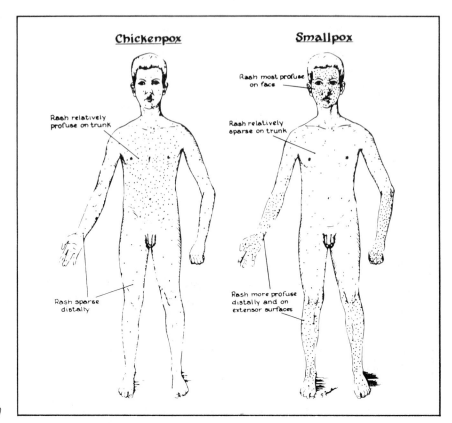

FIGURE 3.2
Signs of communicable diseases. (From McMilan, J., et al. The Whole Pediatrician Catalogue (Vol. 2). Philadelphia: Saunders, 1979, with permission.)

more obvious skin and hair changes. The skin begins to lose its turgor and elasticity. In the face, this change creates wrinkles and sagging of the skin. The loss of skin elasticity for a woman in the upper arms and breasts is common. This loss of elasticity is caused by a decrease of and thinning in the body's subcutaneous tissue. The skin covering the back of the hands and forearms may appear almost transparent.

Many of the changes in the epidermis are the result of years of sun exposure. The skin of the middle-aged person may look thick and furrowed. Light-haired and light-complected people will show these changes earlier than a dark complected person. Black people show the fewest aging changes in the skin.

The appearance of certain kinds of benign skin lesions becomes more likely as a person ages. Most commonly occurring are *lentigos*, (freckles) *seborrheic keratosis* (Chart 3.3), skin tags, increased number of nevi, and *cherry angiomas* (Chart 3.7).

Lentigos, also known as liver spots or age spots, are a collection of melanocytes. They are flat and irregularly shaped. They can be seen most often on frequently exposed areas of the body and are of no significance.

Seborrheic keratosis can be skin-colored, yellow, gray, or brown. They appear attached to the skin. Their surface is wart-like and they are most likely to be found on the scalp, extremities, or trunk.

Cherry angiomas, skin tags, and increased number of nevi may occur anytime during adulthood and are not necessarily related to the middle-aged or elderly person. Cherry angiomas are bright red papular lesions that favor the trunk. Skin tags are often on the torso, but also can be found on the neck. Skin tags are papular, fleshy, and pedunculated in their appearance. A nevus may be flat in a person's youth, but may become raised and fleshy as the person ages. Hair may grow out of nevi.

Elderly people have a tendency to bruise more easily than young and middle-aged adults because of increased capillary fragility. Often the patient will be unable to recall how

CHART 3.2
COMMON INFECTIOUS DISEASES WITH DERMATOLOGIC MANIFESTATIONS

Name	Incubation Period	Subjective	Objective
Rubeola (hard measles)	10–12 days	Rash preceded by fever, cough, cold, lethargy, photosensitivity, some itching with rash	Koplick spots,[a] watery eyes, maculopapular rash—first on face, then behind ears and down trunk and extremities
Rubella (German measles)	14–21 days	May be no symptoms preceding the rash, with the exception of the classic enlargement and tenderness of lymph nodes; mild to moderate itching may accompany rash; no fever	Enlargement of post-auricular, occipital, and posterior cervical nodes; maculopapular rash begins on face and moves to trunk, clears by about third day; afebrile
Exanthema subitum (roseola infantum)	7–17 days	Sudden high fever 3–4 days prior to rash eruption	Few objective signs at this time—possibly slight cold, inflamed pharynx; fever drops and maculopapular rash appears, first on trunk and then on arms and neck; rash usually lasts 24 hours
Erythema infectiosum (fifth disease)	7–28 days (average 16)	None until rash appears and then complaints are present of rash and some itching	Bright red cheeks and the eruption of maculopapular rash on trunk and extremities—rash may last 2–39 days (average 11)
Varicella (chicken pox)	13–21 days	Symptoms 24 hours before rash; slight fever, lethargy, anorexia	Red papules which become clear vessicles on red base; vessicles break and get scabby; rash erupts over 4-day period, begins on face and then goes to trunk and extremities
Scarlatina (scarlet fever)[b]	1–2 days	Sore throat, vomiting, malaise, headache, ↑ temperature	Very red pharynx, probably exudative; strawberry, red tongue; cervical adenopathy; maculopapular red rash, first on skin folds and then on trunk and extremities; rash appears on 1st–2nd day of illness and peels by 3rd–7th day, desquamates

[a] Koplick spots are white spots on the buccal mucosa which precede the appearance of the rash by about 48 hours.
[b] Scarlatina is the only bacterial communicable disease listed; all of the others are viral.

the bruise occurred. In that instance, their history alone will not be adequate.

There is an increased number of skin cancers in the elderly. One example of skin cancer is *actinic keratosis*, which begins as a red macule, and will ultimately form a raised, rough, yellow-brown lesion and is considered premalignant. All skin lesions should be evaluated carefully because some may be premalignant or malignant. Careful recording and referral for any questionable lesion should be done.

Other systemic diseases may affect the integumentary system. For instance, the patient with venous insufficiency and diabetes often has poor peripheral circulation, result-

CHART 3.3
COMMON SKIN CONDITIONS

Category/Name	Definition	Etiology	Clinical Features
Allergic dermatitis Contact	Reaction to external substances which are primary irritants	Contact allergens—i.e., shampoos, soap, clothing, jewelry, lotions, chemicals	Redness → vesicle formation → rupture of vesicle → crusting and scaling of area contacted by irritant
Eczema (atopic dermatitis)	Chronic, recurrent dermatitis	Skin as a target organ of allergic response of chronic or subacute outcome—i.e., milk	Infancy—red, weeping, irritated rash; adult—red, weeping → scaling → hyperpigmentation
Diaper rash	Local irritation with prolonged exposure to urine and stool, over-cleansing	Contact allergen; soap, diaper material	Erythema, oozing vesicles; in diaper area, abdomen, gluteal folds, genitalia, and inner aspects of thighs
Drug rash (dermatitis medicamentosa)	Allergic response to ingestion of drug	Drug allergen	Depends on drug; generally erythematous, macular, or maculopapular rash; vesicles or wheals may form; rashes all over; sudden onset and itching are noted
Nummular Dermatitis	Chronic, recurrent dermatitis. Peak incidence 55–65 years of age.	Unknown, associated with dry skin	Erythematous, coin-shaped eczematous patches. Most frequent on legs, arms, dorsum of hand. Exacerbations most common in winter
Urticaria (hives)	A local edematous response of the skin, often to an allergen; may be acute or chronic	Unknown; allergens frequently are food, drugs, inhalants.	Pink-white wheal which may become bullous; redness around borders; may occur anywhere on the body; much itching

Infectious dermatitis
  Bacterial
    Folliculitis
	Infection in the hair follicle	Exposure to staphylococci	Superficial inflammation; single or multiple pustules at hair follicles, usually buttocks, face, scalp, posterior neck

Furuncle	Deeper inflammation than in folliculitis; one follicle	Exposure to staphylococci	Larger, red, painful, hard pustules which will often drain; posterior neck, buttocks
Carbuncle	Deeper inflammation than folliculitis; more than one follicle	Exposure to staphylococci	Larger, red, painful, hard pustules which will often drain; posterior neck, buttocks
Abscess	Often starts as a folliculitis and develops into a collection of purulent material deep in the skin	Exposure to staphylococci	Deep in the skin; hard, red, tender mass in which purulent material exists but not evident on skin's surface
Impetigo	Very contagious superficial pyoderma; may be associated with poor hygiene	Exposure to staphylococci; B-hemolytic streptococci	Begins with red macules and these become serous vesicles surrounded by erythematous ring; vesicles rupture, leaving yellow, crusty area surrounded by erythematous ring; most often found on face, arms, and legs
Cellulitis	Bacterial infection of dermis and subcutaneous tissue	Exposure to staphylococci; B-hemolytic streptococci; H-influenzae	Tender, erythematous, raised, warm area, well marginated; may be

CHART 3.3 *Continued*

Category/Name	Definition	Etiology	Clinical Features
			associated with lymphangitis
Syphilis	A venereal disease	*Treponema pallidum*	Painless, moist ulceration with raised, firm edge
Primary	Initial lesion is a chancre at site of contact.	*Treponema pallidum*	Painless, moist ulceration with raised, firm edge
Secondary	Appears 6 weeks to 6 months after chancre	*Treponema pallidum*	Scaling papular rash found on soles of feet and palms of hands; generalized macular rash of trunk; mucous patches of oral and vaginal mucosa; flat wart-like white lesions in groin and axilla (condylomata lata)
Viral			
Herpes simplex I (cold sore, fever blister)	A viral syndrome which causes vesicles to occur on the skin and mucous membranes	Viral; often follows sun exposure, stress, fatigue, trauma, other viral syndromes	Groups of small vesicular lesions which erupt and crust within 48 hours
Herpes simplex II (herpes genitalis)	A viral syndrome causing painful vesicular lesions on the genitalia; associated with history of malaise, fever; usually sexually transmitted	Viral; suggestive relationship with cancer of the cervix	Primary occurrence most severe; vesicular eruption on labia, perineum vestibula, or cervix; much pain; recurrent episodes less painful, milder
Herpes zoster (shingles)	Viral syndrome	Same virus that causes varicella (herpes virus varicellae)	History of chicken pox in childhood; unilateral area involved which follows pattern of dermatone; usually face, trunk, lower extremities; painful vesicular eruptions accompanied by erythema
Warts	Viral tumors of the skin	Viral	See specific type
Common wart			Papillary eruption, from pinhead to pea size; may have gray or brown surface; most often on hands
Filliform			Flesh-tone finger-like projections that occur on eyelids, face, neck
Plantar			More painful; flatter than the common wart; surrounded by thickened skin; often mistaken for calloused area; commonly on foot
Venereal (condylomata acuminata)			Cauliflower-white skin, tag-like lesions; multiple, may be found in genitalia, perineum, vestibule, or cervix; itching discharge may accompany
Fungal			
Moniliasis	A fungal infection caused by *Candida albicans*	Increased candida in body, often following antibiotic treatment or while on oral contraceptives; may be active in diabetes, obesity	See Specific type

(Continued)

CHART 3.3 *Continued*

Category/Name	Definition	Etiology	Clinical Features
Thrush	Moniliasis in the mouth	*See* moniliasis etiology	Thick, white, curd-like patches on pharynx or oral mucosa; removal causes bleeding
Vaginal moniliasis	Moniliasis of the female genitalia	*See* moniliasis etiology	Thick, white, nonodorous discharge, white curds in vestibule and on cervix, much itching
Moniliasis of onychia paronychia	Monilial involvement of the nail and surrounding skin	*See* moniliasis etiology	Tender edematous inflammation of the skin around nail's ridge, nails become thickened and discolored
Moniliasis intertrigo and crural areas	A form of moniliasis; common in warm weather, affecting the skin folds and external genitalia	*See* moniliasis etiology	Bright red macules with satellite areas; vesicles and pustules interspersed throughout; occurs mostly in skin folds, under breasts, axilla, and groin; typical diaper rash in infants; will spare scrotum and penis in adult male
Tinea versicolor	Superficial fungus infection	Exposure to fungal agent *Malassezia furfur*	Flat, itchy, yellow, pink, tan patchy areas on shoulder and upper chest and back; some scaling possible
Tinea	Ringworm; a fungal infection (further defined according to body part)	*See* description of specific body part	See description of specific body part
Capitis	A fungal infection/ringworm of the scalp, found mostly in children	*Microsporum audouini* or *M. canis*	Broken hairs and patchy hair loss; inflammation of the areas; some scaling possible; common in ococcipital region
Corporis	Fungal infection/ringworm of the body	*Microsporum audouini* or *M. canis*	Red, scaly, macular, papular, vesicular areas; eventual lichenification erythematous ring surrounding lesion; much itching; occurs on face, neck, trunk, and hands
Pedis (athlete's foot)	Fungal infection/ringworm of the foot	*Trichophyton mentagrophytes* or *T. rubrum*	Fissuring, scaling between the toes, some maceration, much itching; fourth web common; may spread to sole of foot, causing scaling, vesicles, erythema
Onychosis	Fungal infection/ringworm of the nails	*Trichophyton rubrum,* or *T. mentagrophytes*	Particularly in toenails; nail gets white or yellow at borders, infection moves in, and nails get very thick; nail splits (often due to *Candida albicans*)
Infestations Pediculosis	Lice infestation of the body	Exposure to lice	
Pediculosis corporis (body lice)	A body louse that lays eggs near clothing seams	Exposure to lice	Pinpoint small, red, macular lesions; scratch marks obvious, as itching is severe; papules and secondary infection may develop (comes in contact with body only to eat; hard to find lice on body)

CHART 3.3 *Continued*

Category/Name	Definition	Etiology	Clinical Features
Pediculosis capitis (head lice)		Exposure to lice	Not easily seen; nits if present appear as little white specks attached to hair; typical in children; itching and scratching very prevalent; eventually weeping, crusty areas develop on scalp
Pediculosis Pubis (pubic lice)		Exposure to lice, often sexually transmitted	Reasonably easy to see; Looks like gray flecks attached to pubic hair; head often buried in hair follicle; ova attach to hair
Scabies	Infestation of an itch mite in the epidermis; highly contagious	Exposure to itch mites; *Sarcoptes scabies*	Severe itching—worse at night; white-gray winding, linear pattern at the end of which there is a gray-black dot; papules and pustules and vesicles may accompany; most likely to occur on the flexor surface of the wrist, finger webs, axillary areas, nipples, waistline, lower abdomen, genitalia (for pruritic rashes always think scabies!)
Tumors Malignancies Basal cell	Tumor of the skin that arises from epidermis	Malproduction of basal cell; may be highly related to ultraviolet light exposure	History of outdoor occupation or activities; small, smooth-surfaced, well circumscribed areas that may have indentation in the center of the lesion; ulceration may follow; likely to occur on areas exposed to sun
Melanoma	Highly cancerous, can be lethal tumors of the skin and mucous membranes; malignancy of the melanocytes	Unknown	Smooth, isolated, non hairy; pigmented lesions; may be irregularly shaped; darkening and increase in size may occur. May erupt anywhere
Squamous cell	Tumor of the epidermis which in its early form is potentially malignant	Exact cause unknown; high probability that there is a relationship to ultraviolet rays and light skin color	May be preceded by keratoses, leukoplakia; nodular area eventually forming crusty ulceration, commonly on lower lip, tongue, ears, neck, dorsum of hands
Benign Seborrheic keratosis/ senile wart	Seen frequently in elderly	Unknown	Yellow/brown/black, roughened surface; slightly elevated, about 1 cm; usually on upper torso; extremities and scalp
Sebaceous cysts	Blockage of sebaceous gland duct	Same as definition	Usually less than 3 cms; well-defined, round, firm mass attached to skin; may be inflamed
Pigmented nevi	Tumors containing nevus cells	Stimulated growth of nevus cells	Colored or noncolored; raised or flat; associated with hair growth or nongrowth; of varying size, shape, and texture

(Continued)

CHART 3.3 *Continued*

Category/Name	Definition	Etiology	Clinical Features
Miscellaneous dermatitis Acne	Inflammatory response of sebaceous glands	↑ Oil production; secondary to hormonal stimulation	Blackheads, papules, cysts; typically on face, back, chest (any, some, or all)
Psoriasis	Chronic skin condition in childhood which lasts through life, often associated with arthritis; exacerbation and remissions continuous	Unknown: genetic transmission; possibly environment or stress-related	Thick, white, scaly patches surrounded by erythema; when scales picked off, may bleed; commonly on elbows, knees, feet; much itching, often only in scalp
Neurodermatitis	Allergy-like dermatitis; emotional stress acting as a contributing feature; may be contained in one area	See allergic dermatitis; emotional stress; chronic local irritation from neurotic scratching	See allergic dermatitis; may be in one area if repeated scratching takes place there; hyperpigmentation or lichenification
Seborrhea dermatitis	Biochemical imbalance of sebaceous glands	↑ Oil production of sebaceous glands	Greasy scales on scalp, face, eyebrows, nasolabial folds; may spread to body, chest, abdomen, and skin folds; if so, scales are usually salmon colored

ing in thinning of the skin and edema of the legs. This can eventually lead to secondary pigmentation of the areas involved and a resulting venous stasis ulcer. Also anemia, which is common in the elderly, will give the patient's skin a pallor-like appearance.

Fingernails and toenails may change as a person ages. Fingernails may lose their luster; toenails may thicken as a result of poorly fitting shoes, trauma, or a chronic fungus infection (Charts 3.3 and 3.8). An aging person who has problems with mobility may have additional toenail disfigurement because of painful, thickened toenails, or poorly fitting shoes.

In the middle years (earlier for some adults) hair may begin to gray. Often this graying starts with a gradual "salt and pepper" pattern at the hairline. Balding is more apparent in men and is most common among people of European and Near Eastern ancestry. Some men may have a receding hairline as early as their twenties; however, patterns will vary. Because balding is a genetic trait, the amount of hair loss, as well as the time it begins, may reflect family patterns.

As a woman ages, she too, may note a thinning and graying of the hair on the head. In the woman this tends to be a slower process, but may be aggravated by years of stretching the hair on rollers, teasing, blow-

drying, or chemically treating the hair.

Facial hair on an elderly man decreases, but generally increases on a woman as she ages. Under the chin and above the upper lip are places a woman may notice additional facial hair.

Hair covering the extremities will decrease in amount and become straighter in both sexes; this is true of axillary and pubic hair as well. Generally speaking, the amount of body hair, including growth and loss, can often be attributed to genetic disposition and varies greatly among individuals (McDonald & Kelly, 1975).

ANATOMY

There are three layers of the skin: the *epidermis*, the *dermis*, and the *subcutaneous layer* (Fig. 3.3).

Epidermis

The epidermis is the outermost covering of the skin and is considered a protective barrier. There are two components of the epidermis:

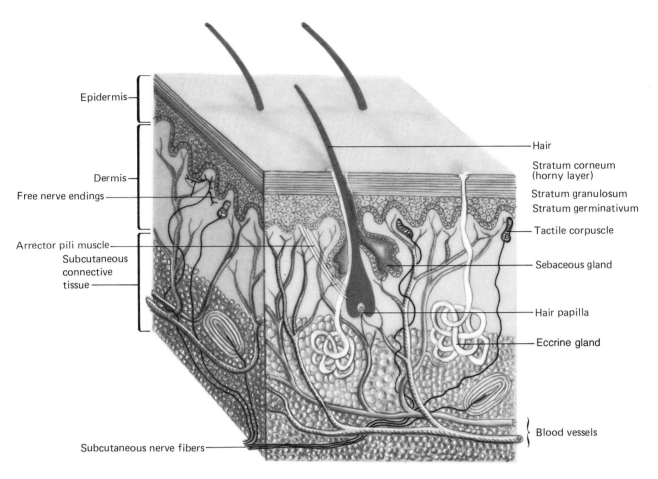

Epidermis

Dermis

Free nerve endings

Arrector pili muscle
Subcutaneous
connective
tissue

Subcutaneous nerve fibers

Hair

Stratum corneum
(horny layer)

Stratum granulosum
Stratum germinativum

Tactile corpuscle

Sebaceous gland

Hair papilla

Eccrine gland

Blood vessels

FIGURE 3.3
Structure of the skin. (From Heagarty, M., et al. Child Health: Basics for Primary Care. New York: Appleton-Century-Crofts, 1980, p. 108, with permission.)

the *horny layer* and the *inner layer.* The horny layer is made up of *keratinocytes.* This is a protein also found in the hair and nails. The horny layer sloughs off continuously and is replenished by new cells. The inner layer contains *melanocytes,* which produce a brown-black pigment called eumelanin and yellow-red pigment called pheomelanin. In the absence of pathology, skin color depends on the relative proportions of the two melanin compounds and on hemoglobin, the red pigment of red blood cells (Quevedo, et al., 1975).

The *epidermal appendages* are the *hair, nails, apocrine glands, eccrine sweat glands,* and *sebaceous glands.* All are indirectly related to the epidermis. The hair and nails are of no particular physiologic value to man. However, in most societies people emphasize them for cosmetic purposes.

There are two types of sweat glands: apocrine and eccrine. They respond to physiologic and emotional stimuli. Apocrine glands are located throughout the dermis and subcutaneous layers (Fig. 3.3). They are found in the axilla, breasts, and genitalia of both men and women and do not begin to function until puberty. The secretion from these glands, called "apocrine sweat," empties into the hair follicles and then onto the skin. Apocrine secretions are thick and milky and are comprised of many organic components. The bacterial action causing the breaking down of these organic components can create distinctive body odors.

The eccrine glands are the most prevalent sweat glands in the integument (Fig. 3.3). They are located throughout the body and are the mechanism of heat dissipation. Both water and salt are secreted by the eccrine glands. Hypothalmic function controls this heat regulating mechanism.

Eccrine "sweat" is basically clear and thin.

It has few organic components and is odorless (Cage, 1971).

Sebaceous glands are also located throughout the body, with the exception of the palms of the hands and soles of the feet (Fig. 3.3). They are most copious on the forehead, scalp, face, and chin. These glands secrete assorted lipids which are collectively called *sebum*. Sebum is a lubricator of the skin surface. The production of sebum is directly related to the amount of androgen in the body.

Dermis

This layer of skin also acts as a protective barrier. It has many blood vessels and nerves that supply the nutritional needs of the skin. The dermis contains *collagen* and *elastin*, which hold the epidermis in place. In an emergency the epidermis can be a storage center for the body's fluid and electrolytes. Neural stimulation to this layer is provided by the postganglionic sympathetic and sensory nerve fibers. The postganglionic nerve fibers control the vasculature in this region, as well as the apocrine and eccrine sweat glands.

Subcutaneous Layer

The body stores its fat in the subcutaneous layer. There are also nerves, sweat glands, and blood vessels in this layer. The distribution and thickness of the subcutaneous tissue varies, but as a rule this layer acts as the body's insulator. There is no subcutaneous tissue in the eyes, penis and scrotum, nipple and areola, or over the tibia.

HISTORY

The review of this system includes general questions regarding any problems with the skin, hair, or nails. The nurse should explore with the patient any tendency toward any of these symptoms:

1. Skin: Dryness, itching, rashes, bruising; existence (either now or in the past) of lesions, moles or lumps; any problem with excess or lack of perspiration.
2. Hair: Any loss or excess, change of growth patterns, texture (described as dry, brittle, coarse, fine), scaliness of scalp; also note use of dyes or chemical treatments.
3. Nails: Biting, splitting, change in appearance (pitting, ridging), markings under nailbeds, or thickening (especially common in toenails).

Remember that if a patient gives a positive response to any of these symptoms, it is important to explore further. A description of the data that are collected when a rash exists illustrates this point. The chronologic story includes answers to the following questions (note that the duration of the problem is recorded in the chief complaint).

1. Location: Where is it? Is it spreading? If so, where is it spreading to and how (i.e., in a linear or circular pattern)?
2. Frequency: Have you had it before? If so, how often?
3. Sequence and chronology: If it has occurred before, describe a typical course of the problem. When did it occur? Was it treated successfully? How was it treated? When did it return again? In terms of the present episode, is it getting progressively worse? Does it heal in one place and appear in another?
4. Quantity: How far does it extend? Is it in more than one place? Where else? Are there several lesions or just one?
5. Quality: Describe the rash. What color is it? Is it raised or flat? Fluid-filled? Crusty? Oozing? If so, describe the discharge. Is there an odor? Does the involved area feel tender or warm to the touch? Are the borders regular or irregular in shape?
6. Setting: Does the patient work or go to school? Does anyone there have a similar complaint? Any recent travel? Camping? Involvement in any new activities?
7. Associated phenomena: Itching? (Is it worse at night?) Is there a fever? Nausea? Vomiting? Diarrhea? Sore throat? Cold? Stiff neck? Any different or unusual foods or restaurants? New soap, perfumes, lotions, or detergent? New clothing or bed linens? Any allergic history or tendencies? Taking any medications? Recent treatment with any medication? What type? Under any stress other than usual?
8. Aggravating factors: What makes it

worse? Scratching, medications, lotions or soaps, bathing, jewelry, exposure to heat or cold, menstrual cycle, pregnancy, sunlight or stress?

9. Alleviating factors: What makes it better? Home treatments, baths, showers, medications, or lotions?

There are other factors worth inquiring about which may contribute information to the history of a skin problem. Looking for a contagious link to the original source is sometimes not as easy as it seems. If a child is in a day-care setting, it is hard to be certain about other exposures. This is also true for the adult who interacts daily with many people. For the elderly who are institutionalized, tracking down the source of exposure might be easier.

Family history may provide some insight about a skin problem. There may be a genetic correlation, or just a familial tendency toward certain skin problems. This family history may be helpful in understanding an infectious processes or skin cancers.

PHYSICAL ASSESSMENT

Examining the skin is often erroneously looked upon as the least significant portion of the physical. The skin can provide the examiner with a significant amount of information. Not only can it be a fair indicator of illness or wellness, but the skin can reveal signs of anxiety or aging. While the condition of the skin can also be a good indicator of general hygiene, the normally sloughing horny layer of highly pigmented patients may appear to be "dirt" to the inexperienced examiner. A very general inspection of the skin begins when the patient enters the room and continues throughout the history taking process. At the onset of the physical examination, the exposed areas of the skin are examined. To preserve modesty, the unexposed skin is inspected and palpated with each body system. For example, the skin on the abdomen is examined at the time of the abdominal exam.

As a rule, all that is needed for this exam is the examiner's hands and eyes and, in some instances, the nose. There are times when equipment is needed (i.e., a Wood's light is used to detect fungal infections. Most fungi will fluoresce under the light. Slide preparations can also be made. A scraping of the involved skin surface and potassium hydroxide are placed on the slide and viewed under the microscope. Fungal growth can be confirmed by this method, too.) Good lighting and full exposure of the area being evaluated are essential. A magnifying glass and a small flashlight may also be of help. The two methods of examination used are inspection and palpation.

Skin

INSPECTION

The skin is inspected for color, lesions, obvious moisture (or lack thereof), edema, and vascular changes. (Obvious changes in turgor and texture are discussed more thoroughly in the section on "palpation.")

Color. Skin color varies from body part to body part and from person to person. An individual's genetic composition is the most dominant factor in his overall coloring. In general, skin tones can range from shades of ivory to deep brown. Different hues of pink, green, and orange are usually apparent and vary among individuals. If a person spends a good portion of his life outside, the exposed areas are likely to be more pigmented than the rest of the body. Vasodilation of the superficial vessels occurs in fevers, sunburns, or blushing and can alter the skin color temporarily. A common characteristic during sexual arousal is a generalized flush over the body, and in a woman the labia will change color markedly. The most common changes in skin color are described in Chart 3.4.

Assessing skin color changes may be more difficult in darkly pigmented individuals. With pallor, dark skin loses the normal underlying red tones, so that patients with brown skin may appear yellow-brown and the patient with black skin may appear ashen gray, particularly around the mouth and on the buccal mucosa. Cyanosis is best detected at the sites of least pigmentation: lips, nail beds, palpebral conjuctiva, palms, and soles. In highly pigmented individuals, just as in lightly pigmented ones, the sclera exhibits yellow pigmentation with jaundice. However, because dark-skinned individuals may normally have yellow subconjunctival fatty deposits, inspec-

CHART 3.4
COMMON CHANGES IN SKIN COLOR

Color/Response	Conditions or Cause	Typical Location
Yellow-orange		
Jaundice	↑ Total serum billirubin (above 2–3 mg/100 ml)	Generalized; sclera, mucous membranes
Carotene (carotenemia)	↑ Serum carotene usually due to excessive intake of carotene-related vegetables (i.e., carrots); typical in infants; pathologic in such conditions as hypothyroidism and diabetes	Palms, soles, around mouth
Bluing		
Cyanosis	↑ Deoxygenated hemoglobin (unsaturated hemoglobin)	Nail beds, lips, mucous membranes, skin
Petechiae (1–3 mm) Ecchymosis (larger petechiae)	Bleeding outside the vessels due to trauma or systemic disease	Anywhere on body
Pallor	↓ Hemoglobin due to anemia, shock, fatigue, startling emotional upset	Generalized, conjunctiva
Albinism	Transmitted metabolic defect of melanocytes, causing lack of pigment	Hair, body, eyes
Vitiligo	Lack of pigment in patchy areas due to an autoimmune or neurogenic etiology	Patchy spots on body
Red		
Erythema	↑ Oxygenated blood to a particular area or all over body as in infection	Local area infected
	↑ Alcoholic intake	Face, cheeks
	Exposure to cold	Areas exposed
	Trauma	Local area involved
Tan-brown	↑ Melanin, as in pregnancy or with oral contraceptives	Face, areola, nipples, linea nigra
	Sun tan	Exposed areas to sun
	Hyperthyroidism, Addison's disease	Diffuse, prevalent in genitalia, areola, recent scars, knees, elbows
Café-au-lait spots (sharply delineated tan-brown patches)	Nonpathologic	One of two small spots on body
	Albright's syndrome, von Recklinghausen's disease (neurofibromatosis)	Spots which vary in size scattered over body

tion of the hard palate should also be made if jaundice is suspected (see Chapter 4). Skin color changes which appear red in lighter-skinned individuals may also be missed in darkly pigmented individuals. In blacks, the characteristic red flush of fever may be visible at the tip of the ears. Inflammation and rashes may best be detected by palpation in combination with patients' verbal reports (Roach, 1972; Williams, 1976; Rubin, 1979).

Lesions. There are many varied causes of lesions. Normal inconsequential markings are usually freckles (*lentigos*), some birthmarks, and some aging spots. However, when something happens to the skin and a lesion occurs, the lesions are classified *primary* or *secondary*. A *primary* lesion is the initial response to some stimulus on the skin (i.e., macule, papule, etc.) (Fig. 3.4, Chart 3.5). The *secondary*

lesion occurs as a response to a change in the primary lesion. For instance, in herpes, vesicular lesions are the primary lesions formed in the initial stage of the disease. After the vesicle drains, a crust forms over the site of the primary lesion and the secondary response of crusting takes place (Fig. 3.4, Chart 3.6).

Lesions should always be described according to their location, number and distribution, color, type (primary or secondary), presence of discharge (including description), and grouping. Skin changes can exist as an isolated lesion or in groups. The most common classifications used to describe groupings are *linear* (occurring in a straight line), *clustered* (groups together), *diffuse* (widespread), *confluent* (blending together), *annular* (ring-shaped, clear-centered) or *circular* (round).

The distribution is also important in describing lesions or a rash. Is the pattern symmetric? Does it only involve sun-exposed areas? Are the intertriginous (skin fold) areas predominantly involved? All of these terms help to classify and accurately describe skin pathology (Chart 3.3). In darkly pigmented individuals, lesions may be difficult to identify by inspection and may necessitate identification by palpation, observation of patients' scratching, or patients' verbal reports. However, in only moderately pigmented skin, a macular rash may be more recognizable if the skin is gently stretched between the thumb and finger (as for administration of an injection). This maneuver decreases the normal red tone and thus brightens the macules. In addition, some generalized rashes can be seen in the mouth, especially on the palate (McDonald & Kelly, 1975).

Moisture. Perspiration is the most obvious moisture seen on the body. The face, axilla, and skin folds are the likely places for it to occur. Dehydration is detected by noting the moisture on the mucous membranes. For instance, in mild dehydration, the mucosa of the oral cavity is likely to look dry. In a more serious stage, the lips may be cracking and look parched and other mucosa of the body may look very dry. Darkly pigmented blacks often have dry skin under normal conditions, not necessarily indicating dehydration. Black skin tends normally to be dry and may appear "ashy" or flaky.

Edema. Obvious areas of swelling are inspected. An edematous area is described in terms of location, shape and color. Edema masks the intensity of skin color because the distance between the skin surface and the pigmented and vascular layers is increased. This increase in distance causes darkly pigmented skin to become lighter. Changes in color indicating pathology, such as pallor of cyanosis, may be obscured.

Vascular Alterations. There are normal and abnormal vascular changes. *Petechiae* and *ecchymoses* are the result of bleeding into the skin. Petechiae are minute lesions which do not blanche when they are pressed. They can be seen on bulbar and palpebral conjunctiva as well as the buccal mucosa. Ecchymoses are larger hemorrhagic lesions also known as "black and blue marks." *Telangiectasis, venous*

stars, *cherry angiomas, hemangiomas,* and *spider angiomas* are other *vascular* markings that occur at different times in the lifespan and are not necessarily pathologic (Chart 3.7). In either situation, the recorded description includes noting location, distribution, color, size, amount, and the presence of pulsations. In highly pigmented individuals, these vascular changes may be difficult to detect (Roach, 1972; Rubin, 1979; Branch & Paxton, 1976).

PALPATION

Inspection and palpation of the integumentary system go "hand in hand." Some features noticed in inspection can be examined by palpation, too. Palpation is used to detect moisture, temperature, texture, turgor, and masses.

Moisture. The moisture seen on inspection should be felt. What appears to be thin and watery may be thick and oily. Fluid oozing from a lesion should be described by its color, amount, thickness, and odor.

Temperature. One of the most traditional ways to detect an elevated temperature is by laying the back of one's hand on the patient's forehead or neck. If there is a fever, a warm or hot sensation can be felt. The examiner must not have cold hands or the results of this gross estimation will be useless. Isolated areas that have been traumatized or are infected or sunburned may feel warm, too. The opposite physiologic occurrence (reduced blood flow) causes a cooler feeling of the skin and may be evidenced in peripheral arteriosclerosis, Raynaud's disease or syndrome, shock, or any circulatory disturbance of significance. For this reason, skin temperature may not be a reliable indicator of disease.

Texture. Skin texture varies on different parts of the body. Normal descriptions include thick, thin, rough, or smooth. A sculptress's hands may be rough and the skin may even be lichenified from contact with harsh materials, whereas the rest of her body will probably be much smoother. People with an overactive thyroid (hyperthyroidism) may notice their skin becoming smoother and softer. Those with an underactive thyroid (hypothyroidism) may have dryer, flaking skin. In both thyroid conditions, the skin changes will be generalized, rather than localized. In darkly pig-

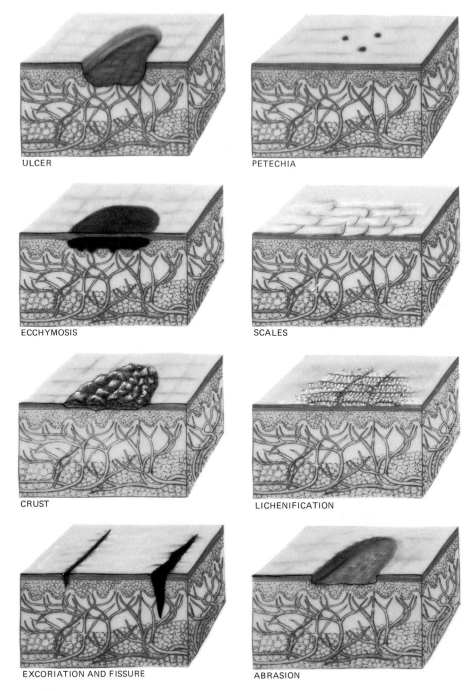

ULCER

PETECHIA

ECCHYMOSIS

SCALES

CRUST

LICHENIFICATION

EXCORIATION AND FISSURE

ABRASION

FIGURE 3.4
Skin lesions. (From Heagarty, M., et al. Child Health: Basics for Primary Care. New York: Appleton-Century-Crofts, 1980, pp. 108–109, with permission.) (Continued on opposite page.)

mented individuals, palpation of skin texture may be the best method of detecting a rash. Some contend that with a little practice, papular rashes can usually be identified by palpating gently with fingertips. However in the case of a macular rash, the nurse may have to rely on the patient's complaints of itching or on evidence of scratching (Roach, 1972).

Turgor. Skin *turgor* is a term used to describe the skin's elasticity. In advanced dehydration, large amounts of weight loss or stretching, or even in normal aging, elasticity of the skin will lessen. To test skin turgor, one gently pinches an area of skin (usually the abdomen, if not too flaccid, or the skin over the radius at the wrist), noting how quickly the skin re-

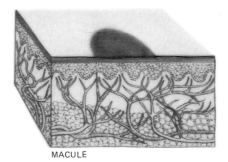
MACULE

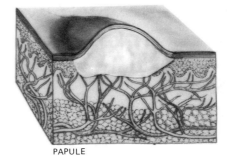
PAPULE

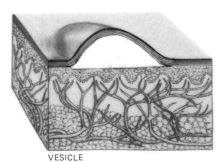
VESICLE

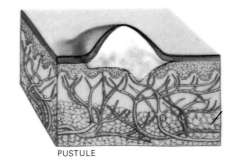
PUSTULE

FIGURE 3.4
Continued.

CHART 3.5
PRIMARY LESIONS

Name	Size	Description
Macule	↓ 1 cm	Flat, circumscribed alteration of skin color (freckle)
Papule	↓ 0.5 cm	Solid, raised area (pimple)
Patch	↑ 1 cm	Flat, discolored area (Mongolian spot)
Nodule	↓ 2 cm	Solid mass in dermal or subcutaneous layer (wart)
Tumor	↑ 2 cm	Solid mass, may extend through subcutaneous layer
Cyst	Varies	Encapsulated, semi-solid, or fluid-filled mass, may extend into dermis and epidermis
Wheal	Varies	Erythematous, smooth, irregularly shaped, flat-topped area
Vesicle	↓ 1 cm	Fluid-filled area below skin surface (varicella)
Bulla	↑ 1 cm	Like vesicle, but larger (blister)
Pustule	Varies	Similar to vesicle and bulla, but pus-filled (acne)

CHART 3.6
SECONDARY LESIONS

Name	Size	Description
Erosion	Varies	Rubbing away of epidermis (abrasion)
Crust	Varies	Dried serum, pus, blood (scab)
Scar	Varies	Healed injury; with fibrous tissue
Keloid	Varies	Overgrowth of scar that extends at least into dermis; fibrous
Scales	Varies	Flakes of skin, especially epidermis (psoriasis)
Lichenification	Varies	Thickening of all layers—an area that is repeatedly exposed to trauma or disease (eczema)
Hyperkeratosis	Varies	Extreme lichenification (callous)
Excoriation	Varies	A linear superficial scratch
Fissure	Varies	Linear furrowing in the epidermis and dermis, may go further (lip-splitting, especially in cold weather)
Ulcer	Varies	Loss of epidermis and portion of dermis (decubitus)

CHART 3.7
VASCULAR MARKINGS THROUGHOUT THE LIFESPAN

Name	Age	Physiologic Cause	Description
Hemangiomas	Birth or old age	Vascular lesions	See specific type.
Nevus flammeus infantile Nevus flammeus infantile (also known as stork bites, capillary hemangioma, telangectatic nevus)	Present at birth, fades by 2 years	Vascular lesion	Small, superficial, flat, irregularly shaped, pink patches over eyelids, especially around nose, forehead, and occiput
Port wine stain	Present at birth, does not usually fade	Vascular lesion	Larger nevus may be dark pink to red; may be found anywhere on body; often on face, scalp or groin; if on face or scalp may be associated with retardation, seizures or glaucoma; often on scalp; if on central face there may be associated neurologic disease
Strawberry	Develops from birth and enlarges through 6 months, may start to resolve by 2 years	Vascular lesion	Raised red lesion, may occur anywhere
Cavernous (mature hemangioma)	May be present at birth and not change in size; does not fade usually	Vascular lesion	Red-blue, spongy, irregularly shaped mass
Cherry angioma (senile hemangioma)	Develops in aging persons	Vascular lesion	Small, nodular, red; most frequently on trunk; may blanch with external pressure
Senile lentigines	Middle age and older	Skin exposure	Sharply circumscribed, light brown flat spots on sun-exposed areas.
Spider angioma	Any age	Can be normal vascular lesion or pathologic indicator (liver disease, pregnancy, ↑ estrogen)	Small, star-like with a solid circular area in the middle; may pulsate when pressure applied; often below waist
Telangiectasia	Middle age	Sun exposure, polythemia, alcoholism	Large or small generalized areas of venous or capillary dilatation, appear as erythematous linear markings
Venous star	Varies	Vascular force on vein	Various sizes, small, blue, star-like; found near veins, often on legs

turns to place. If the elasticity is decreased, the skin will recede very slowly or stand by itself. If the turgor is normal, it will go right back into place. However, with elderly individuals, the skin may normally recede slowly due to the loss of elasticity in the skin.

Masses. Palpating a mass on or under the skin is critical. Any palpable lesion should be felt for temperature, tenderness, size, smoothness of borders, mobility, and consistency. Palpa-tion of a mass may take place when the nurse is assessing a particular system or during the skin exam itself.

Epidermal Appendages

FINGERNAILS AND TOENAILS
The nails are inspected and palpated. They are inspected for color, shape, biting, unusual curvature, thickness, and markings in the nail

beds themselves. In light-skinned patients, healthy nails appear reasonably smooth, convex, and pink over the nailbeds. While pigmentation of the nails is unusual in normal Caucasians, it is not uncommon among blacks, who may normally have brown or black pigmentation along the edge of the nail or in a pattern of longitudinal streaks (Wasserman, 1974).

The nurse should next push on two or more of the nails and look for blanching and the immediate return of the pink color to the nail bed. If the pinkness does not return promptly, she should consider the possibility of a circulatory insufficiency or an anemia. In highly pigmented individuals, the rate of return of the nail bed color may be a more useful indicator than the actual color of the nail. The nails themselves do not change much throughout life unless abnormalities develop (Fig. 3.5; Chart 3.8).

HAIR

The hair on the scalp is inspected routinely in a complete physical and in an acute situation if it pertains to the problem. The hair is observed for color, amount, quality, and distribution. It is also felt for texture.

Most hair changes are due to the aging process. (See discussion earlier in this chapter.) Some changes in hair texture are directly related to systemic disease. In hyperthyroidism, the hair texture often becomes fine and smooth. In hypothyroidism, the patient might report the change in hair texture as being very coarse and dry.

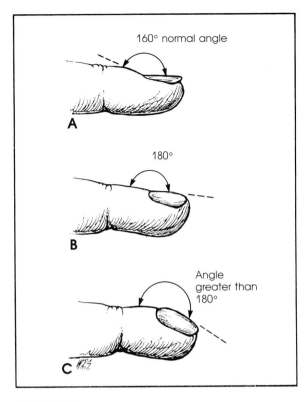

FIGURE 3.5
Clubbing. (**A**) *Normal,* (**B**) *early clubbing,* (**C**) *late clubbing.*

As stated earlier, hair loss can be a part of the aging process or be the result of other causes. Likely causes for abnormal hair loss are chemotherapy, stress, chemical treatments, (hair color, permanents, etc.) or fungal infections.

CHART 3.8
ABNORMALITIES OF THE NAILBEDS

Name	Description
Clubbing	This is the result of advanced heart or lung disease (especially COPD). The fingertips are also likely to enlarge (See Fig. 3.5)
Furrowing (Beau's lines)	This can be the result of systemic problems or traumatic injury. A ridge will appear across the nail that extends to the nail bed
Thickening	This can be the result of chronic fungal infections in the nail beds. *Candida albicans* is one of the most difficult to treat. Removal of the nail is often necessary
Paronychia	This is the result of an infection around the nail, thus causing erythema, edema and tenderness
Linear markings	Some people have hairline type markings under the nail. They are usually white. Their etiology is unknown and they are generally not problematic
Pitting	Single or multiple pinhead-sized lesions in nail; may be closely related to psoriasis.
Spooning	Spoon-shaped nail; may be associated with certain anemias
Splinter hemorrhages	Red-brown vertical linear streaks in the nailbed. May be associated with subacute bacterial endocarditis

Screening Examination of the Skin

Inspection of the skin for:
- color
- lesions
- obvious moisture
- edema
- vascular changes

Palpation of the skin for:
- moisture
- temperature
- turgor
- masses

Inspection and palpation of the hairs
Inspection and palpation of the nails

EXAMPLE OF A RECORDED HISTORY AND PHYSICAL

SUBJECTIVE:

Chief Complaint: "My skin has been itchy for 3 days."

HPH: This 16-year-old female considers herself to be in "good health." Three days ago noticed she was scratching a lot around the elastic waist of her panty hose. She did not pay attention to it. However, as she was about to bathe that evening, she noticed "tiny, flesh-colored bumps" where she had been scratching. The itch increased that night. She applied some calamine lotion but got no relief. The following day, the itching and same bumps appeared on her wrists, between the fingers of her left hand, in the axillary folds, and in the left groin. Last night the itching was so bad "I almost went crazy. I tried dry skin lotions and hot baths. Nothing helped."

Patient has never had this problem before. She has used no new soaps, perfumes, or detergents. No new clothes, night clothes, bed linens. She is taking no medications presently and has taken none in the last 6 weeks. She has eaten no unusual foods or in unusual restaurants. No pets. She did visit some friends last weekend who "found a little puppy and decided to give it a home." No known allergies to foods, medications, or environmental irritants.

OBJECTIVE:

T. 98.6°F orally; P. 80 radial; R. 16; B.P. 124/72 sitting.

Skin: Multiple papules and pustules; white-gray in color in a linear configuration along left flank area at waist, right and left anterior axillary folds, left groin folds, flexor surface of right and left wrist, and between the digits of the left hand. Some crusting and redness along the waist. No edema or discharge in these areas.

Microscopic: Skin scraping of axilla; mite present.

REFERENCES

Bobak, I., & Benson, R. (1984). Maternity Care. The Nurse and the Family (3rd ed.). St. Louis: C. V. Mosby.

Cage, G. (1971). Eccrine and apocrine secretory glands. In T. Fitzpatrick, et al., (Eds.), Dermatology in General Medicine. New York: McGraw-Hill.

McDonald, C., & Kelly, P. (1975). Dermatology and venerealogy. In R. Williams, (Ed.), Textbook of Black-Related Diseases. New York: McGraw-Hill.

Quevedo, W., Fitzpatrick, T., Pathak, M., & Timbow, K. (1975). Role of light in human skin color variation. American Journal of Physical Anthropology, 43, 393–408.

Roach, L. (1972). Color changes in dark skins. Nursing, 2, 19–22.

Rubin, B. (1979). Black skin. RN, Vol. 2, 31–35.

Wasserman, H. (1974). Ethnic Pigmentation: Historical, Physiological and Clinical Aspects. Amsterdam: Excerpta Medica.

Williams, R. (1976). The clinical or physiological assessment of black patients. In D. Luckraft, (Ed.), Black awareness: Implications for black patient care. American Journal of Nursing, 16–26.

Additional Readings

Behrman, H., Labow, T., & Rozen, J. (1971). Common Skin Diseases; Diagnosis and Treatment (2nd ed.). New York: Grune & Stratton.

Branch, M., & Paxton, P. (1976). Providing Safe Nursing Care for Ethnic People of Color. New York: Appleton-Century-Crofts.

Ewing, J., & Rouse, B. (1978). Hirsutism, race, and testosterone levels: Comparison of East Asians and Euroamericans. Human Biology, 50, 209–15.

Fitzpatrick, T., Arndt, K., & Clark, W., Jr., et al., (Eds.). (1979). Dermatology in General Medicine. New York: McGraw-Hill.

Pillsbury, D. (1980). A Manual of Dermatology. Philadelphia: Saunders.

Sauer, G. (1980). Manual of Skin Diseases (3rd ed.). Philadelphia: Lippincott.

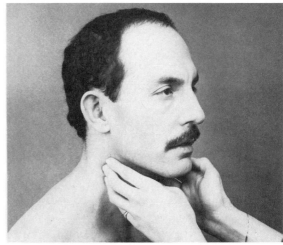

4

The Head, Face, and Neck

Much of the examination of the head, face, and neck is general inspection. Most of this can be done while eliciting the health history. If this is the only time that inspection is implemented, however, it is likely to be superficial and abnormalities may be missed. Close inspection of the head, face, and neck is followed by palpation. To complete the evaluation of the head, face, and neck, include the examination of the eyes, ears, mouth, nose, and sinuses.

DEVELOPMENTAL CHANGES OF THE HEAD, FACE, AND NECK THROUGHOUT THE LIFESPAN

The structures of the head, face, and neck do not change a great deal throughout a person's life, except that they grow proportionately to one's body size. Because of this, many of the features of the head, face, and neck are useful in assessing growth and development. To make accurate assessments, it is important to know what changes to expect and when they should occur.

The structure and shape of the head reveals a great deal about a patient in the early part of his life. The head of the newborn is asymmetric because of labor and delivery. Usually, the asymmetry resolves shortly after birth without any intervention. Three conditions are the result of this birth trauma: *molding, caput succedaneum* and *cephalohematoma* (Fig. 4.1). Caput succedaneum is a soft

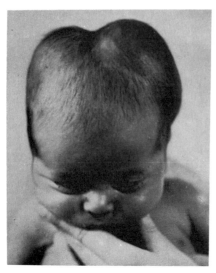

FIGURE 4.1
Cephalohematoma involving both parietal bones in an infant 13 days old. (From Rudolph, A., et al., (Eds.). Pediatrics (16th ed.). New York: Appleton-Century-Crofts, 1977, p. 1827, with permission.)

tissue injury which occurs during birth. It causes edema and ecchymosis of the presenting position of the baby's head during a vertex delivery. Caput succedaneum usually resolves gradually in the first few days of life. Molding, which is an overriding of the parietal bones,

may accompany caput succedaneum. This too, will resolve without treatment during the first few weeks of life (Vaughn & McKay, 1979). The third abnormality of the newborn's head, cephalhematoma, is a subperiosteal hemorrhage which is usually limited to one cranial bone and is often unilateral. A cephalhematoma does not appear until several hours after birth and gradually increases in size. There is no discoloration with a cephalhematoma, but it looks strange and can be frightening to parents. Parents need a lot of reassurance and support if their infant has cephalohematoma. Fortunately, this too resolves without treatment during the first few weeks of life.

The skull is not completely ossified at birth and as a result, there are openings called *fontanelles*, often referred to as "soft spots." There are two important fontanelles: the *anterior* and the *posterior* (Fig. 4.2). The diamond-shaped anterior fontanelle is located at the union of the frontal and parietal bones. The exact size is not as important as its presence so that the brain can grow as it should during the first year of life. The fontanelle is about 3 centimeters long by 4 centimeters wide and closes gradually between 8 months and 2 years of age. The joining of the parietal and occipital bones is the posterior fontanelle. This triangu-

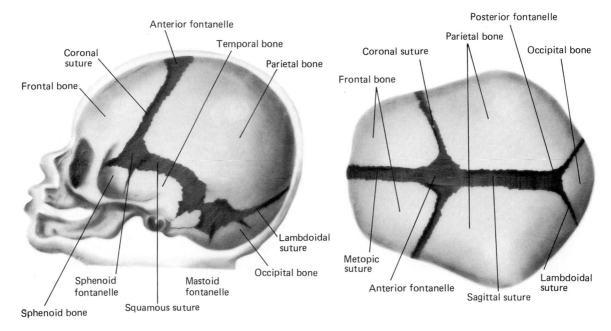

FIGURE 4.2
Fontanelles at birth. (From Heagarty, M., et al. Child Health: Basics for Primary Care. New York: Appleton-Century-Crofts, 1980, p. 119, with permission.)

lar soft spot closes by 3 months of age and may even be closed at birth.

The size of the head is a crucial statistic at birth and during infancy. An average-size baby should have a head measurement of 13 to 14 inches (35 cm.). During the first year of life the head grows about 4 inches. At birth the head is about 2 centimeters larger than the chest. As the child grows, this proportion reverses, but not during the first year of life. Abnormal growth rates can be indicative of serious problems. Some terms commonly used to describe head size are as follows.

- *Normocephalic:* A head size within normal limits.
- *Macrocephalic:* An inappropriately large head for age and body size.
- *Microcephalic:* An inappropriately small head for age and body size.

The hair on a person's head changes significantly throughout the lifespan. The amount and color of a baby's hair is somewhat genetically related. Blond, fair-haired newborns will often be almost bald, or have a very light covering of hair evenly distributed over the scalp. Dark-haired babies are more likely to have more hair. Often this hair falls out during the first few weeks of life and the permanent hair grows in shortly after the temporary hair falls out. Infants have scant and very soft hair, but it gets more plentiful as the baby gets older. The hair of a toddler and preschooler also thickens and increases in quantity.

Hair grows at different rates and differs in quality among individuals. The hair of childhood, adolescence, and young adulthood grows at a relatively consistent rate. As middle and old age approach, many people will notice a loss and a thinning of the hair. Men especially have a problem with *alopecia* (loss of hair). Balding has a genetic predisposition and not much can be done about it. Women may also notice a decrease in the amount and thickness of hair during and after menopause.

Graying is the most common change in hair color as people age. Graying is a result of decreasing melanin in the hair shafts. As the melanin continues to decrease, the gray hair turns to white or pale yellow. There is also decreasing function of the sebaceous glands, making the scalp drier.

The face of a newborn often has the markings of the long laborious birthing process. For the most part, these markings disappear in a few days. A newborn's facial features should be symmetric regardless of the birth markings. Occasionally, a neonate will have temporary paralysis of the facial nerve (cranial nerve VII). This is evidenced by a drooping of one side of the mouth and eye and the infant is unable to open the eye completely. Often this paralysis resolves on its own and may have occurred as a result of the birthing process. If facial features are asymmetric, further evaluation is warranted.

There are not many facial features that change a great deal throughout childhood, except for proportionate growth. However, adolescence brings some significant changes. The appearance of acne on males and females and facial hair on males is synonymous with adolescence. In some cases, acne does not appear until adulthood. For most youths, however, acne resolves in the later teen years or early twenties. The emergence of facial hair on adolescent males is individualized. For some males facial hair appears in the early teen years, for others, not until later adolescence. Fair-haired, fair-complected youths may not have facial hair until late in adolescence. In most instances, the hair above the lip darkens first, then hair appears along the mandible and cheeks. Some dark-haired and dark-complected teenage girls may notice hair on the upper lip darkening, as well as the development of an occasional scattered facial hair. Facial hair can emerge under the chin in these women, too. This hair can be bleached or removed if desired.

The next time one is likely to notice facial changes is during the late-middle and elderly years. Facial hair on both men and women tends to change. Women who are postmenopausal may notice the amount of facial hair increasing. Middle-age and elderly men, on the other hand, will notice a decrease in facial hair and may have to shave less often.

The most prominent facial change that occurs in the elderly years is the decrease of muscle tone. This decrease results in sagging of skin, especially under the chin and around the cheeks. The nasolabial lines that extend from the nose to the outside corner of the mouth become more prominent. Wrinkling of the skin commonly occurs around the eyes, cheeks, forehead, under the chin and neck. The amount of wrinkling is individualized.

The neck changes very little structurally throughout life. However, there are some interesting features of the neck typical to a certain age that are worth noting. The newborn has a very short neck—in fact, in some babies, it looks like the head almost sits directly on the shoulders. In the neonate, the lymph glands are present but difficult to palpate. Even though the newborn cannot hold his head up straight, the neck features should be symmetrical. Even with the floppy head, range of motion should be noted at intervals during the first few weeks of the baby's life. Signs of increasing ability of the baby to hold his head up should also be recorded. An infant should be able to hold his head up when held in a sitting position by 3 to 4 months of age.

Lymph nodes are prominent and easy to palpate in a young child, especially one with a thin neck. Palpable lymph nodes are not necessarily abnormal in this age group, especially if no illness is involved. When there is a question about normal lymph nodes, compare both sides of the neck. Usually, when non-tender, palpable lymph nodes are the same bilaterally, there is no pathology. A single, hard nodule located along any lymph chain should be evaluated further.

In the elderly, the tonsillar lymph nodes occasionally may be felt due to calcification. They are usually smooth, non-tender nodes and are the only enlarged nodes which can be considered normal in an elderly person. Even if these nodes are considered normal, physician consultation is indicated to confirm the diagnosis.

One final comment regarding neck structures concerns the thyroid gland. The thyroid is not usually palpable in children under 9 or 10 years of age, and some authorities feel it is not clearly palpable in adolescents. The area in the general vicinity of the gland must be felt because any palpable mass needs further evaluation.

ANATOMY

The skull is a relatively round, bony structure. It is made up of both the facial and the cranial bones (Fig. 4.3). All the cranial bones of the skull are joined by suture lines. The *frontal*

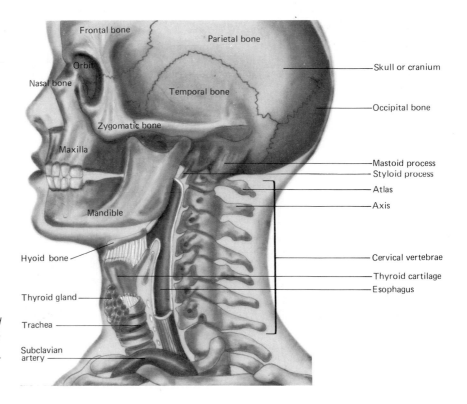

FIGURE 4.3

Major structures of the head and neck. (From Heagarty, M., et al. Child Health: Basics for Primary Care. New York: Appleton-Century-Crofts, 1980, p. 118, with permission.)

bone is the bone called the forehead. It attaches to the *parietal bone* on the anterior aspect of the skull at the *coronal suture line.* The *sagittal suture line* falls in the middle of the parietal bone. Posteriorly, the *lambdoidal suture line* lies horizontally and serves as the connection between the parietal and the occipital bone. The *squamosal suture line* joins the temporal and parietal bones on the lateral aspects of the head. An additional suture line may occur across the occipital bone in American Indian children and between the frontal bones in children of West European descent (Barnicot, 1977). Suture lines, especially the coronal, sagittal, and the lambdoidal, have a ridge-like feeling when palpated at birth, but should be smooth and no longer palpable by 5 to 6 months.

The facial bones are also connected by suture lines, although these are normally not palpable at any time. The facial bones are not movable, with the exception of the *mandible*, the lower jaw. It is the longest bone of the face and contains the sockets for the lower teeth. The upper teeth come out of the *maxillary bone*, which surrounds the nose. Attached to the maxillary bone is the *zygomatic bone;* the two jointly form the lower rim of the orbit of the eye. The maxilla and frontal bone meet as well. Together they surround the *nasal bone*, which is the bony portion of the nose. These are the skull bones accessible to external inspection and palpation.

The neck has a variety of structures that are readily accessible to physical examination. They are the *sternocleidomastoid* and *trape-*zius muscles* (Fig. 4.4), the *trachea*, the *carotid arteries* and *jugular veins*, the *thyroid gland*, the *thyroid cartilage* and the *cricoid cartilage* (Fig. 4.5), and the *lymph nodes of the neck* (Fig. 4.6).

There are two major neck muscles: the sternocleidomastoid and the trapezius. The sternocleidomastoid longitudinally extends from the mastoid process to the clavicle. The trapezius begins at the occipital area and reaches to the shoulder region (Fig. 4.4). The positions of these two muscles are such that they form invisible triangles. The anterior portion of the neck represents the anterior triangle and the posterior triangle involves the posterior region. This description is helpful when trying to learn proper techniques of palpation of the lymph nodes and the thyroid gland.

There are several structures in the anterior portion of the neck with which the examiner must be familiar. The *hyoid bone* is the most superior bony structure in the neck that can be palpated in the midline area. It is the support for the tongue and its muscles. Moving down, the next firm structure that can be felt is the *thyroid cartilage* (often referred to as the Adam's Apple). It is the largest cartilage of the larynx. Below the thyroid cartilage is the *cricoid cartilage.* This cartilaginous landmark is narrower than the thyroid cartilage. Both ascend when a person swallows. The *trachea* lies under these cartilages and is the pipe of respiration. It is about 5 inches in length. The *thyroid gland*, the only endocrine gland accessible to physical examination, is in this same general vicinity. It lies adjacent to the

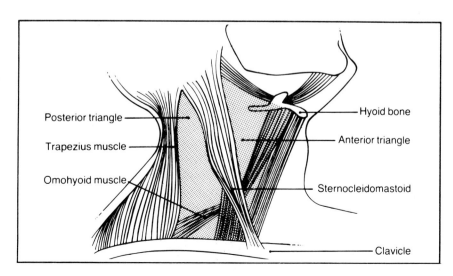

Posterior triangle

Trapezius muscle

Omohyoid muscle

Hyoid bone

Anterior triangle

Sternocleidomastoid

Clavicle

FIGURE 4.4
Anterior and posterior triangle of the neck.

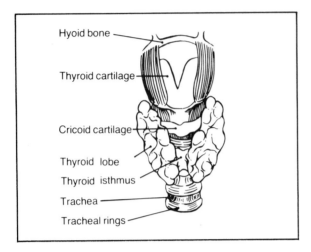

FIGURE 4.5
Major structures of the neck, anterior view.

tracheal rings 2–3–4. The lateral lobes of the thyroid gland are connected by a spongy tissue called the *isthmus*. The thyroid gland and isthmus also ascend with swallowing (Fig. 4.5).

Most of the palpable lymph nodes in the body are located in the neck. The lymph nodes palpable in this region are (Fig. 4.6):

1. Occipital: In the occipital region of the head where the trapezius and the occiput meet.
2. Postauricular: In front of the mastoid process but behind the auricle.
3. Preauricular: In front of the tragus.
4. Tonsillar: 2 centimeters below and inferior to the angle of the mandible in the hollow of loose skin.
5. Submaxillary: Along the mandible halfway from the angle to the chin.
6. Submental: Underneath the chin.
7. Deep cervical: Under the sternocleidomastoid.
8. Superficial cervical: Also under the sternocleidomastoid, but slightly more posterior.
9. Posterior: Below the superficial cervical and along the anterior aspect of the trapezius.
10. Supraclavicular: Above the clavicle, along the base of the sternocleidomastoid.

Circulation of blood to the head and neck is supplied primarily by the *external* and *internal carotid arteries*. The *internal* and *external*

jugular veins are also located in the neck. The twelve cranial nerves are responsible for innervating the head and neck. Both the circulatory and the neurologic aspects will be discussed in detail in later chapters.

HISTORY

There are several questions to ask in reviewing the head, face, and neck. One can usually combine the questions regarding the head and face and then follow with the review of the neck.

A general inquiry about the patient's hair is a good place to begin. What is the texture? (i.e., fine, coarse); How would he describe the amount? (i.e., thick, thin); Has there been any loss of hair, recently or in the past? (all over or one specific area); What is the natural color?; Has the hair been chemically treated? (i.e., permanents, straighteners, or dyes); What is the consistency of the hair? (i.e., oily, dry); and how often does the hair have to be washed? The answers to these questions provide valuable information for the history.

Questions regarding the scalp range from problems with lumps or bumps to itching, scaling, or dandruff. A lump on the head may have been due to traumatic injury. If so, how it was incurred needs to be investigated. A mass on the head may also be some form of a cyst. In either case it is important to get a description of how long it has been there as well as the location, size, associated pain, discharge (describe), and previous history of the problem. Itching, scaling, or dandruff may have various etiologies. Information should be elicited on the area involved, the length of time the problem has existed, and any known cause of the problem (allergy to hair products, incomplete rinsing of shampoos, stress, chronic skin conditions, etc.). If any other abnormalities have occurred in the past, a brief discussion of what the problems were, known causes, symptoms, treatment, and any recurrences should be recorded.

Relevant to the review of this system is any history of loss of consciousness, seizures, dizziness, headache, or recurring headaches, trauma, or facial pain. A loss of consciousness may have occurred for several reasons. A traumatic injury may have caused the patient to

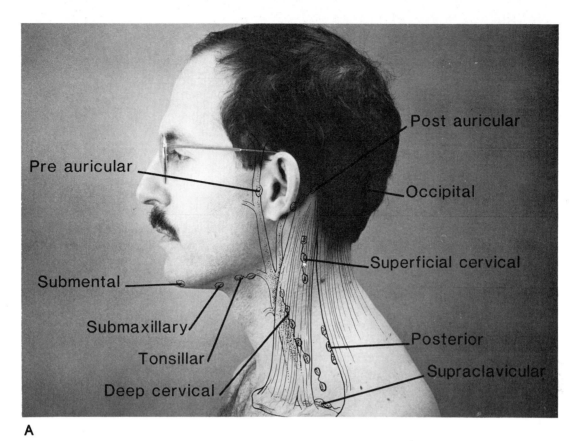

A

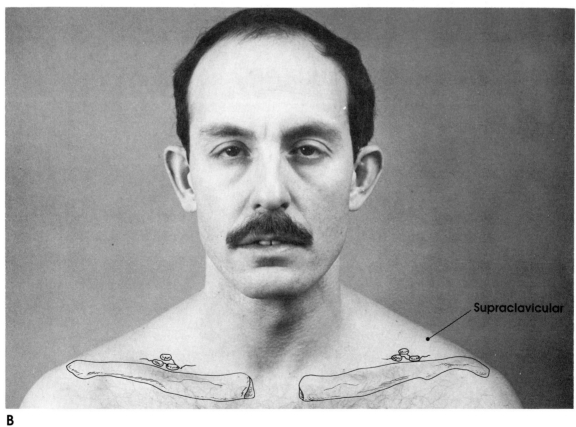

B

FIGURE 4.6
Lymphatics of the neck. **A.** Lateral view. **B.** Anterior view.

become unconscious. If this has happened, the patient should be questioned about the existing circumstances: when and where the incident happened, what activity the patient was involved in at the time, what was done for the patient, how long he thinks he was "out," and any residual effects of the injury.

Seizures may or may not cause a loss of consciousness. If a seizure occurred one time as a result of a high fever when the patient was a child, that is different from a history of seizures through the years. It is important to have the patient describe what he means by the word and what exactly happened to him. People may refer to this as a "spell," so a mutual understanding of what is being described is necessary. Any treatments as a result of the episode(s) should be recorded.

Dizziness can be a symptom and a complicated problem, too. A very helpful question to ask regarding dizziness is: "Do you feel like the room is spinning around you (vertigo) or do you feel light-headed?" Rotational dizziness is due most often to vestibular dysfunction and in this instance the patient will describe the sensation of the room spinning around him. The patient may also describe the sensation that he is spinning, rather than the room.

People who have headaches are often very frustrated. Finding a cause and a successful treatment often follows years of pain and various opinions and treatments. If headaches are a problem, a thorough pain history should be obtained, including location, radiation, duration, intensity, associated activity, aggravating and alleviating factors, accompanying symptoms, and past diagnosis and treatments. Allergies, past history of traumas, stress, and the menstrual cycle may also be related. Gathering data about other family members with headaches may provide very helpful clues about the types of headache the patient has. If the eight areas of investigation are applied, much valuable information can be collected.

Questions regarding the head are basically the same for all ages. One exception is if the parents report a problem regarding the growth of an infant's head. This is unusual and, therefore, not directly asked. If this is or was a problem, other symptoms are usually present as well.

A more specific investigation of the face and its problems includes not only what it is, but also where on the face the problem is located. Common complaints that are likely to

be mentioned are edema; pain; discoloration; unusual movements, such as tics or twitching; and lesions, such as moles and pimples. Remember that positive responses require a more detailed inquiry.

The history regarding the neck follows easily in this systematic approach. The patient should be asked if he has any pain or stiffness or has noticed any lumps in his neck. If he has pain or stiffness, he is then asked where exactly and with what movements the discomfort is associated. If he notices a lump, the nurse should inquire as to how long it has been there; the location, size, and amount of tenderness; and if there has been a recent diagnosis of a systemic infection. This information plus additional questions from the eight areas of investigation will give a more complete picture.

The patient should be asked if he has ever been told he has a thyroid problem. If he has, he may have been told whether his thyroid was overfunctioning or underfunctioning. That knowledge will be very helpful. There may have been blood tests or other diagnostic studies done to confirm the diagnosis. The nurse should find out what the patient specifically recalls about when they were done, what was suspected, and what the results were. Were medications ordered following the tests? If so, what kind and how much did the patient take? Are they still being taken? If not, why not? Were any other treatments implemented, such as surgery or radiation? What was its course and outcome? All these data add to the very important data base that the patient provides.

PHYSICAL ASSESSMENT

For the head, face, and neck, the following techniques of examination are used: inspection, palpation, percussion, and auscultation. Both inspection and palpation are used throughout the exam, while auscultation is only used to check over the major arteries and thyroid for bruits (see Chapter 9). Percussion or palpation is used to assess tenderness of the paranasal sinuses (see Chapter 7). The equipment needed by the examiner is her eyes and hands, good lighting, a stethoscope, a glass of water, and a tape measure.

Because of the nature of the examination of the head, face, and neck, inspection and palpation are discussed together. As always, it is best to begin with a general inspection.

The Head

Inspection and palpation of the scalp and skull are done as part of every screening examination or when a problem is suspected. It is easy to skip over this part of the exam and focus on the eyes, ears, nose, neck, or throat. The examination of the head is as important as that of the other organs and should not be done superficially.

The hair on the head is inspected for texture, amount, and distribution. "Coarseness" and "fineness" are terms used to describe the texture of the hair. The amount and distribution of the hair may vary with age. Hair grows at different rates and differs in quality among individuals.

The scalp is inspected by separating the hair at various spots and taking a thorough look at the skin under the hair. Look for scaliness, lesions, or irregularities. Scaliness on the scalp may be indicative of a common condition such as *dandruff*. This often occurs in the winter months, when skin tends to be drier. *Seborrhea* is another condition commonly found on the head and is a result of an overproduction of sebum (from the sebaceous glands). Seborrhea presents as greasy, scaly patches and is found in places on the body where hair follicles are located. It can be caused by stress and tension in addition to genetic predisposition. This problem can usually be controlled by topical medication or shampoos and by trying to decrease the psychosocial stresses that may be associated with it.

Next the scalp should be observed for lumps, bumps, and lesions. Moles are often found on the head. If they are elevated above the skin surface, combing and shampooing the hair may cause them to bleed. This information may be elicited in the history, but if not, these matters should be investigated when a lesion is found.

A lump on the head may be a sebaceous cyst (see Chapter 3). It will feel like a firm, well-defined mass under the skin surface. These cysts are usually not painful and, if small enough, are not bothersome. Size should be noted for comparative purposes. Traumatic injury may also cause a bump on the head.

These bumps will vary in size, depending on the type of injury incurred.

The skull is inspected and palpated for size, shape, and tenderness. Abnormal skull size is most likely to occur during infancy, unless there is a congenital anomaly (Fig. 4.7).

In order to ascertain the proper size of the baby's skull, the head circumference is measured at all well baby examinations until the age of 2 years. (The exact time to stop measuring head circumference is controversial.) A paper tape or cloth tape with both centimeter and inch calibrations is necessary to measure the head. It is important that the child is still while taking this measurement. It may be helpful to have the parent hold the child's head. The tape is placed around the child's head. The occipital bone and frontal bone are used for landmarks in placing the tape. The tape is placed over the supraorbital ridges anteriorly and the widest portion of the occiput posteriorly (Fig. 4.8). The number is then plotted on a standardized growth chart (Fig. 4.8). As long as the measurement falls within the established norms for the appropriate age, then the head size is considered within normal limits. Any rapid change in head circumference from one evaluation to the next (i.e., rapid acceleration across the growth chart) warrants referral. Because all standardized growth charts currently available in the United States are based on statistical averages for Caucasian children, growth assessment of racially distinct children requires particular attention. For example, the head circumference of newborn children of Asian descent is normally nearly 1 centimeter narrower than that of black or Caucasian children (Alvear & Brooke, 1978). See Chapter 2 for additional information on growth differences.

Next the anterior and posterior fontanelles are inspected and palpated. If they are still open, the nurse should approximate the size. Any bulging or depression of these areas should be noted. A bulging fontanelle may indicate intracranial pressure. In a dehydrated child the fontanelles will appear depressed or sunken. While still palpating the head, the suture lines should be checked. If they are still palpable, a ridge-like sensation will be felt, and nothing more.

The entire scalp is palpated for masses using the pads of both fingers. A systematic approach must be used so that no portion of the scalp is missed. The size, shape, consis-

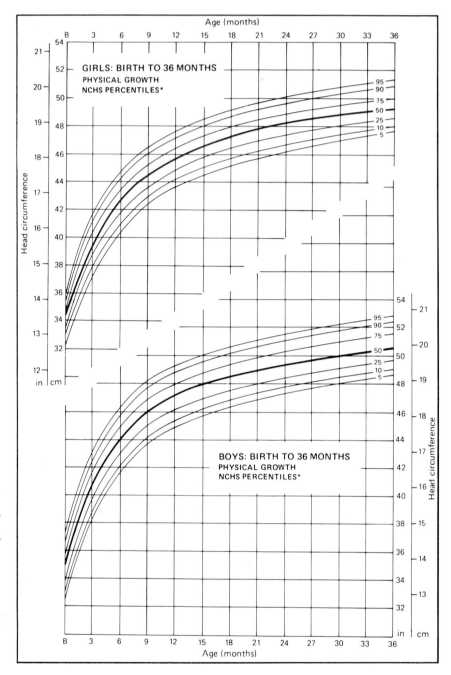

FIGURE 4.7
Head circumference in boys and girls (standardized chart)— birth to 36 months. (Reprinted with permission from Ross Laboratories, Columbus, Ohio, © 1976. Adapted from National Center for Health Statistics: NCHS Growth Charts, 1976. Monthly Vital Statistics Report, Vol. 25, No. 3 Supp. (HRA) 76–1120. Health Resources Administration, Rockville, Md., June 1976. Data from the Fels Research Institute.)

tency, and tenderness of all masses are identified. If there has been a recent injury, tenderness may be palpated over the involved area.

The Face

To inspect the face, the examiner stands directly in front of and at a level even with the patient. She systematically inspects the face of the child or adult for color, facial hair, symmetry, expression, tics, swelling, and any unusual conditions of the skin. Palpation of any lumps, lesions, or other raised abnormalities is necessary. Some facial abnormalities may be due to systemic or localized conditions. The skin may have the classic pallor of fatigue or anemia, or it may have the yellow tones of jaundice. The shape of the face may be "puffy" in advanced hypothyroidism or Cushing's dis-

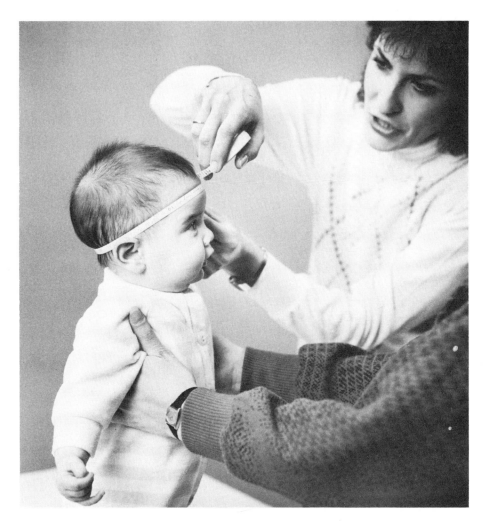

FIGURE 4.8
Measuring the circumference of an infant's head.

ease. Branch and Paxton (1976) point out that in examining black patients this characteristic broadening of facial features with hypothyroidism may be obscured by the health professional's notions about racial characteristics of the face. Periorbital edema may be a clue to kidney malfunction. There are also certain signs that accompany cranial nerve damage. For instance, one side of the face may droop. The condition is known as Bell's palsy and involves the seventh cranial nerve. Ptosis of the eyelid is another manifestation of cranial nerve damage (see Chapter 3). If any acne, moles, or unusual facial hair exists, a thorough description is necessary. When acne is a problem, it is important to keep track of where the lesions are located. In addition lesions should be described by color, size, and type (see Fig. 3.4, pp. 90–91). The nurse should also note whether or not they are blackheads, white heads, or cysts and whether there is permanent scarring. The details are noteworthy if week-to-week or month-to-month change is being assessed. Accurate, detailed descriptions are the only way improvement or deterioration of a condition can be documented.

Acne which does not usually begin until adolescence has several degrees of severity. The more serious types can be treated systemically. The milder forms are approached with topical treatments. In either case the crisis of altered body image is prevalent in the teenagers with the problem.

All lumps, lesions, or other abnormalities

identified on inspection are palpated. At this time, the frontal and maxillary sinuses can be percussed as well (see Chapter 7).

Any facial lesion, especially if it is isolated and elevated, should be described in detail. It should be described in terms of color, location, size, tenderness, discharge, crustation, and type of surface (e.g., pitting in the center).

The Neck

Inspection of the neck begins this portion of the exam. The structures and any abnormalities will be easier to see if the patient raises his chin and tilts his head backward. Good lighting is also necessary. The nurse should look for any asymmetry, swelling, obvious lymph nodes, masses, or lesions and palpate any of these enlargements. She should also note size, tenderness, color, shape, and mobility of any palpable masses.

Palpation of the lymph nodes and thyroid gland follows. A systematic approach for palpation of the lymph nodes is a must! If a meticulous method is not implemented, it is likely that portions of a lymph node chain will be missed. To feel the nodes, the pads of the first two or three fingers of both hands are used. The skin is rolled, not pushed, over the underlying tissue (Fig. 4.9). If the nurse pushes too hard, any palpable nodes will be obliterated. If a gentle but firm technique is used the enlarged nodes will be felt easily. Flexing the neck slightly midline will facilitate the exam. The patient should be asked if there is any tenderness.

The examiner should proceed in the following manner. She should start with the occipital nodes and move to the postauricular

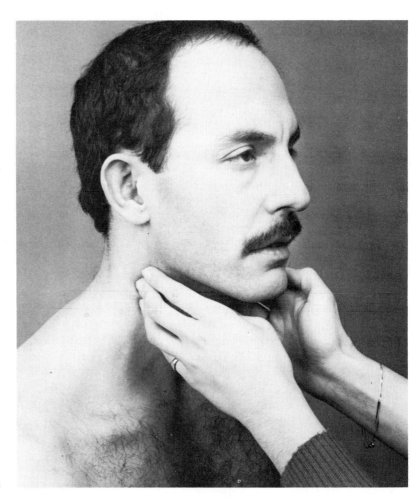

FIGURE 4.9
Palpating the lymph nodes of the neck.

and preauricular nodes. She should follow with palpation of the tonsillar, submaxillary, and submental. In the neck she should feel for the superficial cervical, deep cervical, and posterior cervical nodes. She should complete the exam by palpating the supraclavicular region.

In a well-developed adult, lymph nodes are generally not palpable. In a child, a thin adult, or someone who has recently had mononucleosis they may be easier to feel. However, if while palpating these lymph nodes a lump or lumps are discovered, then the following information must be noted: location, mobility, size, shape (edges well-defined), consistency, discreteness or tenderness (see Chapter 10, page 270, for description of these terms). Tenderness often indicates an acute inflammatory response to a viral, fungal, or bacterial infection. However a hard, immobile, irregularly shaped, nontender node often involves a malignancy.

The Thyroid

The thyroid gland is difficult to inspect and palpate. Health care providers agree that the normal thyroid gland is not normally palpable in children and many adults. However, people with thin necks are likely to have a normally functioning thyroid gland which can be felt. Authorities also feel that a slightly enlarged thyroid gland in adults is not necessarily pathologic.

The thyroid is inspected for enlargement and nodules; palpated for size, tenderness, and masses or nodules; and auscultated for bruits. Palpation of the thyroid gland involves both an anterior and a posterior approach. For screening purposes, only one approach is necessary. When a problem is suspected, both methods should be used to assure accuracy.

In order to inspect and palpate the thyroid and its lateral lobes, one must be able to locate specific landmarks (Figs. 4.4, 4.5, 4.10). The

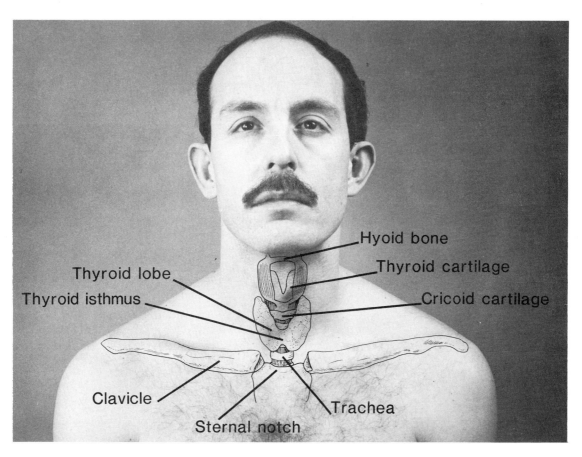

FIGURE 4.10
Major structures of the neck.

hyoid bone is the first landmark. It is slightly inferior and under the mandible. This bone is attached to the tongue's posterior surface. The hyoid has a firm, bony sensation when felt (Fig. 4.5). The firm thyroid cartilage is then found. It sits below the hyoid bone and above the cricoid. The cricoid is a mobile cartilaginous ring that ascends when one swallows. The thyroid isthmus is a soft, spongy band that lies across the trachea below the cricoid (Figs. 4.5, 4.10).

Once the landmarks have been located, inspection of the thyroid can proceed. Good lighting must be available for this portion of the exam. The examiner stands in front of the patient. She asks him to hyperextend his chin slightly and then to swallow. Any obvious enlargement, masses, or asymmetry should be noted. While looking at the trachea, the nurse should note if there is deviation from the midline. Checking for tracheal deviation includes palpation as well.

The patient may want a glass of water. This will make swallowing easier while the examiner is displacing the thyroid during palpation.

ANTERIOR APPROACH

The hyoid, thyroid cartilage, cricoid, trachea, and isthmus of the thyroid gland are palpated to help orient the examiner to landmarks. The examiner should be standing in front of the patient. To palpate the left lobe, the nurse should have the patient flex his head slightly to the left. At this time, the examiner's left thumb is placed next to the patient's right thyroid cartilage, in front of the sternocleidomastoid muscle, her other fingers resting behind the sternocleidomastoid muscle. She then displaces the patient's right thyroid cartilage to his left. (Fig. 4.11). With her right hand, she moves her right thumb which should be on the isthmus, slightly to the patient's left and then gently rests her thumb on the left thyroid

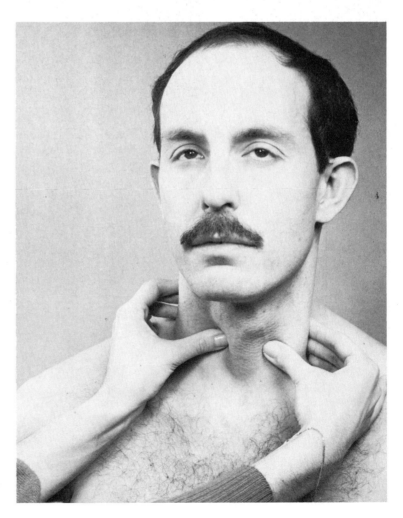

FIGURE 4.11
Proper placement of hands for anterior examination of the thyroid.

lobe. Then the fingers of her right hand are placed a little more firmly behind the sterno-cleidomastoid muscle. The muscle is then pinched slightly between the examiner's right thumb and fingers; this helps to expose the thyroid. The patient is asked to swallow (a sip of water is optional); the thyroid gland will ascend with this motion. The examiner will feel the thyroid gland under her right thumb with this ascension. No enlargement, nodes, or tenderness should be felt. The thyroid gland is normally smooth and sponge-like and should feel this way during palpation. The procedure is repeated with the patient at rest (not swallowing). Then the right thyroid is palpated once with the patient swallowing and then at rest.

POSTERIOR EXAMINATION OF THE THYROID

The nurse stands directly behind the patient and has him relax his neck by bending it slightly towards his chest (Fig. 4.12). The patient is asked to take a sip of water and hold it in his mouth. With her thumbs at the nape of the patient's neck and fingertips of the first two fingers of both hands on the anterior por-

tion of the neck, the nurse locates the cricoid and, directly below it, the isthmus. The patient is told to swallow the water and the examiner feels the isthmus ascend. The nurse palpates and follows the lobes as they curve behind the trachea to check for nodules.

To examine the right thyroid lobe the patient is told to flex his head slightly to the right. With the first two fingers of her left hand in front of the patient's left sternocleidomastoid muscle and her left thumb deep behind the sternocleidomastoid muscle, the examiner gently pushes the thyroid cartilage to the right (Fig. 4.12). The examiner's right hand is on the right side of the patient's neck. The first and second finger of the right hand should be placed in front of the sternocleidomastoid muscle and directly across from the isthmus, while the right thumb rests behind the sterno-cliedomastoid muscle (Fig. 4.12). The muscle is retracted slightly with the fingers. The patient is asked to swallow a sip of water. While the thyroid cartilage is displaced to the right and the patient is swallowing, she will feel the right thyroid lobe ascend under the fingers of her right hand. If an enlargement or irregu-

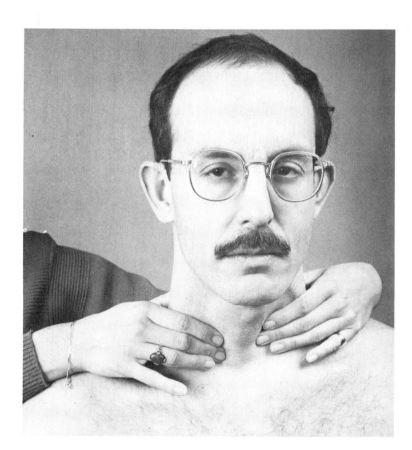

FIGURE 4.12
Proper placement of hands for posterior examination of the thyroid.

larity exists, it will be felt during this ascension. This procedure is repeated with the patient at rest (not swallowing). The left thyroid lobe is then palpated, with the patient swallowing and at rest.

In addition to thyroid enlargement, the nurse should note any tenderness or specific nodules. If the gland is enlarged she should be sure to listen over each lobe with the bell of the stethoscope for bruits (see Chapter 9). This accentuated flow sound may be heard over an abnormal thyroid gland.

Examination of the carotid arteries and jugular veins will be discussed in the chapter on cardiovascular assessment.

Screening Examination of the Head, Face, and Neck

1. Measurement of head circumference (all children 2 years of age and under)*
2. Inspection and palpation of the hair
3. Inspection and palpation of the scalp
4. Palpation of the fontanelles (all children 2 years of age and younger)
5. Inspection of the face
6. Inspection and palpation of the neck
7. Palpation of the lymph nodes
   a. Occipital
   b. Preauricular and postauricular
   c. Tonsillar
   d. Submaxillary
   e. Submental
   f. Superficial cervical
   g. Deep cervical
   h. posterior
   i. Supraclavicular
8. Inspection of the neck structures and thyroid
9. Palpation of the thyroid in either the anterior or posterior position

---

* Some providers only measure through the first year of life.

EXAMPLE OF A RECORDED HISTORY AND PHYSICAL

SUBJECTIVE:

Chief Complaint: "I have had pain behind my left eye for 2 hours."

HPH: This 20-year-old female considers herself to be in "perfect" health. Suddenly, 2 hours ago, while sitting and watching T.V., a "sharp, stabbing, shooting" pain began behind her left eye. She never has had anything like this before. The pain goes from behind her eye straight through to the back of her head. She noticed earlier in the evening that when she was doing dishes she saw "some green rings" in front of her eyes and that the light above the sink seemed unusually "bright."

She took three aspirin when the pain began, "because it was so bad," and vomited them 10 minutes later. She then tried to lie down but was unable to lie still. When she got up to vomit again she felt "very weak and clammy."

She has no dizziness, blurry vision, neck stiffness, ear, or tooth pain. There has been no recent trauma, emotional upset, or history of ↑ B.P. She takes no medications (including birth control pills). She has never had a seizure or loss of consciousness. She has no allergies, sinus problems, or recent upper respiratory illness. Her last menstrual period was 1 week ago and unremarkable.

Her mother and brother have severe headaches. "Now I know what they go through." In the past she has had occasional headaches three to four times/year that are relieved by aspirin. The pain now is "crippling and I couldn't do anything if I had to."

OBJECTIVE:

T. 99°F axillary; P. 72 radial; R. 24; B.P. (R) 140/80 lying, (L) 138/82 lying.

Head: No tenderness over skull. No lesions or masses.

Face: Wrinkling of forehead and squinting eyes. No asymmetry, tics. No tenderness over temporomandibular joint.

Neck: Supple, full range of motion, no palpable lymph nodes.

Ears: Bilaterally—no tenderness with palpation; canal clear; TM— no redness, bulging, retraction, or distortion of landmarks.

Eyes: Left eye—ptosis of lid, some tearing, no redness of sclera, PERRLA;* fundus—no hemorrhages, exudate, A–V nicking, dilated vessels; disc visualized, borders well defined; macula visualized. Right eye—unremarkable (external features → fundus exam)

Nose: Nasal mucosa pink → red. No drainage or polyps. Paranasal sinuses—frontal and maxillary nontender.

Mouth: Dentition—no obvious caries or misplaced teeth; gums— no lesions, bleeding, tenderness, or retraction.

Neurological: MENTAL STATUS—oriented to time, person, place; CRANIAL NERVES—II (vision not tested), III (motorsomatic), V, VI, VII (motor), all intact; MOTOR—walks without difficulty, gait normal; SENSORY—see Cranial nerves above; DEEP TENDON REFLEXES. (See stick figure illustration below.)

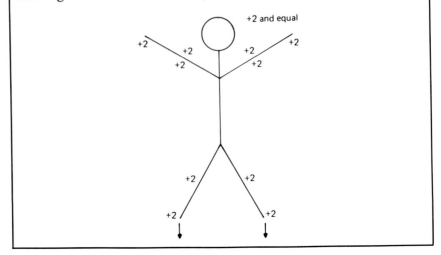

* *Pupils equal, round, and reactive to light and accommodation.*

REFERENCES

Alvear, J., & Brooke, O. (1978). Fetal growth in different racial groups. Archives of Disease in Children, 53, 27–32.

Barnicot, N. (1977). Biological variation in modern populations. In G. Harrison, et al., (Eds.), Human Biology: Introduction to Human Variation, Growth, and Ecology (2nd ed.). New York: Oxford Press, pp. 181–300.

Branch, M., & Paxton, P. (1976). Providing Safe Nursing Care for Ethnic People of Color. New York: Appleton-Century-Crofts.

Vaughn, V., & McKay, J. (1979). Nelson's Textbook of Pediatrics (11th ed.). Philadelphia: Saunders.

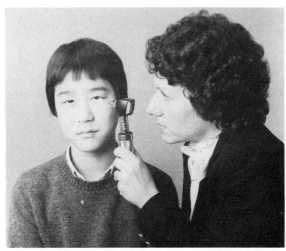

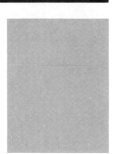

5

The Eye

To maintain the integrity of the eyes, they should be carefully assessed throughout the life cycle. A vision examination is an integral part of every complete physical examination. It is recommended that the eyes be examined at age 6 weeks, 6 months, 1 year, and every year until the age of 12 (Sagaties, 1982). This examination includes visual acuity, tests for ocular motility, examination of the external structures of the eye and a funduscopic examination.

An eye examination is performed as a part of every complete physical examination of the healthy adolescent and adult. Breslow and Somers (1979) recommend that a complete examination be done at age 13, once between the ages of 18 and 24, and at about the ages 30, 35, 40, 45, 50, 55, and 60 and every 2 years thereafter. As with the child, this examination includes visual acuity for far vision, tests for ocular motility, examination of the external structures of the eye and a funduscopic examination. Screening for near vision and glaucoma begins after the age of 40 (Havener, 1984). There are no definitive guidelines for routine screening for the prevention of glaucoma. One suggestion is that screening for elevated intraocular tension, associated with glaucoma, be done on all patients over 40 years of age who have not had a pressure reading taken within the previous two years.

More frequent eye examinations and referral to an ophthalmologist are necessary if the family history is positive for diabetes, hypertension, blood dyscrasia, glaucoma, or other eye diseases. The patient who has a known or suspected systemic disease (e.g., leukemia, sickle cell anemia, hypertension, diabetes) or is on medication known to affect vision (e.g., Myambutol corticosteroids) should be referred for more frequent eye examinations.

DEVELOPMENTAL CHANGES OF THE EYE THROUGHOUT THE LIFESPAN

The nurse should be aware of developmental patterns to adequately assess visual impairment. From the moment of birth the infant is aware of light and dark and responds to bright lights by closing his eyelids. The infant does not have any reflex tearing until 3 to 4 months of age. Random movement of the eyes, due to immature retinal development and inability to fixate centrally, disappears by 3 months of age (Chow, et al., 1984). The 6-week-old infant should be able to fixate on an object and by 8 to 10 weeks the infant can follow and bat at objects. From birth until the age of 4 to 5 years children are farsighted. This gradually decreases and normal visual acuity of 20–20 is reached by 4 to 5 years of age. Chart 5.1 shows the chronological development of the eyes from birth to 4 years of age.

Some school-age children demonstrate *refractive errors* requiring correction with glasses. There are 3 types of refractive errors: *astigmatism, hyperopia* (farsightedness), and *myopia* (nearsightedness). With *astigmatism*, light rays are not sharply focused on the retina because of differences in the curvature of the cornea. *Hyperopia* is a visual defect in which parallel light rays reaching the eye come to focus behind the retina due to a short anterior–posterior diameter of the eyeball. Vision is better for far objects than for near. *Myopia* is a visual defect in which parallel rays come to focus in front of the retina due to a long anterior–posterior diameter of the eyeball. Vision is better for near objects than for far. There can be a progression of all three of these defects as the child grows, even with correction. By young adulthood these changes usually stop and often the same pair of glasses can be worn until middle adulthood.

Strabismus is a congenital condition found in 3 to 5 percent of the pediatric population that affects normal vision. In this condition the visual axes of both eyes are not simultaneously directed to the same fixation point

CHART 5.1
CHRONOLOGY OF VISUAL DEVELOPMENT

Age	Level of Development
Birth	Awareness of light and dark. Infant closes eyelids in bright light.
Neonatal	Rudimentary fixation on near objects (3–30 inches)
2 weeks	Transitory fixation, usually monocular at a distance of roughly 3 feet.
4 weeks	Follows large conspicuously moving objects.
6 weeks	Moving objects evoke binocular fixation briefly.
8 weeks	Follows moving objects with jerky eye movements. Convergence beginning to appear.
12 weeks	Visual following now a combination of head and eye movements. Convergence improving. Enjoys light objects and bright colors.
16 weeks	Inspects own hands. Fixates immediately on a 1-inch cube brought within 1–2 feet of eye. Vision 20/300–20/200 (6/100–6/70).
20 weeks	Accommodative convergence reflexes all organizing. Visually pursues lost rattle. Shows interest in stimuli more than 3 feet away.
24 weeks	Retrieves a dropped 1-inch cube. Can maintain voluntary fixation of stationary object even in the presence of competing moving stimulus. Hand–eye coordination appearing.
26 weeks	Will fixate on a string.
28 weeks	Binocular fixation clearly established.
36 weeks	Beginning of depth perception.
40 weeks	Marked interest in tiny objects. Tilts head backward to gaze up. Vision 20/200 (6/70).
52 weeks	Fusion beginning to appear. Discriminates simple geometric forms (squares and circles). Vision 20/180 (6/60).
12–18 months	Looks at pictures with interest.
18 months	Convergence well established. Localization in distance crude—runs into large objects.
2 years	Accommodation well developed. Vision 20/40 (6/12).
3 years	Convergence smooth. Fusion improving. Vision 20/30 (6/9).
4 years	Vision 20/20 (6/6).

(From Kempe, C., et al: Current Pediatric Diagnosis and Treatment (8th ed.). Los Altos, Calif.: Lange Medical Publications, p. 25, 1984, with permission.)

(Sagaties, 1982). Normally, images viewed fall on corresponding points of the retina in each eye. Images are then passed on to the brain as two sets of nerve impulses that are fused into one. Double vision (*diplopia*) occurs in strabismus because the image viewed falls on noncorresponding points of the retina. In an attempt to avoid double vision the child learns to not use the vision in the deviating eye when eyesight is developing. As a result, this deviating eye permanently loses central visual acuity (*amblyopia*). Imbalance of the muscle alignment of the eyes is the most common cause of strabismus. Caucasians tend to have higher rates of convergent strabismus (esotropia), while divergent strabismus (exotropia) is more common in Orientals (Ing & Pang, 1973). Visual examination of children should be directed toward detecting strabismus. Early detection can result in the prevention of amblyopia and the development of normal visual acuity.

Normal vision can be maintained well into old age. Around the age of 45, however, there is an age-associated change in the crystalline lens of the eye which results in loss of elasticity and ability to accommodate to nearby objects. This ability is almost nonexistent in most persons by the age of 55 years (Kart, et al., 1978). This degenerative change, called *presbyopia,* first becomes apparent to the middle-aged person when he experiences difficulty reading newsprint; he compensates by holding the paper at arm's length. Many people receive reading glasses for the first time when they reach middle age.

Older persons will generally report a need for increased light, an inability to adapt to the changes in light, and a decreased ability to drive at night because of a decreased tolerance of direct lights. These visual changes are thought to occur as a result of the aging process.

Cataract, glaucoma, and *senile macular degeneration* are the most common disorders in the elderly. All three can result in serious impairment of vision. *Cataract* is the most prevalent ocular disorder of old age (Kart, et al., 1978; Yurick, 1981). This condition occurs in 95 percent of persons over 65, but only a small percentage have significant visual impairment (Yurick, 1981). The normally transparent lens of the eye with a cataract becomes opaque due to thickening and sclerosis. This opacity interferes with the passage of light rays to the retina. When a cataract interferes with daily activities the problem is easily remedied by surgical extraction of the lens.

Glaucoma is the most common cause of blindness in people over 40. It is estimated that 1.5 percent of people over 40 develop this eye disease annually (Resler & Tumulty, 1983). Glaucoma is an increase in intraocular pressure due to a disturbance in the circulation of the aqueous fluid. The end result of uncontrolled glaucoma is optic nerve damage and blindness. Ninety percent of people with glaucoma have *open angle* or *chronic glaucoma* (Resler & Tumulty, 1983). In chronic glaucoma pressure builds up slowly and the symptoms often do not present until there is considerable loss of vision. A gradual loss of peripheral vision is often the first indication of chronic glaucoma. In less common *acute narrow angle glaucoma* there is an abrupt rise in intraocular pressure. Symptoms, including intense pain, nausea, and vomiting are dramatic. This type of glaucoma is an emergency situation because vision loss can occur with only one attack (Resler & Tumulty, 1983). There is no cure for glaucoma, but if detected early there are measures for decreasing intraocular pressure and thereby controlling the disease. There is a familial tendency for the development of glaucoma.

Senile macular degeneration is a degeneration of the macular area of the retina. The macular area is that portion of the eye that permits the individual to discriminate detail, such as fine print (Kart, et al., 1978). Persons with this impairment can see only a gray shadow in the center of the visual field, which makes it difficult to see what is straight ahead (Yurick, 1981). Peripheral vision remains intact, therefore, the person is not disabled. There is no definite medical management for individuals with senile macular degeneration, but they can be helped with magnifiers and telescopic lenses. The cause of the condition is unknown, but there seems to be a familial tendency (Yurick, 1981).

ANATOMY

The *orbit* of the eye is a cavity formed by the frontal, maxillary, zygomatic, lacrimal, sphenoid, ethmoid, and palatine bones. The eye occupies the anterior portion of the orbit, the posterior portion being composed of nerves, blood vessels, and adipose tissue, which serve as a cushion to the eye. There are six muscles for each eye which begin at the bones of the orbit and insert in the outercoat of the eye. The four *rectus muscles* are the *superior, inferior, medial,* and *lateral.* These muscles direct the eyeball in the direction which their names indicate. The two oblique muscles are the *superior oblique* and *inferior oblique.* These two muscles rotate the eyeball on its axis. The muscles of the eyes work together to hold the eyes parallel, making binocular vision possible. Cranial nerves III, IV, and VI innervate these muscles.

The anatomy of the eye can be divided into the external structures and the fundus. Included in the external structures are the *eyelashes* and *lids,* the *lacrimal apparatus, conjunctiva, sclera, cornea, anterior chamber, iris,* and *pupils* (Fig. 5.1). The fundus includes the *retina, choroid, fovea centralis, macula, optic disc,* and *retinal vessels* (Fig. 5.2).

The External Structures of the Eye

The eyelids serve to protect the eye. The space between the lids is called the *palpebral fissure.* When the eyelids are open, the upper lid covers a small part of the cornea. The *inner* and *outer canthi* are the points where the upper and lower lids meet. A tarsus plate of dense connective tissue gives shape to the lid. Within the tarsus plate are *Meibomian glands.* Sebaceous glands are located along the lid margins. *Epicanthic folds* are vertical folds of skin cov-

ering the inner canthus. These folds are found in infants all over the world. They are present in up to 20 percent of children of European descent, but generally disappear within the first year of life. They are most common in Oriental individuals, usually persisting for life. Figure 5.3 depicts the anatomical differences between eyes with and without epicanthic folds.

The lacrimal apparatus consists of the *lacrimal gland, lacrimal ducts,* and *lacrimal sac.* The lacrimal gland is an almond-size structure located temporally and slightly above the eye. Its function is to secrete tears which flow over the surface of the eyeball and drain through the puncta at the lid margins into the lacrimal ducts and sac.

The *conjunctiva* is a thin transparent membrane which lines each eyelid and the anterior surface of the eye. It is divided into the *bulbar* and the *palpebral* conjunctiva. Where the eyelids meet the eyeball, the conjunctiva bends around to line the inside surface of the eyelids and becomes the palpebral conjunctiva (Fig. 5.1).

The *sclera* and *cornea* compose the fibrous coating of the eyeball. The sclera is the outer protective, supporting layer of the eye. It is the "white" of the eye viewed through the conjunctiva. In front of the eyeball the sclera bulges and changes from a white, opaque membrane to the transparent cornea. Light enters the eye through the cornea.

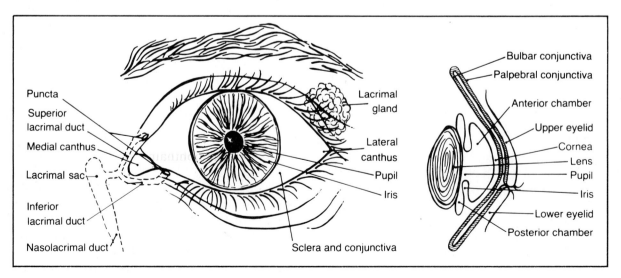

FIGURE 5.1
External structures of the eye.

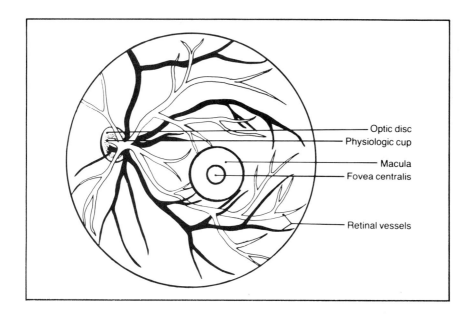

Optic disc
Physiologic cup

Macula
Fovea centralis

Retinal vessels

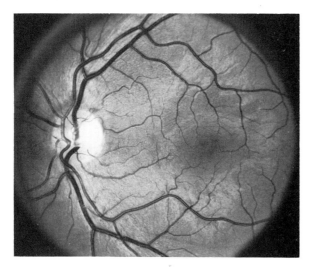

FIGURE 5.2
Fundus of the eye. (Photograph courtesy of Alan Campbell)

The area between the cornea and iris is the *anterior chamber*. It is filled with fluid called the *aqueous humor*. This fluid is drained off into the circulatory system through the *canal of Schlemm*.

The *iris* is a circular muscle that regulates the amount of light entering the eye. The color of the iris varies from person to person, but is usually the same in both eyes. The round hole in the center of the iris is the *pupil*, which allows the entrance of light. Behind the iris and pupil is the crystalline *lens*. This is a transparent structure which bends the rays of light in order to focus an image on the *retina*.

The Fundus of the Eye

The retina is the internal layer of the eye. It is the nervous coat and is only observable with the use of the ophthalmoscope. At the posterior retina the surface shows a slight depression called the *fovea centralis*, which is the region of most acute vision. The area immediately surrounding the fovea centralis is the *macula* (Fig. 5.2). The *optic disc* lies to the nasal side of the macula. The disc is the point of exit for the optic nerve of the eye. The small depression just temporal to the center of the disc is the *physiologic cup* (Fig. 5.2). The disc

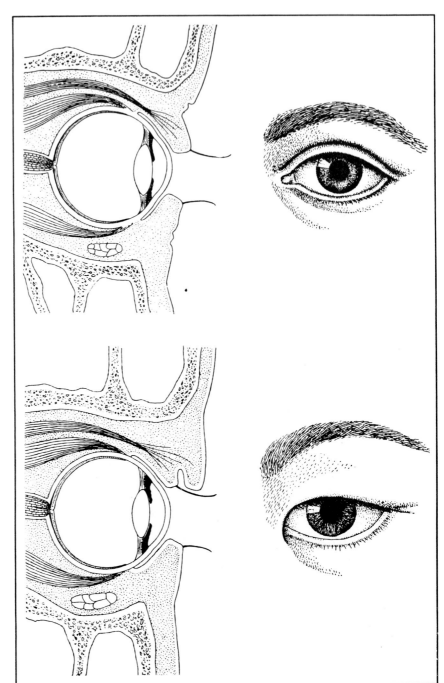

FIGURE 5.3
"Almond" eye of mongoloid races is among latest major human adaptations to environment. The Mongoloid fold, shown in lower drawings, protects the eye against the severe Asian winter. Drawings at top show the Caucasian eye with its single, fatty lid. (From Howells, W. W. The distribution of man. Scientific American, September, 1960, p. 124, with permission.)

has no visual receptors and thus creates a blind spot. The retinal arteries and veins come from the depths of the disc and become smaller as they branch into the periphery of the fundus. The retina lies on the *choroid*, which is the middle layer of the eye. It is a thin, highly vascular membrane.

Visual Pathways

To focus a clear image on the retina, light must first pass through the cornea, anterior chamber, pupil, and lens. Images formed on the retina are upside down and reversed left to right. For example, an object seen in the lower nasal field of vision will form an image on the upper temporal portion of the retina (Fig. 5.4).

The nerve fibers in the retina are preserved in the optic nerves. On entering the cranial cavity the optic nerves unite to form the *optic chiasma,* which are then continued as the *optic tract.* Visual impulses are thus transmitted to the occipital lobe of the cerebral cortex.

The optic nerve fibers from the medial (nasal) halves of the retina cross in the optic chiasma to the opposite side of the brain. The optic nerve fibers from the lateral (temporal) halves remain uncrossed. Therefore, the right optic tract contains fibers only from the left half of each retina. Ultimately, the right occipital lobe receives impulses from the right half of each eye and the left occipital lobe receives impulses from the left half of each eye.

HISTORY

Historical questions are directed by the patient's age and corresponding ophthalmic development to identify visual disturbances. Diseases of a familial nature that affect the ophthalmic system are obtained on all patients regardless of their age.

The Pediatric History

The parent of the infant is asked about the child's ability to fixate on near objects and to follow a moving object. The parents of infants and toddlers are asked if random movement of the eyes (nystagmus) or wandering of the eyes (strabismus) has been noticed. They should also be asked if their toddler has trouble with bumping into objects or holds objects to a very close range. A history is elicited of blinking, squinting, and rubbing the eyes in the toddler and school-age child. Additional symptoms elicited from the school-age-child include headaches, painful eyes, crossed eyes, blurred words when reading, inability to see the blackboard, and double vision. All of these are symptoms of poor visual acuity and warrant further investigation. Problems of a fa-

milial nature include strabismus, cataracts, glaucoma, diabetes, hypertension, and blood dyscrasias.

The Adult History

An overview of the system includes questions regarding changes in visual acuity, blurring of vision, spots before the eyes, lacrimation, photophobia, itching, pain, inflammation, date of the last eye examination, and the use of glasses. Special attention is given to screening for the presence of presbyopia, cataracts, glaucoma, and senile macular degeneration. Middle-age patients are screened for *presbyopia* by asking if they have difficulty discerning objects in the near field of vision. The symptoms of *cataracts,* so common in elderly patients, include blurred and dimmed vision, the need for brighter and brighter light in which to read, and the presence of smoky or cloudy vision. The National Society for the Prevention of Blindness gives the following as danger signals of *glaucoma:*

1. Frequent changes in glasses, none of which are satisfactory.
2. Blurred or foggy vision that clears up for a short period of time.
3. Loss of peripheral vision.
4. Appearance of rainbow-colored rings around lights.
5. Difficulty in adjusting to dark rooms.
6. Difficulty in focusing on close work.

Elderly individuals with *senile macular degeneration* may have a positive history for inability to distinguish what is straight ahead, and difficulty discriminating detail such as fine print.

A family history of glaucoma, cataracts, diabetes, hypertension, and blood dyscrasias is obtained from all adult patients.

PHYSICAL ASSESSMENT

A systematic approach to the examination of the eye includes measuring *visual acuity,* testing *ocular motility,* examining *visual fields,*

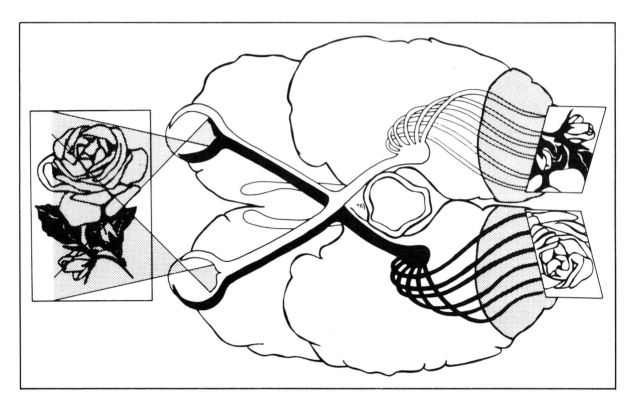

FIGURE 5.4
Left and right visual pathways.

assessing the *external structures* of the eye, *visualizing the fundus,* and *testing for intra-ocular tension.* The equipment needed for this assessment is a Snellen eye chart for near and distant vision, a penlight, an index card (for an eye cover), a wisp of cotton, an ophthalmo-scope and a Schiotz indentation tonometer, for measuring intraocular tension.

Visual Acuity

A good place to begin assessing the eye is by screening for visual impairment. Vision is not very acute at birth, but by 6 weeks visual acu-ity can be estimated by observing the way the infant follows a light. By 2 months the infant should be able to follow the penlight for a few degrees to midline. By 4 months fixation is associated with grasping at the object to bring it to the mouth. Screening for refractive errors is begun about the age of 3 when most children are old enough to cooperate with in-structions necessary to identify pictures on a chart or to use the Snellen *E chart* (Fig. 5.5). Once the child has reached the early school

years refractive errors can be identified by use of the Snellen *alphabet chart* which is used throughout adulthood with patients who are literate (Fig. 5.6).

Adequate vision screening requires that each eye be tested separately and then together first without and then with corrective lenses. A card is used to occlude the eye that is not being tested. The patient is instructed to not push on the card because this pressure on the eye may give a false low acuity if the vision in that eye is assessed immediately after the occluder is removed.

Distant vision is checked on all age groups beginning at the age of 3. *Allen cards* are help-ful with very young children and slow learn-ers. With the client seated and both eyes open, picture cards are shown at a distance of 14 to 20 inches (Sagaties, 1982). The pic-tures most readily recognized are then pre-sented at increasingly greater distances. The greatest distance at which 3 pictures are recog-nized is recorded as the numerator with 30 feet as the denominator (Sagaties, 1982). The child of 3 will usually recognize the pictures at 12 to 15 feet and by 4 years the child will identify pictures at 15 to 20 feet. Findings outside of these norms are considered abnormal.

The Snellen E chart is usually used for 4 to 5 year olds and illiterate adults. By 6 years of age most children can be tested successfully with the *Snellen alphabet chart.* The E chart is placed 20 feet from the patient and he is asked to show with his fingers which way the legs of the E are pointing from the first line down starting from left to right. When the Snellen alphabet chart is used, the patient is asked to identify the letters from the first line down. If a symbol or a letter is missed, the client is asked to repeat the line reading from

right to left. Record on the chart the last line the patient identifies 4 out of 6 symbols or letters. The score is read as a fraction—the numerator is the distance the patient is from the chart and the denominator is the distance the normal eye can read the chart. For example, if the patient's vision is 20/100 he can see at 20 feet away from the chart what a normally sighted person can see at 100 feet away from the chart. The higher the denominator, the greater the vision problem. Generally, if the patient screens 20–40 or worse, a referral is made for follow-up care.

If the patient is unable to read the largest

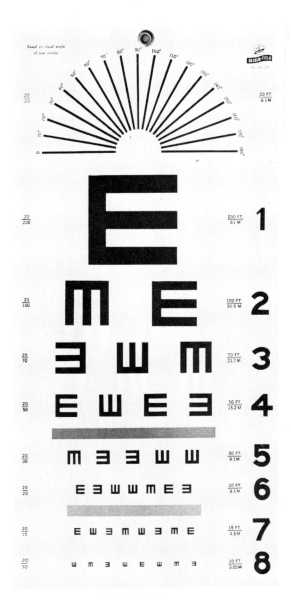

FIGURE 5.5
Snellen E Chart.

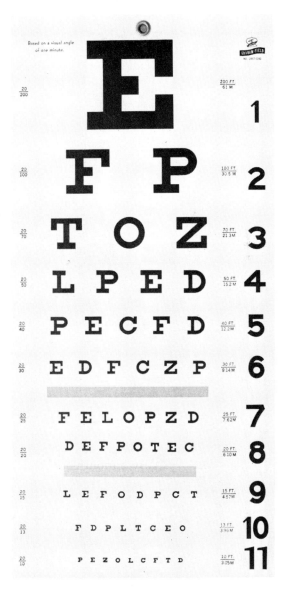

FIGURE 5.6
Snellen Alphabet Chart.

letter on the chart, he should be checked to see if he can count the examiner's fingers. The distance at which the fingers are counted should be measured. When the patient is unable to distinguish finger movement a penlight is directed into his eyes. The eye that cannot distinguish the light is considered totally blind.

Near vision is usually not tested unless the patient has a complaint or is over 40, when presbyopia commonly begins. A gross test of visual impairment can be done by observing the patient read news print. Another test for near visual acuity is the *Snellen pocket screener*. This card is held at a distance of about 14 inches from the eye (Fig. 5.7). The eyes are tested with the glasses on and 3 readings are recorded (right eye, left eye, both eyes together). If the patient is unable to read the largest line the finger test previously described is performed.

The visual acuity test is simple to perform and can detect a variety of problems. In addition to detecting errors of refraction, it tests the function of the second cranial nerve (*optic nerve*).

Ocular Motility

The eyes are assessed for ocular motility which refers to the alignment and coordination of the eyes. *Strabismus,* or faulty alignment of the eyes, must be differentiated from *pseudostrabismus.* Pseudostrabismus results when an epicanthic fold hides a portion of the medial aspect of the eyes, causing the illusion of crossed eyes (Fig. 5.3, p. 122). Pseudostrabismus is a normal finding in the newborn, particularly those of Asian ancestry.

The corneal light reflex test (*Hirschberg's test*) is the test begun in infancy to detect true strabismus. The *cover–uncover test* is an additional method used to evaluate the straightness of the eyes. This test does not become accurate until the infant is 5 months old. Starting at 5 to 6 years through adulthood the *six cardinal positions* of gaze are added as a third measure of ocular movement.

CORNEAL LIGHT REFLEX TEST (*HIRSCHBERG'S TEST*)
The alignment of the eyes is assessed by observing the reflection of light upon the cornea. The examiner darkens the room and has the

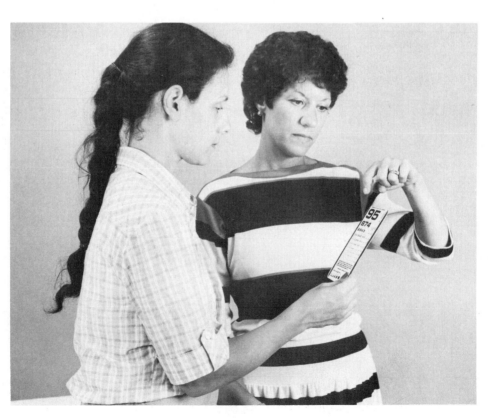

FIGURE 5.7
Near vision testing.

patient look straight ahead as the light from a penlight is directed to the bridge of his nose. Normally the light reflection is symmetrically situated in the same part of the cornea on both eyes (Fig. 5.8). When strabismus is present, the light will be central to the cornea in the fixating eye and either nasal, temporal, superior, or inferior in the deviating eye.

THE COVER–UNCOVER TEST

The cover–uncover test is a sensitive method of determining poor alignment of the eyes. The patient fixes his vision on the tip of a penlight (with the light off) held approximately 5 to 6 inches in front of him. The examiner then covers one of the patient's eyes while observing the uncovered eye (Fig. 5.9A). Nor-

mally the uncovered eye remains stable; if it moves to fix on the penlight, it was not straight before the other eye was covered. After the cover patch is removed, the previously covered eye is observed for movement (Fig. 5.9B). The well-aligned eye will be focused on the penlight. If there is weakness of the muscle, the eye turns out while covered; when the eye is uncovered there is a quick inward movement to bring it back to alignment. Each eye is tested several times to confirm findings.

SIX CARDINAL POSITIONS OF GAZE

Weakness of the extraocular muscles is best detected by moving the eyes through the six cardinal positions of gaze. These positions are used because they specifically identify the de-

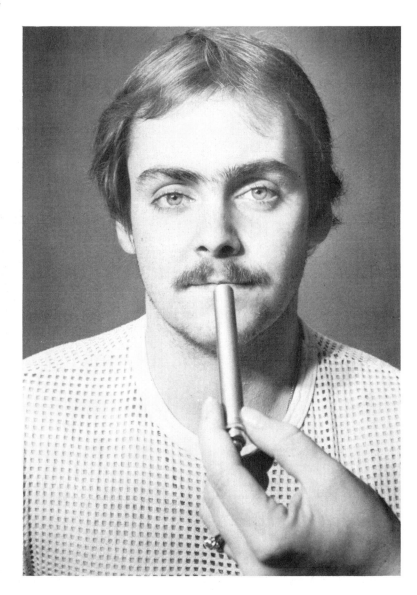

FIGURE 5.8
Corneal light reflex.

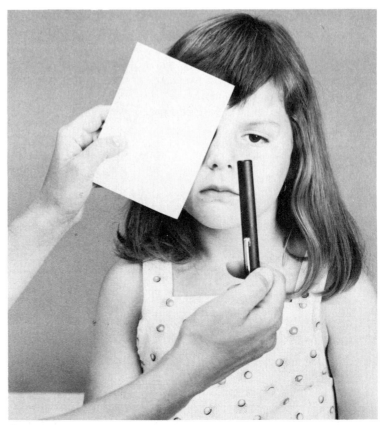

A

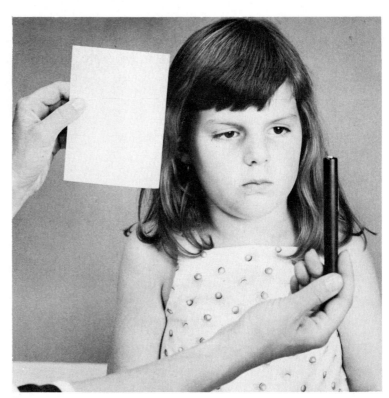

FIGURE 5.9
Cover-uncover test.

B

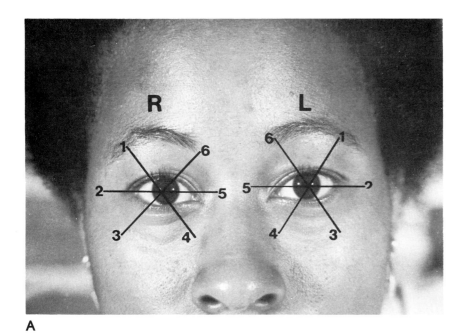

A

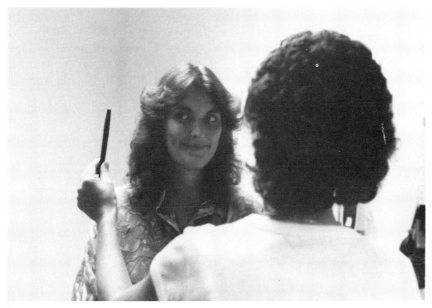

B

FIGURE 5.10
A. Right eye **(R)**. 1. Superior rectus (3rd). 2. Lateral rectus (6th). 3. Inferior rectus (3rd). 4. Superior oblique (3rd). 5. Medial rectus (3rd). 6. Inferior oblique (4th). Left eye **(L)**. 1. Superior rectus (3rd). 2. Lateral rectus (6th). 3. Inferior rectus (3rd). 4. Superior oblique (4th). 5. Medial rectus (3rd). 6. Inferior oblique (3rd). **B.** Testing the cardinal fields of gaze.

bilitated muscle if the eye does not return to position. In addition, the six cardinal fields of gaze test the function of the III (*oculomotor*), IV (*trochlear*), and VI (*abducens*) cranial nerves (Fig. 5.10A).

The patient is positioned directly in front of the examiner, holding his head in a fixed position. He follows the tip of the examiner's penlight (with the light off) with his eyes only. The penlight is held a comfortable distance in front of the patient and the eyes are checked using the six cardinal fields of gaze in a slow, orderly manner.

The patient is asked to gaze briefly at the extreme point of each movement. (Fig. 5.10B). Normally the eyes remain steady at the extreme points. Nystagmus is an uncontrolled and rhythmic movement of the eyes. A few beats of nystagmus on extreme lateral gaze, called *end-position nystagmus*, is a normal finding demonstrated in many patients. Infants up to 3 months of age may have intermittent periods of nystagmus. If any other nystagmus is observed, further investigation and referral are needed. Nystagmus can result from vestibular, neurologic, or ocular dysfunction. Occasionally change occurs in upward gaze among the elderly as a result of atrophy of the elevator muscle due to disease (Yurick, 1981). The penlight is raised above the patient's head and he follows it down below his chin. This is a check for lid lag which tests the function of the *third cranial nerve.*

Visual Fields

Examination of the visual fields, a test of the second cranial nerve (optic), measures the function of the visual pathways. The exam provides a measurement of the retina's ability to receive peripheral stimuli. Assessment of peripheral vision is significant in detecting the insiduous onset of glaucoma. Therefore, it is not usually included in a screening exam until the patient is at least 40. Confrontation testing provides a rough estimate of the visual fields.

The examiner is the control of confrontation testing, and it is assumed that she has good visual fields. The patient and the examiner face one another approximately 2 feet apart, situated at the same level. The patient is asked to cover one eye with a card and to look directly at the bridge of the examiner's nose. The examiner covers her own eye as the control—she covers her right eye, for example, when the patient covers his left eye—and she looks directly at the bridge of the patient's nose. The examiner tests the nasal, temporal, upward, and downward fields by bringing into vision from various points in the periphery a small object or constantly moving finger (Fig. 5.11).

The *nasal fields* are medial to each eye and the *temporal fields* are lateral to each eye. When examining the nasal field of the patient's left eye the examiner extends her left arm for testing. When examining the temporal fields of the patient's left eye the examiner extends her right arm. This avoids having the examiner bring her arm across the field of vision. The pattern is reversed for the right eye. The

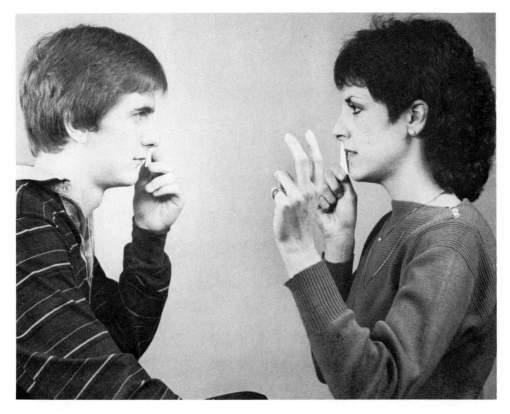

FIGURE 5.11
Testing the right nasal field of vision. (Temporal, upward and downward fields not shown.)

patient tells the examiner when the moving object comes into his peripheral vision. The object should be equidistant from the examiner and the patient so that both see it at the same time. An exception is encountered when examining the temporal field, in which case it is difficult to bring the object far enough peripherally so that it is out of the patient's field of vision. In this case, the examiner should start with the object behind the patient at a point where the examiner is able to see the object. Normally, the visual fields have a full range of vision, without any obvious blind spots.

Confrontation testing does not detect small lesions or early changes in the visual pathways. If the patient complains of decreased peripheral vision, he must be referred for more sophisticated screening. Accurate measurements can be made with the use of the *tangent screen* or *perimeter*.

External Examination of the Eye

A systematic approach to examining the external eye is essential or findings will be missed. A sound knowledge of anatomy is necessary as the examiner moves from the outer structures of the eye to the inner portions. The external structures are assessed in the following order: the *eyebrows, eyelashes* and *eyelids;* the *lacrimal apparatus;* the *orbit;* the *conjunctiva* and *sclera;* the *cornea* and *anterior chamber;* and the *iris* and *pupil.* The techniques of examination include inspection and palpation.

EYEBROWS, EYELASHES AND EYELIDS

The examiner should stand directly in front of the patient to inspect the eyebrows, eyelashes, and eyelids. The eyebrows and eyelashes are inspected for presence, color, condition, and position. Normally, the eyelashes are evenly distributed and curve outward. The eyebrows and eyelids around the eyelashes are a common site for lice.

The eyelids are examined for position, color, edema, signs of infection, and ability to close. Two positional findings to observe for, especially in infants and young children, are *ptosis* and *epiblepharon folds.* Drooping of the eyelid, ptosis, can result from a variety of causes, including congenital underdevelopment of the lid muscle, birth trauma, inflammatory edema, or early impairment of the

third cranial nerve. An epiblepharon or Mongolian fold is a horizontal skin fold in the upper eye and may indicate Down's syndrome or other pathology. This is not to be confused with the vertical epicanthal folds normally occurring in Asian individuals (see Fig. 5.3, p. 122).

Faulty positioning of the eyelids is a common problem in the elderly due to progressive relaxation of the lid muscles. *Ectropion* is an outturning of the lid due to loss of firmness and elasticity of the lid connective tissue. If the lower lid is involved it will droop. This can cause chronic conjunctivitis or a problem with overflow of tears, since it interferes with normal tear drainage. Inversion of the lid so that the eyelashes are in contact with the conjunctiva is called *entropion.* This can lead to corneal irritations due to the lower lashes rubbing on the cornea. Entropion is a common condition among Orientals, regardless of age, and is harmless unless it causes a corneal abrasion.

The eyelids are inspected closely for any color changes. Slightly raised, yellowish plaques observed along the nasal portions of one or both eyelids may indicate a lipid disorder, but plaques can also occur in healthy individuals. This condition is called *xanthelasma.* Edema of the eyelids may point to either trauma, systemic disease, or local disease. Frequently the eyes of the newborn are edematous from the labor and delivery. Some of the causes for edema in children and adults are nephrosis, heart failure, thyroid deficiency, allergy, or an infectious process of the area of the eyelid.

The eyelids can be the site of infection. Oily, scaly lid margins are often associated with *seborrheic blepharitis* which is chronic inflammation of the eyelids. Redness, swelling, and tenderness of the lid margin are typical signs of a *hordeolum.* This is an infection of the hair follicles and glands of the anterior lid margin, usually due to staphylococcus.

If a problem is observed on inspection of the lid or if the history indicates, the lids are palpated. Before beginning palpation of the eyelid, the examiner should be sure that her fingernails are short. The patient should remove his contact lens to prevent injury to the eye. The examiner first places her index finger at the inner canthus of the eye. Using gentle palpation she slides the examining finger across the closed lid, noting any raised areas. A chalazion is a commonly found raised area the eyelid. This is an infection or retention cyst of meibomian glands within the tarsus plate of the eyelid. The cause is unknown.

THE LACRIMAL APPARATUS

The lacrimal gland is inspected for edema and gently palpated (Fig. 5.12A). Normally this gland is not felt. Next, the lacrimal apparatus is inspected between the lower eyelid and the nose for edema and for evidence of increased tearing. These findings indicate blockage of the nasolacrimal duct. *Dacryostenosis* is relatively common in newborns and is caused by a congenital failure of the canalization of the duct. Stenosis of the puncta does occur in some elderly individuals and can interfere with the passageway of tears. The spilling of tears into the lower eyelids can cause reddening and irritation. As individuals age, the tissue laxity of the lids impairs the drainage of the lacrimal sac. A compensatory response to this process is the decreased tear production in the aged. *Dacryocystitis* is secondary to dacryostenosis and occurs because the collection of mucus and tears in the duct causes a bacterial infection. Symptoms include excessive tearing and purulent discharge.

Should the passage of tears from the nasolacrimal duct to the nose be obstructed, finger pressure on the lacrimal sac will cause regurgitation of fluid. The finger tip is placed inside the lower inner orbital rim, not on the side of the nose (Fig. 5.12B). Pressure is applied and the finger is moved inferiorly to observe for fluid.

THE ORBIT

The orbit is first inspected and then palpated. A sunken appearance to the eye is called *endothalmos* and is seen in the malnourished or dehydrated person, or the elderly person with decreased orbital fat. *Exophthalmos*, the outward bulging of the eyeball, is frequently associated with thyroid disease. Normally the lids are positioned so no sclera is visible above the corneas. The outward bulging of the eye will reveal the sclera.

Palpation of the orbit is a gross test of intraocular pressure (Fig. 5.13). The patient is asked to remove his contact lens and look down as the examiner places the tips of both index fingers on the upper lid over the sclera (not over the cornea). Pressure is applied with one finger, pushing the eyeball into the intra-orbital region. The finger is quickly removed as the opposite finger palpates the rebound of the depressed eyeball. A spongy, soft consistency indicates decreased tension, as in dehydration. A hard consistency of the eyeball is indicative of increased intraocular tension, as in glaucoma.

CONJUNCTIVA AND SCLERA

The conjunctiva consists of two components, the bulbar conjunctiva and the palpebral conjunctiva. To separate the lids so that the bulbar conjunctiva can be inspected, the examiner places her thumbs on the patient's lower orbital rims. (Fig. 5.14). The eye should never be pressed when separating the lids. The patient is instructed to look up, and to both sides. Next, the examiner places her thumbs on the patient's upper orbits and asks him to look down and to both sides. Except for a few capillaries, one should see the white of the sclera coming through the transparent conjunctiva.

The sclera may be jaundiced, indicating a liver problem, or excessively pale, as in anemia. In the complexion of blacks, changes that are hard to detect may be initially observed in the eye. The nurse should be aware that many blacks, however, normally have a yellowish discoloration in the subconjunctival fat and sclera which could mislead the nurse into thinking that they are jaundiced. In this case the hard palate should also be assessed for color changes. In the elderly person, the sclera may appear yellow as a result of fat deposits in the subconjunctival layers (Yurick, 1981). The sclera also offers an excellent site for detecting petechiae.

Inflammation of the conjunctiva is called *conjunctivitis*. The signs of conjunctivitis include redness of the conjunctiva, tearing, mucopurulent discharge, and crusting and matting of the eyes. *Ophthalmia neonatorum* refers to bilateral purulent discharge during the first 24 hours of life. The most common cause is the chemical irritation of 1 percent silver nitrate used in the prophylactic treatment against gonococcal infections (Jones & Tippett, 1980). A plugged tear duct can also cause conjunctivitis at birth. Usually external massage works out the plugged duct. Conjunctivitis that occurs 2 or 3 days after birth is usually bacterial. Causes of conjunctivitis in

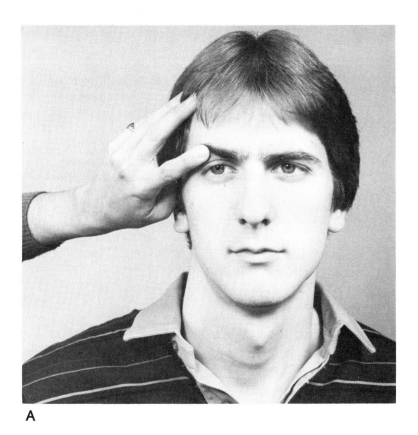

A

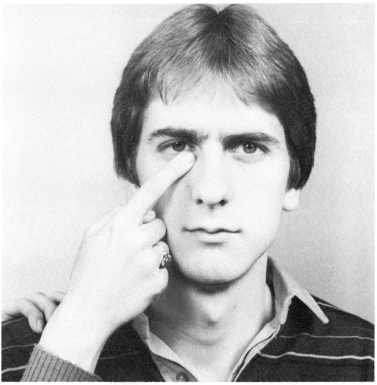

B

FIGURE 5.12
A. Palpating the lacrimal gland. *B.* Palpating the lacrimal duct.

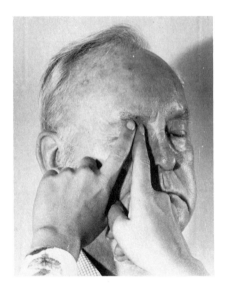

FIGURE 5.13
Palpating for intraocular pressure.

older children and adults are most commonly viral, bacterial, or allergic in origin.

Examination of the palpebral conjunctiva is a difficult skill and is done only if a problem is indicated, such as the presence of a foreign body. This exam involves eversion of the upper lid. The patient is instructed to look down as the examiner grasps the eyelashes between her thumb and index finger and pulls downward and forward (Fig. 5.15A). The upper border of the lid is pushed down with a small cotton swab which everts the eyelid (Fig. 5.15B). When the lid is everted, the swab is removed and the lashes are held to the brow by the examiner's finger so that the palpebral conjunctiva is visualized. To return the lid to place, the upper eyelashes are grasped and pulled gently forward.

THE CORNEA AND ANTERIOR CHAMBER
A thin grayish white ring at the margin of the cornea may be observed when facing the patient. This is called *arcus senilis.* It is a normal finding in elderly patients and is caused by deposits of lipids around the periphery of the cornea. This finding is abnormal in young adults.

The cornea is carefully inspected for signs of *abrasions* and *opacities.* Standing to the temporal (lateral) side of the patient the examiner directs the light of the penlight laterally

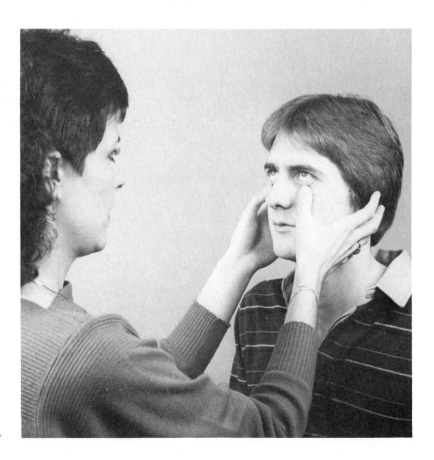

FIGURE 5.14
Assessment of the bulbar conjunctiva.

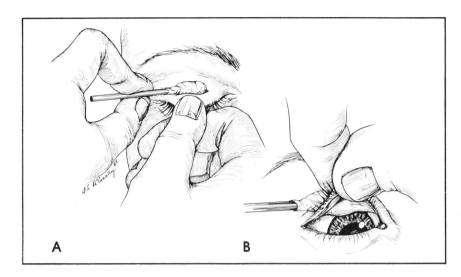

FIGURE 5.15
Assessment of the palpebral conjunctiva. **A.** *Grasping the eyelashes to pull the eyelid downward and forward.* **B.** *Eversion of the eyelid.*

onto the surface of the cornea (Fig. 5.16). Normally the cornea is smooth and transparent; irregularities are detected by noting defects appearing in the light reflections of the normal surface. *Nebulae* (a slight corneal opacity) and small *corneal ulcers* are common in the elderly patient and should not be overlooked.

The anterior chamber is the area of the eye immediately behind the cornea and in front of the iris. In all adults this chamber is inspected for its depth. At the same time that the cornea is being observed with the light from the temporal side, the underlying anterior chamber is examined (Fig. 5.16). Normally no shadows of light will be observed on the iris and both temporal and nasal halves will be flat and illuminated. Illumination will cast a crescent-shaped shadow on the far side of the iris (nasal ward) if the iris is anteriorly displaced. This is due to the bowing forward

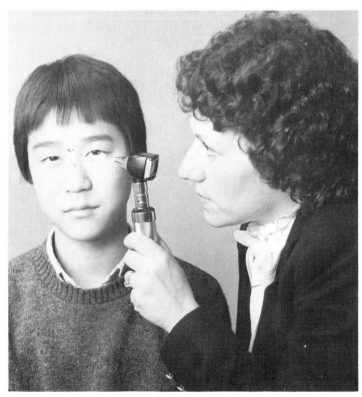

FIGURE 5.16
Assessment of the cornea and anterior chamber.

of the iris with only the temporal half becoming illuminated, the nasal half will be in a shadow. This indicates a shallow anterior chamber and a predisposition to glaucoma.

Corneal sensitivity (cranial nerve V, Trigeminal) is tested by touching a wisp of cotton to the cornea and observing the quick blink of the lid. This test is not routinely done in children because it can be frightening. As the patient is instructed to look straight ahead the examiner brings the wisp of cotton in from behind him when he is unaware. If he blinks after the cornea is touched, one can assume the fifth cranial nerve is intact. Sensitivity of the cornea decreases with age.

THE PUPILS AND IRIS

The pupils and iris are assessed together. The pupils are examined for color, shape, equality, reaction to light, and accommodation. The pupils are normally black in color, round, and equal. If the pupil appears cloudy or discolored, the probable cause is a cataract.

The health of the iris is determined by noting the regularity of the pupil. *Miosis* is constriction of the pupil which can result from drugs such as morphine or pilocarpine (used in patients with glaucoma) or from inflamma-

tion of the iris. *Iritis* is inflammation of the iris caused by local or systemic infections. An irregular, constricted appearance to the pupil results from the edema associated with iritis. Miosis also occurs normally during sleep. *Mydriasis* is enlargement of the pupils, which can be caused by injury, glaucoma, systemic poison, or dilating drops. Miosis and mydriasis occur normally in accommodation to light changes. Approximately 5 percent of the population have nonpathologic unequal pupils, or *anisocoria*. The examiner should, however, be aware that anisocoria can be a result of various central nervous system disorders.

The *pupillary reflexes* include the direct *reaction to light*, the *consensual reaction to light*, and the *reaction to accommodation*. These reflexes are a test of the function of the *third cranial nerve (oculomotor)*. To test the *direct* and *consensual pupillary reactions*, the patient is asked to focus his gaze on the bridge of the examiner's nose. The examiner brings a light in from the temporal side, directing it on the pupil. The pupil receiving increased illumination constricts directly (Fig. 5.17). The light is removed and brought in again so the examiner can observe the reaction in the opposite eye which should *react consensually*

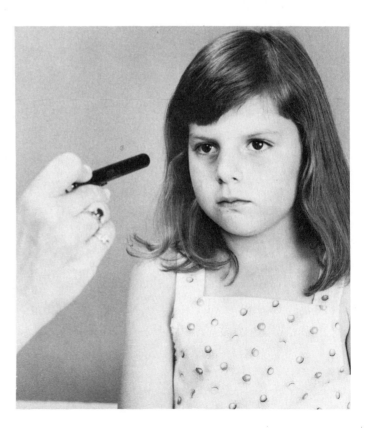

FIGURE 5.17
Assessment of direct and consensual response to light.

by constricting. In monocular blindness, the blind eye will not react directly to illumination and the opposite eye will not react consensually. If the good eye is illuminated, it will react directly and the blind eye consensually.

To *test for accommodation,* the examiner holds a penlight about 4 inches from the bridge of the patient's nose. The patient is asked to look alternately at the top of the penlight and at the far wall directly behind the penlight. The examiner brings the penlight in toward the patient's nose to test for convergence (Fig. 5.18). The examiner observes for pupillary constriction when the patient is looking at the top of the penlight, dilation when the patient is looking at the wall, and convergence of the patient's eyes as the penlight is brought toward the nose. *Argyl Robinson's pupil* is a failure to react to light with preservation of convergence. This is indicative of central nervous system syphilis.

Ophthalmoscopic Examination

That portion of the eye posterior to the lens which is observed through the pupil is called the fundus of the eye. The fundus includes the *retina, choroid, fovea, macula, disc,* and *retinal vessels* (see Fig. 5.2, p. 121). These structures are inspected with the use of an ophthalmoscope.

It takes a lot of time and practice to become proficient in observing the fundus. The purpose here is to explain the technique of using the ophthalmoscope and to describe the normal fundus. The nurse is expected to become familiar with normal findings and to be able to adequately describe abnormal findings.

The ophthalmoscope head consists of the *viewing aperture,* the *aperture selection dial,* the *lens selector dial,* and the *lens indicator* (Fig. 5.19). The lens selector dial is rotated to bring the fundus of the eye into view. The dial rotates through a series of marked numbers called *diopters.* The black numbers have a positive value and the red numbers have a negative value. For clear visualization in the farsighted patient the black diopters are used. For the nearsighted patient the ophthalmoscope will need to be moved into the minus or red diopters.

There are five different viewing apertures on the ophthalmoscope. The small aperture is used for undilated pupils and the large aperture is used for dilated pupils. The green beam is used to examine the optic disc for hemorrhages. The grid is used to locate and measure

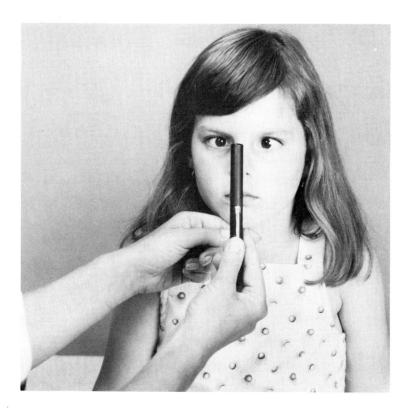

FIGURE 5.18
Assessment of convergence.

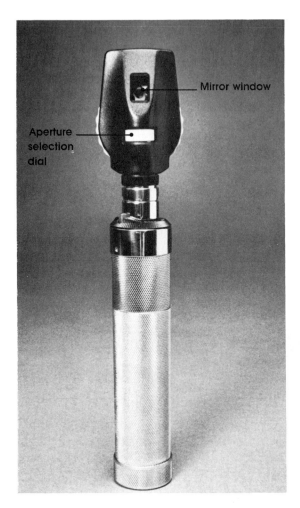
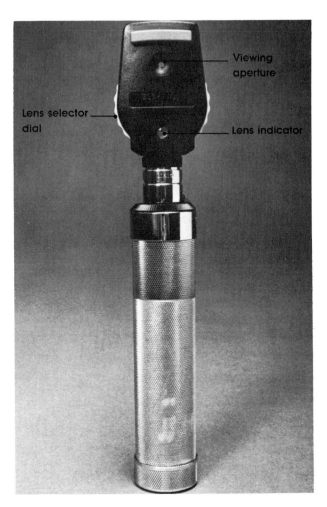

FIGURE 5.19
Left. *Front view of the ophthalmoscope.* **Right.** *Back view of the ophthalmoscope.*

findings. The slit light is used to examine the eye for levels of a lesion. For screening purposes the small and large apertures are the only ones used. The examiner selects the appropriate viewing aperture on the ophthalmoscope by rotating the aperture selection dial and flashing the lights on her hand to determine the proper light source.

To adequately inspect the fundus, the room should be darkened so the pupils dilate. It is easier to examine the eye if the patient takes off his glasses; contact lenses may be left in. The examiner usually keeps her contacts in and may or may not choose to wear glasses. To prevent the eye from moving around during the examination, the patient is instructed to focus in on a specific point on the wall behind the examiner. The viewing aperture is selected and the lens dial is set at +8 to +10 diopters indicated by black num-

bers. This will allow visualization of the structures in front of the fundus as the examiner moves in toward the fundus.

To examine the patient's right eye the examiner takes the ophthalmoscope in her right hand and puts it comfortably to her right eye keeping both eyes open while examining the eye (Fig. 5.20). The examiner's right index finger should rest on the diopter control; her left hand is placed on the patient's head for stabilization. This procedure is reversed for the patient's left eye. The examiner should become proficient with both her right and left eye and her right and left hand when examining the eye. The examiner stands approximately 15 inches from the patient and about 15 degrees lateral and shines the light on the patient's pupil.

An orange glow is observed in the pupil called the *red reflex.* The color of the normal

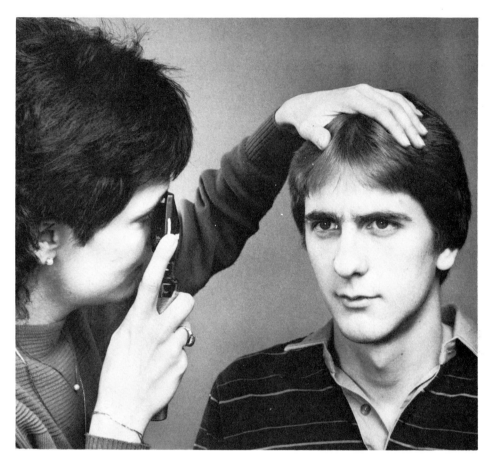

FIGURE 5.20
Ophthalmoscopic examination.

fundus ranges from orange to vermilion. With darker skin colors, the fundus may be brown or purplish (Wasserman, 1974). Any opacities suggest cataracts. The opacities can vary from a pin point to the size of the entire lense. Observation of the red reflex to rule out the presence of a cataract is the only portion of the funduscopic examination that is done on infants and small children. The complete funduscopic examination is done on all children who are old enough to cooperate by holding their eyes on a distant object (Chow, et al., 1984).

As the examiner moves closer to the patient, the dial is moved to successively lower numbers, and possibly into the red numbers, to focus on the retina. Next, the examiner identifies a retinal vessel and follows it toward the nose to focus on the optic disc and cup. In the periphery the vessels are narrow, becoming progressively wider as they reach the optic disc. The order of observation in the examina-

tion is as follows: the *optic disc* and *cup*, the *retinal blood vessels and periphery*, and the *macula*.

THE OPTIC DISC AND CUP

The optic disc is evaluated for color, shape size, margins, and its physiologic cup. The disc is a yellowish pink, round structure. The margins of the disc are more or less regular, frequently with scattered pigment overlying the margins (*pigment crescents*). The margins may be surrounded by a white ring called the *scleral crescent.* Occurring more often in blacks than Caucasians, both of these are normal findings. Just temporal of the center of the disc, the physiologic depression (or cup) is noted. It may be quite large, but normally it never extends completely to the disc margin.

Three serious problems to look for when examining the disc are *papilledema, optic atrophy,* and *glaucoma. Papilledema* (Fig. 5. 21) is edema of the optic disc and thickening of

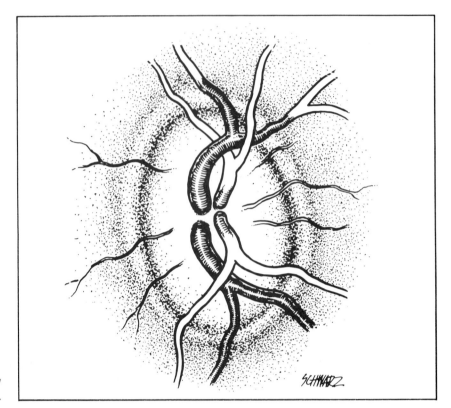

FIGURE 5.21
Papilledema.

the retinal vessels due to increased intracranial pressure. Blurring of the disc margins, elevation of the disc surface and curving downward of the vessels over the borders are signs of this condition.

Optic atrophy results from death of the optic nerve (Fig. 5.22). With the death of the nerve fibers the tiny disc vessels disappear. This results in paleness of the disc. When there is a question of the presence of optic atrophy,

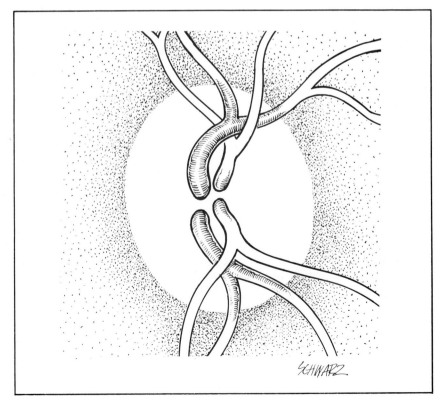

FIGURE 5.22
Optic atrophy.

eyes should be compared

the eyes should be compared. Normally the two discs appear similar. This problem can destroy sight.

Glaucoma results from increased intra-ocular pressure which almost pushes the optic disc backward out of the eye (Fig. 5.23). The nurse will observe a retinal vessel which may disappear at the disc edge and then reappear in the depths of the cup. The disc appears pale due to optic atrophy.

Everything within the fundus is measured in terms of disc diameters (DD). For example, a finding seen in the fundus could be described as 2 DD away from the disc at 6 o'clock.

THE RETINAL VESSELS AND PERIPHERY

In the depths of the disc the central artery and vein will appear. Assessment of the retinal vessels is useful with patients who have hypertension, arteriosclerosis, and diabetes. The retinal vessels are examined for size, color, and arteriovenous crossings. *Arterioles* are normally two-thirds to four-fifths the diameter of veins. A narrow band of light, the arteriolar light reflex, is reflected from the center of the arteries. Normally this light reflex is about one quarter the diameter of the blood column. With hypertension there is a narrowing of the arteriolar blood column and the light reflex. Eventually with hypertension there is a thickening of the vessel wall so that the wall is less transparent. This causes changes of the blood in the vessel, giving it a copper color.

Normal *veins* are darker in color than arterioles and do not have a prominent light reflex. A vein crossing beneath the arteriole can be seen up to the column of blood on either side because of the transparent arteriolar wall. Arterioles and veins may cross and entwine each other, but normal arterioles do not indent or displace veins. Thickening of the arteriolar wall can produce visible changes at the arteriovenous crossing. One change is that the vein appears to stop on either side of the arteriole. This is referred to as *arteriovenous (A–V) nicking* (Fig. 5.24). Occasionally, as a result of arteriolar thickening, the vein appears to taper down on either side of the arteriole.

The blood vessels are followed peripherally in each of four directions. The periphery is an orange color, but is lighter in fair people and darker in black people. It is explored for *hemorrhages, exudates,* and *microaneurysms* (Fig. 5.25). Hemorrhages are typically red or dark in color and are obvious signs of disease.

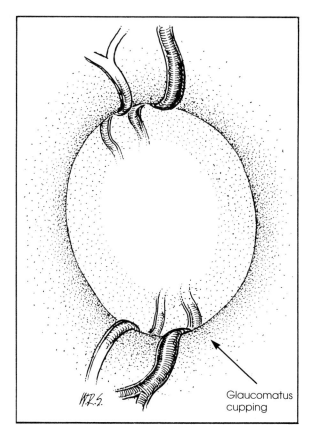

FIGURE 5.23
Glaucomatous cupping.

Hemorrhages are described in terms of location, size, shape, relationship to retinal vessels, and color. Hemorrhages can be *intraretinal* or *superficial.*

Intraretinal hemorrhages are characteristically small. *Deep intraretinal hemorrhages,* commonly found in diabetes, are small irregularly round red spots. *Flame shaped* or *linear red spots* are intraretinal hemorrhages in the nerve fiber. These hemorrhages are commonly found in hypertension.

Superficial hemorrhages are generally large. The three types of superficial hemorrhages are *preretinal, subretinal,* and *choroidal. Preretinal hemorrhages* are located anterior to the retinal vessels therefore they conceal retinal vessels. Characteristically they have a clearly defined horizontal line separating the red cells from the plasma. They are found in blood dyscrasias and subarachnoid hemorrhages. *Subretinal* and *choroidal* hemorrhages are found in senile macular degeneration. Subretinal hemorrhages appear red, but choroidal hemorrhages appear gray or black

142

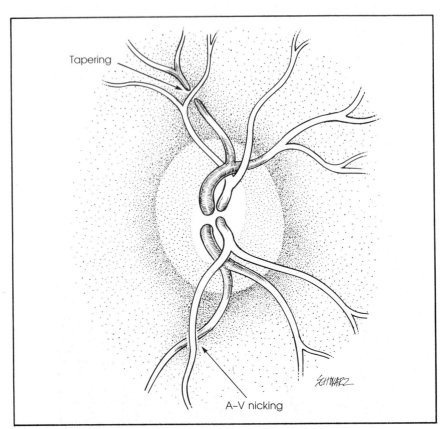

FIGURE 5.24
Arteriovenous (A–V) nicking and tapering.

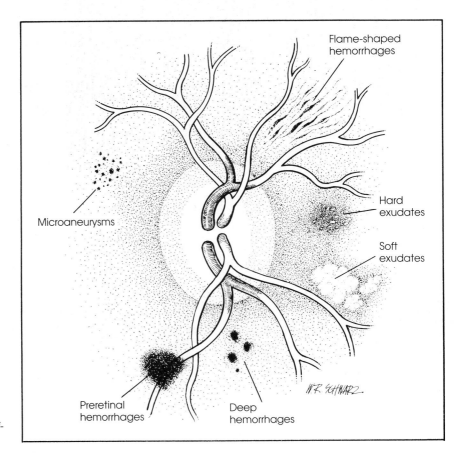

FIGURE 5.25
Retinal background abnormalities.

because they are located deep in the retinal pigment layer.

Exudates are residues of edema and blood substances which are incompletely absorbed due to poor retinal circulation. They can be either soft or hard. *Hard exudates* are arteriolar microinfarctions. These exudates are yellow, small, round spots with well defined borders. They may coalesce into large irregular spots. *Soft exudates* occur in areas of stasis, for example they may accompany venous microinfarction. They are fuzzy, white patches with no definite pattern. Exudates should alert the examiner to explore for the presence of chronic diseases such as diabetes and hypertension. Exudates are described in terms of size, shape, color, and location.

Microaneurysms are tiny, discrete red dots that are commonly concentrated near the macula. They are found in diabetic retinopathy.

THE MACULAR AREA

Last of all, the macular area is examined. This is the sensitive area of vision, and examination requires focusing the light directly on it. This is uncomfortable for the patient, therefore the area can be examined for only a few seconds.

The macula is located approximately 2 DD away from the disc temporally. It is a small circular structure, 1 DD in size. The minute glistening spot of reflected light seen in the center of the macula is a fovea centralis. Macular lesions, including edema, hemorrhages, and exudates, appear much the same as they do throughout the fundus. *Senile macular lesions* appear as small areas of black pigmentation in and around the macula (Fig. 5.26). The degree of pigmentation identified on examination and the patient's actual visual impairment may not correlate. A comparatively small lesion on the macula can seriously interfere with vision, while a large peripheral lesion may cause no disturbance to the patient.

Tonometry Testing

Tonometry is the procedure used in measuring the intraocular pressure, or tension, of the eye. The *Schiotz indentation tonometer* is a tiny, portable tool that is easy to use (Fig. 5.27). Applanation tonometry is a more sensitive measure, but it is more complex and expensive. The Schiotz indentation tonometer consists of a footplate curved to fit the cornea

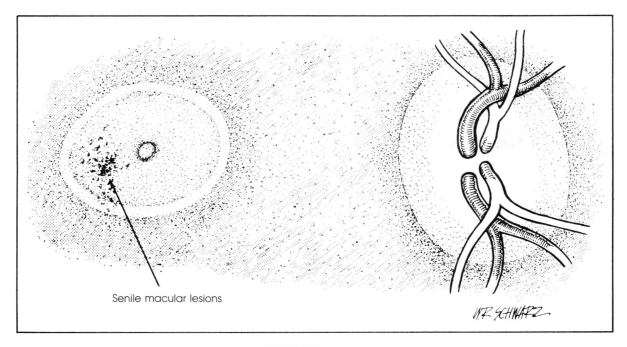

Senile macular lesions

FIGURE 5.26
Senile macular lesions.

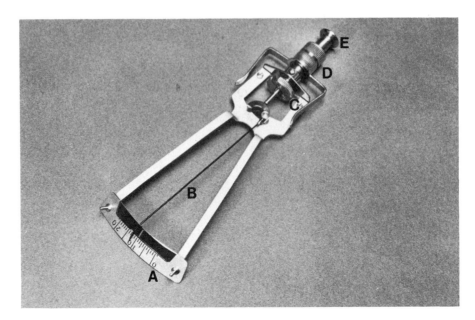

FIGURE 5.27
Schiotz indentation tonometer. **A.** Scale. **B.** Indicator. **C.** Weight. **D.** Plunger assembly. **E.** Footplate.

and a plunger assembly in the center for holding weights. On top of the plunger is a short curved arm with a lever whose larger arm is a pointer for the scale on top of the instrument (Bates, 1982). The pointer rests on 0 when the footplate and the plunger fit flush. As the tonometer indents the cornea, the intraocular pressure is read off the scale. The instrument is not accurate below 3 on the scale, therefore if a 3 reading is obtained the next higher weight must be used. The scale reading is translated to a pressure estimate in mm Hg.

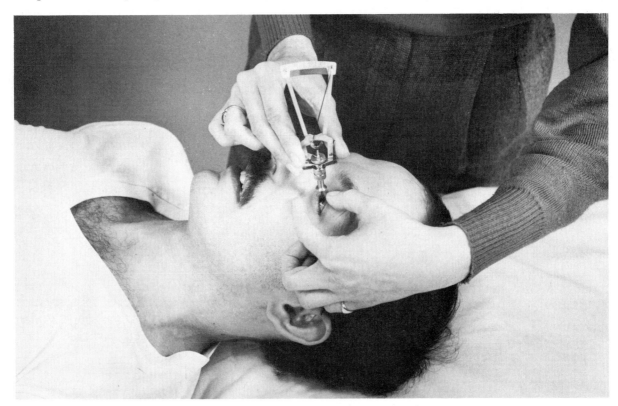

FIGURE 5.28
Screening for increased intraocular pressure.

Normal pressures with the Schiotz are from 10.5 to 20.5 mm Hg.

Prior to beginning the procedure the patient is put in a supine position and a topical anesthetic is applied. He is then asked to fixate on a point directly upward (Fig. 5.28). The examiner retracts the eyelids with one hand and applies the tonometer to the cornea with the other. When retracting the eyelids, care is taken to apply pressure only to the orbital rims. Pressure to the orbit will give a falsely high reading (Rodman, 1984).

If an abnormal reading is obtained, the patient should be referred to an ophthalmologist for more sophisticated testing. Confrontation testing and palpation for intraocular pressure, along with tonometry testing, should be done routinely as a part of every general physical examination on all patients over 40. These 3 measures all screen for presence of glaucoma.

Screening Examination of the Eye

The screening examination of the eyes for infants and toddlers includes:

1. Inspection of the external structures of the eye
   a. Lids
   b. Lashes
   c. Conjunctiva
   d. Sclera
2. Corneal light reflex
3. Pupillary response to light
4. Identification of the red reflex with the ophthalmoscope.

The screening examination of the eyes from childhood through adulthood includes:

1. Near vision (40 years of age and over)
2. Distant vision
3. Inspection of the external structures of the eye
   a. Lids
   b. Lashes
   c. Conjunctiva
   d. Sclera
   e. Cornea
   f. Anterior chamber
4. Pupillary response to light
5. Accommodation
6. Convergence
7. Corneal light reflex
8. Cover–uncover test
9. Six cardinal fields of gaze
10. Palpation of the orbit (40 years of age and over)
11. Confrontation testing (40 years of age and over)
12. Complete funduscopic examination with the ophthalmoscope
13. Tonometry testing (40 years of age and over)

EXAMPLE OF A RECORDED HISTORY AND PHYSICAL

SUBJECTIVE:

Chief Complaint: "Tearing from the right eye began yesterday."

HPH: This 9-month-old white female has been seen regularly for well baby examinations and has been without problems. Yesterday the child's mother noticed that she was rubbing her right eye. Her mother attributed this to the fact that the child had just awakened from a short nap. This morning, when the child awoke, the eye was matted together with a "green, crusty" substance. Her mother cleaned it with clear water and then noticed that the eye was reddened and tearing. The left eye has been clear. The child has had no fever, lethargy, apparent light sensitivity, irritability, runny nose, cough, or exposure to irritants. No one else in the family is experiencing these symptoms. Her father has a history of allergy to ragweed and cats. She has no known allergies.

OBJECTIVE:

T. 99.2°F rectally.

Eyes:

- Lids: Right—tearing, green crusting on lower lid; no edema; left—no tearing, crustation, or edema.
- Conjunctiva: Right—erythematous; left—no erythema.
- Cornea: No clouding, enlargement, or irritation, bilaterally.
- Sclera: White, bilaterally.
- Pupil: Pupils equally round and react to light (PERRLA), bilaterally.
- Alignment: Light reflex equal, bilaterally.
- Iris: Brown, round, bilaterally.
- Lens: No clouding, bilaterally.
- Lacrimal apparatus: No discharge from the inner canthus, no swelling of the lacrimal glands, bilaterally.
- Funduscopic examination: Red light reflex present, bilaterally.

Ears: Canals clear; tympanic membranes pearly gray, landmarks present, bilaterally.

Oral Cavity: Tonsils not enlarged, pharynx without redness or exudate.

Chest: No adventitious breath sounds.

REFERENCES

Bates, S. (1982). Fundamentals for Assessing Primary Care Optometry. Chicago: The Professional Press.

Breslow, L, & Somers, A. (1979). Lifetime health monitoring program. Nurse Practitioner, 4(3), 40, 50, 54–55.

Chow, M., Durand, B., Feldman, M., & Mills, M. (1984). Handbook of Pediatric Primary Care (2nd ed.). New York: John Wiley & Sons.

Havener, W. (1984). Synopsis of Ophthalmology (6th ed.). St. Louis: C. V. Mosby.

Ing, M., & Pang, S. (1973). The racial distribution of strabismus. Hawaii Medical Journal, 32, 22–23.

Jones, M., & Tippett, T. (1980). Assessing the red eye. Nurse Practitioner, 5(1), 10–15.

Kart, C., Metress, E., & Metress, J. (1978). Aging and Health. Menlo Park, Calif.: Addison-Wesley.

Resler, M., & Tumulty, G. (1983). Glaucoma update. American Journal of Nursing, 83, 752–56.

Rodman, W. (1984). Glaucoma screening by the primary care physician. Postgraduate Medicine, 76(1), 224–30.

Sagaties, M. (1982). Screening for strabismus and amblyopia. Nurse Practitioner, 7(4), 19–23.

Wasserman, H. (1974). Ethnic Pigmentation: Historical, Physiological and Clinical Aspects. Amsterdam: Excerpta Medica.

Yurick, A. (1981). Vision in the elderly person and the nursing process. In A. Yurick, S. Robb, B. Spier, & N. Ebert, (Eds.). The Aged Person and the Nursing Process. New York: Appleton-Century-Crofts, pp. 311–48.

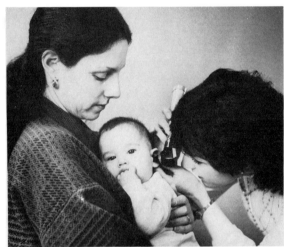

6

The Ear

Although the ear is a relatively small organ, in comparison to the other major organs of the body, there is significant potential for various and serious problems. At different times in one's life, certain pathology or dysfunction may be more likely to occur. For this reason, knowledge of developmental changes and common disorders regarding the ear and hearing helps the examiner anticipate what to expect.

DEVELOPMENTAL CHANGES OF THE EAR AND HEARING THROUGHOUT THE LIFESPAN

When a baby is born, parents and health care providers at the birth inspect the infant very carefully to see if all the "parts" are there and in the correct places. From this quick inspection, the existence of obvious deformities can be established. The ears are very visible and easily inspected for placement, symmetry, and external lesions. The ears of a premature infant are not fully developed. The auricle is less cartilaginous and as a result, is soft and can be folded. The cartilage develops and the infant's ear becomes stiffer and more shapely as the baby grows. The ears of a full term infant might be pressed closely against the head. This is likely to be the result of placement in utero. The infant's ears may appear to be abnormally low with regard to their placement on the head. This child may have a chromosomal disorder (*Down's Syndrome*) or renal disease. In either case, further evaluation is necessary.

Shortly after birth, hearing can be, and is assessed. Babies have a startle response (*Moro reflex*) present at birth that will be elicited in a baby who is startled or hears a loud noise. If the parents report that this response is non-existent, or they feel their child cannot hear, then the nurse should assume that this is true until it can be disproven.

In early infancy, the baby will acknowledge what he hears not only by the startle response, but also by moving his head toward the sound. During the first weeks of life, parents usually report that their child responds to their voices.

During the toddler and preschool years, there is a high incidence of middle ear infections (*otitis media*), due to the juvenile shape of the eustachian tube. Some children get more than three infections a year. Some never get an ear infection. The causes and etiologies of this disease are the source of much research and journal publication. Issues regarding etiology, viral versus bacterial, or allergic versus non-allergic, are considered complex and difficult to establish. Other aspects of the problem concerning the appropriate treatment(s) for ear infections are the subject of much controversy. There are certain conclusions which have been drawn. Most authorities believe that children will outgrow chronicity of the problem between the ages of 5–7 as the eustachian tube takes on a more adult shape. The concern, of course, is what degree of hearing damage has been done as a result of these infections. The degree of scarring on the tympanic membrane will be closely related to hearing loss.

After childhood, there is little change in the ear until the middle and elderly years. Other than non-age related problems, like excess ear wax or traumatic injury to the ears, the next developmental period in which ear dysfunction reflects age is in middle and late adulthood. The most significant problem during these years is hearing loss. This occurs in 60 percent of the population in the United States over 65 years (Libow & Sherman, 1981). *Presbycusis* is the term used to describe the gradual, progressive, permanent, bilateral loss of hearing. This degeneration of the auditory system has multiple causes, for which a chief source is thought to be arteriosclerosis. People with presbycusis lose the ability to hear high pitched sounds such as f, s, sh, and ph. Vowels are lower pitched and better heard by these people.

In addition to high pitched hearing loss, the elderly often find they have reduced speech discrimination and difficulty hearing in a normal environment and an increased sensitivity to loudness. These deficits can easily interfere with a person's comfort and confidence in interacting in his social milieu. Many elderly frequently underestimate their hearing loss and accompanying symptoms until it interferes with socialization and communication. Hearing loss due to neurological deficits is difficult to assess and often not correctable.

Another type of hearing loss, a *conductive hearing loss*, is likely to occur in the elderly, too. This problem involves the external and middle ear and is often the result of otosclerosis or excess cerumen. A conductive hearing loss tends to involve the low frequency sounds. In this type of hearing deficit, correction is often possible (Yurick, et al., 1984).

An additional problem that can be related to hearing loss is *tinnitus* (ringing in the ear). When tinnitus occurs, and it is not a result of too much salicylate ingestion, it is likely to be associated with a hearing loss. The intensity, frequency, and type of sound may all be related to the degree of hearing deficit (Yurick, et al., 1984).

Ear Dysfunction

An accurate assessment of ear dysfunction is crucial at any age because an oversight of a correctable abnormality may cause lifelong damage. In general, ear dysfunction has one of four origins: *acute illness*, a *mechanical problem*, a *neurologic disorder* or *trauma*.

Acute ear problems occur most commonly in children. Although adults can acquire the same types of infections or viruses, youths are much more frequently bothered. The most typical acute ear problems are blockage of the eustachian tubes (serous otitis), middle ear infections (otitis media), and inflammation of the external canal (otitis externa). Further descriptions of these problems can be found at the end of the chapter.

Mechanical dysfunctions have relatively simple explanations. A build-up of cerumen (ear wax) is the most common mechanical problem. This causes an obstruction in the external canal which results in a hearing loss. Such extra growths as tumors, chondromas, and exostoses (the latter two are bony nodules in the canal) can occur, but are less likely and not generally obstructive.

Neurologic disorders will cause some degree of hearing loss. They may be congenital, acquired, or inherited. Congenital hearing losses are often found in children who were exposed to rubella in utero, especially in the earlier months of pregnancy. Babies who are small, premature, and have congenital kidney disease or liver dysfunction run a greater chance of having hearing problems. Acquired hearing losses can come from such diseases as mumps and meningitis and from severe adverse reactions to the administration of drugs—i.e., streptomycin, kanamycin, and gentamycin. Although most inherited hearing problems do not manifest themselves until adulthood, it is important to elicit a good family history as early as possible. If accurate information is given to the provider, earlier intervention can take place and may ultimately prevent severe damage. As individuals age, hearing impairments can result from a combination of age related physiologic changes as well as pathologic conditions that are superimposed. However, it should be remembered that some hearing loss may be part of the normal aging process and cannot be prevented.

Traumatic injury to the ear is most likely to occur in children and adolescents. Children are notorious for inserting unusual objects in their ears. Some foreign bodies can be very destructive, so prompt removal is necessary. Teenagers who are active in contact sports need to be especially protective of their ears. The components of the external ear are relatively close to the surface and can be permanently damaged by a traumatic blow. Another source of traumatic stress to the eardrum involves occupational hazards, such as exposure to loud noises. Men and women exposed to constant loud machine noises have a high potential for hearing loss. Similar damage can be done by frequent, close exposure to loud music.

ANATOMY

The ear is a sensory organ which is divided into three parts: the *external ear*, the *middle ear*, and the *inner ear*.

The external ear includes the *auricle* (pinna) and the external canal (Fig. 6.1). The auricle is a cartilaginous material. The combination of the elastic cartilage and the skin covering the auricle gives it a firm but pliable consistency. There are landmarks to note on the pinna (Fig. 6.2). The *helix* and *antihelix* make up the most obvious curves on the superior aspect. The *tragus* is the protruding fea-

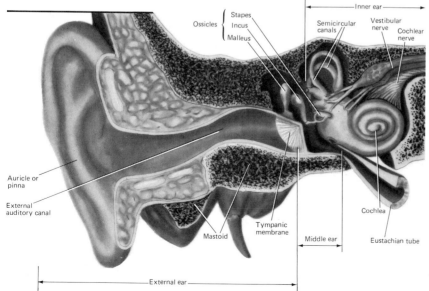

FIGURE 6.1
Structures of the ear. (From Heagarty, M., et al. Child Health: Basics for Primary Care. New York: Appleton-Century-Crofts, 1980, p. 128, with permission.)

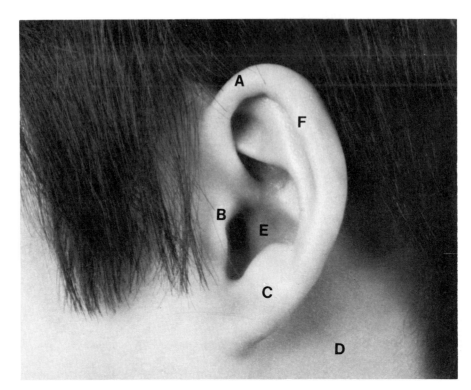

FIGURE 6.2
Landmarks of the ear. **A.** *Helix.* **B.** *Tragus.* **C.** *Ear lobe.* **D.** *Mastoid process.* **E.** *Ear canal.* **F.** *Antihelix.*

ture at the entrance of the external canal. This curved canal, which ends abruptly at the *tympanic membrane*, is about 1 inch (2.5 centimeters) long (Fig. 6.1). In an adult the outer portion of the canal is cartilaginous and the more inferior section is bony. In young children the canal is totally cartilaginous, as bone formation of the nature found in adults has not taken place yet. The skin covering the length of the canal has fine hairs and many glands and nerve endings. The fine hairs are more visible on some people than on others. In fact, in many they cannot be seen at all. These hairs may provide some degree of protection and keep out some foreign substances, but their physiologic function is minimal. The glands are wax producing and secrete cerumen (earwax). This wax is a lubricative and protective substance produced in varying amounts, depending on the individual. Cerumen is classified as wet (sticky) or dry (flaky). Wet earwax, generally found in Caucasian and black patients, is tan or brown. Dry earwax, common among clients of Asian or American Indian descent, is colored a light to brown gray (Mat-

sunaga, 1962).

The confirmation of the existence of several nerve endings is most easily made during the otoscopic exam. When the nerve endings are stimulated, they cause a painful sensation. This is especially apparent in children. Therefore, extreme caution must be taken while examining the ear (see discussion in "Physical Assessment" section). The *mastoid process* is not exactly part of the external ear, but it is an important landmark. It is the bony prominence behind the ear (Fig. 6.2).

The middle ear is an air-filled cavity which begins at the *tympanic membrane*. This membrane is a circular, pearly gray, opaque membrane which lies at an angle (Fig. 6.3). The superior aspect is more anterior than the lower rim of the drum. There are several visible landmarks to note on the eardrum. The *cone of light* is a triangularly shaped reflection that lies diagonally at about 5 o'clock in the right ear and 7 o'clock in the left. At the inferior end of the cone of light, directly attached to the tympanic membrane, lies the *malleus*. This is one of the bones of the ossicles (see

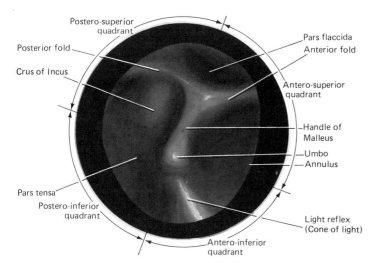

Postero-superior quadrant

Posterior fold

Crus of Incus

Pars flaccida
Anterior fold

Antero-superior quadrant

Handle of Malleus

Umbo

Annulus

Pars tensa

Postero-inferior quadrant

Light reflex (Cone of light)

Antero-inferior quadrant

FIGURE 6.3
Tympanic membrane as seen with the otoscope. (From Heagarty, M., et al. Child Health: Basics for Primary Care. New York: Appleton-Century-Crofts, 1980 p. 129, with permission.)

discussion of the "ossicles" following). There are three portions of this bone that can be seen: the *umbo,* which appears attached to the cone of light; the *handle of the malleus,* which extends to the superior aspect of the tympanic membrane; and the *short process,* which looks like a small circle at the end of the handle. The taut folds which surround the malleus and the cone of light are the *pars tensa* (Fig. 6.3). Along the attic of the eardrum lies another section of taut membrane called the *pars flaccida* (Fig. 6.3).

There are three ossicles in the middle ear: the *malleus,* the *incus,* and the *stapes* (Fig. 6.3). These are the bones of sound transmission. The malleus is the most easily seen of the three. Less frequently, the others can also be viewed; however, the incus is more accessible to inspection than the stapes.

The *eustachian tube* is another portion of the middle ear (Fig. 6.1). It connects the middle ear cavity to the nasopharynx. The tube functions as an air pressure stabilizer between the external atmosphere and the internal air pressure. The eustachian tube does not function as well in children as in adults. As the child gets older, the tube assumes a more mature form and function. It is believed that, for this reason, ear infections decrease as the child matures.

The inner ear houses the end organ receptors of hearing and balance. The *cochlea* is a structure shaped like a seashell that is essential to the transmission of sound (Fig. 6.1). The *vestibule* and *semicircular canals* are the receptors for equilibrium. The inner ear is in-

accessible to examination by inspection. One can evaluate the function of the inner ear with specific hearing and balance testing.

PHYSIOLOGY OF HEARING

A detailed discussion of the physiology of hearing goes beyond the scope of this book. However, a brief review is necessary to understand the physical assessment of the ear.

There are two basic methods of sound transmission: air conduction and bone conduction. In air conduction a sound is heard when:

1. A stimulus is sent to the external canal.
2. That stimulus reaches the tympanic membrane.
3. Most of the sound waves then cross the tympanic membrane to the ossicles.
4. The sound travels from the ossicles to the oval window (the opening to the inner ear).
5. The cochlea, which contains the organ of Corti (the organ of hearing), picks up the vibrations.
6. The stimulus then travels to the auditory nerve in the auditory cortex (the eighth cranial nerve).

In bone conduction, the vibrations are

transferred to the auditory cortex via bone. In this method, the skull bones carry the sound directly to the eighth cranial nerve.

HISTORY

There are two perspectives to explore in the review of this system: present complaints and past problems. In terms of present concerns, the patient should be asked if he has any ear pain, itching, discharge, tinnitus, or change in hearing ability. Investigation of past problems includes a history of ear infections, ear trauma, excess cerumen, or a hearing loss at any time. It is also important to ask about any family history of hearing losses.

If the patient states he has ear pain, the examiner should try to determine its location and quality. Does the pain feel close to the surface or is it deeper in the head? Can the patient elicit the pain by pushing on his ear? Is the pain sharp and stabbing or nagging and aching? Does it stay in one place? Does it come and go, or is the pain always present? Does changing the position of the head make it worse or better? Did any trauma occur? What has been done so far? Has the pain ever occurred before? What was done for it then? Was the problem resolved with the treatment (medication) administered? Were there any symptoms, such as a cold or sore throat, preceding the ear pain? Is there any fever?

If itching is a complaint, the patient should be asked where he feels the sensation. It is also helpful to find out about the patient's showering practices and frequency of swimming. Some people who get water in their ears when showering or who swim on a regular basis may acquire local irritation in the ear canal. For the same reason, the method of maintaining ear hygiene may irritate the canal. Excessive or inappropriate use of "Q-Tips" may cause skin breakdown, which can cause itching. The nurse should inquire as to whether this has been a problem in the past, what was done for it, and whether the problem was resolved. The etiology of this symptom can also be infectious, so asking the patient if he knows anyone with similar symptoms may provide useful information.

When discharge is the complaint, it is necessary to find out what the substance is. Blood will be a pink or red color. Pus is usually white, yellow, or green. The amount of discharge and the existence of any odor is important to note. Pain and discharge will often accompany one another. In the case of discharge leaking from behind the tympanic membrane, the classic story includes a description of severe pain which stopped suddenly after a popping sensation. This was followed by awareness of discharge on the pillow. (In such a case, the tympanic membrane has ruptured.)

If a patient has ringing in the ears, a key area to investigate is aspirin ingestion. Many times a sign of high serum salicylate levels will be tinnitus. A careful investigation of onset, frequency, associated phenomena, medication history (and amount), recent activities (sports, air travel, etc.), and allergy history may shed some light on the cause.

A decrease in hearing can be very disconcerting. The problem usually has an insidious onset. The etiology is probably mechanical or neurologic. Mechanical problems are usually attributed to an earwax build-up and can be resolved easily. The neurologic loss is much more complicated and is often not correctable; thus any information elicited can be helpful. The nurse should inquire about the type of hearing loss (low-pitched or high-pitched sounds), how long it has been going on, the history of noise exposure (certain occupations are especially hazardous in this way—musicians, construction workers, and policemen are at increased risk), and a family history of the same.

In regard to past problems, if frequent ear infections were experienced in the past, further investigation is needed. How often does the patient consider "frequent" to be? Who diagnosed the problem? How was the patient treated? Some people have had their tonsils removed or have had ear tubes inserted to help combat ear infections. If either of these procedures were implemented, the nurse should find out if that ended the problem. Sometimes these turn out to be temporary solutions. The nurse should also inquire as to whether or not there was any permanent hearing loss due to the repeated infections.

If excess earwax has been a long-term concern, the patient should be questioned about what he has done about the problem and how often the treatment is necessary. Some people put mineral oil in their ears (or a similar oil-based solution) to soften the ear wax. Cerumen can be removed fairly easily by flushing the ear with water or by removing the wax manually with a curette.

When a patient states that there is a family history of hearing dysfunction, exact information regarding who it was that has the problem, the specific disorder (if known) and the age of onset is helpful. If there is any known reason for the problem, such as repeated ear infections or trauma, then that should be investigated as well. The patient may know of the treatment that was used (e.g., a hearing aid) and the success or failure of the treatment. Such data are worthy of recording in the permanent record.

Finally, the patient should be asked if he has ever had a hearing test, when the last one was, and what the results were. There are several times in the course of one's life that hearing should be tested. Questioning parents regarding problems in their child's hearing is important at every well-child exam. For the most part, formal hearing testing begins when the child enters school or just prior to that. School programs provide screening with audiometry or require it as part of the school physical. Screening with audiometry should be done during the middle years (45 or older) on a regular basis and throughout the elderly years. More frequent screening, or screening starting earlier in adulthood than middle age, should be done if a problem or a strong family history of hearing loss exists. All of this information can help the nurse anticipate what she might find objectively as she continues the assessment of the ear.

PHYSICAL ASSESSMENT

Inspection and palpation are the techniques of examination used for the ear. Auditory acuity is also evaluated during this portion of the exam.

The examination begins with inspection of the auricles for placement and symmetry, lesions, skin abnormalities, and discharge. The auricles should be level with one another. Where the superior aspect of the pinna attaches to the head, there should be a straight line from the lateral canthus of the eye. Low-set ears may indicate chromosomal abnormalities (mongolism) or renal disease. Typical lesions that appear on the pinna are sebaceous cysts, moles, and tophi (subcutaneous deposits of uric acid on the ear). The cysts may enlarge periodically and will disappear without treatment. Moles may occur around the ear rather than on it, but in any case are observed for change in color, size, or shape. The most likely skin abnormality to occur on or behind the external ear is seborrhea. The skin appears to be flaky and scaling. This is usually seen behind the ear or in the area of the *concha*, the deep depression of the auricle (Fig. 6.2).

Palpation of the external ear precedes inspection with the otoscope (Fig. 6.4). Any tenderness and inflammation can be detected by pulling slightly on the auricle in an up, down, and backward motion; by pushing on the tra-

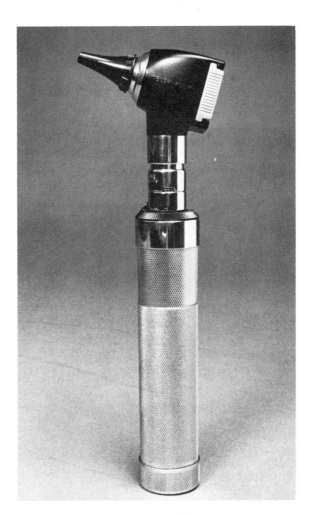

FIGURE 6.4
The otoscope.

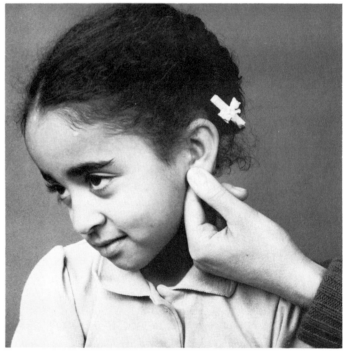

A

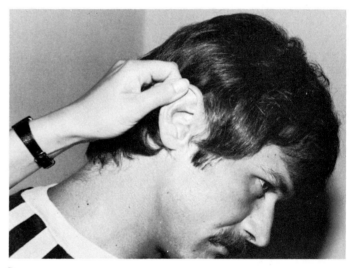

FIGURE 6.5
A. Pulling down on auricle to straighten the external ear canal in the child. B. Pulling up and back on the auricle to straighten the external canal in the adult.

B

gus; and by applying slight pressure to the mastoid process.

Inspection of the remaining parts of the ear requires the use of the otoscope. Because of the sensitivity of the external canal, young children find this exam unpleasant. For this reason, it is recommended to postpone the otoscopic exam until the end of the child's physical.

In beginning the otoscopic exam there are a few helpful points to keep in mind. First, the head of the patient is always tipped slightly away from the examiner. Second, the auricle is pulled in a specific direction, depending on the age of the patient, so that the auditory canal straightens out. In a young child the shape of the canal is such that it is straightened by pulling the auricle down. In an adult, the

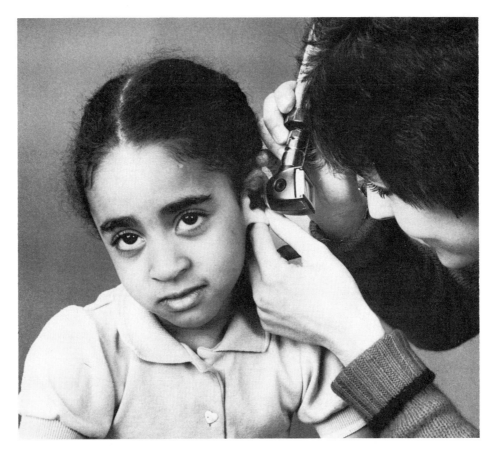

FIGURE 6.6
An alternate method of holding the otoscope that is especially helpful with children.

pinna is pulled up and back (Figs. 6.5A and B). Both these techniques facilitate the visualization of the tympanic membrane. The third point relates to the size of the speculum tip. The largest tip that will fit in the ear without causing discomfort should be used. This helps to assure the examiner maximum visualization of the tympanic membrane.

Now that the patient's head is tipped away from the examiner and the auricle is pulled in the appropriate direction, the otoscope is gently inserted into the ear canal. There are two methods for holding the otoscope. Figure 6.6 shows the instrument held upside down with the examiner's finger between the patient's head and the instrument. This is helpful with squirmy children, as they are not bumped with the otoscope (Fig. 6.7A–C). (Figure 6.8 show suggestions for gaining children's trust for using the otoscope.)

The canal is inspected for cerumen, foreign bodies, inflammation, redness, scaling,

exostoses, and other lesions. At the end of the canal the eardrum is spotted and its landmarks are identified. The most obvious feature is the cone of light. The umbo, the handle of the malleus, and the short process can be viewed as an extension of the cone of light. The pars tensa and pars flaccida are checked for position, lesions, bulging, and retraction. All 360 degrees of the anulus are inspected carefully. The otoscope and the examiner's body will have to be moved slightly to see all these features. The position, color, and gloss of the eardrum are noted in addition to any lesions or unusual markings. The otoscopic exam is not complete until all the landmarks are seen. If cerumen is in the way and there is no way to see around it, then it must be removed before any final assessment can be made.

Pneumatic otoscopy is another technique used to visualize the tympanic membrane and to determine if any pathology exists. In pneu-

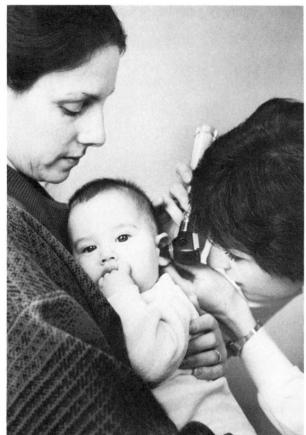

A

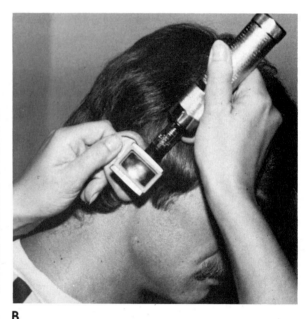

B

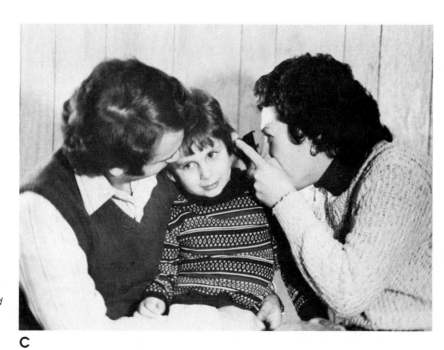

FIGURE 6.7
A-C. Examples of ways to hold
the otoscope while looking in
the ears.

C

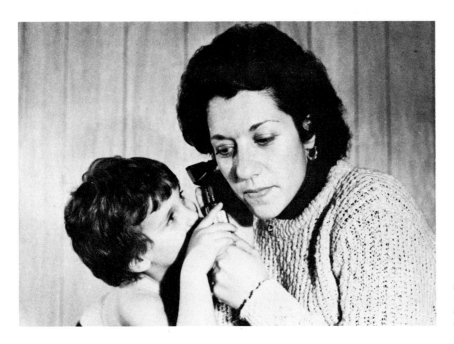

FIGURE 6.8
Gaining trust by helping the child become familiar with the otoscope.

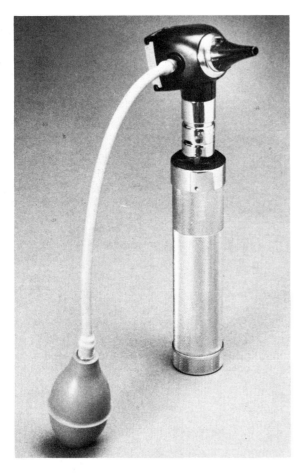

FIGURE 6.9
Equipment used for pneumatic otoscopy.

matic otoscopy, air is squeezed into and withdrawn from the ear canal. This is done with a bulb syringe attached to a rubber tube that is connected to an otoscope. Certain otoscope heads are designed for this (Fig. 6.9). A child may be less afraid of this test if she feels a small amount of the air pressure squeezed on her hand (Fig. 6.10).

The tympanic membrane is inspected initially. If the examiner suspects that there is fluid behind the ear drum, she squeezes the bulb syringe several times in succession and watches for movement of the tympanic membrane (Fig. 6.11). There should be no discomfort for the patient with this inspection. The eardrum moves as quickly as the air is injected and removed; it will move toward the examiner when air is withdrawn and away from the examiner when air is applied. Lack of movement is abnormal. The eardrum with fluid behind it, as in serous otitis, will not move. The healthy tympanic membrane will move easily.

Auditory Acuity

This portion of the physical examination begins when the patient and the interviewer begin talking. If the patient has difficulty hearing

160

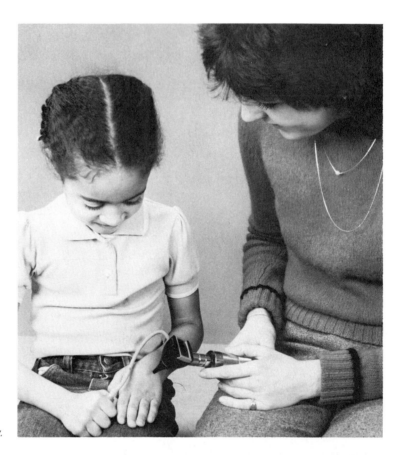

FIGURE 6.10
Helping the child get acquainted with
equipment used for pneumatic otoscopy.

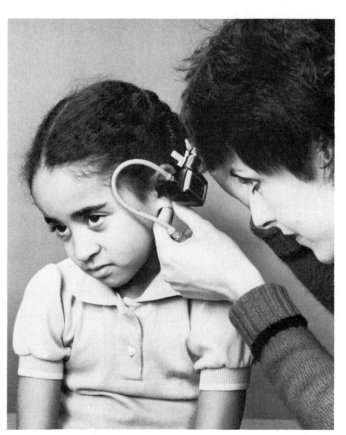

FIGURE 6.11
Examination of the ear using pneumatic otoscopy.

the examiner's voice, then an obvious hearing loss exists. However, there are more specific hearing tests available to confirm any suspicion of a hearing loss or to establish normal hearing patterns.

Gross hearing is tested first. This is done by simply whispering numbers to the patient while standing at his side. One ear is tested at a time. The examiner places 1 or 2 fingers on the tragus of one of the patient's ears, occluding it (Fig. 6.12). The examiner stands 1 to 2 feet to the side of the ear to be examined, which is the unoccluded ear. While occluding the ear (or rubbing the tragus of the occluded ear to produce a muffled sound), the examiner whispers three numbers and asks the patient to repeat them. Non-consecutive numbers should be whispered so that the patient will not anticipate which number will follow. It is also important to be certain that the examiner's lips cannot be read while reciting the numbers. This is accomplished by performing the examination from behind the patient or by standing in front of him and leaning 1 to 2 feet to the side and slightly behind him.

Another method of testing gross hearing is to ask the patient to listen to a ticking watch. The watch is held about 3 inches away from the patient's ear, while occluding the opposite ear (Fig. 6.13). (Many watches today are battery operated and do not tick. A watch that ticks must be used or this test should be eliminated.) The patient then says whether or not he can hear it. The sound of the watch is higher pitched than that of the human voice. Remember to test both ears using both methods.

Assessing the conduction of sound through air and bone comprise the next set of hearing tests. Air conduction is the process by which sound reaches the acoustic nerve as it travels through the canal and the middle ear to the inner ear. In bone conduction, the vibrations are carried via the skull or mastoid process to the eighth cranial nerve. Air conduction is more sensitive than bone conduction. A tuning fork, ranging from 500–1,000 cycles per second is needed to evaluate air and bone conduction.

The Weber Test

The Weber test assesses bone conduction by testing the lateralization of sounds. The tuning

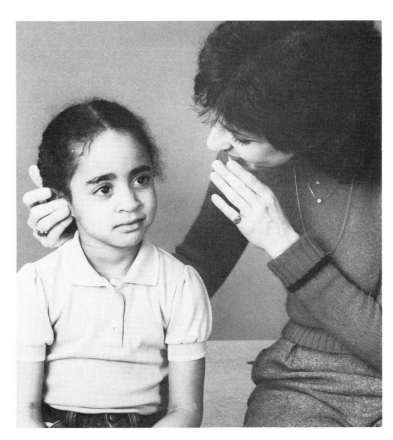

FIGURE 6.12
Testing gross hearing.

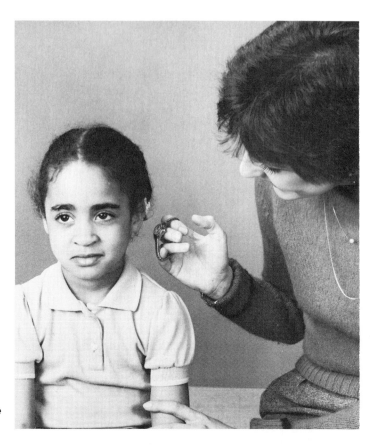

FIGURE 6.13
Another test for gross hearing. Listening to the ticking watch.

fork will vibrate when the examiner taps it against his hand while holding onto it at the base. The vibrating fork is then placed on the top of the patient's head (Fig. 6.14). The patient is asked where he hears the noise. With normal hearing the sound will be heard in both ears or localized in the center of the head. If there is a conductive hearing loss, the sound will be heard better in the poor or damaged ear. A conductive loss represents an inability of the vibration to reach the inner ear. Among other causes, this can be the result of ear canal

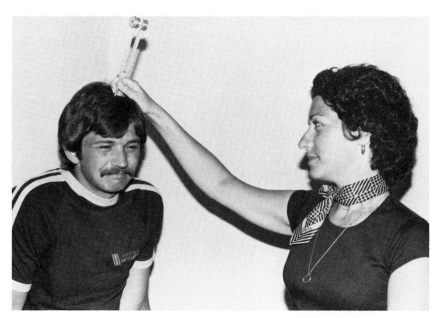

FIGURE 6.14
Performing the Weber test.

blockage (cerumen or foreign body), fluid behind the ear drum, or an obstruction of the ossicles. This type of loss can be imitated by putting a finger in one ear and then speaking. The voice will be louder in the ear with the finger inserted in it. The finger represents a conductive disturbance. Obstruction in the ear canal will obliterate room noise, thus increasing bone sensitivity. When a sensorineural hearing loss exists, there is damage either to the eighth cranial nerve or to the inner ear. In a sensorineural disturbance the Weber will lateralize to the ear without a problem. The ear without any nerve or inner ear damage will always hear better.

The Rinné Test

The Rinné test compares air conduction to bone conduction. It should be remembered that air conduction is more sensitive. In other words, sound vibrations will last longer via air conduction, if there is no disturbance. To perform this test, the vibrating tuning fork is placed on the mastoid process of one ear (Fig. 6.15A). The nurse notes the starting time on her watch. The patient is asked to say when he can no longer hear the vibrations. The examiner notes the number of seconds the vibrations were heard. The fork, which is still vibrating, is then placed in front of the ear canal (Fig. 6.15B). If necessary, the nurse should push the patient's hair away. The patient is asked once again to say when he can no longer hear the sound. The time is also noted. The sound will disappear eventually, although it will take about twice as long to go away as when the fork was on the mastoid process. The same procedure is repeated with the other ear. If air conduction time is longer than bone conduction time (AC > BC), which is normal, the test is considered positive. This is one of the few tests in our classification of terms for which "positive" is the desired result (Chart 6.1).

In the Rinné test a conductive loss will reveal a bone conduction time equal to or longer than air conduction time. In the case of sensorineural disturbance, air conduction time will be greater than bone conduction time because in the damaged ear the nerve will pick up air vibrations more readily than bone vibrations.

Of course, the most precise test is that which measures hearing at various decibels. This testing is called audiometry and can be done without much difficulty with the appropriate equipment. Many ambulatory care facilities and primary care offices have the necessary machine available. If children have it performed in school, and the results are within normal limits, there is no need to repeat it. For adults, annual testing can detect early signs of a hearing loss. If treatment can be initiated to prevent further loss, then the sooner intervention takes place, the better. For the geriatric population audiometry is essential.

ABNORMAL FINDINGS IN THE EAR

The external ear canal is a place in which localized infections or traumatic injury may occur. Disorders in this region are referred to as *external otitis.* Symptoms of this disorder may have a viral, bacterial, allergic, or traumatic (i.e., inappropriate use of "Q-tips") etiology. The chief complaint is often itching or pain. The objective findings may include pain while pushing on the tragus or palpating the auricle. The external canal may be erythematous and inflamed. There may also be flaking of the skin.

In traumatic injuries, which usually occur from overzealous hygiene practices or a foreign body lodged in the canal, the chief symptom is likely to be sudden pain in this area. The otoscopic exam will reveal redness, edema, bleeding, or the foreign body itself.

Any infectious process of the middle ear is called *otitis media.* The two most common forms of otitis media are *acute* and *serous.*

Acute otitis media usually begins with redness on the ear drum or hyperemia of the blood vessels. The next phase may be retraction of the landmarks. Retraction is the result of absorption of air in the eustachian tubes, changing the appearance of the tympanic membrane. This shortens the malleus and the short process and accentuates the pars tensa and pars flaccida. The cone of light will bend. In the most infectious stages of this condition, the tympanic membrane may bulge forward and be vividly reddened. The landmarks will

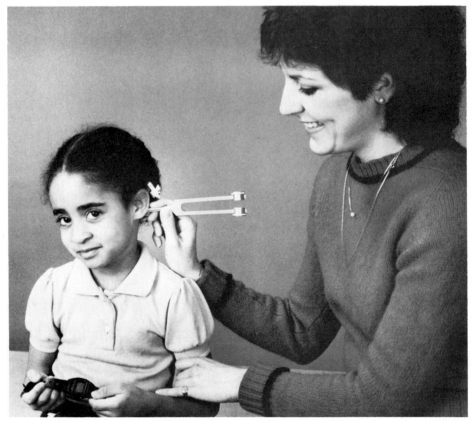

A

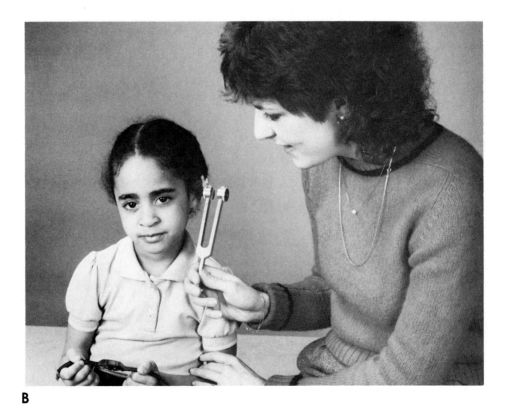

B

FIGURE 6.15
Performing the Rinné test. **A.** *Bone conduction.* **B.** *Air conduction.*

CHART 6.1
*TUNING FORK TESTS FOR NORMAL HEARING, CONDUCTIVE HEARING
LOSS, AND SENSORINEURAL HEARING LOSS*

	Weber (Bone Only)	Rinné (Air-Bone)
Normal	Not lateralized	Positive AC > BC
Conductive loss	Lateralized to poorer ear	Negative BC ≥ AC
Sensorineural loss	Lateralized to better ear	Positive AC > BC

(From DeWeese, D. D., and Saunders, W. H. Textbook of Otolaryngology (5th ed.). St. Louis: C. V. Mosby, 1977, p. 301, with permission.)

be obliterated. This occurs commonly in children and is extremely painful. If the pressure behind the eardrum is too great, a perforation can occur. Perforations usually happen along the peripheral margins. The pain disappears immediately. The appearance of a minuscule hairline will be evident at the site of perforation. Pus or blood may be seen in the canal. Because of the advances of antibiotic therapy, perforations occur much less frequently today. Appropriate intervention usually takes place prior to this occurrence. It is therefore obvious that any reddened ear warrants immediate attention.

If a clear, sterile substance builds up behind the tympanic membrane as a result of a blockage in the eustachian tube, a condition called *serous otitis* exists. The fluid appears amber in color and one can sometimes see a fluid line or bubbles behind the transparent ear drum. This condition usually occurs along with an otitis media or an upper respiratory condition. Patients commonly complain of "voices sounding like my head is in a bucket" or "ear-popping." There is much debate over the method to be used for treatment.

Screening Examination of the Ear

1. Screening test for gross hearing
2. Weber and Rinné tests (in appropriate age groups)
3. Audiometry (if available)
4. Inspection and palpation of the external structures of the ear
5. Inspection of the ear canals and tympanic membranes with the otoscope.

EXAMPLE OF A RECORDED HISTORY AND PHYSICAL

SUBJECTIVE:

Chief Complaint: "I've had ringing in my ears for 1 month."

HPH: This 35-year-old male considers himself in "fair health," but has never had any problems with his ears prior to 1 month ago, when the "ringing in both ears" began. The high-pitched noise is constant "from morning until night," but seems more intense after riding the subway to and from work.

There is no discharge, dizziness, blurry vision, headache, pain, known hearing loss, history of excess earwax, or recent cold, fever, allergies or other acute illness. There is no prior history of this or of any family members with the same problem. Patient has taken no medications or applied any home remedies to relieve the problem.

Patient works in factory, where he has worked for 7 years. The noise level is considered safe by OSHA, although he states some people wear ear plugs anyhow. Patient takes aspirin (10 gr) about three times a week for "my joint stiffness." He does not consider this problem disabling, just a "nuisance."

OBJECTIVE:

T. 98.8°F orally; P. 86 radial; R. 20; B.P. (sitting) (R) 116/72, (L) 120/78.

Left Ear: No lesions, discharge, scaling, or tenderness of external ear. No cerumen or other substances in canal. Tympanic membrane: Light reflex bright and not diffuse. No redness, bulging, or retraction. A white rim appears around anulus. Landmarks visible.

Right Ear: 0.5 cm. flesh-colored, nontender nodule on helix. No discharge. No other lesions, scaling, discharge, or tenderness of external ear. Moderate amount of brown cerumen in canal. Tympanic membrane: Light reflex bright and not diffuse. No redness, bulging, retraction, or scarring. Landmarks are visible.

Rinné: BC > AC bilaterally.

Weber: Lateralization of vibrations to (R) ear.

Gross Hearing: Unremarkable. Can repeat whispered numbers and hear watch tick from 4″ away.

REFERENCES

Libow, L., & Sherman, F. (1981). The Core of Geriatric Medicine: A Guide for Students and Practitioners. St. Louis: C. V. Mosby.

Matsunaga, E. (1962). The dimorphism in normal human cerumen. Annals of Human Genetics, 25, 273–86.

Yurick, A., Spier, B., Robb, S., & Ebert, N., (Eds.). (1984). The Aged Person and the Aging Process (2nd ed.). Norwalk, Conn: Appleton-Century-Crofts.

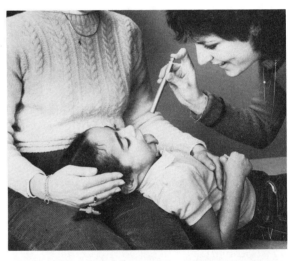

7
The Nasopharynx

The nasopharyngeal region includes the oral cavity, the nose, and sinuses. From a developmental perspective, the nasopharynx is discussed as one system. For the purpose of simplifying the assessment, these regions are divided into two sections: the mouth and throat, and the nose and sinuses.

DEVELOPMENTAL CHANGES OF THE NASOPHARYNX THROUGHOUT THE LIFESPAN

As a system, the nasopharynx does not change a great deal throughout the lifespan, once it has developed. There are certain developmental age-related periods where expected changes do occur.

When a baby is born, he should have no teeth, minimally developed paranasal sinuses, and little saliva. As the neonate becomes an infant, the teeth and salivary glands will emerge and activate; and as the preschooler becomes a school-aged child, the frontal sinuses will develop. Although the newborn is without these findings, there are two other findings typical to this early period that are worth noting. Most infants develop a *sucking tubercle* on the upper lip during the first few weeks of life. This growth is about 0.25 centimeters and looks like a flesh-pink skin tag. It is more prominent on breast fed infants, but can also develop in bottle-fed infants. The tubercle is a normal finding that will disappear when the infant gives up the breast or bottle.

Another interesting phenomenon that occurs in newborns and infants is known as *Epstein's Pearls*. These are small retention cysts that are yellow-white, pearl-like nodules that are most frequently found on the posterior aspect of the hard palate and the gums. Within the first few months of life the cysts resolve spontaneously and require no intervention.

One further feature to note about newborns is that they are all nose breathers. This does not interfere with respiration unless nasal obstruction is a problem. If the nasal obstruction is caused by increased mucus, this must be removed. If there is a true blockage, prompt intervention is necessary.

The major change in the mouth during infancy is the eruption of teeth. Usually the teeth emerge from the gingiva between the fifth to seventh month of life and are complete around the second birthday. There are a total of 20 *deciduous or primary teeth* (see Figs. 7.1 and 7.2). Interestingly enough, teeth form in the sixth week of embryonic life. Each child's teeth erupt at their own rate. Occasionally a child is born with one or two teeth and in other cases, the first teeth may not appear until 12 months of age. Often there will be a family history of late teeth eruption in the family of a child whose teeth come in later than average.

There is little saliva present in the first three months of life; soon the salivary glands develop and begin to produce saliva. Many people think this is a sign of teething. It actually has little to do with the impending emergence of teeth. The drooling comes from the maturation of the salivary gland and ducts; the saliva runs out of the mouth partly because no teeth are present.

The amount and regeneration of tastebuds are of interest because they vary throughout the lifespan. Although the number of tastebuds varies among different populations, they are generally most abundant in infants and children. Tastebuds are also most sensitive to stimuli in infants. As children become adults, the number of tastebuds decreases. By the time a person is beyond middle age, the tastebuds have deteriorated even further. The most important reason to note this is in an attempt to understand a person's sense of taste. Because of the large number of tastebuds children have an acute sense of taste, and to them rich foods (i.e., spinach!) probably taste entirely different than they do to adults. Elderly people suffer from just the opposite problem—

their food does not taste interesting unless it is rich or highly seasoned. It is common to see older people highly salt and season their foods, which can aggravate other problems, such as hypertension.

During the toddler and preschool years, the deciduous teeth are completed. The last of these 20 teeth are the 2-year molars that should be in by 2½ years of age. Also, in the posterior pharynx the tonsillar tissue begins to enlarge. This is usually not pathologic, just a change in the lymphoid tissue itself. During preschool years the tonsils are larger than they are in infancy and adolescence.

Going to the dentist is important during the preschool period; these years are often when hygiene practices are developed and the dental caries (cavities) appear. For this reason, all children should visit a dentist by 3 years of age.

During the school-age period, the primary or deciduous teeth begin to fall out. The *secondary or permanent teeth* (see Figs. 7.1 and 7.2) will erupt from the gums as the primary teeth are lost. The permanent teeth have formed during the sixth month of fetal life. There are 32 permanent teeth and they continue to come in through adolescence. The *third molars* or *wisdom teeth* are the last of the permanent teeth to emerge, making their appearance in most adolescents around 17–18 years of age. These teeth are notorious for becoming impacted or coming in crooked, and eventually may require extraction.

Another physiologic change in the school-age period is the formation of the frontal sinuses. Until this point the only paranasal sinuses that have formed are the maxillary sinuses.

During the young- and middle-adult years, there are not many changes in the teeth. There is, however, a higher incidence of periodontal disease in the adult years that may result in loss of teeth. Annual or semi-annual dental visits are extremely important in the prevention of periodontal disease.

Significant changes in the oral pharynx begin in the elderly years. Changes are observed in the mucous membranes, gingiva, and teeth—the saliva decreases in quantity; the mucosa pales and becomes drier; the gingiva can tend to recede; and the number of taste buds decreases, resulting in a decrease in the ability to taste. If an older person is fortunate enough to have his own teeth, the teeth have usually lost some of their luster and have almost a transparent quality.

One other concern in the elderly is worth mentioning. As the motor and sensory responses decrease in their sensitivity, the gag reflex and ability to cough might be affected. As a result, it is likely that this person may not be able to gag and cough up an irritant, putting the patient at risk for choking.

THE MOUTH AND THROAT

Anatomy

The *lips* begin the region known as the oral cavity (Fig. 7.1). The portion called the *posterior pharynx* terminates the area. The *buccal mucosa* lines the inside of the mouth along the lateral walls. This mucosa extends from the floor to the roof of the mouth. The roof of the mouth consists of the *hard* and *soft palate* (Fig. 7.2). The hard palate is the bony structure directly above the tongue. It is pale pink. The uvula is the short, elongated, pink, finger-like projection attached to the soft palate medially on the *anterior pharynx* (Fig. 7.2). The soft palate, which begins slightly anterior to the uvula, is a deeper pink in color.

The *tongue* is a mass of muscles. *Papillae* are projections covering the dorsal surface of the tongue; they give the tongue its rough surface. There are different sizes of papillae scattered over the tongue. A person's tastebuds are also spread over the tongue and throughout the mouth. Tastebuds detect four different flavors: salt, sweet, bitter, and sour. The bitter sensations are picked up on the posterior portion of the tongue. Sweet tastes are detected on the tip of the tongue. The tastebuds sensitive to salt are located on the lateral aspects of the tongue just behind the sweet region and the sour area is right behind the salt region. There is some overlap of these regions. Knowing these details becomes important if an intracranial lesion is suspected and the examiner is trying to locate its origin. The tongue is attached to the floor of the mouth by the *frenulum*. Under the tongue lies one of two pairs of salivary ducts that are visible in the mouth. (Fig. 7.1). These are called the *submax-*

illary ducts (Wharton's ducts). The other salivary ducts that open into the mouth are opposite the second molar along each maxilla (Fig. 7.3). These are the *parotid ducts* (Stenson's ducts). These ducts are the endpoints of the salivary glands: the parotid and the submaxillary glands. Altogether there are three pairs of salivary glands in the oral cavity. The last one is called the *sublingual,* and its ducts are inaccessible to examination. The sublingual gland is located on the floor of the mouth and helps moisten the oral cavity.

Healthy teeth are important for cosmetic and nutritional concerns. As stated previously, a child has 20 deciduous, or primary, teeth. An adult will have 32 secondary or permanent teeth. Teeth erupt from the gingiva of the maxilla and mandible. There are 2 central incisors, 2 lateral incisors, 2 cuspids, 4 bicuspids, and 6 molars erupting from the gum of the mandible and the maxilla (Fig. 7.2).

Many population differences in dentition have been documented. Gross tooth size of incisors, canines, premolars, and molars varies widely from group to group. Some groups have larger anterior teeth, others have larger posterior teeth. Tooth morphology also differs. For example, the rear surfaces of the incisors of many American Indian and Asian populations are "shovel-shaped." Finally, the number of teeth occurring in any individual is also a population variable. Some people from the Pacific have an entire extra set of molars; American Indians and Asians often have a congenital absence of the third molars.

The posterior section of the mouth begins at the soft palate and uvula. Together these two structures form the anterior pharynx (Fig. 7.2). The arch-like sides that extend to the tongue from the soft palate are called the *anterior pillars*. The *tonsils* and *posterior pillars* comprise the *posterior pharynx*. The portion of the pharynx described above is known as the *oropharynx*.

History

The oral cavity has many functions. It has a sensory division, which is responsible for gustatory and pain responses, and a motor component, which provides the ability to talk, chew, swallow, and gag. From a review of these features it is easy to see that the mouth

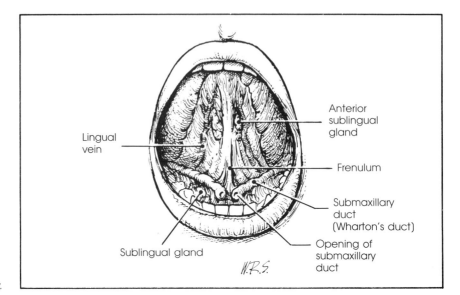

FIGURE 7.1
The oral cavity.

can harbor various problems. Some are simple, acute, and easy to provide care for, such as a sore throat or a broken tooth. Other problems, such as a cancerous lesion discovered under the tongue or on the gum, may be life-threatening.

The subjective review of this system includes questions on everything from the ability to taste, talk, and swallow to the existence of pain.

Just asking a patient if he has pain in his mouth is too general. Taking a more specific direction will provide more information. The patient should be asked whether he has pain

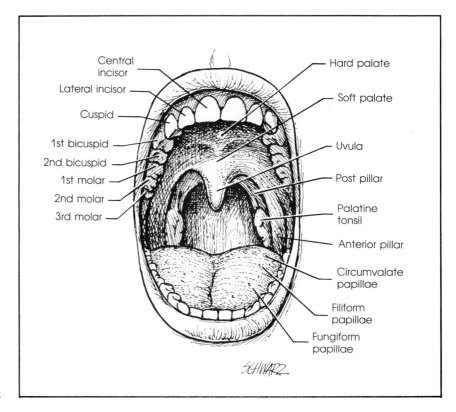

FIGURE 7.2
The teeth and oral cavity.

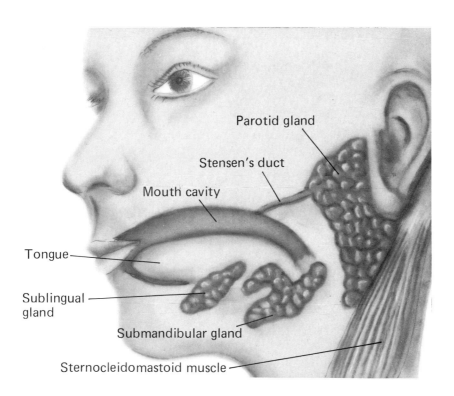

Parotid gland

Stensen's duct

Mouth cavity

Tongue—

Sublingual gland

Submandibular gland

Sternocleidomastoid muscle

FIGURE 7.3
*Position of the salivary glands.
(From Heagarty, M., et al. Child
Health: Basics for Primary Care.
New York: Appleton-Century-
Crofts, 1980, p. 129, with permis-
sion.)*

in his teeth, gums, throat, or tongue. As always, if any of these answers are positive, a thorough history using the eight areas of investigation is necessary.

Specific health-oriented questions that involve the oral cavity should be asked, including questions on the date of the last dental exam, the general condition of the teeth, the presence of caries, and the types and frequency of hygiene measures used (i.e., brushing, flossing, use of a water pick). In addition, certain problems are common to the oral cavity and their existence or nonexistence should be reviewed. These include soreness, bleeding, or ulcerations of the lips, tongue, or gums; halitosis or fruity-smelling breath; hoarseness; a change in the ability to taste; and any recent extractions and the reasons for them. Certain developmental issues regarding the oral cavity may need to be addressed at screening exams.

During infancy and toddlerhood, questioning the parents about teething, use of pacifier, thumbsucking practice, use of bottle in bed, and fluoridation of water is important as these are worthy areas of investigation. In the records of all children, history regarding

the mother's use of tetracycline during pregnancy should be carefully noted. (Implications are discussed later in this chapter.) During late childhood and early adolescence, parents may be concerned about underbite or overbite or missing permanent teeth. Any concerns on the parent's or nurse's part should be referred to a dentist. A dentist may refer the patient to an orthodontist. If a child requires braces, late childhood and early adolescence is the time they are placed on the teeth. When a patient has braces, it is important for nurses to explore comfort, hygiene practices, compliance of routine orthodontist visits, and presence of lesions in the mouth as a result of wiring irritating the gum.

If ulcerations or a history of them exists, then further data are needed:

1. Where are the ulcers (usually) located?
2. How often do they appear?
3. When they occur, is there any association to colds, viruses, menstrual cycle, stress, or time of the year?
4. What treatment is used and how successful is it?

A complaint of *frequent* sore throats may arise during the interview. A precise history of what the patient means by this will give the nurse a better picture. The patient needs to be definite in terms of the number of sore throats that occur in a year's time. The definition of frequency will vary among individuals. Once a common understanding of this word is established, several other questions should follow:

1. Describe the throat pain. Where is the pain? What does it feel like? Is there difficulty with swallowing?
2. Is care usually sought for the problem? Is a throat culture usually obtained? What is the usual diagnosis (i.e., streptococcal vs. viral)?
3. What is the treatment prescribed? Are antibiotics given? If so, what kind? How long are they taken? Do they help?
4. Does the "sore throat" happen in one season more than another? Does it seem worse upon arising? What is the humidity in the room where the patient sleeps? Is there an allergy history? Does the patient smoke? Is occupation or the working environment related?
5. Family history of oral cancer.

After a thorough review of this system and a look at the anatomic structures of the oral cavity, the physical examination can begin.

Physical Assessment

Sharp observation skills, a bright light, and a tongue depressor comprise the basic equipment necessary for this exam. On occasion a glove or finger cot will be needed to palpate a lump or abnormality.

INSPECTION

Inspection is the primary method of examination used for the oral cavity. Any abnormal findings in the anterior portion of the mouth can be palpated, too. The patient who wears dentures is asked to remove them so that the gums can be inspected thoroughly. This is also true for people who wear partial plates. A bright light is necessary to visualize the structures and any abnormalities in the oral cavity.

For the most part, the patient will be in a sitting position for this exam. A child may be more comfortable on a parent's lap; either lying or sitting works well (Fig. 7.4). For a frightened or uncooperative child, laying them on the exam table with the parents holding the child's hands over his head may help expedite the procedure. It is important for the examiner to have control of the child and situation, so no injury occurs.

The correct approach in examining the oral cavity is to start with the outer features and move to the inner aspects: the *lips* to the *posterior pharynx*. The following structures are examined in the oral cavity:

1. Lips
2. Teeth
3. Gingivae
4. Tongue
5. Buccal mucosa
6. Hard palate
7. Anterior pillars
8. Uvula
9. Tonsils
10. Posterior pillars

The lips are inspected for position, color, symmetry, moisture, and lesions (ulcerations or fissures). The most common abnormal findings involve color, texture, and lesions. The normal red color of the lips is likely to change if the patient is anemic, short of breath, or very chilled. Decreased hemoglobin concentration in the blood may cause pallor of the lips. The bluish lip color that is seen on someone who is cold or dyspneic is referred to as *cyanotic.* Because the lips of some black individuals normally have a bluish hue, it is important to know the patient's baseline lip color if this site is to be used in detecting cyanosis.

In the winter months lips may get chapped due to the cold air or wind. This is aggravated by frequent licking of the lips. The lips become dry and rough and the skin appears to be peeling or cracking.

Ulcerations on the lips are often due to a herpes virus (see Chart 3.3, page 81). This relatively painful and annoying lesion will appear as a small vesicle on the edge of the lip. It will ooze and eventually form a crust. Another typical lesion of the lips occurs at the junction of the upper and lower lips. Drying and chapping of the lips, which is common in children, causes lesions and a small fissure

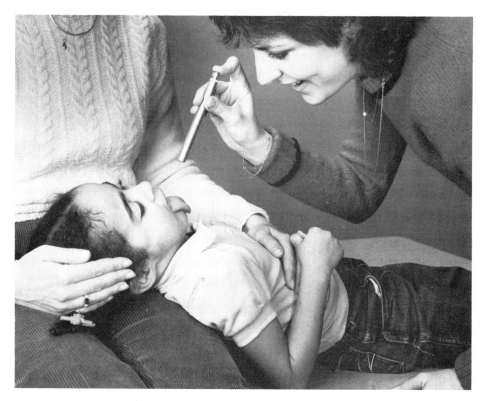

FIGURE 7.4
Gaining the child's trust by examining the child in a familiar person's lap.

results. Such painful lesions are more common in the winter months. Malignant lesions of the oral cavity may also occur on the lips. In malignancy, the history often reveals years of smoking a pipe, cigars, or chewing tobacco. Those who do not smoke are not necessarily immune to this type of cancer, although its incidence is proportionately higher among such smokers.

The teeth are checked for their state of repair, obvious caries, displacement, color, position, and extraction sites. In children it is important to check the deciduous teeth as they are erupting and to note the order in which they are coming in. It is also important to note when these teeth begin to fall out and to make sure that the permanent teeth appear shortly thereafter.

The young child who was treated with tetracycline or whose mother took tetracycline during pregnancy will have yellow staining on the teeth. The degree of damage to the teeth varies with the age of exposure. Another color change is seen with excess flouride intake.

This results in white spotting on the teeth. Excessive iron intake can cause black staining on the teeth.

The importance of good oral hygiene cannot be overemphasized. The earlier a child learns to care for his teeth, the better. Toddlers love to imitate adults and setting a good example is certainly a good way to get them started. If a child sees his parent or sibling practicing good hygiene techniques, then he is likely to do the same. At any age, it is important to reinforce and teach patients about oral hygiene.

The gingivae are examined for color, edema, retraction, bleeding, and lesions. Healthy gums have a pink, moist, and smooth appearance. There is no edema or pulling away of the gums from the teeth (retraction). When the gingivae become red and edematous and the patient states that they bleed easily and feel irritated, *gingivitis* may exist. This is a relatively benign problem if taken care of promptly. If neglected, it can turn into *pyorrhea*. This condition is advanced gingivitis. If untreated, the retraction eventually becomes so marked that the roots of the teeth may be exposed.

Patients taking Dilantin should have regular examinations of the oral cavity, with special attention to the gums. Long-term use of this drug may cause problems, the most common being *gingival hyperplasia.* The gums enlarge and extend to the point of covering portions of the teeth.

With a bright light the nurse should inspect the tongue for color, size, position, lesions, coating, and surface texture. There are some variations in tongue surfaces that should be described:

1. Hairy tongue: In this condition, hairs seem to be growing out of the surface of the tongue. Actually, the hair-like protrusions are brown or black filliform papillae. Hairy tongue is a harmless chronic condition and cannot be cured in most people.
2. Geographic tongue: The tongue in this condition resembles a one-dimensional topographic map. Smooth, reddened areas are located sporadically on the dorsum. These areas have no papillae, thus giving the tongue an irregular texture. Geographic tongue is harmless and does not warrant treatment.
3. Fissured tongue (scrotal tongue): This is a familial condition which is generally not a problem, but occurs in up to 40 percent of some populations. The tongue looks exactly as the name implies, with fissures of various depths on the dorsum of the tongue. Occasionally food will get caught in the fissures and may cause some mild irritation. There is no treatment for this; most problems can be avoided with good oral hygiene.

The tongue and oral mucosa may exhibit hyperpigmentation. Darkly pigmented tongues occur in 10 to 50 percent of Caucasians and in up to 90 percent of black populations (Spuhler, 1950).

To further inspect the tongue and its undersurface, the nurse asks the patient to touch the roof of his mouth with his tongue. The nurse should stand to the side of the patient, because lifting the tongue can result in a spray from his salivary glands. The area under the tongue is examined for lesions, distribution of superficial veins, attachment of the frenulum, and the presence and patency of Wharton's ducts.

Oral cancer is a potentially fatal disease if not discovered early. In its early stages a cancerous lesion may look like a minute ulceration. Therefore, meticulous inspection of the area under the tongue is essential. Many dentists and hygienists consider this inspection part of routine health maintenance. This is certainly a good practice, but the inspection should be done thoroughly during a physical exam. Oral cancer is usually found in this region of the mouth.

Varicosities are another abnormality that can occur under the tongue. These are most likely to be seen in the elderly. They are of virtually no significance and do not require treatment. Some authorities feel they may be related to a deficiency of the cardiovascular system. Last, the patient is asked to extend his tongue. At this time, the tongue is observed for symmetry in shape and with movement.

The buccal mucosa is evaluated for moisture, color, lesions (e.g., canker sores), and pigmentation. Because the buccal mucosa and the tongue may exhibit less pigmentation than any other body areas in dark-skinned individuals, this may be an excellent site for detection of cyanosis or jaundice. However, there are two frequently occuring nonpathologic conditions in the oral mucosa which also lead to color changes. The first is hyperpigmentation of the oral mucous membranes. In Caucasians, the incidence of hyperpigmentation may reach 10 percent by age 50; in blacks, 50 to 90 percent will show mucous membrane hyperpigmentation by the fourth decade. In both groups, there is a higher incidence in darker-hued individuals. A second frequently occurring variation in oral pigmentation results from a condition termed *leukoedema.* This presents on the buccal mucosa as a benign grayish white lesion. This condition is present in nearly 50 percent of Caucasians and 90 percent of blacks (McDonald & Kelly, 1975; Martin & Crump, 1972).

The presence of the parotid ducts should also be noted and can be found opposite the area of the second molar at the level of the maxilla. They look like the top of a straight pin and are the same color as the mucosa.

Canker sores commonly occur on the buccal mucosa. These small white ulcerations are viral in origin and can be very painful. Many people notice that the lesions appear when fatigue, stress, or a systemic infection exist.

If a child presents with a brief history of a cold, cough, and fever, the examiner should check the buccal mucosa for white, patchy, spotty areas. These are called *Koplick's spots* and appear 48 hours before the arrival of the measles (rubeola). The nurse should inquire about the child's immunization status and about how old the child was when he received the MMR (measles, mumps, and rubella) vaccine.

The dome-shaped hard palate is observed for its shape and the presence of any extra bony prominences. In black individuals the color changes of jaundice are especially prominent at the junction of the hard and soft palates. However, instead of the classical yellow hue, the palates of jaundiced blacks are often a muddy yellow or greenish-brown in color (McDonald & Kelly, 1975). Occasionally there may be a bony growth on the roof of the mouth. This is known as *torus palatinus* and is found along the midline of the hard palate. Palatine tori are common in Asian people (up to 77 percent) and less common in blacks and Caucasians (McDonald & Kelly, 1975; Jarvis & Gurlin, 1972). The extent of the extra growth determines whether treatment is required. Rarely is it necessary to do anything about torus palatinus.

Examination of the pharynx begins with inspection of the anterior pillars and uvula. The entire pharynx should be observed for color, edema, petechiae, ulcerations, and exudate. After the anterior pillars are examined, the uvula is visualized for length, deviation from the midline, movement, and symmetry. The patient is asked to say "ah" and the uvula and soft palate should rise (see the section on "Cranial Nerve X" in Chapter 15). Not infrequently, the uvula has an unusual shape. The most common deviation is called a *bifid uvula* and it looks like it has been partially severed in the midline. This may have clinical significance and should be reported, especially when it occurs in children. A bifid uvula may indicate a submucous cleft palate, which implies that there is a deficient muscle of the palate (DeWeese & Saunders, 1982). Incidence of bifid uvula varies dramatically among populations. In American Indians it is seen in 1 of

every 9 to 14 individuals; among blacks it is extremely rare (1 in 300); and in Caucasians the frequency lies in between that of the other groups (Jarvis & Gurlin, 1972).

Observation of the pharynx continues to the tonsils and posterior pillars. To visualize these areas, the examiner should have the patient say "ah" or "eh." Although the "eh" sound is harder to make with the mouth open, it gives the examiner a better look at the posterior pharynx (Fig. 7.4). The use of a tongue depressor may be necessary to see the posterior portion of the oral cavity. If it is needed, ask the patient to open his mouth and place the tongue depressor on the middle of the tongue. It is not necessary to gag the patient, but the tongue depressor must be placed far enough back to see the entire pharynx. If it is necessary to elicit a gag reflex to test cranial nerves IX and X, wait until the end of the exam if possible. Look at the posterior pharynx completely and quickly, so the patient has minimal discomfort. Most patients find the use of the tongue blade uncomfortable and for children, it can be frightening. If an infant or child is crying, the examiner can utilize that time to observe the pharynx. By preschool age, most children can adequately open their mouths for inspection when they receive appropriate instructions.

The tonsils may appear enlarged on examination. This does not necessarily indicate pathology. If a benign state of tonsilar enlargement exists, the tissue will be the same pink color as the rest of the oral mucosa. Enlarged tonsils of this nature are called *hypertrophied*.

PHARYNGITIS

The term pharyngitis has many implications. Obviously, when the word is defined for its actual meaning, it is simply "inflammation of the pharynx." Unfortunately, pharyngitis is not that simple.

A viral pharyngitis may be very minor or it may cause many unpleasant symptoms. Symptoms of a less intense sore throat may cause mild discomfort with swallowing, a low grade fever, rhinorrhea, lethargy, etc. A more severe sore throat may cause marked throat pain and difficulty in swallowing, an erythematous and exudative pharynx, swollen glands, overall weakness, etc. Both can be the description of a viral infection.

The etiology of pharyngitis can be documented by obtaining a throat culture (a strep screen). If this is positive—in other words, if growth on the culture plate occurs—then a diagnosis of a streptococcal (strep) infection can be made.

Many bacterial throat infections are caused by strep and may cause intense soreness and other systemic symptoms. On the other hand, it is easy to be fooled by lack of intense symptoms. However, in general, a strep throat will manifest with a cherry red exudative pharynx, an elevated temperature, and cervical lymphadenopathy (especially in the anterior cervical chain).

The treatment differs for a viral pharyngitis and a strep throat. Antibiotics are warranted for a strep infection. In some instances, antibiotics are given for prophylactic purposes, whether strep exists or not. This is not usually done for a healthy adult, and a great deal of patient education is necessary to help the patient understand the reason for just treating with the supportive measures. It is easy to be deceived by a pharyngitis. Therefore, the patient with more than a minor sore throat irritation should be referred for a throat culture and proper treatment.

PALPATION

The tongue is not routinely palpated unless there is an obvious abnormality on the surface, sides, or under the tongue. If the tongue requires palpation, it is easiest if the patient sticks his tongue out and the examiner holds the tip of the tongue between two pieces of gauze. With the other hand gloved, the examiner palpates the area in question. If other abnormalities appear anywhere in the mouth, the examiner should palpate those as well.

THE NOSE AND PARANASAL SINUSES

Anatomy

The nose has two main functions. It is the air conditioner of the respiratory system and it enables us to use our sense of smell. The nose, in conjunction with the paranasal sinuses, filters, warms, and moistens the air. The sinuses act as voice resonators and also help to reduce the weight of the skull.

To describe the nose anatomically, it is most logical to start with the external structures. The *vestibule* is the first identifiable feature and it is an opening which surrounds the *nares* (Fig. 7.5). The vestibule is separated medially by a skin-covered cartilaginous structure called the *columnella.* This is the bottom of the bony structure which separates the nares, called the *septum.* Both cartilage and bone comprise the septum. The bottom of the septum is cartilaginous. As it progresses up towards the orbital area, it becomes more bony. The lining of the nares is mucosa covered with cilia. The nasal mucosa appears red and more vivid in color than the oral mucosa due to the rich blood supply feeding the area. If this lining lacks the characteristic red color or appears gray-blue and boggy, then there is probably a strong allergy history.

The *turbinates* lie laterally to the septum. These are bony, vascular structures with a meatus in between each turbinate. There are three turbinates: superior, middle, and inferior. There is a corresponding meatus for each turbinate. Each meatus is named for the turbinate above it. The reason one gets a "stuffy" nose with sinus problems or excessive tearing is because the middle meatus drains the sinuses and the inferior meatus drains the nasolacrimal duct (Figs. 7.6A and B).

PARANASAL SINUSES

The eight paranasal sinuses are air-filled cavities with ciliated mucous membrane linings (Fig. 7.6A). Only the *frontal* and *maxillary* sinuses are accessible to physical examination. The *ethmoid* and *sphenoid* sinuses are accessible only with skull films (Fig. 7.6A). The frontal sinuses are located above the eyebrow in each eye. They are separated by the septum. These sinuses are absent at birth and do not

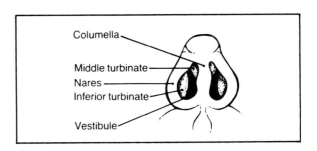

FIGURE 7.5
External structures of the nose.

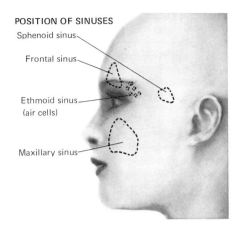

POSITION OF SINUSES

Sphenoid sinus

Frontal sinus

Ethmoid sinus
(air cells)

Maxillary sinus

A

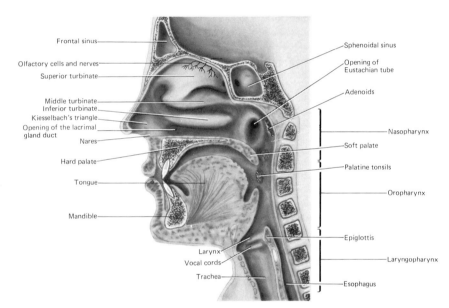

Frontal sinus

Olfactory cells and nerves

Superior turbinate

Middle turbinate
Inferior turbinate
Kiesselbach's triangle
Opening of the lacrimal
gland duct

Nares

Hard palate

Tongue

Mandible

Larynx
Vocal cords
Trachea

Sphenoidal sinus

Opening of
Eustachian tube

Adenoids

Nasopharynx

Soft palate

Palatine tonsils

Oropharynx

Epiglottis

Laryngopharynx

Esophagus

B

FIGURE 7.6
A. Position of the sinuses. *B.* The structure of the nose and pharynx.

develop until 7 or 8 years of age. The maxillary sinuses are the largest of all the sinuses. They can hold up to 20 cc of fluid. These sinuses lie along each maxilla and are present at birth.

History

An overall review for this area includes inquiry about: problems with sinus pain; postnasal drip, nasal obstruction, discharge, or stuffiness; frequent colds; allergies; and epistaxis (nosebleeds) or history of traumatic injury. When the history for any of these problems is positive, further data are required. For instance, if the patient states he has a history

of "nosebleeds," certain information should be elicited:

1. What exactly does the patient mean by a "nosebleed"?
2. How much blood is there? Less than a teaspoon? More than a tablespoon? Does the blood seem to "run" out? For how long? What color is the blood: red, brown? Are there clots? Is only one nostril involved?
3. How frequently do they occur?
4. When was the last episode? What was the patient doing when it occurred? What is he usually doing when they start?
5. What measures are taken to stop the

bleeding? Has treatment been sought in the past? Describe what was done and the outcome.

6. What medicine is the patient taking? How much? How often?

7. Does the patient have any illnesses (i.e., hypertension)?

8. Is there anyone in the family with the same problem?

If allergies exist, an allergy history should be elicited. The nurse should find out what the patient is allergic to, how that was determined (i.e., scratch tests), how the allergy manifests, what treatment is implemented, what time of year seems to be the worst, and what (if any) environment aggravates or alleviates the problem.

To complete the review of the nose and sinuses, the patient should be asked if there is any history of trauma (including an explanation about the course of events) and whether he has noticed change in his ability to smell.

Physical Assessment

The nose is inspected and palpated. The paranasal sinuses are palpated, percussed, and transilluminated. Equipment used for examination of the nose and paranasal sinuses includes a nasal speculum and a head lamp, or else an otoscope with the wide, short speculum tip and a bright penlight. The patient is usually sitting upright for this exam. A child may be most comfortable and relaxed in a parent's lap.

NOSE

The outside of the nose is inspected and palpated. Any unusual skin markings, obvious deviation of the septum (asymmetry), discharge, or flaring of the nares should be noted. If recent trauma has occurred, there may be edema or discoloration as well. The area should be palpated for tenderness, swelling, and structural deviations.

Next, the nasal passages are checked for patency. This is accomplished by the examiner occluding one naris, while the other naris remains unoccluded (Fig. 7.7). With the examiner's opposite hand placed under the open naris, the patient is asked to blow out through his nose. If the naris is patent, the examiner will feel the air against her hand. This procedure is then done on the other nasal passage.

Last, the nasal mucosa, septum, and turbinates are examined. For this portion of the exam, the otoscope with the nasal speculum tip is needed. The examiner places her hand on the patient's head, and her thumb on the patient's nose, gently guiding the head backward. With her hand firmly placed on the patient's head, she can control the degree of movement and stabilize herself as well as the patient. After the patient's head is at the angle desired, the instrument is inserted in the nose about one centimeter along the lateral wall (Fig. 7.8). The septum should not be touched. Like the ear canal, the septum has many nerve endings and is very sensitive when touched.

The anterior aspect of the nose is examined first. The mucosa is inspected for color, lesions, discharge, swelling, and evidence of bleeding. The nasal septum is checked for deviation, lesions, and superficial blood vessels. Adults tend to have short black hairs on the mucosa covering the septum near the nares. In the elderly, there is an increased amount of these hairs. To visualize the turbinates, the examiner tips the patient's head back a little more. This should reveal the turbinates without having to insert the speculum any farther. The examiner should see the inferior and middle turbinates, which are separated by the middle meatus. This area is inspected for edema, polyps, and change in color.

PARANASAL SINUSES

The frontal and maxillary sinuses are palpated and percussed for tenderness. (Remember that the frontal sinuses do not develop in children until 7 or 8 years of age, thus there is no need to examine them until that point.) There are two accepted methods. The first method involves the application of gentle pressure over the frontal sinuses and then the maxillary sinuses (Fig. 7.9). Pain elicited on palpation of any area indicates some degree of irritation. Immediate percussion (see Chapter 2, page 61) is the other method used to detect tenderness.* The examiner simply taps the palmar aspect of the index or second finger lightly over each sinus. Once again, tender areas may be indicative of a blocked sinus.

---

* In this method of percussion no pleximeter is used.

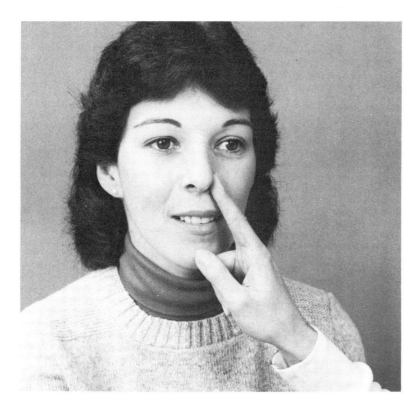

FIGURE 7.7
Testing for nasal patency.

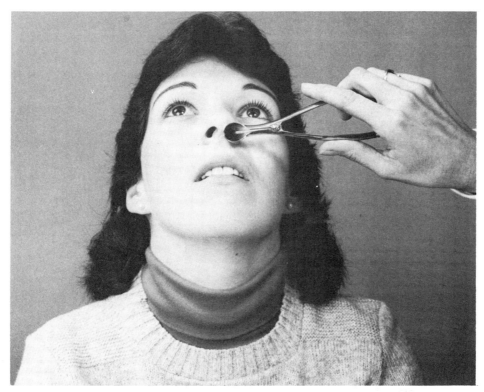

FIGURE 7.8
Inspecting the nasal mucosa.

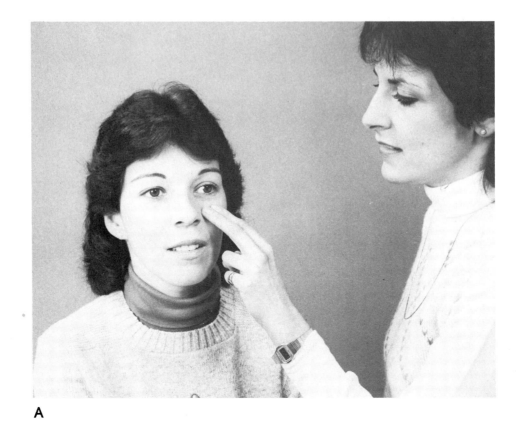

A

B

FIGURE 7.9
*Palpating the sinuses. **A.** The maxillary. **B.** The frontal.*

Transillumination is a technique used to detect abnormalities in the shape and size of the sinuses, but its success and reliability are questionable. Without an extremely dark room and a very bright penlight, the exam is not worth the time it takes to perform. This technique is only performed when the patient presents with a problem. Normally the sinuses are asymmetric in shape and size, so unless there is a question of significant obstruction or inflammation, there will be no findings. It is worth noting that in the elderly, the paranasal sinuses may transilluminate more easily due to the decreased amount of subcutaneous tissue in the face. However, to check for blockage of the maxillary sinuses, the examiner simply places the lit penlight in the patient's mouth. The patient is then instructed to place his lips tightly around the penlight (Fig. 7.10). Both maxillary sinuses will illuminate with

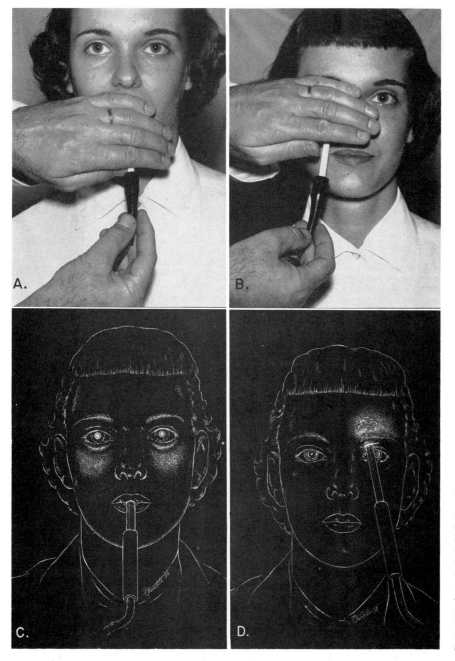

FIGURE 7.10
*Techniques of transillumination of the paranasal sinuses. **A.** The maxillary sinuses. **B.** The frontal sinuses. **C.** Illumination of the maxillary sinuses. **D.** Illumination of the frontal sinuses. (From Saunders, W. E. Ears, nose, and throat. In Prior, J., and Silberstein, J. (Eds.), Physical Diagnosis: The History and Examination of the Patient (5th ed.). St. Louis: C. V. Mosby, 1973, p. 167, with permission.)*

a pink cast. A red reflex will appear in the pupil as well. If either sinus is blocked, the light will not be seen through the cheek.

To check the frontal sinuses, the lit penlight is placed under the eyebrow in the periorbital arch. The examiner must be careful not to burn the patient. These sinuses are tested one at a time. If they are not infected or blocked, their illumination will also give off a pink cast (Fig. 7.10).

Screening Examination of the Nasopharynx

1. Inspection of the lips and oral cavity
2. Assessment of swallowing
3. Assessment of palatal movement
4. Assessment of tongue movement
5. Assessment of nasal patency
6. Inspection and palpation of the nose
7. Inspection of the nasal mucosa and turbinates
8. Palpation (or percussion) of the frontal and maxillary sinuses*

---

* Adults only

EXAMPLE OF A RECORDED HISTORY AND PHYSICAL

SUBJECTIVE:

Chief Complaint: "Sore throat for 2 days."

HPH: (History given by mother and son.) This 11-year-old male considers himself "basically healthy." Woke up yesterday and noticed that he had "difficulty swallowing" and a "burning" pain in the back of his throat. The pain worsened as the day went on. He did nothing for it and went to school. This morning he awoke and the pain was more intense and his right ear hurt "inside" his head. No discharge. Took temperature and it was 100.6°F orally. He also complains of nasal stuffiness and clear drainage of 1 week duration. Today he feels tired, slept most of the day, and has no appetite. He has no dizziness, headache, cough, nausea, vomiting, or diarrhea. Mother gave him two adult aspirin this A.M. He has also been taking throat lozenges every 3 hours or so. He gets about two sore throats every winter. Last winter, he had four sore throats and two were cultured and diagnosed as "strep." He is allergic to penicillin, gets a "rash all over his body." His sister had a strep throat, diagnosed 1 week ago. He feels he cannot go to school as long as he feels this badly.

OBJECTIVE:

T.101°F orally; P. radial 76; R. 18; B.P. (sitting) 110/70.

Ears: Left and right: No discharges and no tenderness with palpation of external ear. Canals clear. Right tympanic membrane: Redness throughout drum; landmarks not visible—retraction. Left tympanic membrane: Unremarkable.

Nose: Clear drainage in each naris. Mucosa red. No inflammation or polyps. Paranasal sinuses (frontal and maxillary) nontender.

Throat: Anterior and posterior pillars red. No tonsils. Exudative patch on left posterior pillar.

Neck: Supple. Enlarged palpable, tender lymph nodes along right anterior cervical chain. Kernig's sign and Brudzinski's sign negative.

Chest: Regular respirations. No retraction. No tenderness on palpation or dullness to percussion. No adventitious breath sounds.

Abdomen: Bowel sounds audible in all four quadrants. Soft. No tenderness or masses on palpation. Liver span 6 cm., nontender. Spleen not palpable or tender.

REFERENCES

DeWeese, D., & Saunders, W. (1982). Textbook of Otolaryngology (6th ed.). St. Louis: C. V. Mosby.

Jarvis, A., & Gurlin, R. (1972). Minor orofacial abnormalities in an Eskimo population. Oral Surgery, 33, 417–26.

Martin, J., & Crump, E. (1972). Leukoedema of the buccal mucosa in Negro children and youth. Oral Surgery 34, 49–58.

McDonald, C., & Kelly, P. (1975). Dermatology and venereology. In R. Williams, (Ed.), Textbook of Black Related Diseases. New York: McGraw-Hill, pp. 513–92.

Spuhler, J. (1950). Genetics of three normal morphological variations: Patterns of superficial veins of the anterior thorax, peroneus tertius muscle and number of villate papillae. Cold Spring Harbor Symposium on Quantitative Biology, 15, 175–89.

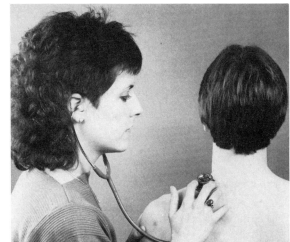

8

The Respiratory System

Every system in the body interfaces with the respiratory system in one fashion or another. For example, the color and quality of the nailbeds and the generalized color of the integumentary system are affected by the O_2–CO_2 balance in the body. The amount of oxygenated blood circulating throughout the body depends not only on the quality of the lung tissue, but also on the "health" of the veins and arteries of the cardiovascular system. Thus the nurse, to make an accurate evaluation of the respiratory system, must understand all its interfacings.

Any degree of change within this system can cause significant problems for the patient. The nurse must be able to quickly assess alteration of respiratory status. In addition to doing a thorough history and physical, she must be able to distinguish between acute and chronic signs. The patient with a chronic obstructive pulmonary disease often depends on the nurse to make decisions and act quickly in order to prevent an acute attack or severe distress.

DEVELOPMENTAL CHANGES IN THE RESPIRATORY SYSTEM THROUGHOUT THE LIFESPAN

Throughout the course of one's life there are structural and physiologic changes that affect the respiratory system. For the most part, these alterations do not affect the quality of respiration. Certainly, if disease is present, the efficiency of this system will decrease. Most of the structural changes occur early in life and in the elderly years. It is among the elderly population that the nurse might be dealing with respiratory decompensation due to the normal aging process.

One of the first tasks a newborn must accomplish is to breathe. Within seconds, the breathing becomes cyclic, rhythmic and consistent. If this respiratory pattern does not occur within seconds after birth, serious problems arise.

The neonate has a round chest. In fact, the lateral measurement of the thorax will be equal to the shoulder to shoulder span. At birth, the chest circumference averages 33 to 35 centimeters (approximately 13–14″). The chest circumference is equal to or one inch less than the head circumference. The chest measurement increases 15 centimeters (6″) the first year. Chest circumference is measured throughout the first year of life and sometimes longer. The shape of the chest will begin to change and become less rotund during the baby's first year of life. The shoulder to shoulder measurement becomes longer while the lateral figure does not change much.

Infants utilize their abdominal muscles for respiration, as opposed to their thoracic muscles. Their musculature is not sufficiently developed for the thoracic breathing that takes over later. The respiration rate of an infant is fairly rapid and can easily be as high as 45+ per minute. Newborns are nose breathers (rather than mouth breathers) and their respiratory rate may be as high as 80 times per minute. The respiratory rate decreases as the child gets older.

The chest wall is thin at birth. As the intercostal muscles develop, the chest wall thickens. Because of the thin wall, breath sounds seem loud and easy to hear. The percussion note of an infant's lung is more resonant (or hyperresonant) than in adults. (See discussion of percussion notes, page 200.) The breath sounds one hears predominantly in this age group are bronchovesicular (see discussion of breath sounds, page 202), again because of the thin chest wall.

As the infant becomes a toddler, the respiratory rate slows down, the breath sounds become less harsh, and the roundness of the chest decreases. Most of these changes are due to the growth of the child and the development of the intercostal muscles. Although the breath sounds are less harsh, they are still mostly bronchovesicular. The child remains an abdominal breather, but is probably no longer breathing solely through his nose. During this time, the circumference of the chest is growing more rapidly than the head circumference.

As the toddler approaches school age, his abdominal breathing will probably become thoracic. During late school age or early adolescence, the respiratory rate slows down and is closer to the rate of an adult (16–20 per minute). In a healthy person, other than the continued development of the musculature of the thorax and the change in respiratory rate, there are not many changes in the respiratory system during childhood, adolescence, and young and middle adulthood.

The next significant physiologic or structural changes seen in the respiratory system occur in the elderly years. The thorax returns to a more round shape again. This is due to the musculoskeletal changes associated with aging—the costal cartilages may calcify, osteoporosis may be present, and the thoracic muscles begin losing some of their tone. The result of these changes often produces a *kyphosis* (an increased convexity of the thoracic spine) (see Fig. 8.8). This kyphotic appearance can give the impression of a barrel chest which may or may not affect the respiratory process. Severe kyphosis can affect respiratory efficiency.

There are also changes in the lung tissue itself. The alveoli function less efficiently because of a decrease in the elastin and collagen. The result is a decrease in the effectiveness of pulmonary diffusion because of the less fibrous alveoli. Additionally, the vital capacity, inspiratory reserve volume, and maximum breathing capacity are decreased as well. The expiratory reserve volume, however, is increased because much air remains in the lung after each breath.

Because of the physiologic changes and environmental contaminants that the elderly have been exposed to (smoking, occupational hazards, etc.) as a population, they are at high risk for respiratory disease. Problems that occur among this population are chronic obstructive pulmonary disease, cancer of the lung, and a generalized decrease in the efficiency of the respiratory system. The gradual decline in efficiency occurs in the vital capacity and the air exchange of the lung tissue. The amount of oxygen circulating in the bloodstream of the young adult can be as much as 60 percent greater than the amount in the bloodstream of the elderly person. In addition, a decreased expansion of the rib cage and loss of muscle tone can decrease the ability of the older person to cough forcefully. Elderly, with chronic respiratory problems, find their symptoms aggravated by cold, dampness, or humidity. Cancer of the lung is the most common site for cancer in males 55 to 74 years of age and second most common site in males over the age of 75 (Steinberg, 1983).

ANATOMY

The respiratory system begins at the nares and ends at the diaphragm, where the lower lobes of the lungs lie. However, for the purpose of this chapter only the thoracic cavity will be discussed, including the area extending from the trachea through both lung fields.

Pathology in the respiratory system is often localized. In order to be able to describe the boundaries of an involved area, certain imaginary and anatomic landmarks must be used.

Landmarks

The chest is assessed laterally, anteriorly, and posteriorly. Imaginary vertical lines are drawn on both aspects from the shoulder to the pelvis. These divide the thorax lengthwise (Fig. 8.1). The most commonly used terms are the *midsternal* line, the *midclavicular* line, the *anterior axillary* line for the anterior aspect of the thorax; the *midaxillary* line and *posterior axillary* line for lateral view; and the *scapular* and vertebral (or *spinal*) lines for the posterior thorax. Actual lines called pigmentary demarcation lines may appear on the anterior chest and arms. These lines are considered normal pigmentary variants and are common in Oriental and American black patients. Figure 8.2 illustrates patterning of pigmentary demarcation lines (Wasserman, 1974; Sebmanowitz & Krivo, 1975).

The other set of landmarks used to describe the chest are not imaginary lines, but bony prominences that help the examiner count ribs and rib spaces (see discussion fol-

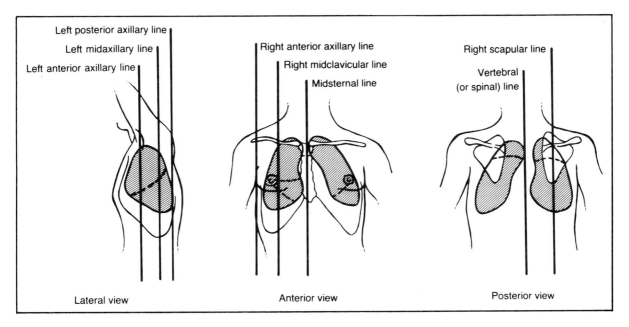

FIGURE 8.1
Landmarks of the thorax.

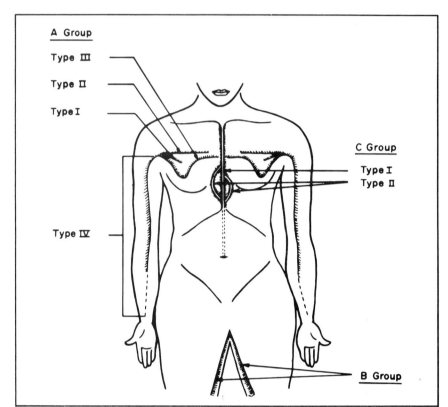

FIGURE 8.2
Demarcation lines of pigmentation (feathered and hyphenated) found in Japanese, after Miura. (Ventral axial lines of inner thigh, to which Group B may correspond, are usually shown in posterior view.) (From Sebmanowitz, V. J. and Krivo, J. M. Comparison of Negroes with Japanese. British Journal of Dermatology, 93, 371–377, 1975, with permission.)

lowing). Counting the ribs aids in mapping out the location of specific organs, consolidations, tumors, etc. This landmark system is also helpful when learning to examine the heart.

ANTERIOR THORAX

The easiest bony landmark to find is the *suprasternal notch* (Fig. 8.3). This U-shaped curve is at the top of the *manubrium*. The ridge-like feature below the manubrium is the *sternal angle* (or *angle of Louis*). This ridge adjoins the second rib. The intercostal space immediately below the second rib is the second intercostal space (also known as ICS). All intercostal spaces are named for the ribs above them. Below the second ICS is the third rib and below that the third ICS, etc.

The body of the sternum is attached to the first seven ribs, shown in Figure 8.3. By using the 2ICS as the starting point, it is not difficult to then locate the next four ribs and their respective intercostal spaces.

The *xiphoid process* is the bony prominence at the bottom of the sternum. The eighth, ninth, and tenth ribs terminate medially at the costal margin. An imaginary angle called the *costal angle* describes the area between the costal margins. The eleventh and twelfth ribs are free-floating and do not articulate with anything anteriorly. The other anatomic features of the rib cage that are important to be familiar with are the *costochondral junctions*. These are located in the middle of each rib (Fig. 8.3). This junction is formed during fetal development and is often a site for an inflammatory response or traumatic injury in the thoracic area.

POSTERIOR THORAX

Of the bony landmarks used to classify boundaries on the posterior aspect of the chest, the spinal column is the most obvious feature. When the patient flexes his head forward, a bony prominence can be palpated at the base of the neck called the *vertebrae prominens*. This is the spinous process of C_7. The easily palpable but not quite as prominent protuberance below C_7 is T_1. Under the scapula lie ribs 2–8. The second rib lies at the most superior aspect of the scapula and the eighth rib lies under the lowest point of the scapula.

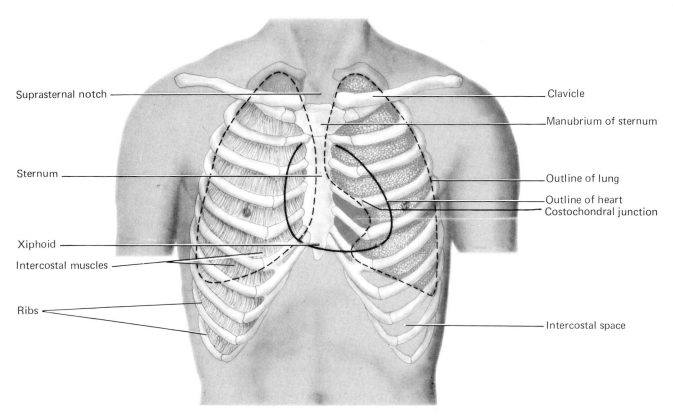

FIGURE 8.3
The thorax: Thoracic cage and position of organs within it. (From Heagarty, M., et al. Child Health: Basics for Primary Care. New York: Appleton-Century-Crofts, 1980, p. 138, with permission.)

LUNGS

After locating all these landmarks, the examiner should be able to picture where the lungs lie. They extend from just above the clavicles (3 cm above) to about the level of the diaphragm shown in Figures 8.3 and 8.4. Anteriorly the lower lobes end at the sixth rib at the midclavicular line (also known as MCL) and at the eighth rib at the midaxillary line. Posteriorly, T_{10}, T_{11}, and T_{12} mark the lower base of the lungs. The precise range is affected by the depth of inspiration (Fig. 8.4).

There are three lobes of the right lung and two lobes of the left. Fissures divide each lung into specific regions (Fig. 8.4). The *oblique fissure* bisects the lung posteriorly at T_3 and extends to the fifth rib anteriorly at the midclavicular line. Since the right lung has upper, middle, and lower lobes, it has an additional fissure. The *right horizontal fissure* separates the right-upper lobe (RUL) and the right-middle lobe (RML). It extends anteriorly from the fifth rib at the midaxillary line to the fourth rib at the midsternal level (Fig. 8.4).

TRACHEA AND BRONCHUS

After air is inhaled, it descends through the *trachea* to the *bronchus* and then to the lungs. The trachea is a long, thin, tube-like structure that lies midline in the neck. The trachea connects to the *main bronchus* (into the right and left bronchus) which bifurcates anteriorly at the level of the *Angle of Louis* (*or sternal angle*) and posteriorly at T_4 (Fig. 8.5). The bifurcated bronchi branch into smaller airway mechanisms called *bronchioles*. From there, the air is carried to the *alveoli*.

HISTORY

The review of this system is not lengthy if there are no present concerns. A general overview of this system includes questions about chest pain with breathing; cough; shortness of breath; night sweats; frequent upper respiratory infections; any history of emphysema,

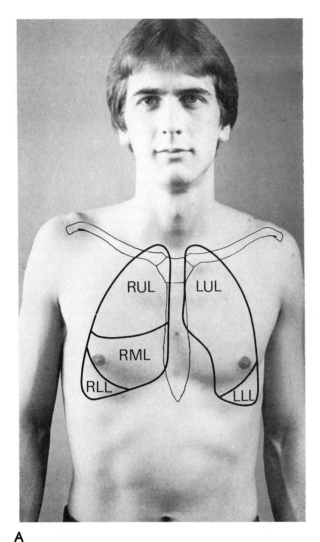

A

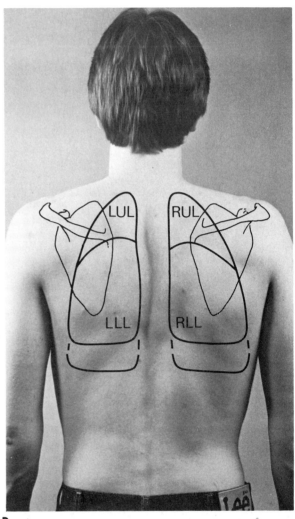

B

FIGURE 8.4
Borders of the lungs. **A.** Anterior view. **B.** Posterior view. (Continued.)

pneumonia, bronchitis, asthma, hemoptysis, or tuberculosis; last tests for tuberculosis (e.g. PPD, monovac) and results; when and why the last chest x-ray was taken and the results, if known; and details about smoking habits. If a patient does smoke, he should be asked what he smokes (cigarettes, pipes, cigars), how much, and for how long. He should also be asked about the presence of a smoker's cough. If this cough exists, a full description is required (i.e., when it occurs, color of sputum, etc.). It is also helpful to note whether or not the patient has ever tried to stop smoking. If so, for how long was he successful and how did he stop (i.e., support groups, hypnosis, nicotine chewing gums, etc.).

The patient is asked if he has ever had a

past history of pneumonia, bronchitis, asthma, tuberculosis, or hemoptysis. If any positive responses are given, the following course of inquiry should be pursued:

1. Who treated the problem?
2. With what medication was it treated?
3. Was a hospitalization necessary?
4. Did the problem resolve quickly or did it linger?
5. Were there any complications?
6. Give a short description about the course of the disease.

The patient should be asked if any other family members have a similar problem or other problems pertaining to the respiratory system

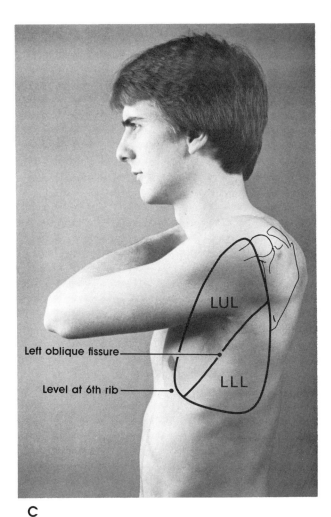

Left oblique fissure

Level at 6th rib

LUL

LLL

C

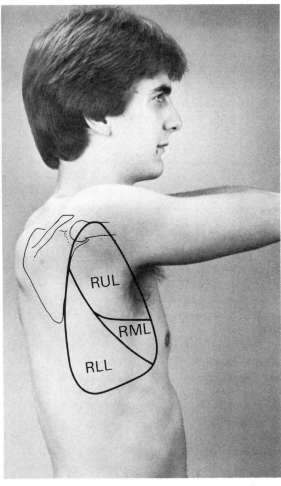

RUL

RML

RLL

D

FIGURE 8.4 (cont'd.)
C. and **D.** Lateral views.

including lung cancer, asthma, emphysema, and tuberculosis.

A frequent complaint involving the respiratory system is a cough. There are several questions to ask regarding this problem:

- *Onset:* When did it begin? Did it start suddenly or gradually?
- *Sequence and chronology:* Has it been consistently present? Did it stop for a period of time and restart? Is it worse at night? Does the cough awaken the patient or keep him from going to sleep?
- *Quality:* Is it high-pitched or low-pitched? Barky? Is it nonproductive or productive? If productive: How much sputum (more or less than a tablespoon)? What color (green, yellow, white, clear)? Does it appear blood tinged (tan or pink—lightly

stained; red, brown, copper—more heavily stained; fresh blood will be bright red, occult blood will be more brown)? Consistency (thick or thin)? Odor (describe)?

- *Setting:* Does it occur at work, home, or school? Where is it most prevalent? What are the ventilation systems like? (This may overlap with *aggravating factors.*)
- *Aggravating factors:* Pollen? Animal dander? Cigarette smoke? Occupational irritants (gases, dust, chemicals, etc.)? Temperature change? Stress?
- *Alleviating factors:* Rest? Medications? Steam? Position? Alteration of the environment? Relief of stress?
- *Associated phenomena:* Chest pain? Fever? Allergies (including dairy products)? A recent cold or postnasal drip? Ear pain or stuffiness? Change in skin color? Nau-

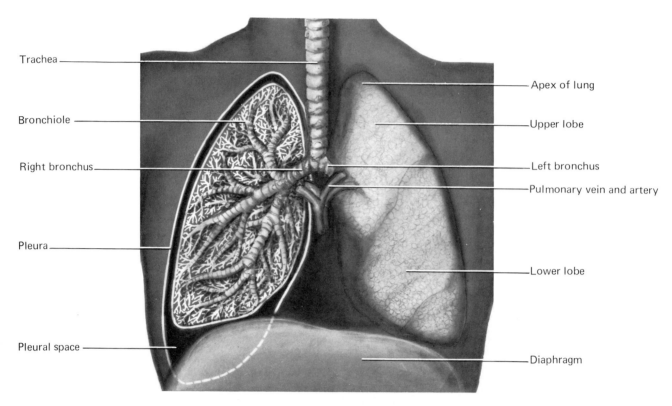

FIGURE 8.5
Structure of the lungs. (From Heagarty, M., et al. Child Health: Basics for Primary Care. New York: Appleton-Century-Crofts, 1980, p. 138, with permission.)

sea, vomiting, diarrhea? Changes in ability and comfort while breathing? Fatigue or weakness?

In children, adolescents, young- and middle-aged adults, the most frequent complaints involve recurrent colds, chronic cough, and allergies. The evaluation of these types of problems follows the same principle of inquiry, using the eight areas of investigation to decipher between relevant and irrelevant data.

PHYSICAL ASSESSMENT

All four techniques of examination are used to assess the respiratory system. Both the anterior and the posterior aspects of the thorax (including the lateral areas and apices of the lungs) are evaluated. For two reasons, the posterior aspect is usually examined first. First, the examiner will have just completed the

head and neck exam, which may have included the posterior approach to the thyroid. Second, the patient is still sitting up and this is the proper position for examining the posterior chest. Assessment of the anterior thorax follows when the examiner returns to the front of the patient. The patient then remains in this position for the cardiovascular exam.

It is important that the total thorax is exposed and that the room is well lit. The only equipment needed is a stethoscope with a diaphragm, a ruler, and a marking pen. Whether examining the anterior or the posterior chest, the order is as follows: inspection, palpation, percussion, and auscultation.

Examination of the Posterior Thorax

INSPECTION
The skin should be examined for lesions, rashes, moles, discoloration, and edematous areas. If any physical abuse has taken place in either a child or adult, one might see some ecchymotic areas or other signs on the thorax.

While marked bruising may indicate pathology or child abuse, bruising of a Vietnamese child's posterior thorax is a common result of the folk treatment *Cao Gio* (Fig. 8.6). This practice is commonly used for treating colds and consists of stroking a child's oiled back with the edge of a coin (Yeatman, et al., 1976).

The thoracic contour should be assessed next. The examiner should note any irregularities in shape, whether congenital or from newly developing problems.

The *anterior–posterior* diameter (A–P diameter) should be visually estimated. This is done by comparing the shoulder-to-shoulder breadth to the lateral span. In Caucasian adults, the average A–P ratio is approximately 1:2. In infants this ratio is equal. By 5 or 6 years of age this ratio is the same as that of an adult. The chest circumference of a child is often measured through the first year of life. (The usefulness of serial chest circumference measurements throughout the first year

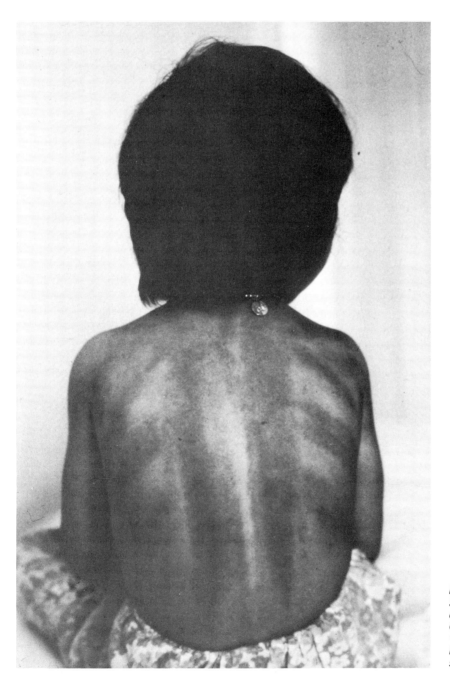

FIGURE 8.6
Symmetrical purpura caused by coin-rubbing. (From Yeatman, G. W., et al. Pediatrics, 58(4):617, 1976. © American Academy of Pediatrics, 1976, with permission.)

of life is questionable. There is questionable reliability and therefore is not always a component of the well child exam.) Precise measurements can be taken with a tape measure. The tape measure is placed around the thorax, using the nipples as landmarks (Fig. 8.7). As a person ages, major changes in the A–P diameter will most likely be signs of pulmonary disease. There are special terms used to describe abnormalities of the chest contour. Irregularities in chest contour are either congenital or the result of significant respiratory dysfunction. A *barrel chest*, (Fig. 8.8A–E and Chart 8.1) for example, is present in the neonate and early infancy and occurs again as a result of the aging process during the elderly years; these are expected findings. A barrel chest can also represent an abnormal process. The patient with a long term disease such as emphysema will often have a barrel-shaped chest and this finding should be recorded. *Pectus carinatum* (pigeon chest) and *pectus excavatum* (funnel chest) (Fig. 8.8A–E and Chart 8.1) are usually congenital. For the most part, they do not effect respiratory status. With severe pectus excavatum, there may be pressure placed on the heart, which could affect the quality of the cardiovascular and respiratory systems.

The rate, rhythm, regularity, and quality of respiration are observed next. The rate is also counted at this time (Chart 8.2). If any irregularities are noted, they are described (Chart 8.3). Respirations should be regular and unlabored. Men and children breathe diaphragmatically, whereas women breathe using costal muscles.

PALPATION

The thoracic cavity is palpated for tenderness, masses, lesions, extent of thoracic expanse, and vocal fremitus. First, using the pads of the fingers, the ribs and intercostal spaces are palpated in a "Z" pattern across and down the posterior chest. Next the lateral aspects of the chest are palpated. Any specific areas of chest pain should always be palpated to see if pain can be elicited or if there is a mass. Any unusual lesions or rashes should be felt for consistency and elevation. The exact location, size, color, shape, and mobility should be described thoroughly.

Assessing the *thoracic expanse* is neither difficult nor time-consuming and reveals significant information about the symmetry of breathing. To palpate thoracic expanse, the examiner places her thumbs around the posterior costal margins at the level of the tenth rib. Thumbs should be placed equidistant from the spinal column to measure symmetry (Fig. 8.9). The patient is then asked to take a deep breath. The examiner observes the movement of her thumbs while the patient inspires. The thumbs should separate symmetrically. The regularity of breathing can also be watched while doing this test.

Vocal fremitus is defined as palpable vibrations through the lung fields. These vibra-

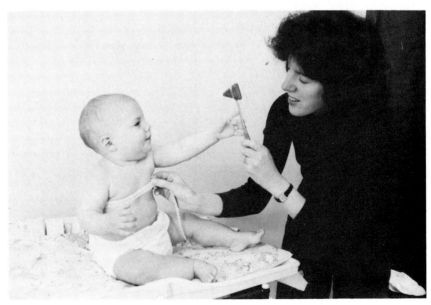

FIGURE 8.7
Measuring chest circumference on an infant.

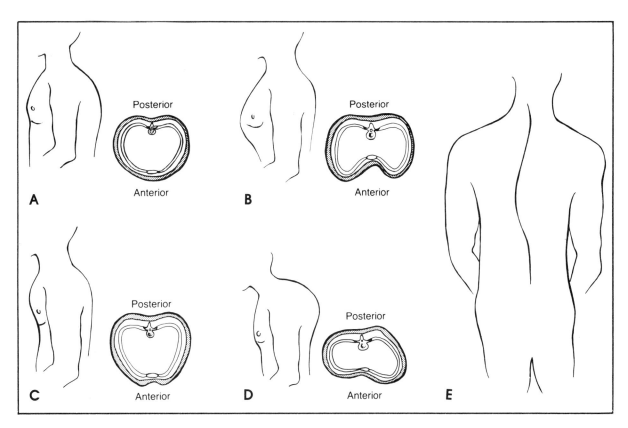

FIGURE 8.8
Abnormalities of the chest contour: ***A.*** *Barrel chest,* ***B.*** *Pigeon chest,* ***C.*** *Funnel chest,* ***D.*** *Kyphosis,*
E. *Scoliosis.*

CHART 8.1
ABNORMALITIES OF CHEST CONTOUR

Abnormality	Description
Barrel chest	The A–P diameter is about equal; typically seen in emphysema
Pigeon chest (pectus carinatum)	The sternum juts anteriorly and the chest looks like that of a chicken
Funnel chest (pectus excavatum)	The sternum points posteriorly; this may cause abnormal pressure on the heart, which could affect function
Lumbosacral deformities (kyphosis and scoliosis)	May cause other defects, depending on the degree (see Chapter 14)

CHART 8.2
NORMAL RESPIRATORY RATES

Adult	12–20/min or 16–20/min
Older child	12–20/min
Toddler	24–30/min
6 months–2 years	Up to 30/min
Newborn	Up to 45/min

CHART 8.3
DESCRIPTION OF ABNORMAL RESPIRATORY PATTERNS

Irregularities	Description
Tachypnea	Rapid superficial breathing ↑ 20
Bradypnea	Slow deep breathing ↓ 12
Apnea	Cessation of breathing
Hyperventilation	Fast, deep, and constant breathing: offsets O_2–CO_2 imbalance, causing dizziness, etc.; often a stress-related reaction
Kussmaul's	Deeper than normal respiration; often seen in acidosis
Cheyne–Stokes	Often in a critically ill patient; regular episodes of apnea occur within a regular breathing pattern
Stertorous breathing	Rattly snoring type of respiration; often heard in the terminal states
Dyspnea	A subjective complaint of difficulty in breathing
Orthopnea	A subjective complaint; air gets "stuffy" when patient is sleeping and he feels a need to sit up or sleep on extra pillows

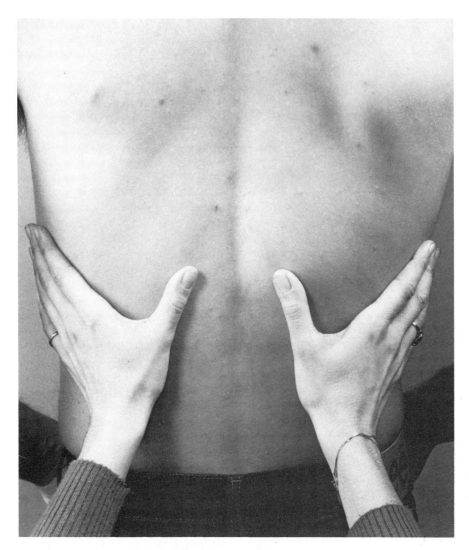

FIGURE 8.9
Palpating for thoracic expanse.

tions are most easily felt when the patient says a word like "99" and the palmar aspects at the base of the fingers of the examiner's hands are placed along either side of the spinal column (Fig. 8.10). The ulnar side of the hand may also be used. One or both hands may be used. The goal is to compare corresponding parts of the thorax (Fig. 8.10). If two hands are used at the same time, they are placed over corresponding regions along each side of the spinal column. It is important to compare the vibrating response felt simultaneously. If only one hand is used, it is moved from one side to another comparing the corresponding regions. (Fig. 8.10). The upper lobes are palpated first, including the area over the apices; then the mid-thoracic area, to the level

of the diaphragm, and last the lateral flank areas above the diaphragm. The vibrations will be strongest around the tracheal bifurcation and the major bronchus. Although this is a gross test, symmetry of fremitus is expected in the normal, healthy lung.

In an infant, palpation for vocal fremitus is not carried out routinely. However, if it is necessary and an abnormality is suspected, it can be done when the baby cries. Fremitus is altered under the following conditions:

1. A low voice, an obstructed bronchus, chronic obstructive pulmonary disease (COPD) and pleural effusion result in *decreased fremitus.*
2. Pneumonia, large airways, a consoli-

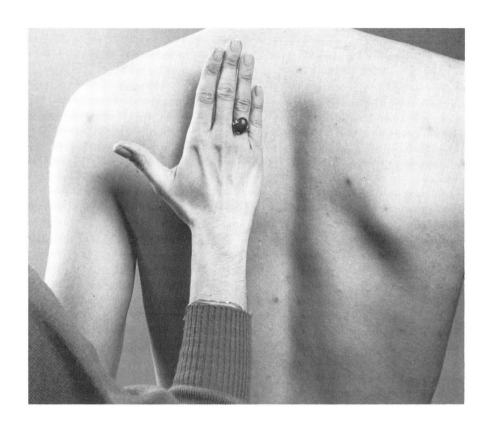

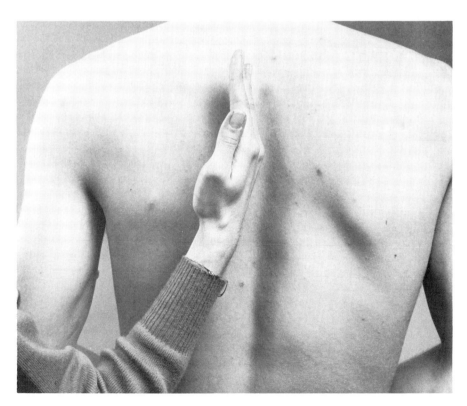

FIGURE 8.10
Alternate methods of palpating for vocal fremitus.

dated area, or other inflammatory processes result in *increased fremitus*.

The level of the diaphragm can be estimated where vocal fremitus stops. Determining the level is also the first step in measuring *diaphragmatic excursion*. (See following discussion.)

PERCUSSION

As described in Chapter 2, percussion is used to determine whether an underlying area is filled with air, fluid, or a solid material. Using the *indirect* or *mediate method* to percuss the thorax (Fig. 8.11), percussion is begun on the posterior thorax. It is important to start at the apices and move toward the lower and lateral aspects of the posterior thorax. The examiner moves from side to side always comparing corresponding areas. (Fig. 8.12). It is considered improper technique to percuss down one

side of the thorax and then the other. Percussion is repeated two or three times over each area. The examiner proceeds at 3-to 5-centimeter intervals down the thorax. The percussion sounds over corresponding areas are compared.

The five notes of percussion are *flat, dull, resonant, hyperresonant* and *tympanic* (Chart 8.4). Percussion notes are relatively consistent throughout the age groups. In infants, however, one finds the lung fields more hyperresonant than resonant. This is due to the close proximity of the lungs to the chest wall, as well as to the large amount of the surface area of the baby's body that the thorax occupies.

In addition to this general orientation, the *posterior* thorax is percussed for diaphragmatic excursion. This span estimates the elevation and lowering of the diaphragm during breathing. (The examiner should keep in mind that the diaphragm descends with inspiration

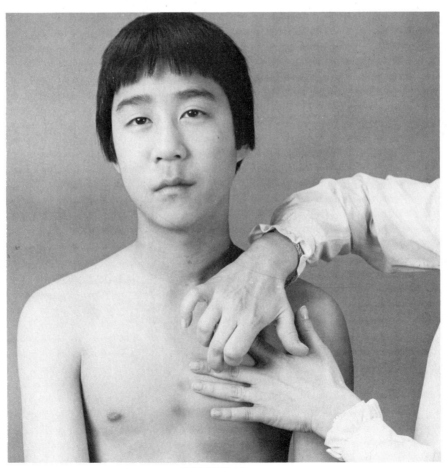

FIGURE 8.11
Indirect percussion.

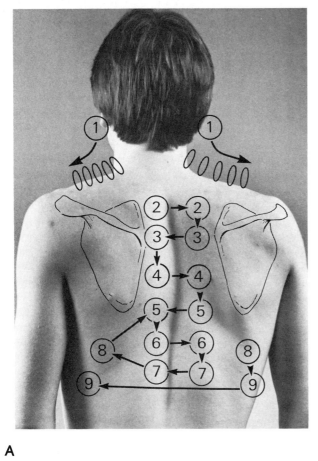

A

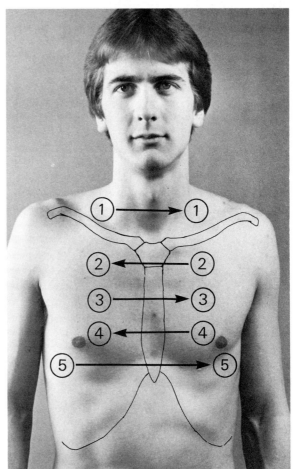

B

C

FIGURE 8.12
Sequence of percussion sites.

CHART 8.4
THE FIVE PERCUSSION NOTES

	Relative Intensity	Relative Pitch	Relative Duration	Example of Location
Flatness	Soft	High	Short	Thigh
Dullness	Medium	Medium	Medium	Liver
Resonance	Loud	Low	Long	Normal lung
Hyperresonance	Very loud	Lower	Longer	Emphysematous lung
Tympany	Loud	*	*	Gastric air bubble or puffed-out cheek

* Distinguished mainly by its musical timbre.
(Adapted from Bates, B. A Guide to Physical Examination (3rd ed.). Philadelphia, J. B. Lippincott, 1983, with permission.)

and ascends with expiration.) The procedure is as follows:

1. The patient takes a deep breath and holds it. This moves the diaphragm downward.
2. The examiner begins percussing downward from an area of resonance along the midscapular line from the bottom of the scapula at about 3 centimeter intervals (Fig. 8.13A).
3. The point where the percussion note changes from resonance to dullness is noted and marked with a pen.
4. The patient is then asked to expire forcefully and hold his breath. This maneuver moves the diaphragm upward (Fig. 8.14A and B).
5. The examiner begins percussing upward from 3 centimeters below the line marked with a pen (Fig. 8.13B). She percusses from dullness until she hears resonance again and marks the spot with a pen.
6. The distance between these points is measured and recorded.

The procedure is repeated on the opposite side. The average span of the diaphragm is 3 to 5 centimeters. It is normally slightly higher on the right side because of the presence of the pancreas.

AUSCULTATION

Auscultation is used to determine the existence of air, fluid, or solid mass in the lung. Any presence of the latter two will obstruct air flow to some degree, thus creating various auscultatory sounds. An overall decrease in air exchange will cause a lessening in the volume of the breath sounds. This can be the re-

sult of a disease process or the aging process in general.

To determine the status of the lungs, the examiner listens for normal breath sounds, adventitious (abnormal) breath sounds, and voice sounds. To auscultate the posterior thorax, the examiner simply places the diaphragm of the stethoscope on the chest (Fig. 8.15) at the points in Figure 8.12. The patient is asked to breathe in and out through his mouth slowly and deeply (more deeply than normal). Many consecutive deep breaths can cause light-headedness. The patient should be given a chance to rest between breaths, if necessary. The examiner must listen through an entire cycle of inspiration and expiration (Fig. 8.15).

An array of breath sounds can be heard throughout the lungs. They will seem louder and more "raspy" in infants and young children. The sounds are named for their location over a specific region of the lung. They are evaluated in terms of their intensity, quality, pitch, duration, location, rate, and rhythm.

The three normal breath sounds are: *vesicular, bronchovesicular,* and *bronchial* (or tubular). Vesicular sounds are heard over most of the lung as a soft, low-pitched sound in which inspiration is longer than expiration. Bronchovesicular breath sounds are heard most clearly where the bronchi and trachea are close to the chest wall and along the scapular area. They are heard as a medium-pitched sound in which inspiration and expiration are about equal. Bronchial breathing produces a loud, high-pitched, blowing sound in which expiration is longer than inspiration. This is heard over the trachea; if it occurs anywhere else in the lung fields, it is always indicative of disease.

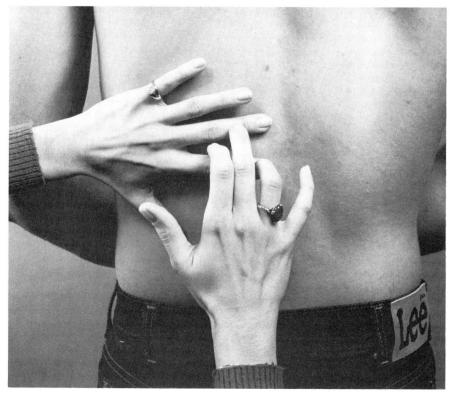

A

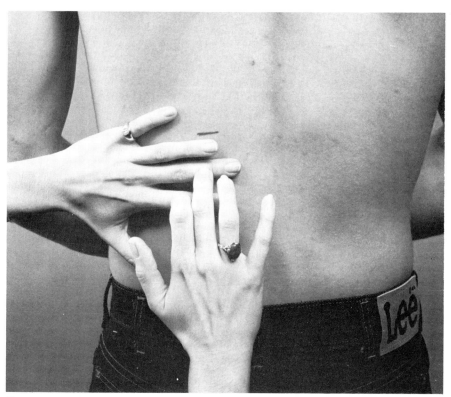

B

FIGURE 8.13
A. Percussing down along the thorax to locate the lower border of the diaphragm *B.* Percussing upward to locate the upper border of the diaphragm after the patient forces the air out of his lungs.

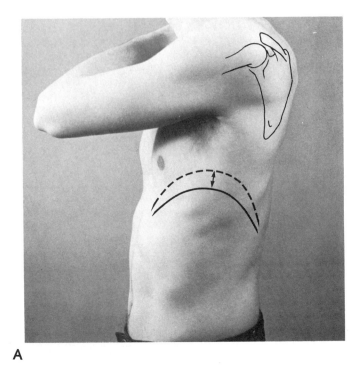

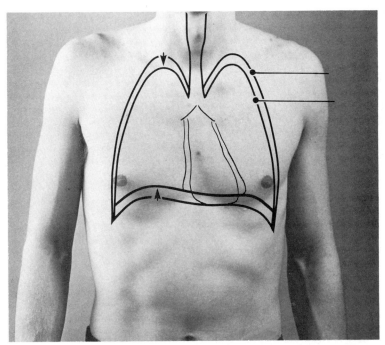

FIGURE 8.14
Movement of the diaphragm during inspiration and expiration. **A.** *Lateral.* **B.** *Anterior.*

Adventitious breath sounds are often heard along with normal breath sounds. The most common abnormal sounds are: *rales, rhonchi,* and *friction rubs.*

Rales are noises that are created when air is traveling through vessels that have abnormal moisture in them (Fig. 8.16). These are noncontinuous noises that do not usually disappear with coughing. They are most frequently heard during inspiration. Rales are divided into three categories: *fine, medium,* and *coarse.* The gradation depends on the

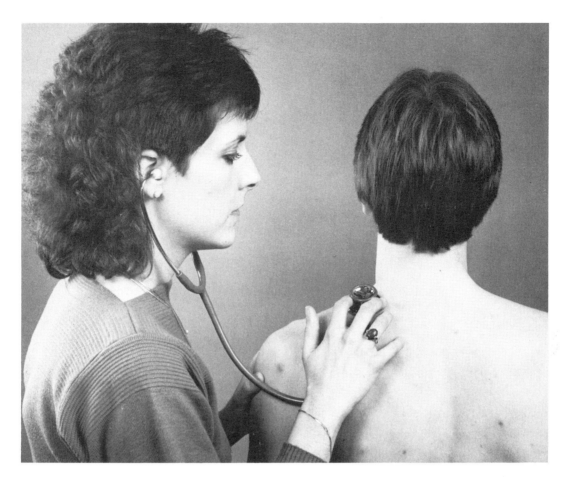

FIGURE 8.15
Auscultating the upper left lobe of the posterior thorax.

amount of moisture and the airway involved. The larger the airway, the louder the rale will be.

Fine rales sound like two hairs rubbing

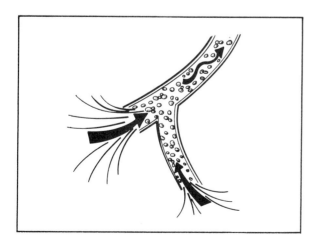

FIGURE 8.16
Air traveling through moisture.

together next to the ear. They usually represent moisture in the alveoli. Fine rales can be heard in disease processes involving the alveoli, such as pneumonia or congestive heart failure.

Medium rales are slightly louder than fine rales. The sound is similar to that of opening a can of soda. These can be heard over the bronchioles, which are larger airways.

Coarse rales are the loudest of the three. They will be heard over the trachea and bronchi. Coarse rales have a gurgling, bubbling quality. They may change in intensity with coughing. Coarse rales usually represent extremely thickened secretions. This type of rale is often equated with the "death rattle" of critically ill or comatose patients.

Rhonchi are adventitious sounds that are the result of air passing through airways that are narrowed or defective, as shown in Figure 8.17. The alteration of the vessel contour by either internal or external compression cre-

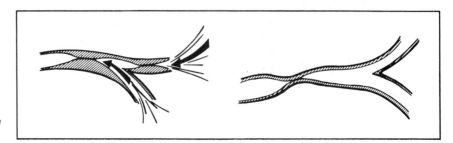

FIGURE 8.17
Air traveling through a narrowed lumen.

ates these abnormal sounds. Rhonchi are due to the presence of exudate, inflammation, asthma, emphysema, or a solid mass. Rhonchi are more easily heard during expiration, although they may be audible during both phases. Rhonchi are characteristically alternated with coughing, especially if there are secretions in the airways in addition to a change in the vessel contour.

There are two types of rhonchi: *sibilant* and *sonorous*. Sibilant rhonchi are musical, high-pitched, and wheezy in nature. Sonorous rhonchi are lower-pitched and sound like snoring (Prior & Silberstein, 1981).

The third adventitious breath sound is the friction rub. It is typically found in the anterior thorax and is outlined in detail on pages 206–207.

One other abnormality that can affect what the examiner hears in the chest is the loudness of the breath sounds. It has already been said that the normal aging process can cause a decrease in breath sounds. This decrease can also be produced by the existence of emphysema, obstruction, pneumothorax, pleural thickening, or any fluid in the pleural space. Although the sounds may be diminished, one may still be able to hear adventitious breath sounds. The sensations palpated with vocal fremitus can be auscultated, too. This is not usually done for screening purposes, but is implemented when pathology is suspected.

The stethoscope is placed in the same places as when listening for breath sounds. The patient is then asked to repeat certain words. The choice of sounds selected varies according to what is being evaluated. The words will be the loudest at the upper and middle lobes along the spinal column.

There are three abnormal voice sounds: *bronchophony, egophony,* and *whispered pectoriloquy.* Bronchophony is increased voice resonance, with the increase primarily in intensity and to some degree in clarity. For this test the patient is asked to repeat "99." The nurse listens over the designated areas. The exact syllables are distinctive and can be heard clearly. In the normal lung the auscultated sounds are muffled. Often accompanying bronchophony are increased fremitus, a dull percussion note, rales, and bronchial breathing. This combination of positive findings over a specific area probably indicates a consolidation.

Egophony is an increased version of bronchophony. The major difference is in the bleating quality of the voice sounds. The patient is asked to say a word with the end syllable having an "ee" sound to it, such as "Tennessee." The noise heard through the stethoscope will be an "a," so that "Tennessee" will sound like "Tennessā." This is most often heard in pulmonary consolidation.

Whispered pectoriloquy indicates a clear interpretation of what the examiner hears through the stethoscope when the patient whispers. The words will sound distinct, clearly like whispers to the examiner as she listens through the stethoscope. This is the most obvious of the three tests and it always indicates consolidation.

Physical Examination of the Anterior Thorax

Inspection
Skin*
Thoracic contour*

Rate and rhythm of
 breathing*
Palpation
 Lesions*
 Tenderness*
 Thoracic expanse

The thumbs of the examiner's hands are placed along the costal margins, while the rest of the hand lies on the lateral aspects of the rib cage. The rest of the procedure is identical to measuring the thoracic expanse on the posterior aspect.

 Vocal fremitus

The procedure is the same as for the posterior thorax. However, in a woman with breast tissue, fremitus will only be palpable in certain areas.

 Pleural friction rubs

This is a pathologic condition in which the inflamed pleural surfaces rub over one another. The auscultated sound is similar to the noise made by two pieces of leather being rubbed together. It is most easily found in the anterolateral chest where the thoracic expansion is greatest. The mapped boundaries of decreased fremitus, increased fremitus, or a friction rub should be recorded specifically.

Percussion
 General orientation

The procedure is the same as for the posterior chest. The area around the heart and liver will produce a dull note. The gastric air bubble (see abdomen, page 290) will be tympanic. Diaphragmatic excursion is not percussed on the anterior thorax.

Auscultation
 Normal breath sounds*
 Adventitious breath sounds*
 Friction rub

This is the same as with palpation, except the rubbing sensation is heard, not felt.

Voice sounds*

* Unless otherwise indicated, the exam is the same as posterior thorax.

CHART 8.5
COMMON CONDITIONS OF THE RESPIRATORY SYSTEM

Condition	Age	Etiology	Subjective (Symptoms That May Be Present)	Objective (Signs That May Appear)
Bronchiolitis	Usually under 1 year	Viral (always first episode of wheezing in an infant)	↓ Appetite No previous history of asthma Dyspnea Fever Audible wheezing	Cyanosis ± Wheezing Retraction ± Nasal flaring ± Low grade temperature Lethargic ± Tachypnea Voice sounds (auscultated), normal or ↑ Crackling rales Possible friction rub
Croup	6 mos.–5 yrs.	Usually viral	Barky cough—worse at night Hoarse Afebrile or low grade temp. Difficult breathing URI[b] symptoms may precede More comfortable sitting	Barky, nonproductive cough Hoarse ± Afebrile or low-grade temp.[a] Labored breathing Inspiratory stridor
Bronchial asthma	Pediatric	Usually allergic (can be infectious, exertional, or from environmental irritants or stress)	Known history of allergy or family history of allergy Cough SOB[b] Dyspnea Wheezing Abdominal or chest pain associated with labored breathing	Prolonged expiratory phase Expiratory wheezes SOB and tachypnea Hyperresonance in lungs Rales Intercostal retracting Use of respiratory accessory muscles ↑ A–P diameter Rhinorrhea Eczema
	Adult	(See Etiology, Bronchial asthma, above)	Recurrent eczema, etc. See Subjective, Bronchial asthma, above)	(See Objective, Pediatric above)
Pneumonia	Any age	Viral, mycoplasmic (common in school-age children, adolescents, and young adults)	Insidious onset Malaise, fever (low grade) Headache, myalgia Cough after 2–3 days of symptoms; usually nonproductive or small amount Chest soreness on inspiration	Low grade temp. Nasal rhinorrhea Mild to moderate red throat Minimally red ear drums Cervical lymphadenopathy Fine to medium rales Rhonchi and/or wheezes over involved area
		Bacterial	Preceded by URI symptoms Shaking chills Elevated temp. Chest pain Cough, productive, "rust-colored" sputum Malaise, weakness, anorexia, myalgias	Elevated temp, rapid pulse and respiration Warm, moist skin Shallow, labored breathing Possible cyanosis Dullness to percussion Possible bronchial breathing Fremitus, normal or ↑
Bronchitis (acute)	Any age	Usually viral (may be bacterial)	Cough, productive, less than 1 tablespoon, mucopurulent Substernal chest pain Labored breathing URI symptoms preceding and associated	Temperature ↑ 101 Malaise, rhinorrhea Normal or resonant percussion note Rhonchi, wheezing, or both Normal or prolonged breath sounds Normal voice sounds and fremitus

CHART 8.5 (Continued)

Condition	Age	Etiology	Subjective (Symptoms That May Be Present)	Objective (Signs That May Appear)
Bronchitis (chronic)	±50	Diagnosis made on subjective data: productive cough at some time of the day for 3 months of the year for 2 or more consecutive years	Smoker for years Dusty occupation Productive cough—sputum on arising and produced again 1–2 times during day Mild dyspnea	Normal rate of respiration No distress at rest May be cyanotic Resonant percussion note Coarse rhonchi Wheezing Normal voice sounds and fremitus Normal or prolonged expiration
Emphysema	±60	Unknown	↑ Dyspnea with ↓ activity Minimal cough SOB History of chronic bronchitis, dusty occupation, smoking	SOB Rapid and shallow respiration Barrel-shaped chest Hyperresonant percussion note ↓ Breath sounds ↓ Voice sounds and fremitus Possible wheezes at the end of respiration
Congestive heart failure	Adult	Myocardial deterioration, often due to ASHD[b] and hypertension	Dyspnea with exertion Rapid, shallow breathing SOB Paroxysmal nocturnal dyspnea Orthopnea Ankle edema Nocturia	SOB Pallor Moist, clammy skin S_3-gallop rhythm Tachypnea Bilateral rales, especially in lower lobes Neck vein distension Bilateral dependent edema in the lower extremities

[a] A high fever may indicate epiglottitis.
[b] URI, upper respiratory infection; SOB, shortness of breath; ASHD, arteriosclerotic heart disease.

There are various acute and chronic conditions that affect the respiratory system. Chart 8.5 describes some of the more common respiratory illnesses in terms of the etiology, subjective, and objective data.

Screening Examination of the Respiratory System

1. Assessment of respirations
2. Inspection of the anterior, posterior, and lateral thorax
3. General palpation of the anterior, posterior and lateral thorax
4. Palpation tactile fremitus of the anterior, posterior and lateral thorax*
5. Percussion of the anterior, posterior, lateral and apical thoracic areas*
6. Auscultation of the anterior, posterior, lateral and apical thoracic areas

---

Adults only

EXAMPLE OF A RECORDED HISTORY AND PHYSICAL

SUBJECTIVE:

Chief Complaint: "My baby has been wheezing for about 2 hours."

HPH: The mother of this 2-year-old states that the baby is in "fair health." He has a 12-month history of this problem. The first episode occurred one day when he went to the baby sitter's and they had a new dog. Baby's mother was called home from work and found the child breathing "fast and hard" and could hear "gurgling" when he "breathed out." She took him to the emergency ward and they gave him "a shot to help him breathe." A prescription was given for "Theophylline Elixir," 1 teaspoon every 6 hours for his wheezing. "The doctor told me he has asthma." The mother states she uses the medicine once a month when "his breath gets short."

Today he was brought in because the same hard breathing started and 1 teaspoon of the medication did not help. The mother noticed his "rib cage was moving funny" and he got "very pale." His wheezing was worse than usual." He had a new terry cloth outfit on and was playing outside in the grass. There was no nasal flaring; no runny nose or previous cold; no animals around; and no new soaps, foods, or linens. There has not been any allergy testing, but dogs and cats do bring on symptoms. No foods bother the patient.

His father had a history of asthma as a child. His mother states that the problem is "frightening and seems to be getting worse."

OBJECTIVE:

T. 99°F (rectal); P. 146 (radial); R. 52; B.P. 90/54 (sitting)

Skin: Pale and diaphoretic. No cyanosis of lips, hands, feet, earlobes. No rashes or lesions.

Nose: No rhinorrhea or nasal flaring.

Chest: Intercostal retractions and use of accessory muscles to breathe. Respirations are rapid and shallow. Bilateral hyperresonance over lung fields. Expiratory wheezes audible in both lungs—middle lobes. Prolonged expiratory phase. No rales. No change in fremitus or voice sounds.

REFERENCES

Prior, J. & Silberstein, J. (1981). Physical Diagnosis: the History and Examination of the Patient. (6th ed.). St. Louis: C. V. Mosby.

Sebmanowitz, V. J., & Krivo, J. M. (1975). Pigmentary demarcation lines: Comparison of Negroes with Japanese. British Journal of Dermatology, 93, 371–77.

Steinberg F. (1983). Care of the Geriatric Patient (6th ed.). St. Louis: C. V. Mosby.

Wasserman, H. (1974). Ethnic Pigmentation: Historical, Physiological, and Clinical Aspects. Amsterdam: Excerpta Medica.

Yeatman, G., Shaw, C., Barlow, M., & Bartlett, G. (1976). Pseudobattering in Vietnamese children. Pediatrics, 58, 616–18.

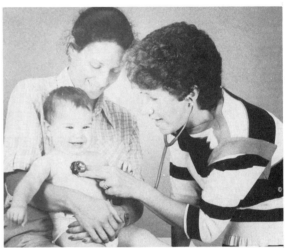

9

The Cardiac and Peripheral Vascular System

The heart is the physiologic pump of the body—such a sterile, technical statement! In truth and in legend, it is much more. Artists and philosophers have for centuries devoted much of their writing to the heart; it was even viewed by some to be the soul. The heart is often personified and seems to possess its own essence. Anyone reading this chapter has experienced and voiced the expressions, "a heartful of love," "a broken heart," and so on.

This chapter deals with the assessment of the cardiac and peripheral vascular system. The heart is the unquestioned star. It should be pictured as a unique instrument expressing and reflecting the integrity of its holistic system. It will function inadequately when one of its arteries is occluded. The "heavy" heart of the unhappy, tense, or depressed person has just as important an effect on the whole system of the person.

Assessment of the cardiovascular system is made at periodic intervals throughout the lifespan. The goal is to identify cardiac risk factors and to detect coronary heart disease and hypertension as early as possible. At every well examination, starting in infancy and continuing through old age, the patient is screened for cardiac risk factors in his personal and family history, for symptoms related to the cardiovascular system, and for objective signs of cardiovascular disease on physical examination. Additional screening measures may be appropriate at specified intervals. These measures include serum cholesterol levels, blood pressure screening, electrocardiogram, and stress testing.

The levels of serum cholesterol are important predictors of risk of developing coronary heart disease. There is no doubt that cholesterol levels can be lowered by diet or drug treatment (Levy, 1980). Epidemiologic studies and animal studies have shown that lowering cholesterol will result in reduced incidence of heart attack. Until recently, however, there was still no proof that lowering cholesterol levels in man diminished coronary heart disease (Podell, 1984). Consequently the value of screening for preventive purposes was unknown. In 1984, the Lipid Research Program published the first well-designed study demonstrating that treatment of patients at risk for coronary heart disease on the basis of their elevated levels of serum cholesterol is accompanied by a significant reduction in coronary heart disease events. Based on these new data definitive guidelines for cholesterol screening may soon be generated. At present laboratory screening is not routinely done on all children. However, a child who has a family history of increased cholesterol levels or premature ischemic heart disease (before age 65 years), or a child who presents with unexplained abdominal pain or is overweight, is encouraged to have serum cholesterol level obtained (Chow, et al., 1984). Lipid researchers recommend a baseline cholesterol screening be done on everyone in early adulthood. Breslow and Summers (Lindberg, 1980) suggest that this baseline be done at age 18; and starting at age 30, that testing be repeated every five years through life. More frequent testing is required if the individual is at risk for cardiovascular disease or develops symptoms.

The incidence of hypertension in the United States is approximately 15 percent (BP 140/90 or greater) (Lindberg, 1980). Prevalence rates increase with age and the rate is greater in the black population than in the white population. Findings of major clinical trials indicate that identification and treatment of hypertension can result in decreased cardiovascular morbidity and mortality (Stamler & Stamler, 1984). The Joint National Committee on Detection, Evaluation, and Treatment of High Blood Pressure (1984) encourages health professionals to measure blood pressure at each patient visit. The committee recommends that those persons who do not have regular contact with the health care system find an opportunity to have their blood pressure checked every 2 years. All blood pressures should be charted on grids so that changes can be monitored.

The use of a resting electrocardiogram to screen asymptomatic, healthy individuals is not adequate. This method is not sufficiently sensitive and its high rate of false negatives can give inappropriate reassurance (Hake, 1978). A resting electrocardiogram and an exercise electrocardiogram, however, are recommended for certain individuals prior to beginning an exercise program. This screening should be conducted on all individuals considering an exercise program who have a family or personal history of cardiovascular disorders, have present or previous signs or symptoms of cardiovascular diseases, or are over 35 years of age (Pender, 1982).

DEVELOPMENTAL CHANGES OF THE CARDIOVASCULAR SYSTEM THROUGHOUT THE LIFESPAN

During the life cycle the cardiac system undergoes many age-related changes. The heart rate of an infant and young child is rapid with comparison to the rate at later stages of development. The average pulse rate for the neonate through the first year of life is 120 beats per minute. The average pulse rate for a 2-year old is 110 beats per minute with a range from 100 to 120. By school age the heart rate begins to slow down. The normal pulse rate for an 8- to 10-year-old child is from 80 to 84. The normal adult heart rate through old age ranges from 60 to 100 beats per minute. Arterial changes in old age may cause the pulse to be normally slightly irregular.

When stressed by exercise the young person's heart beats fast and there is an increase in the strength of muscle contractions. At old age the heart rate is not able to increase in response to physical activity as it did in young adulthood. In addition, after activity it takes longer for the heart rate of the elderly individual to return to basal levels.

Blood pressure, as well as the heart rate, varies with age. The average blood pressure from infancy to the age of 4 is 85 mm Hg systolic and 60 mm Hg diastolic. By the time the child reaches school age the average blood pressure is 100 mm Hg systolic and 65 mm

Hg diastolic. The average blood pressure level for adolescents (115 mm Hg systolic and 72 mm Hg diastolic) is slightly lower than the average blood pressure level for adults (120 mm Hg systolic and 80 mm Hg diastolic). Although these figures represent average blood pressure readings there are wide variations in normal blood pressure range in children and adults. Serial blood pressures must be done to identify an upward or downward trend.

At present, agreement has not been reached with regard to the level of blood pressure that defines hypertension in children (Joint National Committee on Detection, Evaluation, and Treatment of High Blood Pressure, 1984). Chart 9.1 gives the recommended categorial scheme for arterial blood pressure for use in persons aged 18 or older.

There is also disagreement in the literature as to what is the normal range of blood pressure for the elderly. The vascular changes and changes in general health status that accompany aging can cause an increase in the systolic or diastolic readings. As the individual becomes older it is difficult to determine at exactly what point an elevated blood pressure becomes pathologic. Thirty-five percent to 50

CHART 9.1
CLASSIFICATION OF BLOOD PRESSURE IN THE ADULT

Range, mm Hg	Category[a]
Diastolic	
<85	Normal BP
85–89	High normal BP
90–104	Mild hypertension
105–114	Moderate hypertension
≥115	Severe hypertension
Systolic, when diastolic BP is <90	
<140	Normal BP
140–159	Borderline isolated systolic hypertension
≥160	Isolated systolic hypertension

[a] A classification of borderline isolated systolic hypertension (systolic BP, 140 to 159 mm Hg) or isolated systolic hypertension (systolic BP, > 160 mm Hg) takes precedence over a classification of high normal BP (diastolic BP, 85 to 89 mm Hg) when both occur in the same person. A classification of high normal BP (diastolic BP, 85 to 89 mm Hg) takes precedence over a classification of normal BP (systolic BP, < 140 mm Hg) when both occur in the same person.
(From Joint National Committee on Detection, Evaluation and Treatment of High Blood Pressure. The 1984 report of the Joint National Committee on detection and treatment of high blood pressure. Archives of Internal Medicine, 144, 1047, 1984, with permission.)

percent of those persons 65 to 74 will have a blood pressure of more than 160 mm Hg systolic and 90 mm Hg diastolic (Lebow & Sherman 1981). The Joint National Committee on Detection, Evaluation and Treatment of High Blood Pressure (1984) now states that an elevated systolic blood pressure, diastolic blood pressure, or both increase the risk of cardiovascular morbidity and mortality in the elderly. Elderly individuals who have a diastolic blood pressure of 90 mm Hg or greater derived benefit from treatment. Data do not exist to confirm the benefit of treating isolated systolic hypertension in the elderly.

As the individual continues to age it is often difficult to identify normal degenerative changes from pathologic conditions. Cardiac disease is the most common cause of death in the elderly and is the most common cause of curtailed physical activity. The incidence of both *coronary artery disease* and *hypertension* increase with age. These diseases result from a mix of genetic and environmental factors. Although the genetic component of cardiovascular disease is fixed, early identification of contributing environmental factors can result in interventions that may decrease the risk.

Coronary artery disease is a condition in which there is a narrowing of the cardiac vessels that supply blood to the heart. Narrowing of the vessels (*atherosclerosis*) is due to the accumulation of collagen, calcium salts, and lipids on the interior walls (Yurick, 1980). The reduction in the size of the lumen impairs blood flow and increases the load of the left ventricle. Atherosclerotic changes can begin early in life. For many years the changes remain silent; however, eventually the reduced blood flow can become significant enough to cause angina pectoris or myocardial infarction. Risk factors that contribute to the development of atherosclerosis include a stressful lifestyle, high serum cholesterol, obesity, lack of exercise, and smoking. Males in general are at greater risk than females.

The collection of calcium and salt deposits in the vessel wall result in decreased elasticity of the arterial walls. This age-related condition, referred to as *arteriosclerois*, contributes to reduced arterial blood flow. As a result of both atherosclerotic and arteriosclerotic changes the blood flow through the coronary arteries of the elderly adult may be as much as 35 percent lower than in the young adult.

Like coronary artery disease, hypertension results from an interplay of both genetic and environmental factors. The prevalence of hypertension is greatest for blacks and increases across all races with age. Additional risk factors include smoking, obesity, high sodium diet, and stress. Arteriosclerotic and atherosclerotic changes contribute to the increase in the elderly person's blood pressure. These changes decrease the diameter, elasticity, and capacity of the arteries and thereby increase the peripheral resistance. Hypertension results in reduced blood flow with impaired circulation to the brain, heart, and kidney. Secondary effects appear in the form of cardiovascular accident, myocardial infarction, congestive heart failure, and renal failure. The rate of blood pressure increase is related to the original blood pressure. Identification of a tendency toward an elevated blood pressure during early life allows time for interventions to be implemented that

may be effective in preventing or delaying the development of hypertension.

ANATOMY AND PHYSIOLOGY

The Heart

The heart is examined through the anterior chest wall. Figure 9.1 depicts the heart and its location in the chest. The heart is located in the center of the chest, under the sternum, and somewhat to the left of the midline. The upper portion is called the base and the tip is the apex. The apex is about 8 centimeters to the left of the sternum, at the level of the fifth intercostal space, in the midclavicular line. The heart almost appears to lie on its side. It is divided into four chambers—the right and left atria and the right and left ventricles. The part of the heart most accessible to examination is the *right ventricle*. The left ven-

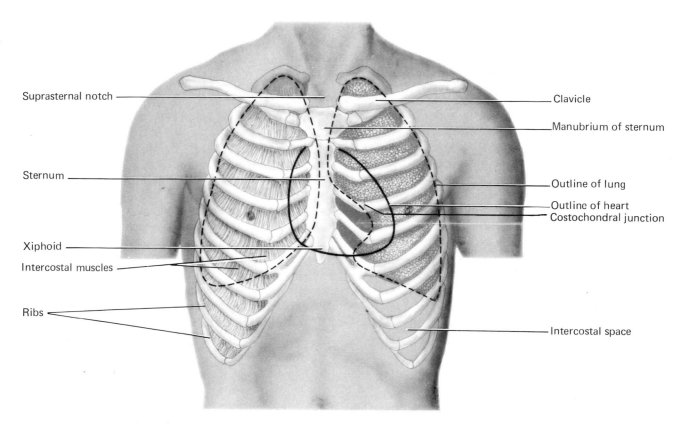

FIGURE 9.1

The thorax: thoracic cage and position of organs within it. (From Heagarty, M., et al. Child Health: Basics for Primary Care. New York: Appleton-Century-Crofts, 1980, p. 138.)

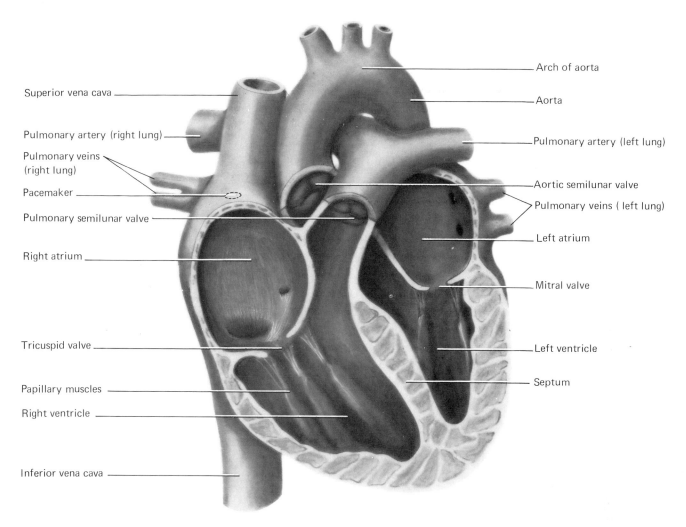

Superior vena cava

Pulmonary artery (right lung)

Pulmonary veins (right lung)

Pacemaker

Pulmonary semilunar valve

Right atrium

Tricuspid valve

Papillary muscles

Right ventricle

Inferior vena cava

Arch of aorta

Aorta

Pulmonary artery (left lung)

Aortic semilunar valve

Pulmonary veins (left lung)

Left atrium

Mitral valve

Left ventricle

Septum

FIGURE 9.2
The heart and great vessels. (From Heagarty, M., et al. Child Health: Basics for Primary Care. New York: Appleton-Century-Crofts, 1980, p. 144.)

tricle presents a much smaller surface to the examiner. It projects a tip that rests at the apex. The *left ventricle* is of critical importance, as it forms the *left border* of the heart and *produces* the *apical impulse* or *point of maximum impulse* (PMI). The *right border* of the heart is formed by the *right atrium.* Neither the right nor the left atrium is directly accessible to examination.

THE CARDIAC CYCLE

Blood flows from one chamber to the other through valves (Fig. 9.2). The tricuspid valve is located between the right atrium and the right ventricle and controls the flow of blood between the two. The corresponding valve on the left is the mitral valve, which controls blood flow from the left atrium to the left ven-

tricle. Because of their positions, these valves are also called atrioventricular valves.

Blood leaves the left ventricle to enter the aorta via the aortic valve. Similarly, blood passes to the pulmonary artery from the right ventricle via the pulmonic valve. The pulmonic and aortic valves have a half-moon appearance and for this reason are often called the semilunar valves.

Closure of the valves is responsible for the first and second heart sounds. In order to adequately explain heart function and sounds, it is necessary to begin with a description of pressure within each chamber and the role the varying pressures play in valve closure. Events in the cardiac cycle are described as they occur in the left side of the heart. This is done for three reasons:

1. The left side of the heart carries the greatest workload.
2. It is therefore often the first to become deficient.
3. The whole process is easier to understand if it is explained in this manner.

Blood flows into the left atrium from the pulmonary veins. As the left atrium fills with blood, its pressure eventually becomes greater than the pressure in the left ventricle. When that happens, the mitral valve opens, the left atrium contracts, and the blood is pumped into the left ventricle. As the pressure builds in the left ventricle, the mitral valve closes. *Closure of the mitral valve is responsible for the first heart sound.* The pressure in the left ventricle continues to rise. When the pressure in the left ventricle exceeds the pressure in the aorta, the aortic valve opens and blood is ejected into the aorta. As the pressure in the aorta builds, the aortic valve closes to prevent regurgitation of blood back into the left ventricle. *Closure of the aortic valve is responsible for the second heart sound.*

Events on the right side of the heart occur in a similar manner, but at much lower pressures. *The manner in which myocardial depolarization occurs and the effects of respiration on heart sounds cause events on the right side of the heart to occur slightly later than those on the left.* This is an important fact to remember and will be helpful later in the chapter in determining pathologic sounds.

Heart sounds are given names. S_1 refers to the first heart sound—i.e., closure of the mitral and tricuspid valves. S_2 refers to the second heart sound—i.e., closure of the aortic and pulmonic valves. There are two additional S sounds which may or may not be normal. S_3 (*third heart sound*) is the sound that correlates with the phase of rapid filling of the left ventricle as it occurs in early diastole; its atrial cause is unknown. It is a normal sound when heard in children and young adults. S_4 (*fourth heart sound*) is the sound that marks atrial contraction. This sound is termed an atrial gallop and can be normal.* It is more often related to increased resistance to ventricular filling following atrial contraction and is produced by cardiac pathology.

---

* *"Normal," as used here, means "nonpathologic" rather than "usual."*

SYSTOLE AND DIASTOLE

Flow of blood through the heart has been discussed and related to varying pressures in the chambers of the heart. The first and second heart sounds have been explained. Figure 9.3 depicts these events occurring in a circle as S_1 and S_2 follow each other in a continuous repetitive sequence.

Now that S_1 and S_2 have been explained, they can be related to systole and diastole. *Systole is the period of time occurring between S_1 and S_2.* The circle can then be shown as in Figure 9.4.

It is important to remember that systole and diastole are periods of time and that particular events occur during each period. Normally, the ventricles contract during systole and relax during diastole. The pressure curve is therefore highest in systole, as the pressure in the ventricle rises to a peak of 120 mm Hg. Pressure falls to almost zero in diastole as the ventricle relaxes. Late in diastole there is a small rise in pressure represented by the extra volume of blood sent into the ventricles by atrial contraction (Fig. 9.5).

LOCATION OF HEART SOUNDS

Figure 9.6 depicts the point at which sound is best heard as compared to the location of the valve responsible for the sound.

From Figure 9.6 it is easy to see that the *sound is not heard directly over the valve producing it.* The most obvious theory to explain this occurrence is that the valve closes with force, the blood is ejected forward, and the sound is heard along the trajectory of the ejected blood. Thus:

1. Closure of the *mitral* valve is heard in the left fifth intercostal space just medial to the midclavicular line.
2. Closure of the *tricuspid* valve is heard in the left fifth intercostal space close to the sternum.
3. Closure of the *aortic valve* is heard in the right second intercostal space close to the sternum.
4. Closure of the *pulmonic valve* is heard in the left second intercostal space close to the sternum.

Erb's point is located in the third intercostal space close to the sternum. Murmurs of

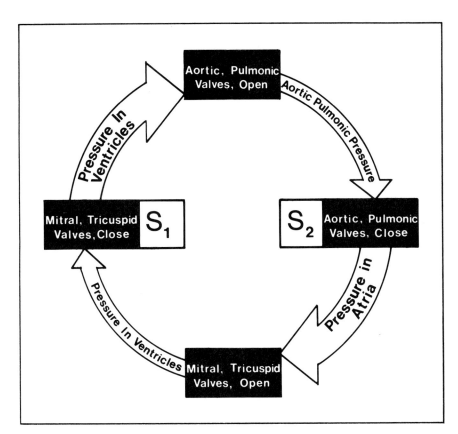

FIGURE 9.3
Events occurring in the cardiac cycle.

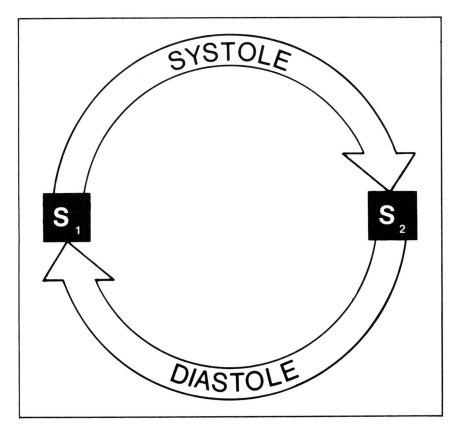

FIGURE 9.4
Diagram depicting systole and diastole in relation to the first and second heart sounds.

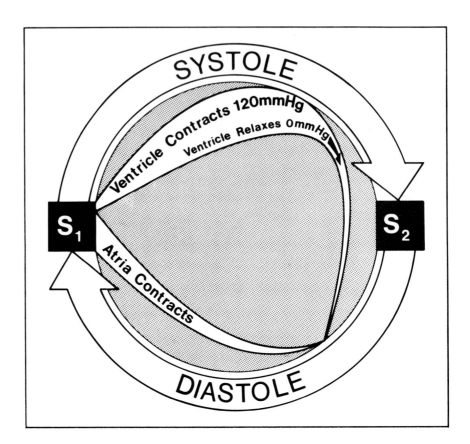

FIGURE 9.5
Pressure changes within the heart during systole and diastole.

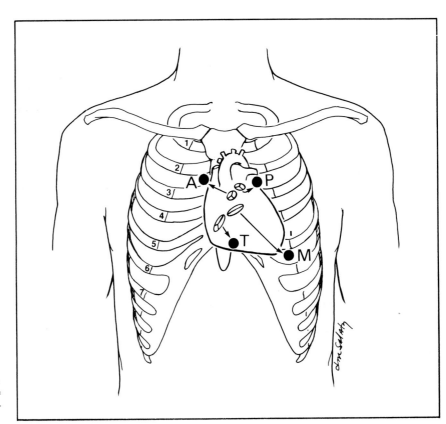

FIGURE 9.6
Transmission of sounds with the closure of the heart valves. **A** = aortic; **P** = pulmonic; **T** = tricuspid; **M** = mitral.

aortic and pulmonic origin can often be heard in this area.

S_1 and S_2 are audible all over the precordium. Figure 9.6, however, helps in understanding why *S_2 is loudest at the base and S_1 is loudest at the apex.* This knowledge is important and will help during auscultation as the examiner attempts to place abnormal sounds heard within systole and diastole.

VARIATIONS IN HEART SOUNDS

First Heart Sound. Pressure is greatest on the left side of the heart; therefore sounds produced by the left side of the heart are longer and louder. Events on the left side slightly precede those on the right. Usually both components of S_1 are heard as one sound, but they are sometimes heard with a slight split. This can be normal but is not heard as frequently as the splitting of S_2 sounds. An S_1 split is obvious in the tricuspid area. Pathologically, the tricuspid sound is more pronounced with pulmonary hypertension. Although the mitral sound is usually loudest, it may be unduly exaggerated with mitral stenosis. However, a very stenotic mitral valve that moves very little may produce a muffled sound. If the mitral sound is increased, it will be heard in the mitral area.

A louder S_1 with or without splitting may be produced extracardially by the increased metabolic states in exercise, fever, thyrotoxicosis, and anemia.

Second Heart Sound. The ejection time of the right ventricle is slightly longer than the left; therefore the pulmonic valve closes slightly after the aortic. This normal variation is increased during inspiration because of the decreased intrathoracic pressure which facilitates an increase in venous return to the right side of the heart. This further delays pulmonic valve closure and produces what is known as a *physiologic splitting* of S_2. That is to say, the splitting of S_2 varies with respiration, is increased with inspiration, and decreases or disappears (the split disappears, not S_2) with expiration. The splitting is most evident in the pulmonic area.

S_2 is further divided according to the two sounds responsible for it. Thus A_2 refers to the portion of S_2 produced by the closure of the aortic valve, while P_2 represents the closure of the pulmonic valve. it is not unusual to see just "A_2" or "P_2" written when an author wishes to discuss one of the components of S_2.

Abnormal splitting of S_2 occurs with essential hypertension in which the aortic sound becomes very loud and most pronounced in the aortic area. S_2 is abnormally increased in the pulmonic area with pulmonary hypertension and congestive heart failure.

The normally split S_2 may be varied abnormally with a widened, fixed, or paradoxic splitting. A widened splitting is associated with right bundle branch block (delayed pulmonic valve closure). Atrial septal defects produce a fixed splitting of S_2, which means that the split does not vary with respiration. Paradoxic splitting, a reversal of normal splitting (splitting of S_2 is normally increased with inspiration), occurs with left bundle branch block.

Third Heart Sound. As previously described, S_3 is produced during the phase of rapid blood flow from the left atrium to the ventrical in early diastole. It is a normal sound in children and young adults. In the older person, an S_3 may signify myocardial failure. S_3's closeness to S_2 produces a triple sound like a galloping horse and is sometimes called a ventricular gallop. *The sound of S_3 is best heard at the apex with the bell of the stethoscope, with the patient lying in the left-lateral decubitus position.*

Fourth Heart Sound. S_4 immediately precedes S_1 and is heard in late diastole. It is marked by atrial contraction and can normally be heard in a young person with a thin chest wall. In the elderly, with an absence of cardiovascular symptoms, an S_4 can be considered part of normal aging. It is, however, less often a normal sound than S_3. Pathologically, S_4 results from an increased resistance to filling of the ventricles and is associated with hypertensive cardiovascular disease, coronary artery disease, or aortic stenosis. An S_4 may also be associated with hyperthyroidism or anemia.

Because S_4 falls so closely in diastole to S_1, the sound produced is a triple sound again, akin to a galloping horse; thus its additional title of *presystolic* or *atrial gallop.* As with S_3, *S_4 is best heard at the apex with the bell of the stethoscope.* Figure 9.7 depicts S_3 and S_4 as they are related to the cardiac cycle.

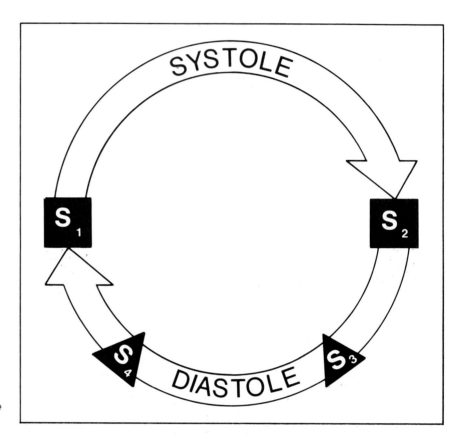

FIGURE 9.7
Occurrence of S_3 and S_4 in the cardiac cycle.

Other Heart Sounds. There are three basic extra heart sounds: the *midsystolic click* of a prolapsing mitral valve (Barlow's syndrome), the *opening snap* of mitral stenosis, and the *aortic click*. An extra cardiac sound is also produced by a pericardial friction rub.

The midsystolic click occurs as a click or snap in mid-sytole and is caused by the ballooning into the left atrium of the mitral valve. This ballooning stretches the chordae tendonae producing a snapping sound. Prolapsing mitral valve is extremely common in women and particularly in young women. It is occasionally associated with an arrhythmia, but is considered benign and is not associated in any way with increased mortality.

An opening snap results from the opening of a stenotic mitral valve at the beginning of diastole and is usually the result of long term sequelae of rheumatic fever. It is best heard at the apex in the left lateral position.

The aortic click occurs as a stenotic aortic valve opens at the beginning of systole. It is usually heard in the second right intercostal space immediately after S_1 and it is always considered pathologic. Figure 9.8 depicts the occurence of S_3, S_4, clicks, and snaps in the cardiac cycle and displays where they are best heard.

When the pericardial sac becomes inflamed, the surfaces rub together, producing a scraping sound much like two balloons being rubbed together. A pericardial friction rub is a distinct, unforgettable sound, not easily confused with heart sounds or murmurs, which does not vary with respiration and is best heard at the apex and sternum.

MURMURS

Murmurs are "whooshing" sounds occurring in various stages of systole or diastole. They are related to one of three factors: (1) an increased rate of blood flow, (2) a forced forward flow through an incompetent valve, or (3) a back flow through an incompetent valve, a septal defect, or patent ductus arteriosus.

There are eight characteristics of mur-

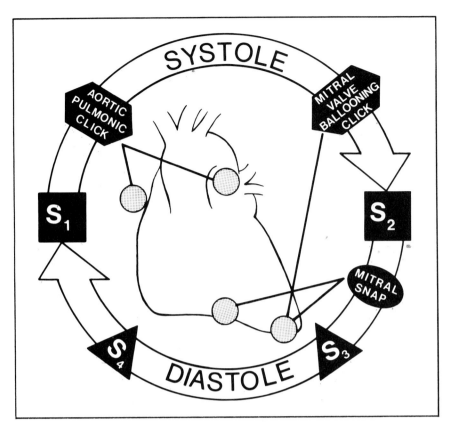

FIGURE 9.8
Occurrence of S_3, S_4, clicks, and snaps in the cardiac cycle, with auscultatory areas included.

murs. These eight are critical to commit to memory as they are always included in a written objective description. More important, however, if a murmur can be described according to the eight characteristics, it can lead the examiner, step by step, to the most probable cause of the murmur. It is not unusual for the student to be unsure of what she hears. After methodically working through all eight characteristics, however, the light often dawns. The examiner can distinguish functional from abnormal murmurs and have a very good idea of the cause of the abnormality. The eight characteristics of murmurs are:

1. Timing
2. Frequency or pitch
3. Location
4. Intensity
5. Radiation
6. Quality
7. Effect of respiration
8. Effect of position

Timing. Murmurs are described according to the cardiac cycle in which they are heard.

They are, therefore, systolic or diastolic murmurs. In addition, they are described according to the period of time they are heard in the cycle—i.e., early, mid, late, or holo or pan (heard throughout the cycle). For example, a systolic murmur might be: (1) early systolic, (2) midsystolic, (3) late systolic, or (4) holosystolic or pansystolic.

Frequency or Pitch. Frequency or pitch varies from high to medium to low.

Location. The point at which the murmur is the loudest is described in terms of location over the particular cardiac area (e.g., aortic area) or particular interspaces and in terms of centimeters from the midsternal, midclavicular, or axillary line.

Intensity. Loudness of the murmur is described according to a scale varying from I (softest) to VI (loudest).

- *Grade I:* Very faint, heard only after the listener has listened carefully.

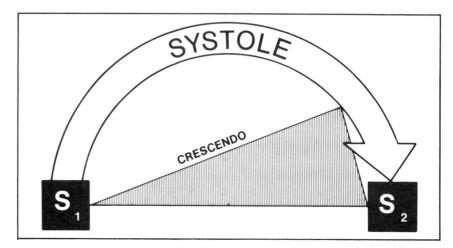

FIGURE 9.9
The crescendo murmur.

- *Grade II:* Quiet, but heard immediately with the stethoscope.
- *Grade III:* Moderately loud, not associated with a thrill (a thrill is a fine vibration palpated with the ball of the hand).
- *Grade IV:* Loud, may be associated with a thrill.
- *Grade V:* Very loud, may be heard with the stethoscope partly off the chest; associated with a thrill.
- *Grade VI:* May be heard with the stethoscope off the chest; associated with a thrill.

The intensity of the murmur is written as a Roman numeral fraction. For example, if the listener hears a Grade II murmur it is written as Gr II/VI. The numerator represents the existing murmur and the denominator represents the maximum possible grades.

Loudness of the murmur is also described according to the pattern of intensity. Words are borrowed from music to describe the varying intensity. The most frequently used terms are crescendo (building to a climax) and decrescendo (starting at a climax and dropping off). *It should be remembered that the crescendo or decrescendo intensity will occur in one of the cardiac cycles.* It is helpful to picture this variation in intensity as being like the vibrations of a tuning fork or to picture what such variations might look like on a tracing from an echocardiogram. A systolic crescendo murmur, for example, would look like the tracing in Figure 9.9. A decrescendo murmur would then look like Figure 9.10.

As in music, there are variations in this theme. Murmurs can be crescendo–decrescendo (also known as diamond-shaped). The crescendo–decrescendo murmur would look

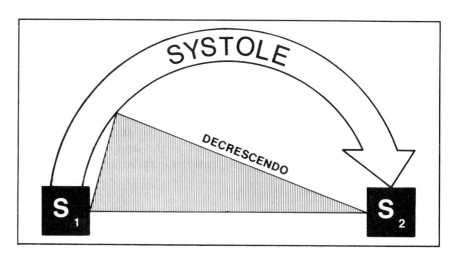

FIGURE 9.10
The decrescendo murmur.

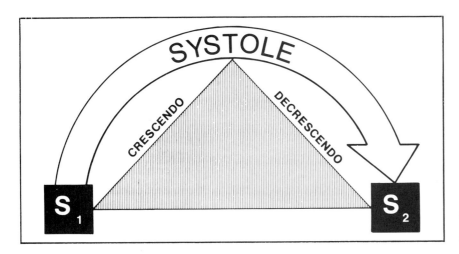

FIGURE 9.11
The diamond-shaped or cre-scendo–decrescendo murmur.

like the tracing in Figure 9.11. Finally, murmurs can have a consistent intensity that is heard throughout systole or diastole. The term for this type of murmur is pansystolic or holosystolic. The pansystolic murmur would look like Figure 9.12. Similar variations occur and can be described in diastole.

Radiation. It is important to describe where the murmur is loudest, but the murmur must also be described in terms of radiation of the sound. The examiner should indicate whether or not the murmur radiates into the neck over the carotid arteries (unilaterally or bilaterally), down the left sternal border, or to the axillary line.

Quality. Descriptive terms should be used to give the murmur a character. Examples of such terms are: musical, blowing, harsh, and rumbling.

Effect of Respiration. The examiner should note whether the murmur increases, decreases, or disappears with inspiration or expiration.

Effect of Position. The examiner should determine whether the murmur increases, decreases, or disappears when the patient is in the sitting or supine position. Aortic sounds are increased when the patient is in the sitting position, leaning forward, and mitral sounds are accentuated when the patient is supine and lying on his left side.

Nonpathologic Murmurs. All diastolic murmurs are considered pathologic, but many systolic murmurs are not. It is estimated that 30 to 50 percent of infants and young children have innocent murmurs (no demonstrable pathology). There are several theories that explain this phenomenon, but the most plausible is

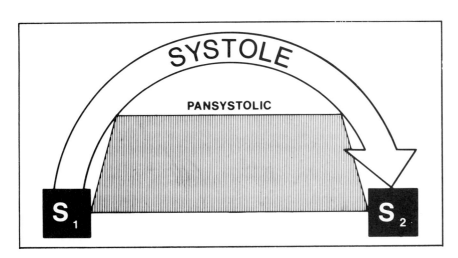

FIGURE 9.12
The holosystolic or pansystolic murmur.

that the chest wall is thinner and the sounds have higher pitches in children.

The term "functional" is sometimes used interchangeably with "innocent" to describe murmurs. Generally, however, innocent murmurs refer to those found in childhood. Functional murmurs occur in the abscence of structural changes in the heart and disappear when the causative factor is remedied. The following paragraph gives examples of functional murmurs.

Pregnant women after the eighth week of pregnancy have an increasing circulating blood volume. It is, therefore, not abnormal to detect a murmur in the second and especially the third trimesters. Fever and acute infections will also sometimes produce murmurs that resolve with the infection.

Innocent and functional murmurs have particular characteristics in common that help to distinguish them from abnormal sounds. They are:

1. Usually systolic, except for the venous hum.
2. Usually of short duration.
3. Usually loudest at the lower-left sternal border or at the second- or third-left intercostal space.
4. Varying in loudness and presence from visit to visit.
5. Usually soft (no more than Grade II/VI and localized).
6. Rarely transmitted.
7. Of varying loudness with changes in position.
8. Heard best in the recumbent position, during expiration, and after exercise, except for the venous hum.
9. Associated with normal heart sounds.
10. Accompanied by normal pulses, respiratory rate, and blood pressure (Caceres & Perry, 1967).

The venous hum was mentioned twice in the list above. Venous hums are normal, murmur-like sounds that are often confused with abnormalities. They are produced by blood flow through the jugular veins. They are heard under the clavicles, in the neck, and to the right and left of the sternal border. The murmur that is produced is low-pitched, ranges as high as Grade III–IV/VI and is continuous throughout the cardiac cycle. It may vary with respiration and disappear in the supine position. It can be eliminated by tilting or rotating the head, occluding the veins in the neck with the examiner's thumb, or performing the Valsalva maneuver. The Valsalva maneuver is performed by asking the patient to exhale forcibly while holding his mouth and nose closed. It increases intrathoracic pressure and impedes venous return to the heart.

Systolic murmurs in elderly persons are of little significance if there are no other signs or symptoms of cardiac disease. This change is due to the increase in the rigidity of the aortic valve that impedes its closure.

The Peripheral Vascular System

ARTERIES AND PULSES

Pressure changes in the left ventricle as it contracts are transmitted as pressure waves to the root of the aorta. These pressure waves are then transmitted to the peripheral arteries, where they can be palpated as pulses. The pressure waves of the arteries travel much faster than the circulating blood within them. It takes the red blood cell about 2½ seconds to go from the left ventricle to the dorsalis pedis area, whereas the pressure transmitted by the contraction of the left ventricle will be palpated over the dorsalis pedis pulse in considerably less than ½ second. The arteries expand and contract in rhythm as they transmit pressure waves. All arteries exhibit a pulse throughout, but these pulses are normally palpated only when the artery is close to the skin and overlying a bone. Arterial pulses are evaluated according to five characteristics:

1. Condition of the wall
2. Rate and rhythm
3. Quality or amplitude
4. Type or contour
5. Equality

Condition of the Wall. This is checked first because other characteristics will be affected if the condition of the wall is altered. The arterial wall is normally elastic. Abnormally, it may be described as thickened, hard, rigid, beaded, inelastic, or calcified.

Rate and Rhythm. Rate is termed normal, rapid, or slow. The definition of the rapid and slow pulse varies, but a rate above 100 is gener-

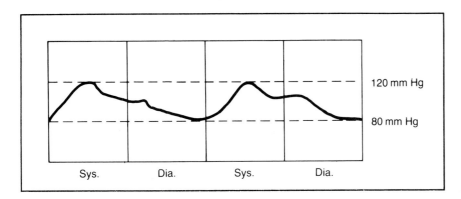

FIGURE 9.13
Amplitude of the normal pulse.

ally agreed to be rapid (tachycardia), and a rate below 60 is termed slow (bradycardia).

Rhythm is described as regular or irregular. An irregular pulse is caused by a cardiac arrhythmia. The physiology of arrhythmias is beyond the scope of this book, but the most frequent causes are atrial fibrillation; atrial flutter, with varying heart block; second degree heart block, with varying dropped beats; sinus irregularity; and premature beats. An irregularity in pulse will be palpated in the peripheral arteries as missed beats. That is to say that the actual heart rate will not be palpated peripherally because of the irregularity. The difference between peripheral arterial rate and actual heart rate is termed *pulse deficit.*

Quality or Amplitude. Arterial pressure waves can be depicted graphically. As the pressure is transmitted, it produces a wave that reaches its peak as the ventricle contracts in systole and falls to its low point as the ventricle relaxes in diastole. Pulse quality or amplitude is the extent of the divergence between systolic and diastolic pressure waves. On a graph the normal amplitude would appear as it does in Figure 9.13.

Amplitude of the pulse is regularly described as strong or weak. The strong pulse appears in Figure 9.14. The weak pulse is depicted in Figure 9.15.

Strong pulses are most often associated with increased cardiac output. Frequent causes are stress, fear, fever, and increased physical activity. A weak pulse will have two basic causes: (1) partial occlusion of an artery (the weak pulse will be palpated distally to the occlusion), and (2) any abnormality reducing cardiac output, such as endocardial lesions, myocardial disease, pericardial disease, or shock.

In addition to defining pulses as weak or strong, they are given a rating on a scale of 0 to 4:

- 0: No pulses
- 1: Pulse is thready, weak, and difficult to palpate; it may fade in and out and is easily obliterated with pressure.
- 2: Pulse is difficult to palpate and may be obliterated with pressure, so light palpa-

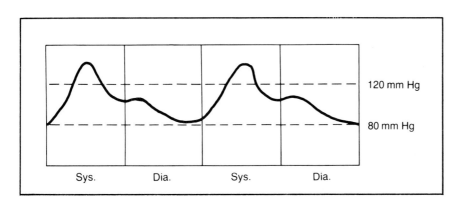

FIGURE 9.14
Amplitude of the strong pulse.

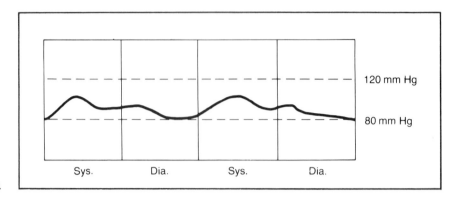

FIGURE 9.15
Amplitude of the weak pulse.

tion is necessary; once located, it is stronger than 1.

• 3: Pulse is easily palpable, does not fade in and out, and is not easily obliterated by pressure; *this is considered to be the normal pulse.*

• 4: Pulse is strong or bounding, easily palpated, and not obliterated with pressure; in some cases, such as aortic regurgitation, it may be considered pathologic (Miller, 1978).

There are two abnormalities associated with pulse amplitude that are worthy of mention. *Pulsus alterans* is an alteration of a weak and strong beat (Fig. 9.16). It occurs with abnormal heart function, particularly left ventricular heart failure. *Pulsus paradoxus* is a change in arterial pressure with respiration. Arterial pressure is decreased with inspiration and returns to full amplitude in expiration (Fig. 9.17). Pulsus paradoxus occurs when one of the following conditions exists:

1. Impairment of return of venous blood to the right ventricle during inspiration (pericardial effusion, constrictive pericarditis).

2. Gross exaggeration of diaphragmatic and rib cage movements during inspiration (tracheal obstruction, asthma, emphysema).

3. Normal forced expiration.

Type or Contour. Contour or type of pulse is defined as the speed of the rise of the pressure wave in systole, the duration of the summit, and the speed with which the wave falls back to the diastolic level. There are three variations in contour from the normal pulse.

Plateau pulse occurs with endocardial lesions and is manifested by a decreased amplitude, a slower rise in systole, a longer summit, and a more gradual fall in diastole. It is classically associated with aortic stenosis (Fig. 9.18).

A *waterhammer pulse* is felt as a knock-like sensation and is characterized by increased amplitude, a rapid rise in systole, a high momentary peak, and a sudden fall in diastole. It is classically associated with aortic insufficiency (Fig. 9.19).

Pulsus bisferiens was created just to confuse us all and is a combination of aortic stenosis and aortic insufficiency. The resultant wave is a combination of a rather rapid rise

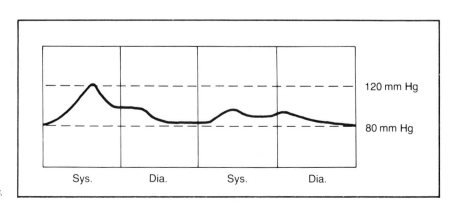

FIGURE 9.16
Pulsus alterans.

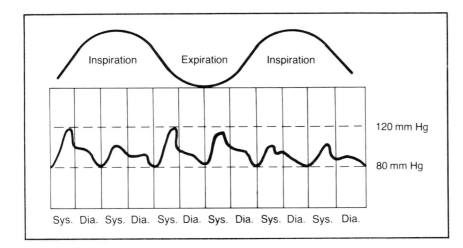

FIGURE 9.17
Pulsus paradoxus.

to a summit with a double impulse at the summit and a weak falling off to the diastolic level (Fig. 9.20).

Equality. All of the pulses are compared to each other for equality and symmetry. Inequality is related either to an abnormally placed artery or to an obstruction.

VEINS AND PULSES

Venous pulses and waves are evaluated at the external and internal jugular veins. Pressure in the venous system is significantly lower than in the arterial. Extent of venous pressure is dependent upon the relative force with which the left ventricle contracts. Pressure is also affected by blood volume, the ability of the right atrium to receive venous blood and pass it to the right ventricle, and the right ventricle's subsequent ability to eject blood into the pulmonary system. When any of these variables are altered, venous pressure will be affected—it will fall when blood volume or left ventricular force decreases and it will rise

when blood flow to the right atrium is impeded. *Congestive heart failure is the most frequent cause of increased venous pressure.*

Figure 9.21 depicts the location of the external and internal jugular veins. The external jugular veins are the most superficial and most visible and lie above the clavicle close to the insertion of the sternocleidomastoid muscles. Visualization of the internal jugular veins is more difficult, as they lie deep to the sternocleidomastoid and are quite close to the carotid arteries. Visible pulses from the internal jugular veins are seen in the surrounding soft tissues. Measurement of internal jugular pressure is more accurate than measurement of external jugular pressure.

The internal jugular pulse is composed primarily of two waves, *a* and *v*, that give information on right atrial pressure. The *a* wave is produced by atrial contraction and has a quick rise and fall. The *v* wave occurs during ventricular contraction but is produced by a build-up of pressure in the right atrium. It rises slowly and falls rapidly after

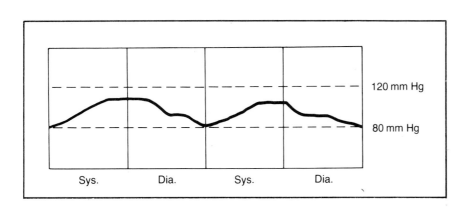

FIGURE 9.18
Plateau pulse.

230

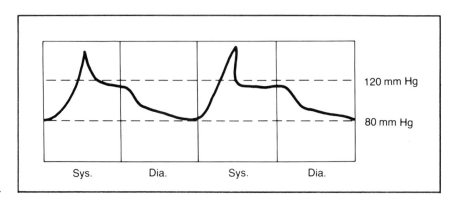

FIGURE 9.19
Waterhammer pulse.

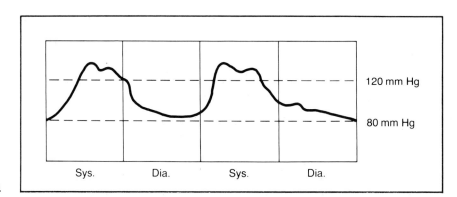

FIGURE 9.20
Pulsus bisferiens.

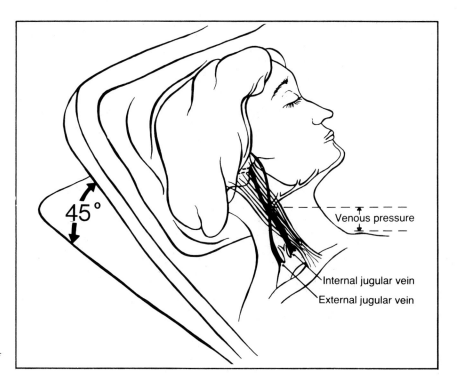

FIGURE 9.21
Location of the external and internal jugular veins.

the fall of the carotid pulse. The descent of the *v* wave is what is actually noted, and this is sometimes referred to as the *y* descent. Figure 9.22 depicts the relationship of the *a* and *v* waves and the *y* descent to the cardiac cycle. The *c* represents a reflection of the carotid artery. The *a* wave amplitude is increased in patients with tricuspid stenosis, pulmonary stenosis, or pulmonary hypertension. The *v* wave amplitude is increased with an incompetent tricuspid valve.

HISTORY

The Pediatric History

The cardiac history of the child is elicited to identify children with congenital heart defects. Approximately, 8 to 10 per 1,000 live-born children have congenital cardiac disorders (Chow, et al., 1984). Some of these defects are detectable at birth or in early infancy and others are not evident until later childhood. Identifiable defects are referred for medical evaluation.

Symptoms of congenital heart disease in children include anorexia, falling asleep after drinking a few ounces of milk, continuous squatting, sleeping in the knee–chest position, decreased exercise tolerance, cyanosis, dyspnea, delayed development, and frequent respiratory infections. It is particularly important to help the parent recall information related to exercise and behavior. The following questions may be helpful in prompting the parent's memory:

1. Does the child play as long as the other children or does he sometimes come home without being called?
2. Does he squat in the middle of play?
3. Does he run easily and go up and down stairs without difficulty?
4. Does he seem to play with the same energy as his siblings or peers do?
5. Does he seem to be growing as fast as his siblings or peers?

Additional data to obtain from the parent/child include any previous history of mumps, group A β-hemolytic streptococcal infections, kidney disease, rheumatic fever, or maternal rubella during pregnancy.

Pertinent family history is important for all age groups. It is presented here to conclude the history for the child and to introduce necessary information for the adult.

The family history should include information on incidence of heart attack (including age of occurrence), hypertension, high cholesterol levels, type II hyperlipoproteinemia (familial hypercholesterolemia), stroke, obesity, congenital heart disease in siblings or other family member, rheumatic fever, and coarctation of the aorta (Chow, et al., 1984).

The Adult History

The goal of the adult cardiovascular history is to detect underlying cardiac disease and to identify cardiac risk factors. Symptoms to be reviewed that indicate cardiovascular disease include: dyspnea, orthopnea, paroxysmal nocturnal dyspnea, edema, cough, hemoptysis, chest pain, wheezing, palpitations, syncope, claudication, fatigue, history of high cholesterol and a history of hypertension (duration and levels of elevated blood pressure). Of significance is a past history of heart murmur, rheumatic fever, kidney disease, heart failure, heart attack, or varicosities, with or without thrombophlebitis. The examiner should be

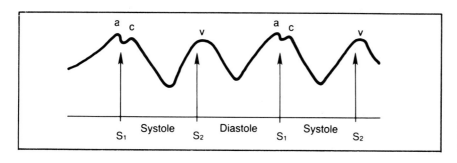

FIGURE 9.22
Pulse waves of the internal jugular pulse.

alert to a history of diseases that involve the heart, including diabetes mellitus, obesity, lung disease, endocrine and metabolic disorders, and syphilis.

Data collected regarding the patient's habits and lifestyle can point to potential risk factors. The nurse should inquire about the patient's smoking, alcohol use, eating (sodium and cholesterol intake), and exercise patterns. She should identify areas of stress and anxiety in the patient's work and family relationships. It is also important to determine the patient's perception of his psychological well-being and satisfaction with self.

The patient is asked for the names of all prescribed and over-the-counter medications he is taking. The nurse should be alert to medications that may raise the blood pressure including oral contraceptives, steroidal anti-inflammatory agents, antihistamines, appetite supressants, and tricyclic antidepressants. All patients are asked if they have ever had a cholesterol level drawn and the results are requested. The cardiac history for the elderly includes what has already been presented for the younger adult. In addition, a review of the cardiac medications should be included. The evaluation and management of the patient is directed toward functional abilities to continue one's lifestyle and patterns of living with minimal interference.

During the history the elderly patient should be questioned regarding signs and symptoms of peripheral vascular problems, because these are common in the aged. Coldness and loss of hair on the extremities, paresthesia, and taut skin are symptoms of an arterial problem. Symptoms of a venous problem are edema, cyanosis, inflamation and ulcerations of the lower extremities.

Cardiovascular disease is one of the chief hazards to life for those over 50 (Mezey, et al., 1980). Frequently, the patient will have already experienced stress or damage to the cardiovascular system. The history then will be concerned with symptoms indicating change or increased damage. Particular symptoms to watch for are increased respiratory effort, fatigue, and edema of the extremities. It is important to determine if these symptoms represent a change or are relatively stable. A change is often expressed by the patient as an inability to maintain his daily routine.

The family history of cardiovascular disease for the adult is the same as for the child.

PHYSICAL ASSESSMENT

Assessment of the cardiac and peripheral vascular system includes:

1. Blood pressure
2. Peripheral pulses
3. Examination for phlebitis
4. The heart
5. Great vessels of the neck

Necessary equipment includes a sphygmomanometer, a stethoscope with a bell and a diaphragm, a penlight, and a centimeter ruler. The blood pressure is usually taken at the onset of a complete physical exam and the peripheral pulses are integrated with examination of the skin and musculoskeletal system. The great vessels of the neck may be checked at the time the patient first assumes the recumbent position. Examination of the heart follows examination of the lungs.

Blood Pressure

To obtain an accurate blood pressure reading, it is important to obtain an appropriately-sized cuff. The cuff should not be more than 20 percent wider than the diameter of the patient's limb and should be long enough to completely encircle it. A bag that is too narrow or short will produce readings that are falsely high. A large cuff will result in falsely low readings. If the patient is very obese, it may be necessary to use a thigh cuff on his arm.

In an initial screening, the blood pressure is taken in two positions (supine or seated, and standing) and verification is obtained in the contralateral arm. If the femoral pulses are decreased or absent, or if there is a family history of *coarctation of the aorta,* a blood pressure should be obtained from the thigh. The thigh blood pressure is equal to that in the arm before one year of age. After the first year, systolic pressure is slightly higher in the lower extremities because larger muscle masses in the thighs produce an increased resistance to compression of the artery. If the pressure in the thighs is lower than the arms, coarctation of the aorta should be suspected.

To avoid erroneous measurement, a patient's blood pressure should not be taken after any stressful situation such as walking up several flights of stairs. To take the blood pressure, the patient should be in a relaxed position with his arm flexed. The patient is asked to remove his clothing from the arm to be measured. Constriction of the upper arm by a rolled sleeve affects the validity of the reading. If the blood pressure is taken in only one arm, the same arm should be used each time, as the pressure will normally vary 10 to 15 millimeters between the right and left arm. The nurse should wrap the cuff around the

arm so that it is 2 to 3 centimeters above the antecubital area. She should then palpate the brachial artery and place the diaphragm of the stethoscope over it in the antecubital area and below but not underneath the cuff (Fig. 9.23). The next step is to inflate the cuff 30 to 40 mm Hg above the level at which the radial pulse disappears and then slowly deflate the cuff. The tappings and murmurs heard while taking the blood pressure are called Korotkoff sounds. Three sounds are read. The first sound, a sudden tapping, is the systolic blood pressure. The next reading is at the point where the sounds become muffled. The third reading is the diastolic reading where the sound disappears.

Information on hypertension and cardiovascular disease has led to an increased effort

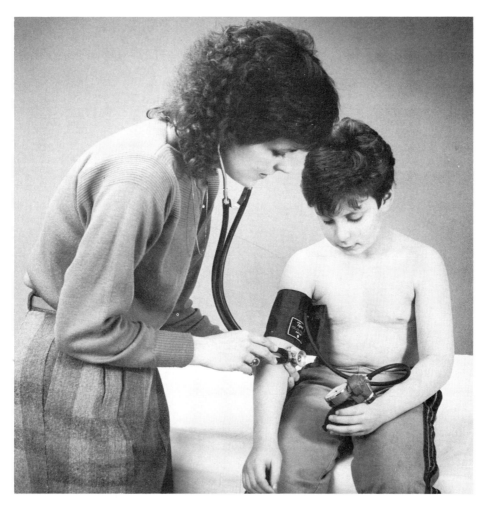

FIGURE 9.23
The pediatric blood pressure.

to monitor blood pressure in children. Cuffs are available for infants and small children. Because hypertension is more frequent in blacks and appears in this population at considerably earlier ages, particular attention must be given to obtaining the blood pressures of black patients. Figure 9.24 gives the percentiles of blood pressure in male children and Figure 9.25 gives the percentiles of blood pressure in female children. Refer to Chart 9.1 for the recommended categorical scheme for arterial blood pressure for use in persons aged 18 and over.

In infants and young children, however, the blood pressure may be difficult to hear due to the smallness of the extremity and poor cooperation. The blood pressure can be estimated by use of the *flush technique.* The child's arm is elevated to drain the blood from it. The cuff is applied and an ace bandage is wrapped from the fingers to the antecubital space. The examiner then inflates the cuff and removes the bandage. The arm is lowered to

the child's side as the cuff is gradually deflated. The point where the arm flushes is recorded as the median between the systolic and diastolic pressure.

The pediatric cuff should be used with toddlers and small children. The cuff must cover two-thirds of the upper arm and there should be no gap where the cuff encircles the arm. For toddlers and preschoolers it is often helpful to first practice on a doll or stuffed animal. This gains their attention and cooperation.

There are variations in blood pressure due to age, exercise, pain, crying, emotional upset, and some drugs (i.e., estrogens and antihistamines). Before a blood pressure is considered elevated it should be taken on several different days, at several different times of day, and in different environments (i.e., home, school, work). The nurse should note the difference between the systolic and diastolic recordings. This is called the pulse pressure and is normally 30 to 40 mm Hg. A widened pulse pressure can be due to age, systolic or diastolic

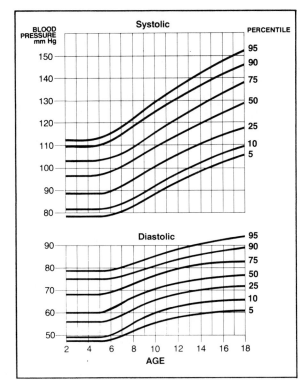

FIGURE 9.24
Percentiles of blood pressure in seated males.
(From "Report of the task force on national blood pressure control in children" by the National Heart, Lung, and Blood Institute, 1977. Pediatrics, 59, 803, 1977. © by the American Academy of Pediatrics. Reprinted with permission.)

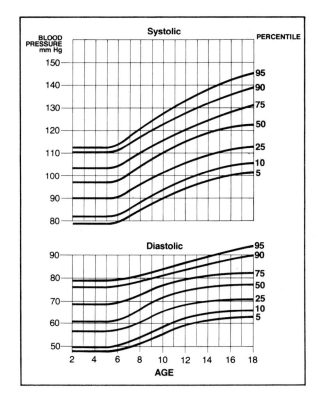

FIGURE 9.25
Percentiles of blood pressure in seated females.
(From "Report of the task force on national blood pressure control in children" by the National Heart, Lung, and Blood Institute, 1977. Pediatrics, 59, 803, 1977. © by the American Academy of Pediatrics. Reprinted with permission.)

hypertension, aortic regurgitation, patent ductus arteriosus, AV fistulas, coarctation of the aorta, and emotional stress. A narrowed pulse pressure can be found with tachycardia, severe aortic stenosis, pericardial effusion, and ascites.

In addition to a lowered blood pressure, the patient should be examined for other manifestations of hypotension. These include a decreased mental status, agitation and lethargy, tachycardia, tachypnea, dilated pupils, orthostatic changes, and pallor.

Peripheral Pulses

Palpable arteries of the body include the temporal, external carotid, brachial, radial, ulnar, abdominal aorta, femoral, popliteal, dorsalis pedis, and posterior tibial. Palpation of the carotid artery is discussed along with the great vessels of the neck and palpation of the abdominal aorta is covered in the examination of the abdomen. The peripheral pulses are taken with the patient in the supine position, using the index and middle fingers. The pulses are palpated bilaterally for condition of the wall, rate and rhythm, quality or amplitude, type or contour, and equality. Condition of the wall is evaluated by flattening the artery with digital compression and rolling the vessel back and forth. Pulses are auscultated with the bell in the carotid, aortic, kidney, and femoral areas for bruits.

PULSE RATE

Pulse rate varies normally with age and exercise. In addition, normal average rates vary by race. Black newborns have higher heart rate levels during sleep than white newborns (Schachter, et al., 1976). As one ages there is a slight decrease in rate. Chart 9.2 includes a list of normal pulses for the various age ranges.

Tachycardia is an increased heart rate occurring in a variety of instances, including exercise, excitement, fever, anemia, hyperthyroidism, and heart disease. Bradycardia is a slow heart rate, which can be normal in athletes.

PULSE RHYTHM

Pulse rhythm is the feel of the vessel as blood flows with the beating of the heart. In the normal person the rhythm is regular. In the eld-

erly, arrhythmias may be felt in the absence of overt cardiac disease; but arrhythmias are apt to be precursors to cardiac disease, therefore, any irregularity in the pulse rhythm of an elderly patient requires further investigation. *Atrial fibrillation, atrial flutter,* and *ventricular tachycardia* are the most common arrhythmias found in the elderly. Atrial fibrillation is a grossly irregular rhythm that can be detected by palpating the radial pulse. It most commonly occurs with mitral stenosis, arteriosclerotic heart disease, and hyperthyroidism. Atrial fibrillation can occur without any cause and be transient. Atrial flutter is a rapid, regular, transient pulse, with a ventricular rate of 140 to 150 beats per minute. Ventricular tachycardia is rarely seen in a healthy individual. It has a slightly irregular rhythm with a pulse rate between 140 and 220 beats per minute. This serious arrhythmia is associated with severe organic heart disease. Any irregularity found on palpation should be confirmed by auscultation of the heart and when findings are grossly abnormal, an electrocardiogram is necessary.

PALPATION OF THE PULSES

Figure 9.26 depicts the areas for palpation of the arterial pulses.

Temporal Pulse. This pulse overlies the temporal bone and is palpated anterior to the ear. The temporal artery is the only palpable artery of the head and is normally tortuous. It should always be palpated when headache is a complaint.

Brachial Pulse. This pulse is palpated in the groove between the biceps and the triceps muscles. The brachial pulses are usually pal-

CHART 9.2
NORMAL PULSE RATES

Age	Pulse Rate
Newborn	70–170
11 months	80–160
2 years	80–130
4 years	80–120
6 years	75–115
8 years	70–110
10 years	70–110
Adult	60–100

(Adapted from R. Behrman and V. Vaughn (Eds.). Nelson Textbook of Pediatrics (12th ed.). Philadelphia: W. B. Saunders, 1983, p. 1100, with permission.)

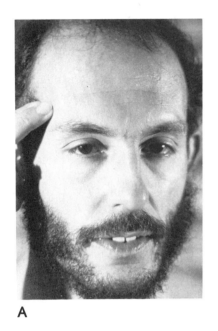

A

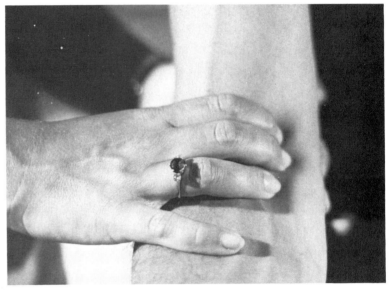

B

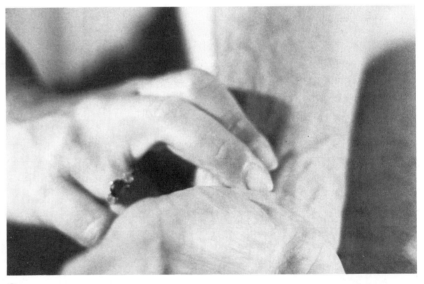

C

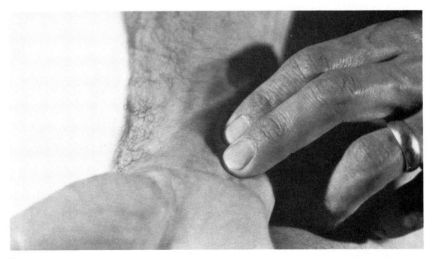

D

FIGURE 9.26
Palpating the arterial pulses: **(A)**
The temporal pulse, **(B)** *the bra-chial pulse,* **(C)** *the radial pulse,*
(D) *the ulnar pulse.* (Continued.)

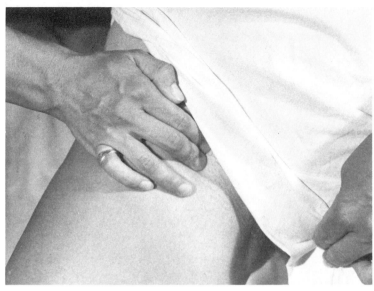

E

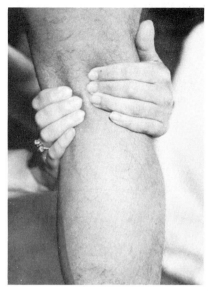

F

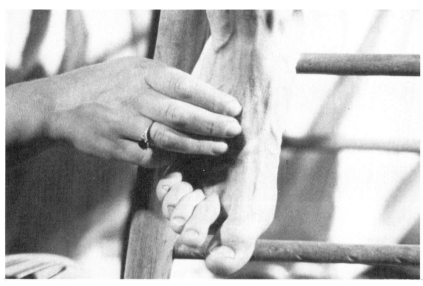

G

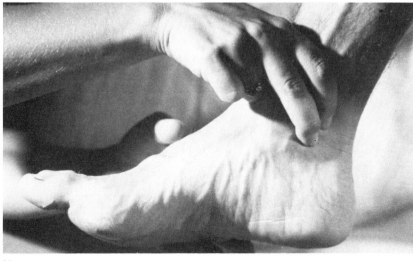

H

FIGURE 9.26 *(Cont'd.)*
(E) the femoral pulse, (F) the popliteal pulse, (G) the dorsalis pedis pulse, (H) the posterior tibial pulse.

pated only when arterial insufficiency is suspected. Just below the elbow the brachial artery branches into the radial and ulnar arteries.

Radial Pulse. The radial artery extends down to the radial side of the forearm to the wrist. The radial pulse is the most commonly palpated and is located on the flexor surface of the wrist laterally.

Ulnar Pulse. The ulnar artery extends down the ulnar side of the forearm and wrist. It then divides into two branches, which anastomose with branches of the radial artery to form the arterial arches of the hand. The ulnar pulse is found on the flexor surface of the wrist medially. It is usually palpated only when arterial insufficiency is suspected.

Femoral Pulse. The femoral artery arises at the level of the inguinal ligament and extends downward through the thigh. The femoral pulse is palpable at the inguinal ligament midway between the anterior-superior iliac spine and the pubic tubercle. It is especially important to identify this pulse in infants and children. Its absence or diminution in relation to the radial pulse may indicate coarctation of the aorta.

Popliteal Pulse. The popliteal artery is a continuation of the femoral artery and is located behind the knee. To palpate the popliteal pulse, the patient should be asked to slightly flex his knee. The examiner then places the fingertips of both hands deeply into the popliteal fossa. This is often a difficult pulse to locate.

Posterior Tibial Pulse. The posterior tibial artery reaches down the posterior aspect of the leg around the medial malleolus to the side of the foot. The posterior tibial pulse is palpable behind and below the medial malleolus. It may also be congenitally absent.

Dorsalis Pedis Pulse. This pulse is felt in the groove between the first two tendons on the medial side of the dorsum of the foot. It is congenitally absent in approximately 10 percent of the population. The criteria for estimating pulses have already been described. (After palpating the pulses, it is sometimes helpful to draw a figure that depicts at once the relative equality of the pulses. A stick figure is used, as displayed in Figure 9.27.)

Examination of the Extremities

Close examination of the extremities will indicate the quality of the arterial and venous systems. The legs, being the most distal extremities, are the most likely to show signs of arterial–venous disease.

INSPECTION

With the patient supine, the extremities are first inspected for color, hair distribution, ulcerations, and swelling. Shiny, taut appearing skin on the legs and diminished hair distribution are characteristics of arterial disease. Evidence of venous disease may be noted by the presence of brown pigmentation near the inner aspect of the ankles, ulcerations of the foot, and cyanosis of the foot. The calves are inspected for signs of *phlebitis,* an inflammation of a vein. The characteristic signs of phlebitis are redness and swelling which may not be apparent in highly pigmented individuals. The ankles are inspected for edema which may be due to localized injury as well as systemic disease. In a standing position the patient's legs are examined anteriorly and posteriorly for varicosities. The size and distribution of the varicosities should be noted.

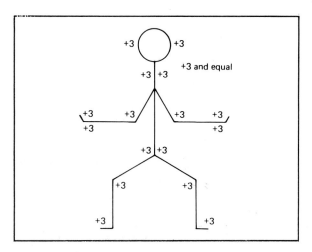

FIGURE 9.27
A stick figure used to record location of arterial pulses.

PALPATION

Following inspection, the extremities are palpated in the supine position for the presence or absence of peripheral pulses, temperature, edema, and phlebitis. Palpation of the peripheral pulses has been discussed previously. A decreased or absent peripheral pulse may be the initial sign of arterial disease. Next using the dorsum of the hand the examiner palpates the lower extremities bilaterally for temperature. In the presence of arterial disease the extremities will be cool. A feeling of significant warmth in the calf is indicative of inflammation as in phlebitis. The lower extremities are palpated for edema bilaterally over the shin, over the dorsum of the foot, and behind the medial malleolus. The thumb is pressed firmly on the skin for at least 5 seconds.

To check for phlebitis the calves are pushed from side to side to test for tenderness. In the presence of deep vein phlebitis of the leg, forceful dorsiflexion of the foot produces pain in the calf muscles. This is called a positive Homan's sign.

The Heart

Examination of the heart includes inspection, palpation, and auscultation. Percussion of the cardiac borders is not the most accurate technique for determining the size of the heart, but it is a technique that was used in the past. Now it is rarely used. Inspection and palpation give much of the information obtained from percussion, so it is imperative to develop these skills.

INSPECTION AND PALPATION

The techniques of inspection and palpation will be described together because they have a close relationship. For example, a movement observed over the precordium can often also be palpated. For adequate inspection and palpation of the anterior chest wall, the patient should be supine with his head elevated 30 to 45 degrees. To observe pulsations that are visible on the chest, light must come from the side, so that rays are tangential to the skin. The examiner should observe from the patient's right side.

The entire precordium is inspected for visible cardiac impulses. In a systematic manner the examiner inspects and palpates the aortic area, the pulmonic area, the right ventricular area, and the left ventricular or apical area. Figure 9.28 depicts the areas on the chest wall in both the child and adult to be closely inspected and palpated.

The entire precordium is palpated, using the palmar surface of the hand at the base of the fingers (Fig. 9.29). This area is the most sensitive to vibrations. When a pulsation is identified by either inspection or palpation, its exact timing in relation to the cardiac cycle is determined. This is done by simultaneously auscultating or palpating the carotid artery to locate the pulse in either systole or diastole.

Aortic Area. Examination of the aortic area involves assessment of the function of the aortic valve. Normally, the aortic area is quiet to palpation. The presence of valvular aortic stenosis will often produce a thrill. A *thrill* is a palpable vibration caused by blood flowing through a narrowed opening. In patients with hypertension the accentuated valve closure can be palpated as a thrill.

Pulmonic Area. The pulmonary artery and valve are assessed in two areas. The first area is immediately to the left of the sternum in the second intercostal space and the second area is in the third intercostal space, just to the left of the sternum (Erb's point). In the presence of pulmonic valve stenosis, it is possible to palpate a thrill. There is also accentuated pulsation in this area due to the abnormally sharp closure of the pulmonic valve in pulmonary hypertension. These thrills and pulsations should be timed in relation to the cardiac cycle.

Right Ventricular Area. The right ventricular area is observed and palpated for any general lift or heave, and for thrills. Normally, the right ventricle is not strong enough to produce a visible impulse. *Lifts* or *heaves* occur with *right ventricular hypertrophy. A systolic thrill* is associated with a ventricular septal defect. This is a congenital problem resulting in the mixing of blood from the two ventricles. When there is increased cardiac output, as seen with anxiety, anemia, fever, pregnancy, or hyperthyroidism, slight outward pulsations may be observed to the left of the sternum.

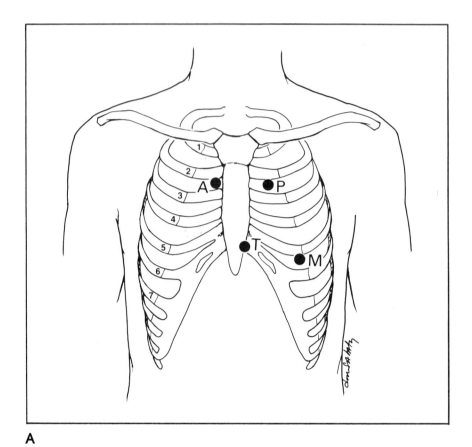

A

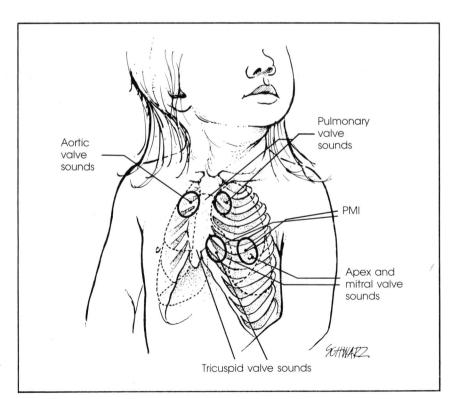

Aortic valve sounds

Pulmonary valve sounds

PMI

Apex and mitral valve sounds

Tricuspid valve sounds

B

FIGURE 9.28
A. Points of inspection, palpation, and auscultation on the adult's precordium. **B.** Points of inspection, palpation, and auscultation on the child's precordium.

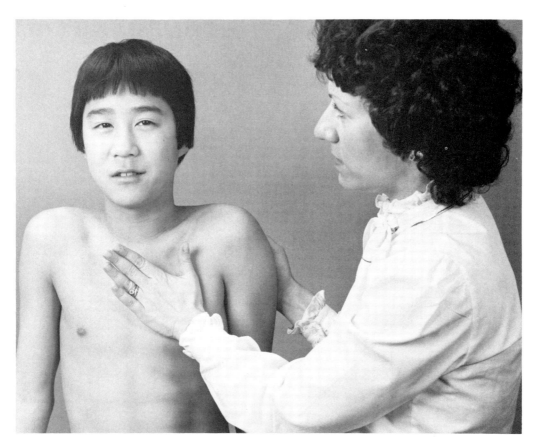

FIGURE 9.29
Palpation of the precordium with the palmar surface of the hand.

Left Ventricular Area. The apical impulse (PMI) is assessed in the apical or left ventricular area. Using the tips of the index and middle fingers, the impulse can only be palpated in a small area less than 2 centimeters in diameter (Fig. 9.30). The amplitude of the impulse is normally light or absent and the impulse normally lasts no longer than half the duration of systole. The impulse will be longer and more forceful in amplitude than normal with left ventricular hypertrophy and will last longer throughout systole.

Description of Cardiac Impulses. Once the impulse is located, it is described in terms of location, size, character of impulse, and distance from the sternal border. In adults, the apical impulse is palpated in the fifth intercostal space in the midclavicular line. In children under 7, it is located in the fourth intercostal space. The impulse may normally be located lateral to the midclavicular line in association with a high diaphragm in pregnancy. In the elderly patient with kyphosis the apical impulse may be displaced. In left ventricular hypertrophy the impulse will be displaced to the left and below its usual location.

Epigastric Area. Figure 9.31 depicts the examination of the epigastric area. The palm of the hand is placed on the epigastric area. The examiner then slides the fingers under the rib cage to the left of the base of the sternum. The fingers are immediately under the right ventricle, and under the palm of the hand is the pulse of the abdominal aorta. An increased amplitude of the abdominal aortic pulse may indicate the presence of an aortic aneurysm or aortic regurgitation. However, epigastric pulsation can occur following exertion.

AUSCULTATION
To auscultate the heart, the examiner needs a stethoscope with a diaphragm and a bell (Fig. 9.32). The diaphragm detects high-pitched sounds and is pressed snugly against

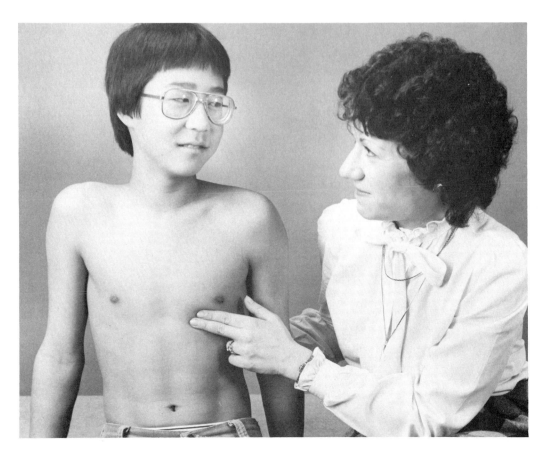

FIGURE 9.30
Palpation of the PMI with the fingertips.

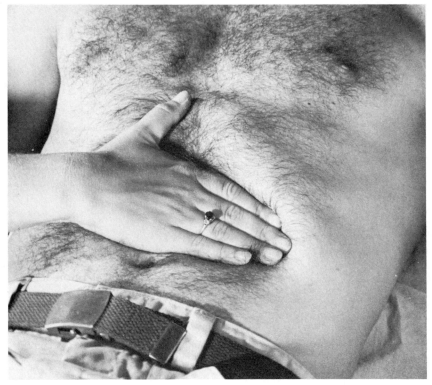

FIGURE 9.31
*Palpating toward the epi-
gastric area.*

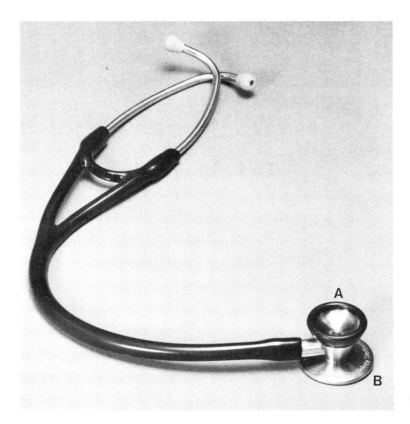

FIGURE 9.32
*The stethoscope. **A.** Bell. **B.** Diaphragm.*

the skin. The bell detects low-pitched sounds and is applied lightly to the skin. If the bell is applied snugly, it will form a diaphragm. The examining room should be free of distracting noises. The patient is examined in the sitting, recumbent, left-lateral, and leaning forward positions. The heart sounds of a thin person sound sharp and clear, while those of an obese person are often distant and muffled. The entire heart is auscultated first with the diaphragm and then with the bell in the sitting and recumbent positions. The diaphragm is used in the leaning forward position and the bell in the left lateral position.

Children can be easily frightened by the stethoscope. It is always difficult to auscultate the heart of a crying child. Referring to the stethoscope as a telephone and allowing the child to handle the equipment can facilitate a trusting interaction and afford the examiner the opportunity to listen in a quiet atmosphere (Fig. 9.33). Auscultating the young child's heart sound while the child is sitting on his parent's lap helps in gaining cooperation.

A systematic approach to auscultation of the heart is essential. The same order used in inspection and palpation is repeated, using the bell and the diaphragm and with the patient in the sitting and supine positions. The examiner starts in the aortic area and proceeds to the pulmonic area, the right ventricular area, and the left ventricular or apical area. The stethoscope moves in a sliding progressive fashion across and down the sternum and out to the axillary area. Figure 9.28 (page 240) depicts the areas of auscultation in children and adults. This can be compared with Figures 9.34 and 9.35, which show the examiner auscultating the chest.

The examiner must be familiar with the events of the cardiac cycle. *She must identify the rate, rhythm, heart sounds, and extra sounds in systole and diastole.* While auscultating the heart, she should concentrate on each event, blocking out the other events. To identify S_1, she must palpate the carotid artery while auscultating. S_1 just precedes the carotid impulse and is synchronous with the onset of the apical impulse. As mentioned earlier, S_1 is normally more intense than S_2 at the apex. An increased intensity of S_1 may accompany exercise, anemia, hyperthyroidism, and mitral stenosis. A diminished S_1 is present in first degree heart block and in mitral regurgitation.

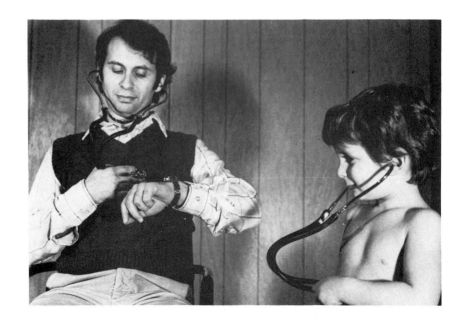

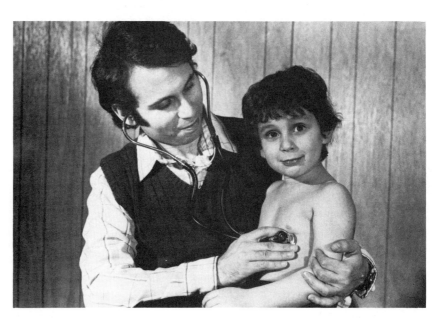

FIGURE 9.33
Allowing the child to become familiar with the equipment creates happy feelings for all concerned.

If S_1 varies in intensity, there may be complete heart block. Splitting of S_1 is heard best in approximately the fifth intercostal space along the left sternal border. If the split is wide or heard in an area other than the tricuspid area, the patient should be referred.

Next, the examiner should concentrate on the second sound, noting its intensity and splitting. Normally, S_2 is louder than S_1 at the base. If there is an increase in the pulmonic component (P_2) of S_2, pulmonary hypertension should be considered. Arterial hypertension may produce an increase in the aortic component of S_2. Splitting is best heard in the pulmonic area. if the sound is split, it is described in terms of its degree of splitting and its relationship to inspiration and expiration. As mentioned previously, S_2 is normally more apparent during inspiration and diminishes or disappears during expiration. If the split is wide, fixed, or paradoxical, the patient should be referred.

Extra Sounds. Once S_1 and S_2 have been identified, the examiner listens for extra sounds in systole and diastole. The extra sound to listen

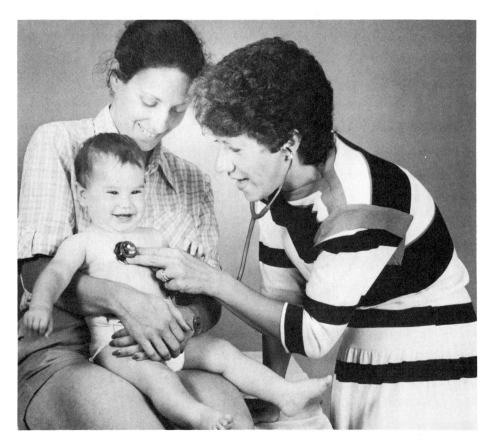

FIGURE 9.34
Modification to approach of the auscultation of the child's heart.

for in systole is an ejection click due to the opening of a diseased semilunar valve. An aortic ejection click, the most common finding, is due to the opening of a stenotic aortic valve. It is heard at both the base and apex of the heart. Pulmonic ejection clicks are heard best at the second left interspace. Sounds to listen for in diastole are an opening snap, S_3, and S_4. The opening snap is the first sound heard in diastole, occurring close to S_2. It is due to the opening of a diseased atrioventricular valve.

S_3 can be differentiated from the opening snap because it occurs slightly later in diastole. S_4 is heard just before S_1 in late diastole, producing a presystolic gallop.

Sounds that can be heard in systole and diastole are venous hums, pericardial friction rubs, and murmurs. As the final portion of auscultation, the examiner listens for murmurs. Murmurs are described according to the eight characteristics presented earlier. For the student, however, a helpful hint is worthy of

note here. As she listens in each area, she should concentrate first on identifying heart sounds. Her thinking should then proceed as follows:

Q. Do I hear S_1 and S_2?
A. Yes.
Q. Which is loudest?
A. S_1 (then I must be listening at the apex).
Q. Do I hear another sound?
A. Yes.
Q. Is it heard in systole or diastole?
Q. Is it crescendo, descrescendo, diamond-shaped or pan?
Q. Is it high- or low-pitched?
Q. What grade is it?
Q. Is it harsh, musical, blowing, or rumbling?
Q. Does it increase, decrease, or show no change with respiration?
Q. Does it radiate, and to where—up the sternal border, into the neck, or to the axillary line?

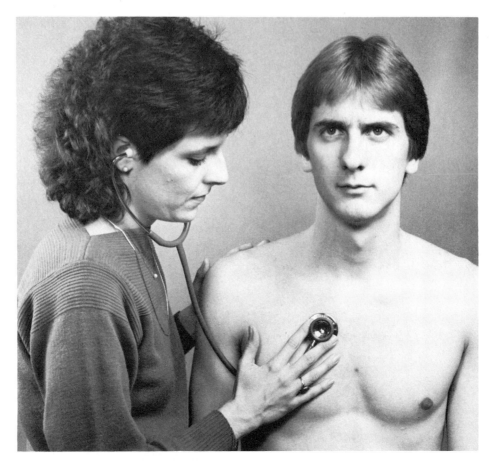

FIGURE 9.35
Auscultation of the aortic area of the heart.

Q. Is it louder with the patient sitting up or lying down?

In this manner she can come very close to identifying murmurs. There are two additional methods that are helpful if abnormalities are suspected of being of aortic or mitral origin.

Aortic murmurs, especially those of aortic regurgitation, are best auscultated with the patient sitting up and leaning forward. The patient is asked to exhale and hold his breath. The examiner auscultates with the diaphragm of the stethoscope and listens in the aortic area and down the left sternal border. Figure 9.36A depicts the examiner auscultating in this manner.

S_3 and mitral murmurs are best elicited with the patient lying on his left side. The examiner auscultates with the bell of the stethoscope in the apical area (Fig. 9.36B).

Chart 9.3 depicts the signs of extra heart sounds.

Great Vessels of the Neck

The great vessels of the neck, including the carotid arteries and jugular veins, are assessed as a part of the cardiac exam. They reflect on the status of the heart. The carotid arteries are examined for the characteristics of their pulsations. The jugular veins are assessed for pulse waves and pulse pressure.

CAROTID ARTERIES
The techniques utilized in the examination of the carotid arteries are inspection, palpation, and auscultation. The arteries are observed for abnormally large and bounding pulses. The pulses are then palpated for rate, rhythm, and character, as are all of the peripheral pulses.

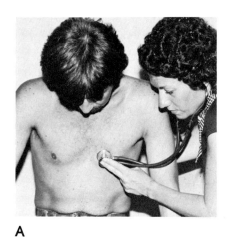

A

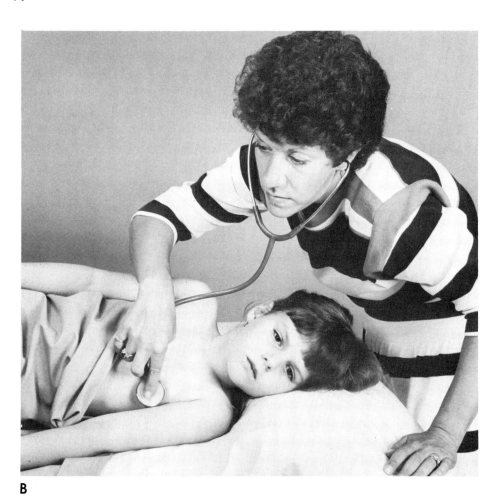

B

FIGURE 9.36
A. A patient leans forward as the examiner listens for an aortic murmur. *B.* The patient lies on her left side as the examiner listens for a mitral murmur.

CHART 9.3
SYSTOLIC AND DIASTOLIC MURMUR

Type of Murmur	Diagnosis	Auscultation	Other Physical Examination
Systolic Murmurs: Left Second Interspace	Innocent murmur	A systolic murmur, variable with respiration. Commonly heard between the left sternal border and apex in the third to fourth intercostal space or in the pulmonary area. Increases in intensity with position change. Poorly transmitted and usually does not radiate (McEvoy, 1980)	Likely in normal thin chest, straight spine, or pectus excavatum. Never associated with thrills
	Physiologic murmurs	Disappear with treatment of primary condition	Signs of thyrotoxicosis, anemia, fever, etc.
	Atrial septal defect	S_2—wide, fixed split S_1—split, accentuated tricuspid closure sound Middiastolic rumble at lower-left sternal border	Right ventricular lift Pulmonary artery lift
	Pulmonary stenosis	Ejection click S_2 split, P_2 delayed and soft	Thrill Right ventricular lift Venous a wave prominent
	Partial anomalous pulmonary venous return	S_2 accentuated Not fixed split	
	Idiopathic dilatation of pulmonary artery	Ejection click	
Systolic Murmurs-Right Second Interspace	Aortic stenosis	Early systolic murmur transmitted to neck Rarely may be maximal at apex $S_2(A_2)$ soft with rigid valve Ejection click with mobile valve	Left ventricular lift Slow-rising pulse Narrow pulse pressure Systolic thrill S_4 gallop Paradoxical splitting of S_2
	Aortic regurgitation	Decrescendo diastolic murmur Early systolic murmur Middiastolic murmur at apex (Austin Flint)	Wide pulse pressure Fast-rising pulse Left ventricular lift
	Mitral regurgitation	Holosystolic murmur, not transmitted to neck, heard better at apex and axilla	Left ventricular lift
	Aortic sclerosis	Short systolic murmur	Age: usually over 50 years Evidence of atherosclerosis
	Bicuspid aortic valve	Short systolic murmur Early decrescendo diastolic murmur Ejection click	Common in youths Associated congenital abnormality, coarctation, ventricular septal defect
	Aortic dilatation or aneurysm	Short systolic murmur Diastolic murmur may be present Tambour S_2 Lift in right second interspace	Signs of syphilis or Marfan's syndrome
	Flow murmur secondary to increased pulmonary blood flow—e.g., in atrial septal defect, ventricular septal defect, or patent ductus arteriosus	S_1 normal S_2 fixed split in atrial septal defect Murmurs of primary lesion	
	Tricuspid stenosis	Diastolic murmur heard best near sternum Increased by inspiration	Big a waves, jugular venous pressure
	Aortic regurgitation (transmitted)	Decrescendo diastolic murmur Lower-left sternal border Onset with S_2	Signs of aortic regurgitation Left ventricular lift

CHART 9.3 (*Continued*)

Type of Murmur	Diagnosis	Auscultation	Other Physical Examination
	Aortic regurgitation (Austin Flint)	S_1 normal or soft OS absent Middiastolic rumble Presystolic rumble	Peripheral signs of aortic re-gurgitation Left ventricular lift
Diastolic Murmurs: Second Interspace Right and Left (Base)	Aortic regurgitation	Murmur descrescendo heard right-second interspace and third-left interspace S_2 may be of decreased intensity, but normal; S_2 does not exclude severe aortic regurgitation	Left ventricular lift Peripheral signs of wide pulse pressure
	Pulmonary regurgitation	$S_2(P_2)$ loud if pulmonary regurgitation secondary to pulmonary hypertension Murmur left-second interspace, not to right of sternum In absence of pulmonary hypertension normal Murmur rough and scratchy crescendo–decrescendo	Right ventricular lift Peripheral signs of aortic re-gurgitation absent
	Diastolic component of continuous murmur (transmitted)	Characteristic continuous murmur heard elsewhere—e.g., under left clavicle or over neck	

(*Adapted, from Harvey, A., et al. (Eds.). Principles and Practice of Medicine (21st ed.). Norwalk, Conn.: Appleton-Century-Crofts, 1984, pp. 206, 208, 210, 212.*)

Last of all, they are auscultated for bruits indicating local obstruction or transmitted cardiac murmurs.

The patient should be comfortable, with his head and neck elevated on a pillow 15 to 30 degrees. Relaxation of the sternocleidomastoid muscle is facilitated by turning the head toward the side being examined. The patient's clothing about his neck and upper chest is removed so the examiner can easily inspect the area. The arteries are gently palpated by hooking the index and middle finger in the groove at the medial edge of the sternocleidomastoid muscle. Figure 9.37 depicts this maneuver.

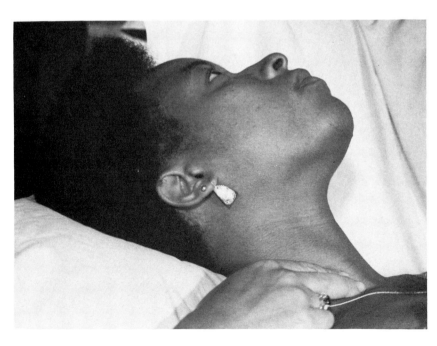

FIGURE 9.37
Palpating the carotid artery.

One side is palpated at a time, taking care to avoid the carotid sinus, which is located at the level of the thyroid cartilage just below the angle of the jaw. Massage of the carotid sinus may produce slowing of the heart rate. The arteries are auscultated with the bell of the stethoscope. The patient is asked to hold his breath as the examiner listens for the presence of bruits (Fig. 9.38).

JUGULAR VEINS

The internal jugular vein gives the best estimate of right heart function. It reflects changes in pressure from the right atrium. Examination for jugular venous distention is not routinely done in infants and children without cardiovascular disease. For screening purposes the adult patient is examined in the recumbent position and at an elevation of 45 degrees.

Inspection. The patient is placed in a recumbent position and asked to turn his head away from the side being examined. Using a tongenital light the examiner looks across the sternocleidomastoid muscle and observes the *a* and *v* waves of the internal jugular vein and the *c* wave of the carotid artery (Fig. 9.39). The *a* wave will be almost synchronous with S_1. The *v* wave is almost synchronous with

S_2. The internal jugular vein lies very deep in the sternocleidomastoid muscle, so only the pulsations transmitted through the soft tissues are seen. They may be seen in the suprasternal notch, around and behind the acromioclavicular joint, or just behind the sternocleidomastoid muscle. In most people, the venous pulsations can be observed in the supine position. The head and neck should then be raised to 45 degrees and supported with a pillow to relax the sternocleidomastoid. When the patient is elevated to 45 degrees, the pulsations should not be observed more than 2 centimeters above the manubrium of the sternum. Normally, the pulsations are not observed when the patient is in a sitting position. The *a* and *v* waves are differentiated from those of the *c* wave of the carotid artery. Chart 9.4 depicts the characteristics that identify the a, v, and c waves.

Measurement. After identifying the pulse waves, the examiner should measure the pulse pressure at an elevation of 45 degrees. Figure 9.40 depicts this maneuver. This can be done by using either the internal or external jugular veins. The examiner should note the distance between the end of the sternal angle of Louis to the highest level of jugular pulsations. This is accomplished by placing a centimeter ruler

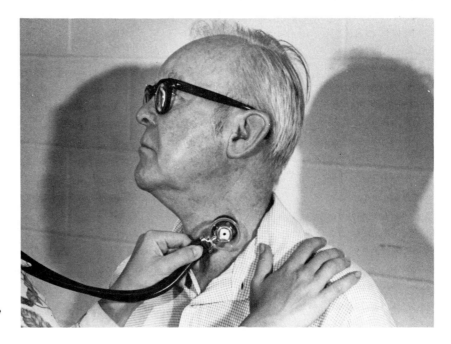

FIGURE 9.38
Auscultating for bruits over the carotid artery.

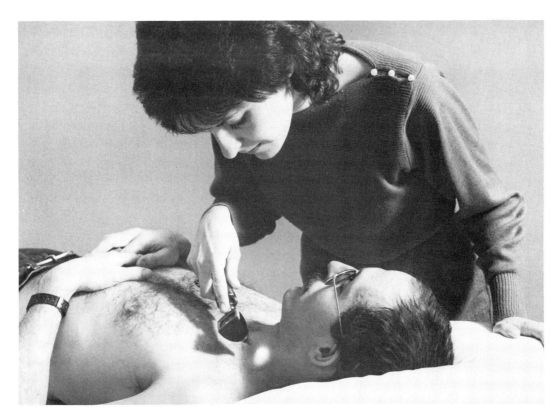

FIGURE 9.39
Observation of the internal jugular vein (observation at a 45° angle not pictured).

vertically at the end of the sternal angle of Louis. Another straight edge device is placed horizontally from the point above which the veins are distended to the ruler. A perpendicular angle is formed. The measurement of ve-

nous pressure is the point where the straight edge touches the ruler. Normally at an elevation of 45 degrees this reading should not be greater than 2 centimeters. If the venous pressure is elevated at this level, the patient should also be examined sitting erect and another measurement taken. Congestive heart failure is the most frequent cause of abnormally increased venous pressure.

Hepatojuglar Reflux. If the presence of congestive heart failure is suspected and cannot be determined by the methods already described, the *hepatojugular* reflux may be employed. Figure 9.41 depicts this maneuver. To perform the maneuver, pressure is applied over the right-upper abdominal quadrant for 30 to 60 seconds. The examiner watches for an increase in the jugular venous pressure during this maneuver. A rise greater than 1 centimeter above the previous level is abnormal.

This completes the examination of the cardiac and peripheral vascular systems.

CHART 9.4
DIFFERENTIAL CHARACTERISTICS OF JUGULAR AND CAROTID PULSES

Internal Jugular Pulsations	Carotid Pulsations
Rarely palpable	Palpable
Soft undulating quality, usually with 2 or 3 outward components (a, c, and v waves)	A more vigorous thrust with a single outward component
Pulsation eliminated by light pressure on the vein just above the sternal end of the clavicle	Pulsation not eliminated
Level of pulsation usually descends with inspiration	Pulsation not affected by inspiration
Pulsations vary with position	Pulsations unchanged by position

(From Bates, B. A Guide to Physical Examination (3rd ed.). Philadelphia. J.B. Lippincott, 1983, p. 187, with permission.)

252

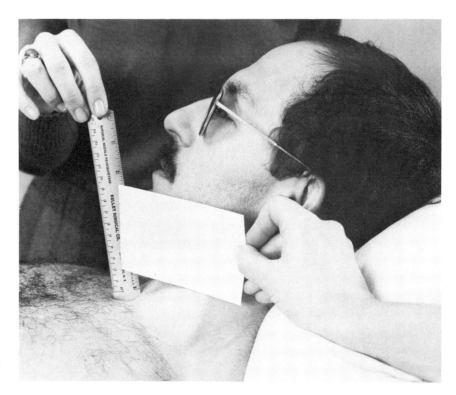

FIGURE 9.40
Measuring the venous pulse
pressure.

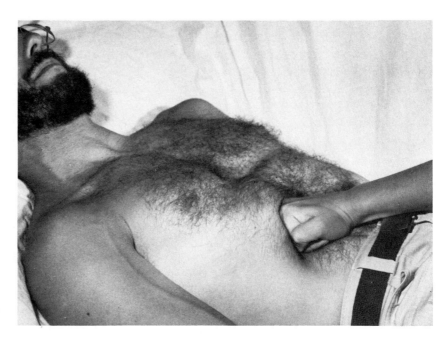

FIGURE 9.41
Elicitation of the hepatojugular
reflux.

Screening Examination of the Cardiovascular System

The screening examination for the cardiovascular system includes:

1. Two blood pressures in the supine and standing positions with a third blood pressure taken in a corresponding extremity
2. Inspection of the neck veins at a 45° angle
3. Auscultation of the carotids with the bell
4. Bilateral palpation of the peripheral pulses
   a. Brachial*
   b. Radial
   c. Femoral
   d. Popliteal*
   e. Posterior tibial*
   f. Dorsalis pedis*
5. Inspection of the lower extremities for edema and varicosities
6. Palpation of the lower extremities for temperature
7. Palpation for edema over the shin, dorsum of the foot and behind the medial malleolus
8. Inspection and palpation of the precordial area
9. Palpation of the PMI
10. Auscultation for cardiac sounds in the aortic, pulmonic, tricuspid and apical areas using the diaphragm and the bell with the patient in the sitting, supine, left lateral recumbent and leaning forward positions
11. Apical pulse

---

* Adults only

EXAMPLE OF A RECORDED HISTORY AND PHYSICAL

SUBJECTIVE:

Chief Complaint: "Shortness of breath for 4 weeks."

HPH: Patient is a 48-year-old male who describes himself as being 5' 9" tall, weighing 150 lbs, and feeling well until 4 weeks ago. At that time, he began to exercise and jog because, "I should be in better shape and my wife gave me a jogging outfit for my birthday." Since that time, he has noticed fatigue and increasing shortness of breath during jogging. "It's working the wrong way—instead of running more each day, I'm walking more." Patient feels he has followed instructions carefully and has done proper exercising, gradually increasing walking and running. The weather has averaged 50° F and he does not feel that weather has been a factor. Three of these jogging outings have ended in fits of nonproductive coughing that lasted 2 to 3 minutes. He has noticed a dry cough that is more prevalent at night and thinks it began also within the past few weeks. He has taken no medications or treatment and relieves his shortness of breath by stopping his running. Prior to jogging he was not physically active and took occasional walks in the neighborhood. He does not smoke and drinks about four beers at social events 3 to 4 times a month. He has no pain, fever, nausea, or headaches. He had measles and chicken pox as a child and was in the hospital for about 2 weeks when he was 14 for rheumatic fever. He was checked 6 months after discharge by his physician and told he was in good health. Visits to the doctor since then have been only episodic for such conditions as flu or colds. He denies edema of the legs, varicose veins, a history of murmur, increased blood pressure, orthopnea, and palpitations. He has had no other illness or hospitalizations. There is no family history of cardiovascular or respiratory diseases.

OBJECTIVE:

B.P.:	Left	120/100/80	Right	118/84/86	sitting
		120/104/82		122/86/80	lying
		120/100/80		126/82/84	standing
P. 76				128/90/88	leg/lying
R. 18					

General: 5'9", 142 lbs, male in no acute distress. Physical appearance is pleasant. Talks freely and expresses symptoms and feelings clearly.

Lungs: No visible deformities or respiratory irregularity. All lung fields clear of palpable fremitus. No dullness to percussion. Breath sounds clearly audible without adventitious sounds. Expansion of diaphragm equal and symmetrical.

CV and PV:

PULSES: 3 + and equal; elastic, regular rate and rhythm.

CV: No lifts or thrills visible or palpable. No pulsations noted or palpated in the epigastric area. S_2 louder than S_1 at the base. S_1 is louder than S_2 at the apex, but S_2 is unusually loud. In addition, there is a fixed snapping of S_1 and an early diastolic opening snap that does not vary with respiration. There is also a middiastolic rumbling murmur that is low and grade III/VI. It is loudest at the apex and radiates slightly toward the lower-left sternal border. It is best heard with the patient lying on his left side, auscultating with the bell. The PMI is visible and palpable in the 5th ICS, 8 cm from the left sternal border. It is about 1 cm. wide and gives a short sound synonomous with that of S_1. *Carotid artery*—no bruits auscultated. *Jugular veins*—external and internal jugular veins are 2 cm. above the sternal angle with the head of the bed elevated 45 degrees. The *a* wave is synchronous with S_1, as the *v* wave is with S_2. *Extremities*—no edema of hands or feet. No varicosities or calf tenderness in either leg.

REFERENCES

Caceres, C., & Perry, L. (1967). The Innocent Murmur. Boston: Little, Brown.

Chow, P., Durand, M., Feldman, M., & Mills, M. (1984). Handbook of Pediatric Primary Care. New York: John Wiley & Sons.

Hake, J. (1978). Health maintenance and disease prevention. In C. Leitch, and R. Tinker, (Eds.), Primary Care. Philadelphia: F. A. Davis, pp. 39–54.

Joint National Committee on Detection, Evaluation, and Treatment of High Blood Pressure (1984). The 1984 report of the Joint National Committee on detection, evaluation, and treatment of high blood pressure. Archives of Internal Medicine, 144: 1045–56.

Lebow, L., & Sherman, F. (1981). The Core of Geriatric Medicine: A Guide for Students and Practitioners. St Louis: C. V. Mosby.

Levy, P. (1980). Declining mortality in coronary heart disease. Arteriosclerosis, 1(5): 312–24.

Lindberg, S. (1980). Periodic preventive health screening schedule for adult men and women. Nurse Practioner, 5(5), 9–13, 21.

Lipid Research Clinics Program (1984). The lipid research clinics coronary primary prevention trials results. II. The relationship of reduction in incidence of coronary heart disease to cholesterol lowering. Journal of the American Medical Association, 25(3): 365–74.

McEvoy, M. (1980). Functional heart murmurs. Nurse Practitioner, 6(2): 34–36.

Mezey, M., Rauckharst, L., & Stabes, S. (1980). Health Assessment of the Older Individual. New York: Springer.

Miller, K. (1978). Assessing peripheral perfusion. American Journal of Nursing, 78, 1674.

Pender, N. (1982). Health Promotion in Nursing Practice. Norwalk, Conn.: Appleton-Century-Crofts.

Podell, R. (1984). Coronary disease prevention proof of the anticholesterol pudding. Postgraduate Medicine, 75(6): 193–6.

Schachter, J., Lachin, J., & Wimberly, T. (1976). Newborn heart rate and blood pressure: Relation to race and to socioeconomic class. Psychosomatic Medicine, 38, 390–8.

Stamler, J., & Stamler, R. (1984). Intervention for the prevention and control of hypertension and atherosclerotic diseases: United States and international experience. The American Journal of Medicine, February, 13–36.

Yurick, A. (1980). The nursing process and the activity of the elderly person. In A. Yurick, S. Robb, B. Spier, & N. Ebert, (Eds.), The Aged Person and the Nursing Process. New York: Appleton-Century-Crofts, pp. 405–450.

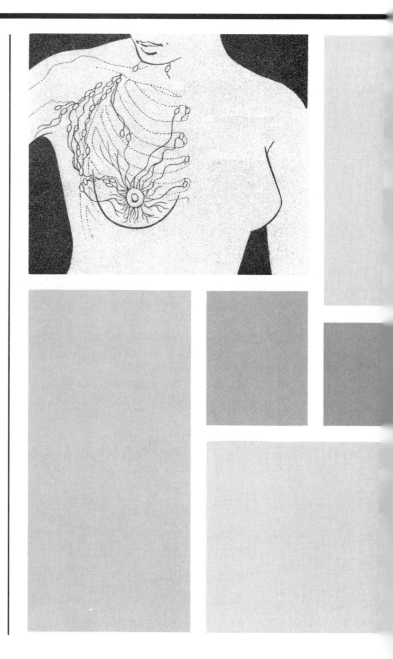

10

The Breast

The breast is a very significant part of the human body, especially for a woman. To the preadolescent female (10–12 yrs.), the breast development indicates approaching menarche and womanhood. To the new mother, the breast may be a means of feeding her new baby. For all women the breast can be a very sensuous part of their bodies. Unfortunately, the breast is a common place for disease which provokes fear in women. Problems can be either acute or neoplastic, including benign or malignant lesions.

Estimates show that 1 out of 11 American women have a chance of developing breast cancer at some point in life (American Cancer Society, 1985). It is the leading cause of death in women aged 35 to 54 (American Cancer Society, 1985). The 5-year survival rate for women who have localized breast cancer is 96 percent. If the cancer has spread to the lymph nodes or beyond, the survival rate is 70 percent (American Cancer Society, 1985).

The Health Insurance Plan of Greater New York began a study in 1964 to examine the effects of annual physical examination and mammograms on women between the ages of 40 and 65 (Guidelines, 1980). Findings indicated that the proportion of women who detected their own cancers in the interval between examinations increased with breast self-examinations. Therefore, breast self-examination results in earlier diagnosis at a time when treatment is most effective. It is further estimated that 90 percent of women seeking medical attention for breast lumps discover their masses through self-examination (Graham & Kalinowski, 1981). Despite these findings, a Gallup survey done in 1977 indicated that only 24 percent of American women do a breast self-examination on a monthly basis (American Cancer Society, 1979). Fear of detecting cancer seems to be the main reason women are reluctant to practice this technique. However, only 25 percent of women who seek advice from a health care provider for a breast mass have cancer (Townsend, 1980). The monthly breast exam remains one good way to detect underlying disease early, thereby increasing the chances for a good prognosis. Recently, it has been suggested that breast self-examination be taught routinely to preteenage girls when they learn about menstruation (Beaman, 1982). This would encourage young girls to view breast self-examination as a normal part of womanhood.

Women should not rely merely on an annual breast check by their health care providers. However, the importance of a professional examination including a mammogram for women over 35 cannot be minimized. Results of a 5-year study by the Breast Cancer Detection Demonstration Project indicated that mammography was impressively high in detecting cancers that were not found on physical examination (Baker, 1982).

The following guidelines are provided by the American Cancer Society for detection of breast cancer in asymptomatic women (American Cancer Society, 1985):

1. Women 20 years of age and older should perform breast self-examination every month.
2. Women 20 to 40 should have a physical examination of the breast every three years, and women over 40 should have a physical examination of the breast every year.
3. Women between the ages of 35 and 39 should have a baseline mammogram.
4. Women 40 to 49 should have mammography every 1 to 2 years, depending on physical and mammographic findings as well as other risks.
5. Women over 50 should have a mammogram every year when feasible.

The American Cancer Society does not provide guidelines for examination of the male breast. However, it is an important part of the screening examination on all male patients.

DEVELOPMENTAL CHANGES OF THE BREAST THROUGHOUT THE LIFESPAN

Neonates, both male and female, are often born with enlarged, firm breasts. The bilateral breast enlargement is a result of the mother's hormones, which transfer across the placenta. This normal physiologic response usually disappears in 4 to 6 weeks.

Development of the breast is the first visible sign of puberty in girls, occurring 1 to 2 years prior to menses. Enlargement of the breast buds begins between the ages of 8 and 13 and development is generally completed between the ages of 13 and 18.

Transient breast enlargement may occur in approximately 50 percent of boys aged 10 to 16. This enlargement may be restricted to the nipple area or extended to the subcutaneous fat deposits. The condition, called gynecomastia, is caused by the hormonal changes of puberty and generally dissipates within a year or two without treatment.

During pregnancy the breast may double or triple in size. The changes related to the first trimester will be primarily subjective, including tingling and tenderness. Some enlargement occurs, but the real increase in size begins after the second month when the nipple and the areola become darker. Surface veins appear bilaterally. As pregnancy progresses, colostrum may be expressed from the nipple.

After a woman has had one or more pregnancies and her breast size has increased and decreased one or more times, it is realistic to expect a lessening in the firmness of the breast tissue. In addition, if a woman is overweight, more subcutaneous tissue may form, causing enlargement. Both of these changes can cause breasts to become pendulous.

As a woman approaches menopause and her estrogen level decreases, the breast may shrink and the firmness of the breast may lessen. Throughout life, alteration of breast tissue takes place, and this can provide clues to physical as well as emotional well-being.

Breast enlargement does occur in some elderly males with decreased testosterone levels and is considered a normal part of aging. However, gynecomastia in the adult male may be associated with liver disease, lung cancer, or other pathology so this finding should always be referred for further investigation.

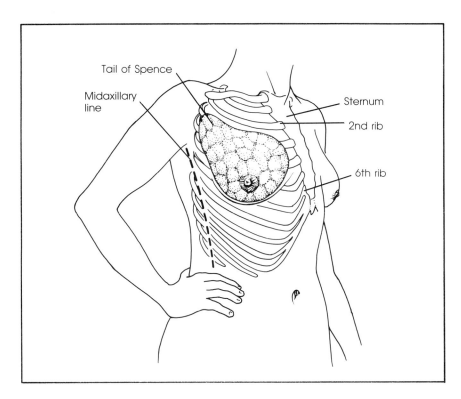

FIGURE 10.1
Location of the breast on the chest wall.

ANATOMY

The breasts are *modified sebaceous glands* that lie directly over the muscles of the chest. Each breast extends from the second rib to the sixth rib and from the sternal border to the anterior axillary line (Fig. 10.1). There are multiple fi-

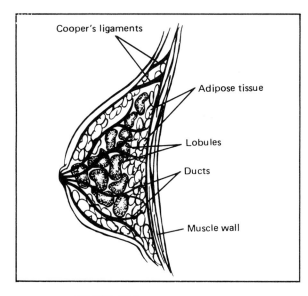

FIGURE 10.2
Anatomic structures of the breast.

brous bands which begin at the subcutaneous layer of connective tissue immediately beneath the skin of each breast. These bands, called *Cooper's ligaments,* run deeply through the breast to attach loosely to the fascia over the muscles of the chest wall (Fig 10.2). When these ligaments become stretched due to lack of good support the breast becomes pendulous.

The largest portion of the glandular tissue of the breast is located in the upper–outer quadrant. There is a portion of breast tissue which extends from this quadrant into the *axilla* called the *tail of Spence* (Fig. 10.1). Approximately 50 percent of breast tumors are located in the upper-outer quadrant in the tail of Spence.

The primary components of the breast are the *milk-producing glands* and *ductal system, the nipple,* and the (*drainage system*).

The Milk-producing Glands and Ductal System

Each breast contains 10 to 20 *lobes* which consist of many smaller *lobules.* Within each lobule (Fig. 10.2) there are between 10 and 100 *milk-producing glands.* The duct system drains the lobules and these ducts branch and join each other. There is one terminal duct

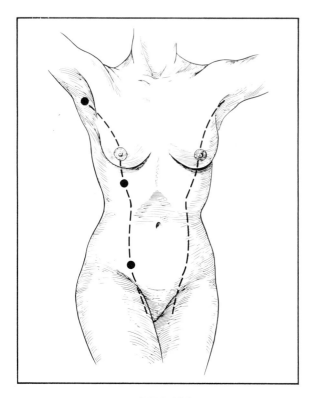

FIGURE 10.3
Milk lines.

for each lobe that exits on the surface of the nipple. The remainder of the breast consists of fat, which determines the size of the breast. This is related to heredity and nutritional factors.

The Nipple

The nipple is located slightly below the center of each breast. At the tip of each nipple there are 10 to 20 perforations—the openings of the ducts. The nipple is surrounded by the *pigmented areola. Sebaceous glands* on the areola present as small, round elevations called *Montgomery's tubercles.*

In embryonic development there are *ridges* that extend from the axilla to the groin (Fig. 10.3). These ridges usually disappear, except at the site of the normal breast and nipple. Occasionally this ridge does not atrophy, and a woman may have a *supernumerary breast* or *nipple.* The most frequent locations are in the axilla and below the normal breast. A supernumerary nipple consists of a small nipple and areola. It is less common for glandular tissue to be present.

The Drainage Pattern

There are two normal patterns of venous drainage in the mammary region visible on the anterior chest. In the first or *transverse* type, the superficial veins radiate laterally from the pectoral venous plexus toward the axillary and costoaxillary regions. In the second type, the veins radiate in a fan-like pattern downward and laterally into the breast from the point where the anterior jugular vein turns beneath the sternocleidomastoid muscle. Classification as to pattern type is determined by the drainage of the mammary region. The pattern is constant, and the only known alterations in pattern are due to breast tumors (Spuhler, 1950). Knowledge of the lymph drainage of the breast is important to understanding the spread of cancerous cells. Depending on the location of a lesion in the breast, metastases may occur to the axillary nodes, to the supraclavicular and infraclavicular nodes, or even to the opposite breast.

Most of the lymphatic drainage of the breast is to the nodes of the axilla. There are four lymph node groups in the axilla (Fig. 10.4). The lateral axillary nodes are in the inner aspect of the upper part of the humerus, along the axillary vein. The central axillary nodes are located deep in the apex of the axilla close to the ribs. The anterior pectoral nodes are behind the lateral edge of the pectoralis major. The subscapular nodes are under the anterior edge of the latissimus dorsi muscle.

HISTORY

The Female Patient

The major purposes of the history are to alert the nurse to any symptoms of underlying breast disease; to assess normal developmental changes; and to identify risk factors for breast cancer. The general screening questions asked of all adolescent and adult patients include the following:

1. Do you presently have any breast masses or have you ever noticed any in the past?
2. Do you ever have any breast pain or tenderness? How does this relate to your menstrual cycle?
3. Have you noticed any discharge from

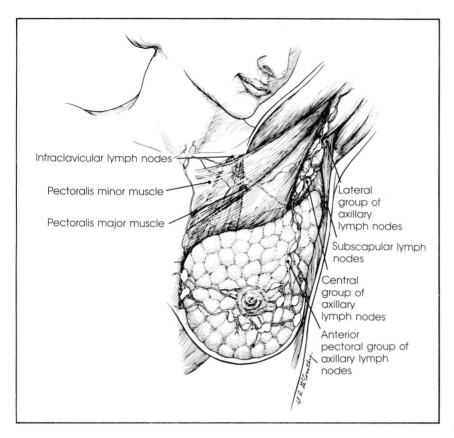

FIGURE 10.4
Axillary and infraclavicular lymph nodes.

your nipples or rash around your nipples?

4. Do you practice a monthly self breast examination? What technique do you use? At what time during the month do you conduct the examination?
5. Have you ever had breast surgery? Type?
6. Have you ever had a mammogram? Results?

DEVELOPMENTAL CHANGES

Normal breast changes occur in women during adolescence, pregnancy and during the postmenopausal period. Changes specific to these developmental stages need exploration. Questions to be addressed in a sensitive manner with the young female include:

1. Have you noticed your breasts changing?
2. When did this begin to happen?
3. What changes have you noticed?
4. How do you feel about these changes?

The breasts change rapidly beginning in very early pregnancy. This can be startling to the woman who has not been alerted to these changes. The following questions are asked of the pregnant patient:

1. Have you noticed any breast tingling or tenderness?
2. Have your breasts enlarged?
3. Do the veins on your breasts appear more prominent?
4. Are your nipples inverted? Do your nipples appear more erect? Have you noticed that the area around your nipple has become darker?
5. Can a thick, yellowish fluid be extracted from the nipple?

Finally, during the peri- and postmenopausal periods, a woman may again notice developmental changes in her breasts. With the decrease in natural estrogen the breasts lose their firmness and homogeneity. When the estrogen decline is rapid as well as marked, she may also notice some shrinkage. The middle-aged and elderly woman should be asked if she has noticed changes in her breast size and consistency. This provides the opportunity to clarify any concern the woman may have regarding these natural occurrences.

RISK FACTORS

When evaluating a well female patient or a patient presenting with a problem related to the breast, the family and past history should be carefully reviewed for risk factors related to *breast cancer.* The risk is increased for the patient who reports a history of breast cancer in her mother, sister, aunt, or grandmother. The increased risk associated with a family member treated postmenopausally is 2 times the risk of disease in the general female population (Senie, et al., 1983). The risk is 9 times greater when the relative developed breast cancer prior to menopause (Townsend, 1980). The risk seems to be greatest when mothers and sisters have had cancer, but it is now thought that any history of breast cancer in female relatives increases risk (Sheahan, 1984). If the patient has a history of cancer in one breast, she is at a 5 times greater risk of developing cancer in the second breast than the woman who has never had cancer (American Cancer Society, 1976).

There seems to be a higher incidence of breast cancer in the woman who has had an early menarche (before 13), as well as in the woman who has prolonged menstrual activity (more than 35 years) (Sheahan, 1984). The woman who had her first child after 35 or who has never had children is also at greater risk. The results of studies on the relationship between benign breast disease and the subsequent development of cancer are conflicting. At present, a history of fibrocystic disease, especially proliferative fibrocystic disease, is considered a possible risk factor (Senie, et al., 1983). Ethnic or racial background may be related to the incidence of breast cancer. American Caucasian women seem to have a greater chance of getting breast cancer than women from Japan or China (Rhodes, et al., 1974). However, recent studies of migrants show that environmental factors may influence the frequency of the disease. When Japanese women move to the United States, their chances for breast cancer increase (Senie, et al., 1983). Also, the incidence of breast cancer among women who move from the low-risk areas of Asia and Africa to high-risk areas of the United States and northern Europe consistently increases (Larson, 1983).

The medication history is reviewed for drugs that cause breast side effects. Drugs that may alter hormone balance and cause nipple discharge include oral contraceptives, phenothiazine, digitalis, diuretics, and steroids (Round table, 1975). Some medications show a relationship to cancer, especially in women who have other risk factors. These drugs include phenothiazine, Rauwolfia alkaloid, and methyldopa (Anthony, 1978). Exogenous estrogens taken for birth control or for the treatment of menopausal symptoms have caused cystic breast changes in some women, but at present there is no association with the development of cancer. One study reported a slightly higher frequency of breast cancer in women who ingested diethylstilbestrol, a drug commonly used from 1945 to 1960 in the treatment of threatened or habitual abortion and other high-risk pregnancy problems, than that of women who had not taken the medication (Prenatal diethylstilbestrol, 1983). However, the difference was not statistically significant due to the small number of women studied. The surveillance of these women is continuing (Prenatal diethylstilbestrol, 1983).

The Male Patient

General questions to be reviewed with all male patients regarding breast changes include:

1. Have you noticed any breast masses?
2. Have you noticed any breast enlargement?
3. Have you noticed any discharge from your nipples or rash around the nipples?

PHYSICAL ASSESSMENT

The Female Patient

A good time for the examiner to give instructions for the breast self-examination is while the examiner is inspecting and palpating the breasts. Verbal instructions should be supplemented with reading material and the patient's understanding should be evaluated by a return demonstration. Inspection and palpation are the techniques used in the examination of the breast.

INSPECTION

The examination of the breast begins with inspection which requires good lighting. The patient is seated with the arms relaxed at her sides and her gown lowered to the waist. The patient should be properly exposed for adequate visualization. First, the *axillary area, clavicular area, breasts, nipples,* and *areola* are generally inspected. Then each area is assessed individually.

Inspection of the Axillary and Clavicular Areas. The axillary and clavicular areas are inspected for swelling and evidence of rash or infection. The nodes located in these areas may become enlarged with cancerous spread from the breast. Axillary nodes can also become enlarged when there has been a recent infection in the corresponding hand or arm. The axillary areas often normally appear swollen during pregnancy and lactation.

Inspection of the Breasts. The breasts are inspected for development, symmetry, superficial appearance and dimpling. Tanner (1962) has identified *five stages of breast development* (Fig. 10.5). The first stage is the infantile stage—from the immediate postnatal period to the onset of puberty. The second is the bud stage where the breast and papilla are slightly elevated and the areola's diameter is increased. During the third stage the breast is further enlarged. At the time of the fourth stage, in addition to further breast enlargement, the areola forms a secondary mound above the breast. The fifth stage is the one of adult size and contour. Breast development before 9 years of age or no breast development after 14 years of age requires further investigation.

One breast may grow more rapidly than the other. However, by the average age of 15 the breasts will have reached their full (nonpregnant) size and will be relatively symmetrical. It is not unusual for normal breasts to be slightly unequal in size. However, a recent increase in the size of one breast may denote inflammation or underlying tumor. There may also be a difference in size due to underlying *cystic formation.*

The superficial appearance of each breast is examined for *redness, edema,* an *increased superficial vascular pattern,* and *dimpling.* Redness of the breast may indicate inflamma-

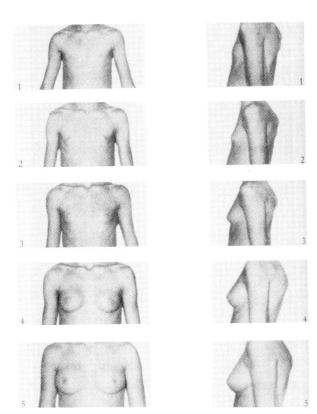

FIGURE 10.5.
Standards for breast development rating during adolescence. (1) Infantile stage. (2) Bud stage. (3) Further breast enlargement. (4) Areola forms a secondary mound. (5) Adult breast. (From Tanner, J. Growth at Adolescence (2nd ed.). Oxford, England: Blackwell Scientific Publications, Plate 7, 1962, p. 37, with permission.)

tion or involvement of the superficial lymphatics by a neoplastic process. When the breasts are edematous the follicular openings are more pronounced and may denote inflammation or neoplasm. Edema associated with cancer is caused by the mechanical blocking of the lymphatic channels in the skin by cancer cells. The appearance of the skin in this situation is described as being like *orange peel* or *pig skin* (Fig. 10.6B). The *subcutaneous veins* over the breast may be visibly dilated, indicating an accessory blood supply to a neoplasm (Fig. 10.6B). This should be differentiated from the bilaterally increased vascular pattern normally seen in pregnancy.

One of the most important parts of the breast examination is inspecting for *dimpling* or *retraction* (Fig. 10.6A). When Cooper's ligaments are invaded by cancer they become fibrotic, causing retraction of the skin over the lesion. To bring out the dimpling that may be missed on simple inspection, the patient is asked to raise her hands over her head, press her hands against her hips and to lean forward, holding the hands of the examiner (Fig. 10.7). Any maneuver that causes a contraction of the pectoral muscles is a good way to bring out retraction.

Inspection of the Nipples and Areola. The nipples and areola are examined for *color, lesions, discharge* and *position.* In Caucasian patients, the nipple and areola are normally pink but become brown with pregnancy. In darkly pigmented individuals, the nipple area is usually darker than other skin surfaces and becomes even darker with pregnancy. Unilateral nipple

erosion, scaling, fissures, and crusting may indicate *Paget's disease*, which is a malignant condition (Sheahan, 1984). If the ulceration is bilateral, it may be due to an eczema-like lesion that occasionally develops in this area. Any ulceration of the nipple should be viewed with suspicion and the woman should receive further evaluation.

Discharge from the nipple usually does not indicate any underlying cancer but is of great concern to patients. It may be related to medication the patient is taking (see "Breast History"). Serosanguineous nipple discharge may be due to a *benign indraductal papilloma* which most frequently occurs in women between the ages of 35 and 45 years (Graham & Kalinowski, 1981). *Chronic cystic mastitis* is a disease along the ductal system, producing a discharge that ranges from clear to blue-yellow. A sticky, multicolored nipple discharge, called *mammary duct ectasia*, may occur around the time of menopause. A yellowish nipple discharge is normally present during pregnancy. Although discharge is usually a benign condition, 30 percent of patients over the age of 60 who have a nipple discharge and no palpable mass are found to have cancer (Sheahan, 1984). Any patient, with the exception of a pregnant woman, who presents with a nipple discharge should receive further evaluation.

The position of the nipples is carefully noted. The nipples are normally pointing in the same direction. *Inversion* of the nipple is a common variant of the normal and is usually a long-standing feature. Recent development of inversion in a previously erect nipple may

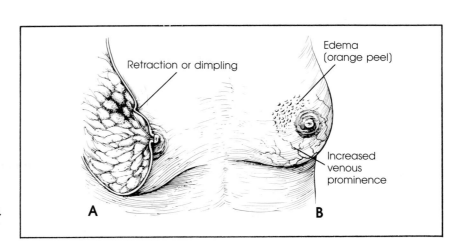

FIGURE 10.6
Abnormalities of the breast. **A.** *Breast retraction or dimpling.* **B.** *Edema or orange peel and increased venous prominence.*

Retraction or dimpling

Edema (orange peel)

Increased venous prominence

A

B

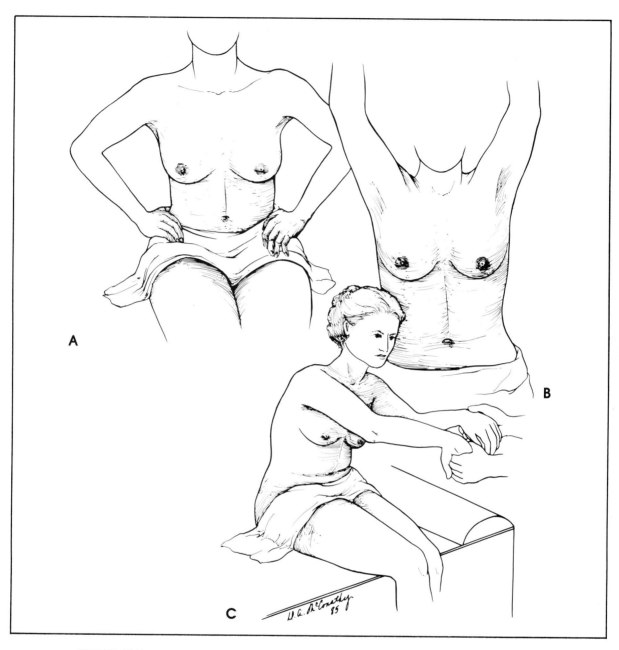

FIGURE 10.7
*Inspection of the breasts. **A.** Arms pushing into the hips. **B.** Arms elevated. **C.** Leaning forward.*

be due to retraction. *Retraction* occurs normally in the aged and is due to subcutaneous fat loss. The nipple can be easily everted in this case. Retraction also occurs in the presence of a malignancy. In this case the nipple cannot be everted. Retraction or deviation of the nipples is observed as the woman puts her hands over her head, presses her hands on her hips and leans forward (Fig. 10.7).

PALPATION
Examination of the breast includes palpation of the epitrochlear, axillary, and clavicular nodes and the breasts, including the nipples. Following presentation of the approach taken to the palpation of these areas will be a discussion of the appropriate terms used for describing breast masses. Finally, characteristics of common breast masses will be presented.

Palpation of the Epitrochlear, Axillary, and Clavicular Nodes. The epitrochlear, axillary, and clavicular nodes are palpated while the woman is still sitting. Standing at the patient's left side, the left epitrochlear node is palpated in the depression above and posterior to the medial condyle of the humerus (Fig. 10.8). The nodes of the axilla are palpated with the woman's arms at her sides, so the muscles are relaxed. To facilitate this relaxation, the examiner can support the patient's left arm with her right arm and palpate with her left hand (Fig. 10.9). For the right-handed examiner, the hands are reversed with the examiner supporting the patient's left arm with her left arm and palpating with her right hand. The axilla is palpated inside the anterior axillary fold (anterior pectorial nodes), deep in the posterior axillary fold (subscapular nodes), and high in the axilla (central nodes) (Fig. 10.10). When performing the examination of the deep axilla, the examiner milks the axillary contents downward along the thorax between the axillary folds. The axilla is also palpated along the humerus (lateral nodes) (Fig. 10.11A). The examiner then moves to the patient's right side to palpate the right epitrochlear and axillary nodes. Enlargement of the axillary nodes may indicate metastases of cancerous cells, but women who have had a recent infection in the corresponding hand or arm will normally have enlarged nodes (Graham & Kalinowski, 1981). Standing in front of the woman and slightly to the side, the supraclavicular and infraclavicular areas are palpated bilaterally with both hands or one side at a time (Fig. 10.11A and B).

Palpation of the Breasts and Nipples. If the woman has noticed a mass, or if there are any suspicious areas on inspection, the breast should be palpated with the patient in both the sitting and the supine positions. If no problems have been elicited or observed, the breasts need only be palpated with the patient in the supine position. When the examiner is right-handed she stands on the patient's right side to examine both breasts. The left-handed examiner stands to the patient's left side. Placing a pillow beneath the woman's scapula on the side to be examined and having her raise her hand behind her neck will stretch the pectoral muscles on that side, shift the breast me-

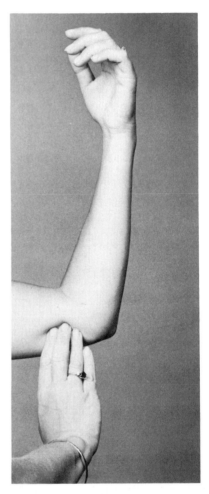

FIGURE 10.8
Palpation of the epitrochlear nodes.

dially, and thin the breast over the chest wall. This makes palpation easier. When the woman has noted a mass, the examiner should palpate the opposite breast first. This allows for comparison and forces the examiner to consciously examine the normal tissue before zeroing in on an abnormality.

To palpate the breast, the examiner uses the palmar surfaces of the first three fingers in a rotary motion to compress the breast tissue gently, but firmly against the chest wall. The use of the finger tips for palpating should be avoided because they are less sensitive and tend to push any underlying mass away from the examiner's touch. Only one hand should be used while palpating (Fig. 10.12A and B).

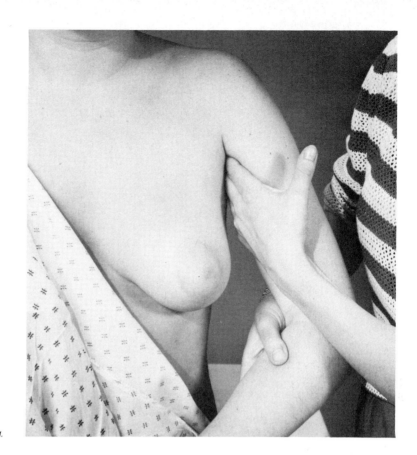

FIGURE 10.9
Positioning for palpation of the axilla.

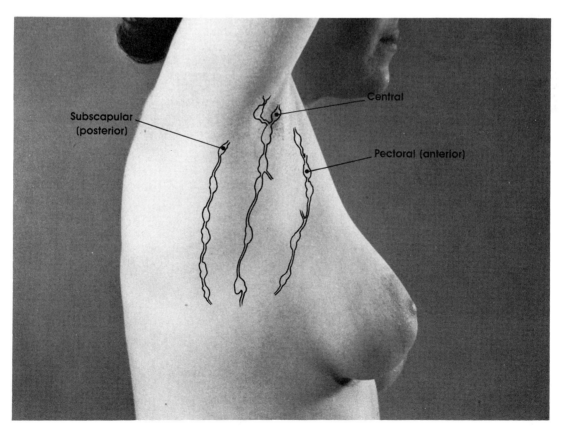

FIGURE 10.10
Location of the subscapular, central axillary, and anterior pectoral nodes.

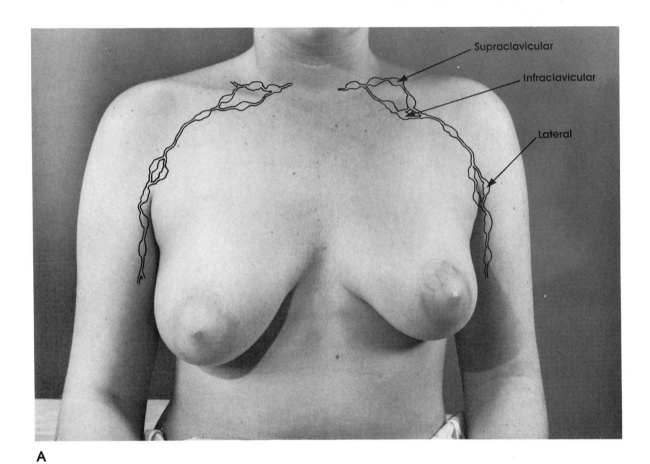

A

B

FIGURE 10.11
A. Location of the clavicular and lateral axillary nodes. *B.* Palpation of the infraclavicular nodes.

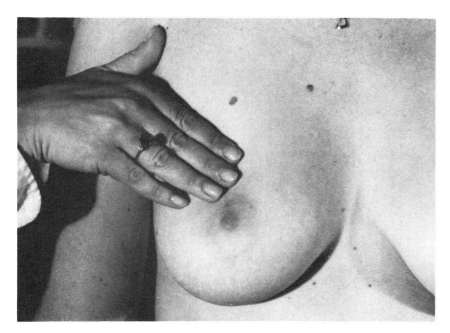

A

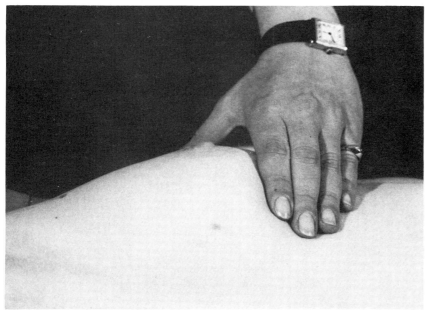

B

FIGURE 10.12
Palpating the breast.

When a two-handed technique is used, it is easier to miss breast tissue. However, when there is a large amount of breast tissue one of the examiner's hands can be used to support the breast tissue while palpating with the other hand.

One approach to palpation is to envision the breast as a wheel with spokes. Starting at the nipple, the examiner palpates up the spoke of the wheel to the breast periphery and then palpates down to the nipple repeating this pattern until the entire breast is covered. Alternate methods include palpating in increasingly larger circles starting at the nipple or palpating in a linear pattern across the breast. Establishing a consistent, systematic approach is of extreme importance in developing one's skill in palpation. Due to the high incidence of cancerous lesions located in the tail of spence this area of the breast should always receive special attention and be palpated separately. Finally, the nipples are examined by palpating for tissue elasticity and by compressing the nipple between the thumb and index finger, noting discharge.

When the breasts are very large, they may be more difficult to palpate and more time must be taken. When there is a large amount of breast tissue, it is often hard to distribute the breast tissue evenly over the chest wall with the patient in a supine position. In this case the bimanual technique is used in addition to palpation in the supine position. This technique is best implemented with the woman in a sitting position. The breast is palpated between the palmar surfaces of the fingers of both hands while the hands are gently and slowly rotated. Again, it is important to establish a systematic pattern for palpation.

Normal breasts vary greatly in their feel to palpation. They differ according to the age of the woman, where she is in her menstrual cycle, the amount of subcutaneous fatty tissue, and the presence or absence of pregnancy. In young women the breasts are soft and have a homogeneous feel while those of older women are commonly stringy and nodular. Just prior to menstruation, the breasts become engorged, lobular, and sensitive. When breasts contain a lot of fatty tissue, changes are not as distinct because of the distance of much of the tissue from the examining fingers. Large breasts often have a palpable *inframammary*

fold or ridge. This is a ridge of dense tissue at the junction of the mammary tissue to the chest wall at the inferior edge of the breast. This normal finding can provoke fear when found during a breast self-examination if not pointed out to the woman at the time of her professional examination. During pregnancy, the breasts are firmer and larger and the lobulations become more distinct.

Breast Masses. When a mass is located on palpation, it is described according to the following criteria:

1. **Location:** The location of the mass is described according to the quadrant in which it is palpated. The breast is divided into four quadrants including the upper-inner, upper-outer, lower-inner and lower-outer and the tail of Spence (Fig. 10.13). An alternate method of localizing findings on the breast is to describe their locations in terms of time zones on a clock and to give the distance in centimeters from the nipple. For example, a lesion may be located at 1 o'clock, 2 centimeters from the nipple. Description of the location is further facilitated by drawing a picture of the involved breast noting the lesion.

2. **Size:** The size of the mass can be described in terms of centimeters or by comparison to the sizes of such common items as a pea or a walnut.

3. **Consistency:** This refers to the texture of the mass. Descriptive terms include cystic or fluid filled, soft, firm and hard.

4. **Tenderness:** When a mass is tender it is often associated with the hormonal changes of the menstrual cycle, particularly with the increased estrogen levels just prior to the onset of menstruation.

5. **Contour:** This refers to the shape of the surface of the mass. The surface is described as regular, smooth, irregular, or rough.

6. **Mobility:** It is essential to note if the mass moves freely or if it is fixed to the chest wall.

7. **Discreteness:** This refers to how easy or hard it is to determine the margins of the mass. The margins are either clearly delineated or indistinct.

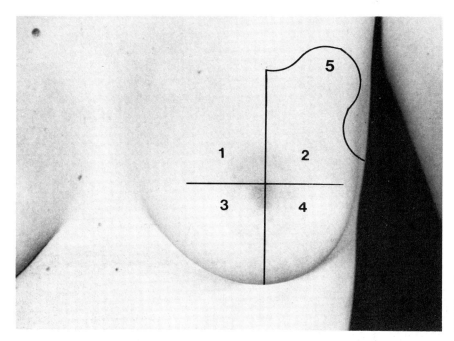

FIGURE 10.13
The breast quadrants. (1) Left-up-per-inner. (2) Left-upper-outer. (3) Left-lower-inner. (4) Left-lower-outer. (5) Tail of Spence.

Following are some of the typical characteristics of the masses found in breast tissue:

1. *Cystic masses* are the most common finding in the examination of the breasts of women between the ages of 20 and 55 and are found in about 35 percent of lesions coming to surgery (Sheahan, 1984). These masses are most commonly located in the upper-outer quadrants of the breast, are mobile, often tender, round, may be hard or soft and have a well-delineated border. Usually multiple cysts are found bilaterally. Frequently, one breast is more affected than the other. When this condition occurs it is referred to as fibro-cystic disease. The cause is not known although an estrogen-related factor is believed to exist because the disease is less prevalent and regresses after menopause. The cysts change with the menstrual cycle getting larger and more tender pre-menstrually. It can be difficult to differentiate a benign lesion from a cancerous one with the use of the common diagnostic techniques of palpation and mammography. Diagnosis is confirmed by aspiration or biopsy.

2. A *fibroadenoma (adenofibroma)* is a mobile, usually nontender, round mass with a well-delineated border. It is usually solitary and unilateral. The mass does not change with the menstrual cycle. This is a breast tumor which occurs in women from the age of 15 to 50 years, with a median age of 20 years (Graham & Kalinowski, 1981). It appears suddenly and can become very large. A biopsy should be done for confirmation of diagnosis followed by excision of the mass.

3. A *cancerous mass* is irregular, is not usually tender, may be fixed to the skin or underlying tissue, and is not clearly delineated from surrounding tissues. Usually there is a single lesion in one breast. The most common location is the tail of Spence.

The Male Patient

Inspection and palpation of the epitrochlear, axillary, and clavicular nodes are the same as for the female. Due to the small amount of breast tissue in the male breast, the breast examination does not require all of the maneuvers involved in the examination of the female. Those aspects of the examination that may be eliminated include eliciting breast retraction with the patient's hands over his head, hands pressing into his hips, and leaning over. With these exceptions, the examination of the male breast follows the same procedure as for the female breast.

Screening Examination of the Axillae and Breasts

The screening examination of the axillae and breasts includes:

1. Inspection of the axillae and clavicular areas
2. Palpation of the axillae in 5 locations
   a. Humerus
   b. Anterior axillary line
   c. Midaxillary line
   d. Posterior axillary line
   e. Deep axilla
3. Palpation of the infraclavicular, supraclavicular, and epitrochlear nodes
4. Inspection of the breasts sitting
   a. Hands on lap*
   b. Hands over head*
   c. Hands pressing into hips*
   d. Hands suspended and leaning forward*
5. Palpation of the breasts and tail of Spence in the supine position

---

Adult females only

THE BREAST SELF-EXAMINATION

The best time for a breast self-examination differs according to the woman's menstrual status, the presence of the uterus or ovaries, and pregnancy. The menstruating woman should do the exam on the last day of her menstrual period every month. At this time her estrogen level is at its lowest and she should not have the breast swelling and tenderness that comes with the increase in estrogen levels later in the cycle. A woman who has had a hysterectomy and is still premenopausal should examine her breasts each month after breast tenderness and swelling are gone. The woman who has had an oophorectomy and the postmenopausal woman should check her breasts at the same time every month. She is encouraged to associate the time of her examination with another regularly occurring monthly event, such as pay day, or she could use the date of her birth as a reminder. For example, if she was born on 6/20, she should check her breasts on the 20th of every month. One problem with the very elderly woman is that the tactile senses in the fingertips diminishes and the range of motion of the upper extremities decreases resulting is a less-accurate breast self-examination. A pregnant woman is not immune to cancer and must continue with her monthly breast exam. The pregnant woman is not menstruating and has no cyclic breast changes, therefore, the examiner should suggest mnemonic devices such as those given to the postmenopausal woman.

A frequent comment from patients is that they are concerned that they will not notice changes in their breasts, stating "My breasts always feel so lumpy." One suggestion is to have them keep a record describing the consistency of their breasts using terms such as smooth, sandy, gravely, etc. Once confidence is gained they can rely on their memory from month to month. For the woman who is especially fearful of performing the exam, suggest that her partner or another close family member or friend do the exam for her.

EXAMPLE OF A RECORDED HISTORY AND PHYSICAL

SUBJECTIVE:

Chief Complaint: "I felt a lump in my breast yesterday."

HPH: This 24-year-old female considers herself to be in excellent health. Yesterday, when she was taking a shower, she noticed a nonpainful lump "about the size of a peach pit" in her right breast. She says it feels "hard and round, and it moves easily." She has not noticed any changes in her skin or discharge from her nipple. She does a breast self-exam every 2 months or so. She has never had anything like this before. Her last menstrual period began 1 week ago (10/23). There is no family history of breast cancer or any other breast disease. She is seeking consultation today because, "I'm afraid that I have cancer."

OBJECTIVE:

T. 98.6° F; P. 74 radial; R. 14; B.P. 126/74 (sitting).

Breasts: No evidence of lesions, moles, rashes, redness, or discharge in either breast. Bilateral symmetry on inspection. No dimpling. *Right breast:* A nontender, round, hard, well defined, movable mass about 2.5 cm. in the RUQ at about 11 o'clock, 3 cm. from the nipple. No other lumps or tender areas. *Left breast:* No tenderness or masses palpable. Breast tissue soft throughout.

Lymph nodes: No enlargement or tenderness of the axillary, supraclavicular, infraclavicular, or epitrochlear nodes bilaterally.

REFERENCES

American Cancer Society (1976). 1976 Cancer Facts and Figures. New York: American Cancer Society.

American Cancer Society (1979). 1979 Cancer Facts and Figures. New York: American Cancer Society.

American Cancer Society (1985). 1985 Cancer Facts and Figures. New York: American Cancer Society.

Anthony, C. (1978). Risk factors associated with breast cancer. Nurse Practitioner, 3, 31–32.

Baker, L. (1982). Breast cancer detection demonstration project: Five-year summary report. New York: American Cancer Society.

Beaman, M. (1982). Breast cancer health beliefs and practice of breast self-examination. Unpublished master's thesis. University of Illinois at Chicago.

Graham, S., & Kalinowski, B. (1981). Problems of the breast. In C. Fogel, and N. Woods, (Eds.), Health Care of Women—A Nursing Perspective. St. Louis: C. V. Mosby, pp. 332–60.

Guidelines for the cancer-related checkup. (1980). Ca-A Cancer Journal for Clinicians, 30(4), 195–237.

Larson, E. (1983). Epidemiologic correlates of breast, endometrial, and ovarian cancers. Cancer Nursing, 6(4), 295–301.

Prenatal diethylstilbestrol exposure. (1983). Clinical Pediatrics, 22(2), 139–43.

Rhodes, G., Glober, G., & Stemmermann, G. (1974). A review of some tumors of interest for demographic study in Hawaii. Hawaii Medical Journal, 33, 283–84.

Round table. (1975). Odds and options in breast cancer risks. Patient Care, 9(7), 20–57.

Senie, R., Rosen, P., & Kinne, D. (1983). Epidemiologic factors associated with breast cancer. Cancer Nursing, 6(5), 367–71.

Sheahan, S. (1984). Management of breast lumps. Nurse Practitioner, 9(2), 19–22.

Spuhler, J. (1950). Genetics of three normal morphological variations: Patterns of superficial veins of the anterior thorax, peroneus tertius muscle, and number of vallate papillae. Cold Spring Harbor Symposia on Quantitative Biology, 15, 175–89.

Tanner, J. (1962). Growth at Adolescence (2nd ed.). Oxford, England: Blackwell Scientific Publications.

Townsend, C. M. (1980). Breast lumps. Clinical Symposia, 32(2), 3–14.

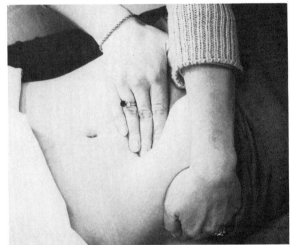

11

The Abdomen

The evaluation of the abdomen can be straightforward if there are no problems, or it can be more involved and time consuming if concerns are present. There are a multitude of assessments to consider when a patient has abdominal complaints. These range from mild viral infections to emotional stresses to malignant disease. If the nurse is a good investigator, she can do much of the work during the history. The completeness and quality of the history may be more revealing than the findings of the physical exam of the abdomen.

DEVELOPMENTAL CHANGES OF THE ABDOMEN THROUGHOUT THE LIFESPAN

The abdomen and its structures change significantly throughout one's life. The skin, musculature and organs change structurally from infancy to the elderly years. In the neonate and young infant, the abdominal organs are relatively easy to delineate because the musculature has not developed. The liver edge, spleen tip, kidneys and diastus rectus (separation of the abdominis rectus which is not a significant problem in infancy) are often easily palpable in the neonatal or early infant period.

A toddler's abdomen is oval shaped and protrudes significantly when he is standing. This is a classic finding of toddlerhood lost as the youngster approaches school age. The exam of the toddler's abdomen will often depend on whether he is ticklish. If he is very ticklish, he will guard, and the exam will be difficult to conduct. Gaining the child's trust and making the exam fun (when possible) is usually most helpful for this age group.

The musculature of the child's abdomen becomes more evident in the school-age child. For this reason, the abdomen is beginning to get harder to examine. The school-age child is generally not afraid of being examined, so it is easier to get this age group to trust the provider and to relax. This relaxation facilitates the exam.

Defining organ structure and feeling masses may be the hardest to assess in adolescents and young adults. During the adolescent and young adult years, these young people often have such sound abdominal musculature, especially athletes, that eliciting abdominal masses or irregularities (i.e., hernias) may be difficult. Tenderness, even in this population, is relatively easy to locate.

The musculature begins to decrease in middle adulthood. Often this will depend on what kind of athletic shape the person is in, or how many pregnancies a woman has had. If there is less subcutaneous tissue and adipose tissue, it will be easier to define organs and palpate masses. In very obese people, the abdominal exam may reveal nothing more than tender areas.

The elderly often have very soft abdomens. A thorough and precise exam is necessary because there is a relatively high incidence of abdominal cancers in the elderly and the masses are often palpable.

There are certain health concerns related to the gastrointestinal system (which includes many of the abdominal organs) that are more likely to occur at one developmental period than another. For this reason, the nurse needs to be aware of what problems may occur at certain ages and assess them accordingly. As an example, anorexia nervosa and bulimia are more common during adolescence and young adulthood than the school-age years.

To think of these health issues in a developmental sequence, one must first consider those most prevalent at the beginning of life. A prime concern during the neonatal and infant period is feeding disorders. These often manifest early in the neonatal period and go on throughout infancy. The two common problems that may occur during this time are *pyloric stenosis* and *milk intolerance.* Both

may have vomiting and poor weight gain as predominant symptoms. In both disorders, the vomiting occurs shortly after eating, but in pyloric stenosis the vomiting is classically projectile. As a rule, pyloric stenosis becomes evident after two weeks of life and before two months. A milk allergy can become evident shortly after feeding is initiated.

During toddlerhood, a developmental task which has the potential of becoming a health issue is toilet training. Often bowel control precedes bladder control. In most cases children accomplish this without difficulty. Some children, however, become afraid of moving their bowels and therefore, try to retain their stools. This not only causes serious discomfort but can materialize into a fairly significant problem. Appropriate intervention is essential after a thorough investigation confirms the existence of bowel withholding.

School-age children, adolescents and young adults are often the victims of stress-related illnesses. For the school age child who has unpleasant feelings and fears about going to school, a phenomena called *school phobia* can arise. This often presents as abdominal pain occurring upon waking or the night before a school day. The child has real pain, and this should be acknowledged. The source of anxiety behind the pain should be carefully and thoroughly investigated.

Two stress-related illnesses that often occur in the adolescent and young adult are *bulimia and anorexia nervosa.* Bulimia is an eating disorder characterized by binge eating and purging (either by forced vomiting or excess use of laxatives). Bulimics tend to be very secretive. Anorexia nervosa is also an eating disorder manifested by severe and constant dieting. This self-imposed starvation causes cessation of menses and symptoms of severe malnourishment. Both symptoms occur in varying degrees. Both require extensive counseling as well as medical management. Bulimia and anorexia nervosa can be very debilitating and ultimately life-threatening without appropriate intervention.

Peptic ulcers are common stress-related occurrences in adulthood. People who present with symptoms of peptic ulcer disease often cannot initially identify a stress-related issue in their lives. Symptoms are not always specific, but the patient may complain of dyspepsia; epigastric pain; pain that occurs after meals; pain that awakens the patient at night; or pain relieved by taking foods or antacids. Working with this patient to identify stress-related causes can be as important as the medical regime that has been prescribed. Ulcer disease can start with mild discomfort of an irritated mucosal lining or acid hypersecretion but can develop to a life-threatening condition—gastrointestinal bleeding. A precise history is very important in this situation. *Ulcerative colitis,* an ulcerative disease of the colon, is another potentially serious illness that often begins in young adulthood. The patient may have a gradual change in bowel habits, lassitude, anorexia, and rectal bleeding. Rectal bleeding is the chief complaint. Some patients may also notice blood, pus, or mucus in the stools. This disease can also proceed to a fulminant state rather quickly. The rectal discharge and bleeding may be life threatening. In this case, more dramatic interventions are required.

Middle-aged adults and the elderly can be victims of abdominal cancers. Many of these malignancies—colon, pancreas, and liver have a poor prognosis. Many people have few if any, early symptoms. Often by the time the signs and symptoms appear, like blood in the stool, jaundice, a palpable mass in the abdomen, or weight loss, it is too late to control the progression of the disease. Therefore, because the incidence of these types of abdominal malignancies is higher in this age group, appropriate screening is necessary. Screening can be done fairly easily by testing for occult blood in the stool on an annual basis, or more often if indicated. (See discussion of this procedure in Chapters 12 and 13.)

Elderly people can suffer from constipation. Much of this problem is related to diet, lack of exercise, and medications. It is important to assess the actual meaning of constipation to the patient. Some people believe that they are constipated if they do not have a bowel movement once or twice daily. Although this may not be the health provider's definition of constipation, it is, nonetheless, a serious concern and discomfort to the patient. Supportive measures such as change in the diet, increased exercise, and increased fluid intake should be offered.

Many other illnesses occur with the gastrointestinal system. The previously discussed problems are an example of a way to look at gastrointestinal problems in a developmental mode.

ANATOMY

Because the abdominal region has many underlying organs, the area is divided by two systems of imaginary landmarks (Figs. 11.1A and B). This region has certain boundaries, and these should also be described, in order to help clarify the imaginary landmarks. The *xiphoid process* is the superior boundary and the *symphysis pubis* is the inferior marking of the first imaginary landmark. Drawing a line through the umbilicus across the abdomen makes it easy to divide the abdomen into four quadrants. Specific organs lie in each designated region (Chart 11.1).

The other imaginary method of dividing up the abdomen resembles a tic-tac-toe board. This nine-region division has smaller sections and is most helpful for describing midline findings. (See Figure 11.1 for demarcation of areas.) The terms *epigastric, umbilical,* and *hypogastric* are most frequently adopted from this particular method. The *kidneys* are not often described within the two imaginary systems, but are referred to as being in the *costovertebral region.* This landmark is named for the meeting of the spinal cord and the twelfth rib.

The organs of the abdominal region are involved in many systems of the body. The specific organs of the gastrointestinal system that lie in this area are the *stomach,* the *pancreas,* the *liver,* the *gallbladder,* and the *small* and *large intestines* (Fig. 11.2). The stomach begins at the end of the *esophagus* and extends to the beginning of the small intestine. The *cardiac sphincter* is at the esophageal entrance, and the *pyloric sphincter* is at the duodenal entrance. The stomach is an organ for the motility of food, hydrochloric acid secretion, and the enzymatic digestion of foods.

The pancreas lies behind the stomach. It contains the endocrine hormones insulin and glucagon. Exocrine hormones and pancreatic enzymes are also located there.

The liver lies under the diaphragm and extends across the right-upper quadrant and slightly into left-upper quadrant. It secretes

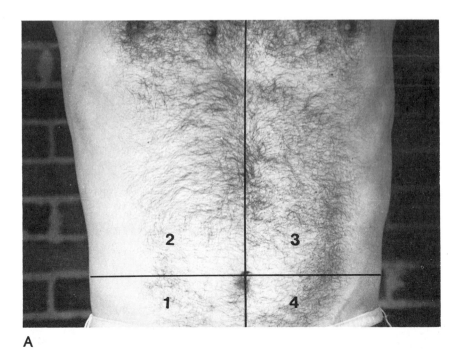

A

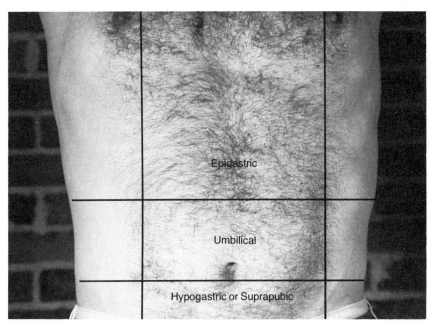

B

FIGURE 11.1
*Imaginary landmarks of the abdomen. **A.** Four quadrants: (1) Right-lower quadrant (RLQ), (2) Right-upper quadrant (RUQ), (3) Left-upper quadrant (LUQ), (4) Left-lower quadrant (LLQ). **B.** Nine region division.*

bile, which aids in the digestion of fat. Liver cells function in iron metabolism, plasma protein production, detoxification of plasma substances, metabolism of hemoglobin breakdown products, and in other capacities. The liver is essential to life.

The storehouse for bile is the gallbladder, which lies behind the liver. This organ is not essential to life and can be removed without permanently damaging the digestive system.

The small intestine is made up of three branches and is responsible for the most absorption in the gastrointestinal tract. The three components making up the 18 feet of the small intestine are the *duodenum,* the *jejunum,* and the *ileum* (Fig. 11.2). Located on the wall of

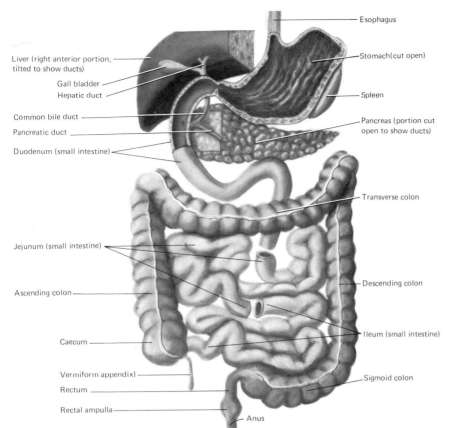

Esophagus

Liver (right anterior portion, tilted to show ducts)

Stomach (cut open)

Gall bladder

Hepatic duct

Spleen

Common bile duct

Pancreatic duct

Pancreas (portion cut open to show ducts)

Duodenum (small intestine)

Transverse colon

Jejunum (small intestine)

Descending colon

Ascending colon

Caecum

Ileum (small intestine)

Vermiform appendix)

Rectum

Sigmoid colon

Rectal ampulla

Anus

FIGURE 11.2
The gastrointestinal system. (From Heagarty, M., et al., Child Health: Basics for Primary Care. New York: Appleton-Century-Crofts, 1980, p. 156.)

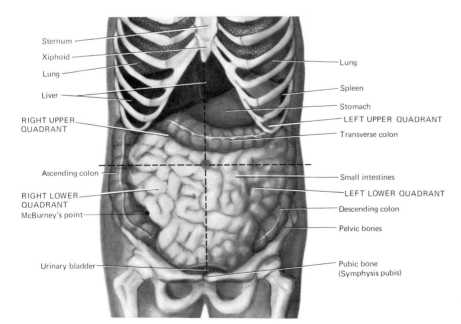

Sternum

Xiphoid

Lung

Lung

Liver

Spleen

Stomach

RIGHT UPPER QUADRANT

LEFT UPPER QUADRANT

Transverse colon

Ascending colon

Small intestines

RIGHT LOWER QUADRANT

LEFT LOWER QUADRANT

McBurney's point

Descending colon

Pelvic bones

Urinary bladder

Pubic bone (Symphysis pubis)

FIGURE 11.3
The gastrointestinal system: the abdomen. (From Heagarty, M., et al., Child Health: Basics for Primary Care. New York: Appleton-Century-Crofts, 1980, p. 156.)

CHART 11.1
ORGANS IN THE ABDOMEN

Right-upper Quandrant	Left-upper Quandrant
Liver	Left lobe of liver
Gallbladder	Stomach
Pylorus	Spleen
Duodenum	Upper lobe of left kidney
Head of pancreas	Pancreas
Pancreas	Left adrenal
Right adrenal gland	Splenic flexure of colon
Upper lobe of right kidney	Section of transverse colon
Hepatic flexure of colon	Section of descending
Section of ascending colon	colon
Section of transverse colon	

Right-lower Quadrant	Left-lower Quadrant
Cecum	Lower portion of left kidney
Appendix	Sigmoid colon
Lower portion of right kidney	Left ovary
Right ovary	Left fallopian tube
Right fallopian tube	Left ureter
Right ureter	Left spermatic cord
Right spermatic cord	Section of descending
Section of ascending colon	colon

Midline
Bladder (if not distended)
Uterus (if not enlarged)

(Adapted from Malasanos, L., et al., Health Assessment (3rd ed.). St. Louis: C. V. Mosby, 1986, p. 363, with permission.)

the small intestine are villi, which control the small intestinal absorption of carbohydrate, protein, and fat.

The large intestine is different than the small intestine. There are no villi and it is a much wider organ. The large intestine has three branches. They are the *ascending colon,* the *descending colon,* and the *transverse colon* (Fig. 11.3). The function of the large intestine mainly concerns the absorption of water and the storage of feces.

Portions of the reproductive system also lie in the abdominal region. In the female these include the *uterus,* the *right* and *left ovaries,* and the *fallopian tubes.* In the male the *left* and *right ureters* and the *left* and *right spermatic cords* are found in the abdomen.

Somewhat accessible to examination in the abdomen are the *kidneys.* Although they belong to the genitourinary system, they are examined as parts of the abdomen. They lie behind the muscles of the posterior abdominal wall. The upper borders reach the diaphragm at about T_{12}. The lower borders are located

in the area of L_3. The right kidney is usually lower than the left due to liver placement.

The *adrenals,* which lie directly on top of the kidneys, are parts of the endocrine system but are discussed along with the abdominal anatomy. These small but extremely potent glands have a major role in the production of the corticosteriods, epinephrine, and norepinephrine.

HISTORY

Although there are some questions in the review of systems that are age related, most of the general history pertaining to this system can be elicited by asking the following questions:

1. Presence or concern about pain? (See discussion that follows these questions).
2. General bowel habits.*
   a. Times per week normal for patient?
   b. Character of stool: color, consistency, amount?
   c. Pain with bowel movements?
   d. Changes that affect bowel habits (i.e. travel, menses, stress, etc.)?
3. Constipation?
   a. What is meant by the word constipation?
   b. How often do episodes occur?
   c. Related to diet, stress, medication?
   d. Previous diagnostic work-up?
   e. What makes it worse? What makes it better?
4. Hemorrhoids?
   a. Past or present history?
   b. Know whether they are internal or external?
   c. Associated with bleeding?
   d. Treatments used? Successfully? Unsuccessfully?
5. Diarrhea?
   a. What is meant by diarrhea (exact specifics required like color, consistency, explosive, etc.)?

---

* In the pediatric history, it is important to inquire about bowel control in children. Parents should be asked if their child had difficulty in achieving bowel control and at what age he successfully did so.

b. How often do episodes occur?

c. Associated with fever, mucus or blood in stool?

d. Related to diet, use of milk products, stress or medication usage?

e. Diagnostic studies done in past?

f. Treatment(s) used in past?

6. Change in appetite, increase or decrease?
7. Change in thirst, increase or decrease?
8. Food intolerances?

   a. What are they?

   b. How do they manifest themselves?

   c. Age of onset?

   d. Treatment used to alleviate symptoms?

9. Heartburn? (See questions for constipation)
10. Presents a past history of excessive belching?
11. Presents a past history of excessive flatulence?
12. Previous or other gastrointestinal problems not addressed in above questions?

    a. Description of episodes including diagnostic studies, diagnosis, and treatments?

13. Previous history of jaundice, gastrointestinal bleeding?

    a. Description of episodes including diagnostic studies, diagnosis, and treatments?

If a positive response is given to the question of abdominal pain, then a thorough pain history must be elicited. If the history is taken in appropriate detail, many causative factors can be eliminated. Asking the patient to tell you first about the pain in general, will give some, but not all information. After listening to the patient's description, complete the history with the following information about the pain:

- *Onset:* When did the pain first begin?
- *Frequency:* How often does it occur?
- *Sequence and Chronology:* Is it always there? Does it come and go? Describe a typical episode. Does it wake you out of a deep sleep? Is this the first occurrence, or is there a past history of the same pain? Describe past episodes.
- *Location:* Where is the pain? Can it be pointed to with one finger or is it more generalized? Does it move around? From where to where?
- *Quality:* Describe the pain. Is it sharp? Dull? Stabbing? Nagging? Aching?
- *Intensity:* Does it peak? When? Is it the same all the time?
- *Associated Phenomena:* Nausea, vomiting, diarrhea? Constipation, flatulence? Belching? Fever? Rectal bleeding? Blood or mucus in stools? Hematemesis? Difficulty swallowing? Frequent urination, burning, itching?* Vaginal or penile discharge?* Date of last menstrual period? Other menstrual irregularities? Pain with, or before menses or ovulation?* Weight loss?
- *Aggravating Factors:* Foods? Medications? Position? Activities? Stress (occupational, environmental, or people-related)? Eating, drinking, and smoking habits?
- *Alleviating Factors:* Treatment used? Hot water bottle? Heating pad? Medications? Rest? Change in position? Relief of stress?
- *Miscellaneous:* Exposure to anyone with the same kind of symptoms? Foods eaten in the last 24 hours? Where (restaurants, picnics, etc.)? Recent change in job, school, home environment? Allergies (or past history of lactose intolerance)?

There are nine major sites to check in the localization of abdominal pain (Judge & Zuidema, 1982): Sometimes a guide such as this may be helpful in locating causes. Use this list only as a guide—it is not absolute by any means.

1. **Esophageal:** Midline retrosternal with radiation to the back at the level of the lesion.
2. **Gastric:** Epigastric; radiation occasionally to the back, particularly the left subscapular area.
3. **Duodenal:** Epigastric; radiation to the back, particularly the right subscapular area.
4. **Gallbladder:** RUQ or epigastric; radiation to right subscapular or midback areas.
5. **Pancreatic:** Epigastric; radiation to midback or left lumbar areas.
6. **Small Intestine:** Periumbilical.

*A more complete review of symptoms may be indicated

7. Appendicular: Periumbilical, migrating to RLQ.
8. Colonic: Hypogastrium, RLQ or LLQ; sigmoid pain may radiate to the sacral region.
9. Rectal: Deep pelvic location.

A physiologic change in the elderly that the nurse should be alert to is an elevated pain threshold masking the severity of the abdominal pain. In addition, the patient may have trouble localizing the pain or may inaccurately describe and remember the duration of the discomfort. The nurse needs to be sensitive to the existence of this problem. It will affect the accuracy of her subjective data.

One final note about historical information regarding this system. Acute gastrointestinal problems can occur anytime in one's life. A virus can happen suddenly and be gone in 12 or 24 hours. Food poisoning can begin a few hours after ingesting the toxin. Gastrointestinal bleeding can be insidious or suddenly life threatening. Without an accurate history, much time and energy can be wasted and, in some cases, cause the patient serious consequence. It is critical never to assume anything. People who have rectal bleeding can have anything from constipation to colon cancer. For this reason, all the previously mentioned areas of investigation *must* be included in the interview when the patient responds affirmatively to any question regarding the gastrointestinal system.

PHYSICAL ASSESSMENT

All four techniques of examination are used to perform the abdominal exam. However, this is one system in which the order is different. As always, inspection begins the examination. In this case, auscultation follows inspection. If percussion and palpation precede auscultation, then the bowel sounds will be falsely stimulated.

Among the items required for the abdominal exam are a relaxed patient with an empty bladder, good lighting, a stethoscope, a marking pen, and a ruler (tape measure).

The patient should be as relaxed as possible. Any stress or fear will tighten up the abdominal muscles and make the exam more difficult. Some hints to help the patient and the examiner follow:

1. The patient's abdominal area should be completely exposed.
2. The examiner should place a pillow under the patient's knees.
3. The patient should place his arms at his side or across his chest.
4. The nurse may converse with the patient during the exam to facilitate relaxation.
5. The patient's face should be watched not his abdomen, because any distress signs will appear on the face.
6. The nurse can palpate with the patient's hand under her own if the patient is ticklish, gradually easing his hand away.
7. Tender areas under suspicion should be examined last.
8. The left-handed examiner should stand at the patient's left side and the right-handed examiner should stand at the patient's right side. This provides for ease of movement as the examiner reaches across the patient to palpate the abdomen. The examiner remains on the same side throughout the entire examination.

Inspection

For inspection of the abdomen, the patient is supine and the examiner is positioned at the patient's side level with the abdomen. When inspecting the abdomen, the examiner observes shape, symmetry, skin, and movement. The shape is usually described as flat, round, protruding, or sunken. A sunken abdomen is often the result of dehydration. A protruding belly may have several causes: pregnancy, distension, obesity, or a tumor. Rounded "tummies" can be noted in infants, toddlers, and young children. Extreme roundness in a young child may indicate malnutrition. (If this is being considered, a comprehensive diet history should be elicited.) A flat abdomen is usually the result of appropriate weight and muscle tone. In our society this is a highly valued commodity.

An abdomen is normally symmetrical. Asymmetry can occur as a result of pregnancy or other masses, a hernia, obstruction, or fluid.

The skin is inspected carefully. If a scar or scars exist, several features about it should be noted: where it is exactly (from what point to what point), how long and wide it is (exact measurements are appropriate), and when and how it occurred (old scars are silver or skin-toned, while new scars are pinker in color). It is helpful to draw a picture of the abdomen with the placement of the scar when recording the data. *Striae* are stretch marks, which can result from a rapid weight gain, as in pregnancy, or a large weight loss. Red striae indicate recency. As with scars, silver striae show age. Purple striae may indicate Cushing's disease and can often be found on people who have a long history of cortisone usage.

The skin should also be inspected for lesions, moles, and rashes of any type. The location, color, and size of these should be recorded. If a mole is changing color or size, it is important to know at what rate that is occurring. If a record is made of the location, color, and measurements, then future comparisons can be made. This is especially important when a malignancy is suspected.

The umbilicus is observed for its position, shape, redness, irritation, discharge, or the presence of hernias. An *umbilical hernia* (Fig. 11.4) is one that protrudes through the umbilicus. In infants, in whom such hernias occur most often, this defect may be the result of inadequate closing of the abdominal wall. Large umbilical hernias that can be seen during inspection may be larger than 6 centimeters. The visibility may be magnified by the child's crying or straining. Umbilical hernias in adults are not very common. The cases that do occur are seen primarily in the obese and in pregnant women. The patient is asked to raise his head and shoulder while keeping his legs flat to demonstrate the presence of an umbilical hernia.

In the newborn, the remains of the mother's umbilical cord on the baby's umbilicus are present for the first 2 weeks of the baby's life. At around that time the stub should slough off. This is a common site of infection for the newborn. The cord and umbilicus should, therefore, be observed for erythema, swelling, discharge, and odor. Any or all of these signs may indicate infection and call for a referral.

Movement in the abdomen occurs with respiration, peristalsis, and pulsations. Abdominal breathing can be observed while inspecting the abdomen. Up to the age of 7, children are primarily abdominal breathers. Men are much better abdominal breathers than women. Most women employ only their thoracic muscles, and the result is superficial breathing techniques. Men, on the other hand, use both thoracic and abdominal breathing muscles. Using both sets of muscles provides for the most efficient air exchange.

Pulsation from the aorta may be observed in the epigastric area. This pulsation is most likely to be seen in thin adults or children. Peristalsis may or may not be visible. It too,

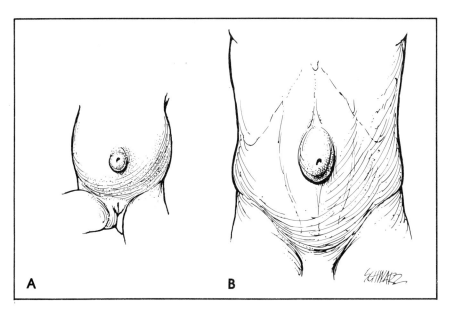

FIGURE 11.4
Umbilical hernia in an (**A**) *infant and* (**B**) *adult.*

is most evident in thinner people. To see peristalsis the examiner's eyes should be level with the patient's abdomen and she should be watching across the abdomen for a wave-like movement.

Auscultation

As mentioned previously, the abdomen is auscultated before it is percussed or palpated. The purpose of auscultating this area is to listen for active bowel sounds and bruits. The diaphragm of the stethoscope is used for auscultating bowel sounds. The examiner must hear this irregular, tinkly noise in all four quadrants. Such noises normally occur every 5 to 20 seconds. Bowel sounds are described with the terms *hypoactive, hyperactive,* and *audible.* Before concluding that they are inaudible, one must listen for 3 to 5 minutes. The examiner can flick the abdominal wall with her fingers to stimulate intestinal movement.

Absence of bowel sounds means decreased intestinal motility. One reason may be a *paralytic ileus,* which occurs postoperatively or as a result of such electrolyte disorders as hypokalemia. Other causes could be gangrenous bowel or appendicitis. Any obvious decrease in bowel sounds warrants immediate attention.

Increased bowel sounds, or *borborygmi,* can be the result of laxative ingestion or of anything else that might increase gastric motility. Increased bowel sounds, along with flatulence, abdominal cramping, and diarrhea, are common symptoms among lactase-deficient individuals who consume a sufficient quantity of milk. Gastroenteritis will also often cause an increase in bowel sounds, among other objective findings.

The bell of the stethoscope is used to auscultate for abdominal bruits. A bruit is an abnormal flow sound (see Chapter 9, page 249), that is often the result of a dilated, stenosed, or obstructed vessel. Bruits in the abdomen are auscultated over the aorta, and bilaterally over the iliac, renal, and femoral arteries (Fig. 11.5). The bell of the stethoscope is usually used for this purpose.

A loud bruit heard over the aorta, just above the umbilicus may indicate an aortic aneurysm. Arterial insufficiency in the lower extremities may be detected by listening over the iliac and femoral arteries for a bruit. Renal bruits may be heard in the patient with stenotic kidney vessels. A patient with cardiovascular disease or a long-standing history of hypertension should be evaluated carefully for these abnormal sounds. On a rare occasion, a bruit can be heard over the liver. When the bruit can be detected, it usually indicates a malignancy of the liver.

The friction rub is another abnormal

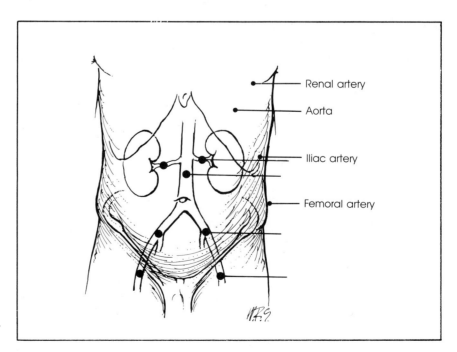

FIGURE 11.5
Sites to auscultate for abdominal bruits.

Renal artery
Aorta
Iliac artery
Femoral artery

sound that can be heard in the abdomen. This is a grating sound that resembles two pieces of leather riding over one another. Such sounds are rare, but are most commonly heard over the liver or spleen and are related to infection or malignancy.

Percussion

Percussion of the abdomen is utilized to detect the presence of fluid, air, or solid tissue. This technique is also used to outline the borders of the liver and of the spleen and to assess the fullness of the bladder. A tympanic percussion note is heard throughout the air-filled areas of the abdomen. The solid areas give a duller sound.

The abdomen is percussed in an organized and thorough manner. Percussion may elicit a painful response over tender areas. If it is possible to determine where the tenderness is from the history, then the examiner should avoid percussing and palpating the tender area until the end of the abdominal exam. Evincing pain early in the exam might cause the patient to guard, which will make the evaluation more difficult.

GENERAL ORIENTATION

The examiner percusses over all four quadrants, including the flank region. The percussion note of tympany is dominant, although dullness will be found over masses, stool, or a distended bladder. Tenderness may be elicited as well.

When percussing over all four quadrants, the examiner should include the flank region. It is important to establish a pattern of percussion and stick to that pattern. One suggested method is to percuss from the top of the abdomen down along 3 or 4 imaginary lines covering the entire surface of the abdominal area. Another method is to start at the side furthest from the examiner and percuss along 3 to 4 imaginary lines across the abdomen. More detailed percussion may be required for obese individuals because of the increased surface area.

PERCUSSION OF THE LIVER BORDERS

This is not a difficult procedure if the examiner can picture the underlying organs (Fig. 11.2). The liver can be percussed along the right mid-clavicular line and the midsternal line. The midclavicular (MCL) measurement alone is an acceptable estimate if there are no related problems. When in doubt, the measurement at the midsternal line should be used, too.

It is helpful to remember that the lower border of the liver normally lies just above the right costal margin and the upper border sits approximately between the fifth and seventh intercostal spaces along the midclavicular line.

The examiner should begin by percussing upward at the level of the umbilicus along the right MCL (Fig. 11.6). Tympany will predominate here. Somewhere around the costal margin, the tympanic note will change to one of dullness. The point at which the change in percussion notes occurs is the lower edge of the liver. (Note: percussion over a rib will also sound dull.) This point should be marked with a pen.

Next the examiner percusses down from the right nipple along the MCL from lung resonance to the first note of dullness. Once again, if a rib is not being percussed, the point of dullness denotes the upper border of the liver (Fig. 11.7). The examiner should mark this point and measure the span (Fig. 11.8). The average width of the liver at the MCL is 6 to 12 centimeters in the adult. (The liver span of a child varies depending on the age and size of the child.)

In measuring the span at the midsternal line, the same procedure is followed. The average span along the midsternal line is 4 to 8 centimeters. These distances may be greater in men and taller people.

Accuracy may be obscured if dullness exists due to right pleural effusion or a consolidation in the right lung. Excess air in the colon may increase the tympanic area in the right-upper quadrant and also distort correct measurements of the lower border. Liver displacement can occur as a result of pregnancy, abdominal or flank tumors, or ascites. These conditions, too, will affect the measurement of the liver span.

PERCUSSION OF THE SPLEEN

The spleen can be percussed most easily if it is enlarged (as in mononucleosis). However, a slight change in the percussion note can be heard over the normal spleen somewhere between the sixth and tenth ribs close to the left

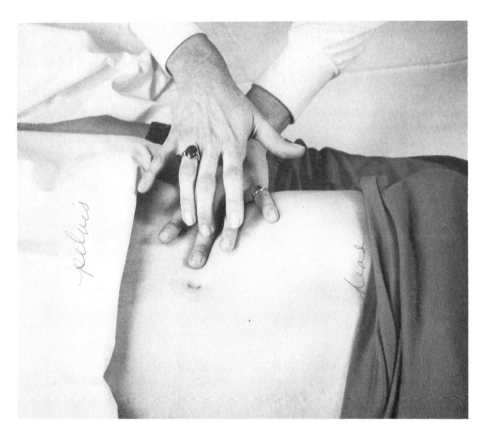

FIGURE 11.6
The place to begin percussion to locate the lower border of the liver.

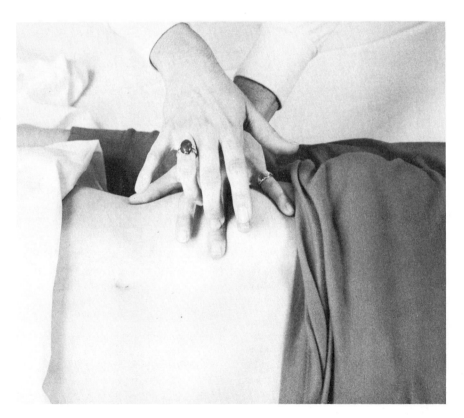

FIGURE 11.7
Trying to locate the upper border of the liver.

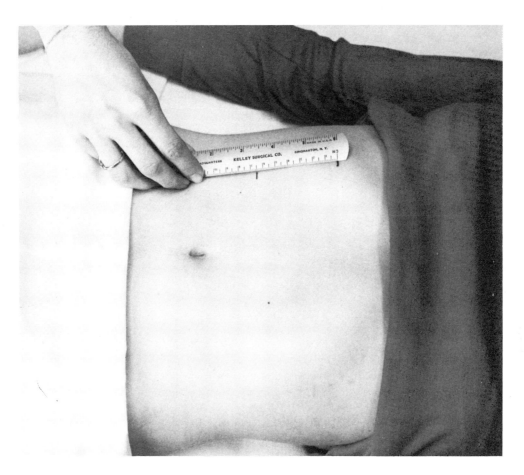

FIGURE 11.8
Measuring liver span.

midaxillary line (Fig. 11.9). As with the liver, the note will change from tympany to a duller tone.

PERCUSSION OF THE STOMACH
The tympanic sound of the gastric air bubble is elicited in the lower left anterior rib cage (Fig. 11.10).

PERCUSSION OF ASCITES
The accumulation of serous fluid floating in the abdominal cavity is known as *ascites* or *ascitic fluid.* Through percussion, the general level of this fluid can be assessed.

On inspection, an ascitic abdomen looks distended, especially in the flank areas. The degree of distension depends on the extent of the ascites. When the patient is in the supine position, the fluid sinks towards the flank and posterior regions of the abdominal cavity.

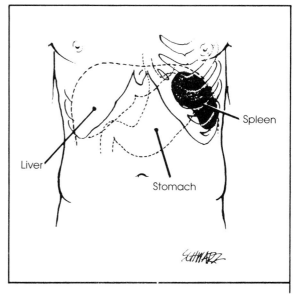

FIGURE 11.9
Areas of splenic dullness.

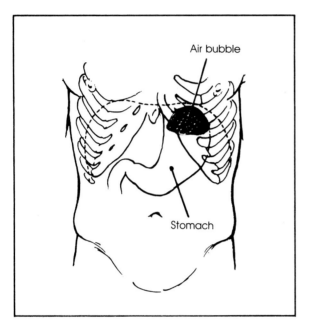

FIGURE 11.10
Gastric air bubble.

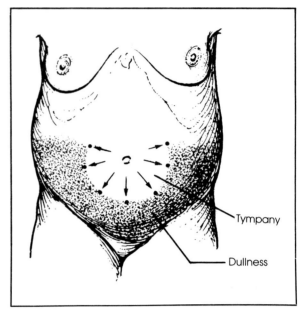

FIGURE 11.11
Assessing possible ascites with the patient in supine position.

Therefore, when the examiner is percussing for the fluid borders, she will find dullness in the lateral areas of the abdomen. The percussion note of tympany will be found where no fluid exists. The borders of where the fluid line lies should map out in a U-like shape around the umbilicus. The distance this line is to the umbilicus should be measured and recorded. This measure will help determine if there has been an increase or decrease in the ascitic fluid. (Fig. 11.11).

A less precise method of measuring ascites requires that the patient lie on his side. The fluid will move to the side on which the patient is lying (Fig. 11.12). Again, the examiner percusses to define where dullness ends and tympany begins. There will be an imaginary vertical line along the abdomen at the fluid level. This distance should be measured from the umbilicus to ascertain if there are changes in the degree of ascites.

Palpation

Palpation is used to detect tenderness, distension, and fluid; to outline abdominal organs; and to determine the presence and location of masses. Two types of palpation are performed: *light* and *deep*. Light palpation is uti-

lized to assess superficial pain, organs, and masses. Deep palpation is used to distinguish inferior organs or to elicit deep pain. In either method the examiner should always observe the patient's face, not his abdomen, while palpating. It is important to remember that pain will be evinced by a change in facial expression or by muscle guarding. In the elderly patient, organs may be more readily palpated

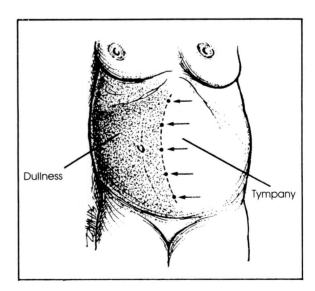

FIGURE 11.12
Assessing possible ascites with patient on right side.

due to loss of abdominal musculature as the person ages.

For light palpation, the palmar surfaces of the fingertips are used (Fig. 11.13). The examiner depresses her hand lightly and systematically over the entire abdomen (if the patient is ticklish, the examiner should slide the patient's hand under her own). The examiner should follow the same pattern for palpation as she did for percussion. The examiner feels for tenderness, muscle tone, abdominal stiffening, or masses. If a sensitive area is discovered, she should postpone examining it until the end, as is done with percussion.

When resistance is met during light palpation, the nurse can determine if this is a tender area by observing the patient's face and asking him directly. If the patient seems entirely relaxed and pain-free and a point of resistance is met, one can suspect involuntary resistance. If the involuntary response is confirmed, the nurse should suspect peritonitis.

Sometimes malingering is suspected. In this case, while auscultating the four quadrants for bowel sounds, the examiner should apply some light pressure to the diaphragm of the stethoscope. If a painful response has been elicited during light palpation, then the same response should occur during the application of pressure over that spot. This maneuver mimics light palpation.

Next, deep palpation is begun. Once again, all four quadrants are surveyed thoroughly and systematically. This portion of the exam may cause some discomfort, therefore, helping the patient to relax is very important. Deep

abdominal breathing will help the patient to relax. Here, too, tender areas should be palpated last.

The same portion of the examiner's hand is used for deep palpation as for light palpation. However, this time much more pressure is applied. In fact, many examiners use two hands. In this method, one hand is superimposed on the other and the top hand is used to exert pressure (Fig. 11.14). This bimanual approach is thought to allow for deeper palpation and better delineation of organs and masses. As with any mass that is discovered, the examiner should note its size, location, mobility, contour, consistency, and tenderness.

When a painful area is discovered, a test for *rebound tenderness* needs to be done. The examiner depresses her hand deeply into a remote area from the involved area and then lets go quickly. If the pain is increased with the release of the hand, as opposed to increasing with the deep palpation, the test is positive. This tests for peritoneal inflammation and is commonly used to aid in the diagnosis of appendicitis. The patient with appendicitis will have rebound tenderness in the right-lower quadrant, known as *McBurney's Point*. This point is to the left of the iliac crest. When palpating over McBurney's Point, the patient with appendicitis will experience pain when the pressure is withdrawn. If the history indicates that peritoneal inflammation is a possibility, and if among the objective findings is right-lower quadrant rebound tenderness, then proper referral is needed quickly.

If a patient presents with right-upper quadrant pain or other indicators (i.e., the history) that the gallbladder may be acutely inflamed, (acute cholecystitis) one should test for *Murphy's Sign*. This is elicited by having the patient take a deep breath while the examiner places her palpating hand under the right costal margin. Both the liver and gallbladder will descend with inspiration. It is important, therefore, for the examiner to get her hand under the rib cage to elicit gallbladder tenderness when the patient inspires. A sudden sharp gasp is the usual response as the patient inspires and the gallbladder is touched. Because the liver and gallbladder descend together, the same response may occur if the pressure is placed directly on the liver. The gallbladder is compressed slightly as a result of the liver

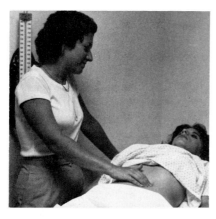

FIGURE 11.13
Light palpation of the abdomen.

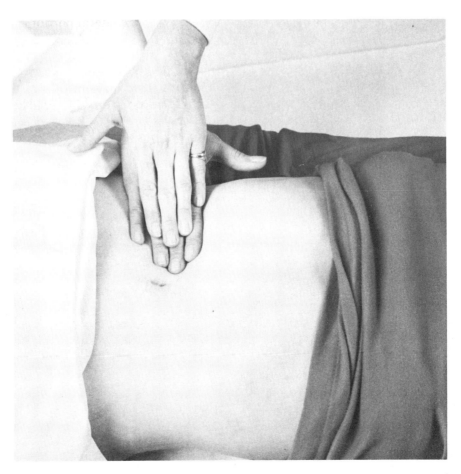

FIGURE 11.14
Deep palpation of the abdomen.

palpation. Both can give a positive Murphy's Sign.

In children under 6 months of age, it is not unusual to palpate an umbilical hernia. This may or may not have been seen on inspection. This type of hernia can be felt by pressing down inwardly with one finger on the umbilicus. If a fingertip can be admitted, a small hernia is present. It will often resolve spontaneously without treatment by 1 year of age, especially if it is small. An average size ranges from 1 to 5 centimeters. Appropriate referral is indicated for an exceptionally large hernia or one that does not disappear. An adult can get an umbilical hernia. Its appearance is similar; there is a bulge around the umbilicus. In most adults, however, the hernia does not encircle the umbilicus. The bulge may be just around the lateral and superior aspects.

A condition which occurs in early infancy is called *pyloric stenosis.* This is characterized by the age of onset (from 2 weeks to 2 months of age) and consistent projectile vomiting. When this malfunction is suspected, two classic physical findings are present, visible peristalsis and an olive-sized and shaped mass. The peristaltic waves are best seen with a bright light shining horizontally across the baby's abdomen. The waves are most visible in the epigastric area immediately after the baby has been fed. The classic olive-like mass is found below the right costal margin and lateral to the rectus muscle. These findings warrant immediate referral for treatment.

In some infants and adults, especially a woman who is very pregnant or obese, the rectus abdominis muscle may separate causing a palpable groove along the muscle on exam (Fig. 11.15). This separation feels like a ridge along the sternal line from the xiphoid to the symphysis. The finding is most likely felt when the patient is asked to look at his

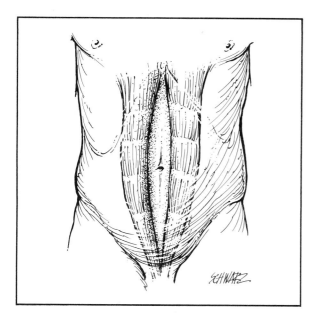

FIGURE 11.15
Diastus rectus.

umbilicus when in the supine position. This deviation is called *diastus rectus* and causes no problems.

Specific Organs that Undergo Deep Palpation

THE LIVER

Palpation of the liver is used to detect enlargement and tenderness. There are two commonly used methods. In both methods, the examiner should be standing on the patient's right side, if she is right-handed and to the left if she is left-handed. The following describes the approach to be used for right-handed examiners. The positions must be reversed for the left-handed examiner.

In the first approach, the examiner's left hand is placed on the posterior thorax at about the eleventh or twelfth rib (Fig. 11.16). She then pushes upward with that hand to brace the upcoming anterior palpation. The right hand is placed at about a 45 degree angle to the right of the rectus muscle along the rib cage. The procedure is explained to the patient and he is told that he might experience some discomfort or queasiness when his liver edge is felt. The patient is then asked to inspire deeply (inspiration causes the liver edge to descend). When the patient inhales, the exam-

iner slides the lateral portion of her hand (or the fingertips) under the costal margin (Fig. 11.16). If the patient breathes deeply and the examiner applies enough pressure, the liver edge will whisk by her hand during the patient's inspiration. The liver edge as it slides by will give a firm, blunt sensation to the examiner's hand under the rib cage. It may be necessary to ask the patient to take two or three deep breaths before the liver edge can be palpated. It is important for the examiner not to retract any pressure, but to continue to palpate deeper as the patient inspires again. The liver is normally palpable 1 to 2 centimeters below the costal margin in the first year of life. Some livers are harder to palpate than others. This is especially true of obese, tense, or very physically fit people. In patients with lung disease, however, who have large lungs and low diaphragms, the liver may be of normal size but displaced so it frequently can be palpated 1 to 2 centimeters below the right costal margin.

The second method uses the same basic principles. This approach involves the superimposition of the examiner's left hand over her right hand along the right costal margin (Fig. 11.17). This method gives the examiner more anterior pressure, but the posterior pressure is lost. Either method is acceptable. The method chosen should provide the most accurate information. When the liver is not palpable, but there is a concern about the existence of liver tenderness, one further test can be done. The examiner places the palm of one hand along the right costal margin, where the liver edge should be located. With the examiner's other hand in the shape of a fist, a light blow is delivered to the hand placed on the patient. If there is pain with this maneuver, one can assume there is liver tenderness. If the patient is unsure, repeat the test on the patient's left side to see if he can detect a difference in the responses.

THE SPLEEN

The spleen should not be palpable in a healthy adult, but it can occasionally be felt in a small child. Palpation of the spleen follows liver palpation. The examiner reaches across the patient's abdomen and places her left hand on the left posterior thorax under the area of the spleen (Fig. 11.18). The patient is asked to roll slightly to the right to facilitate the exam. The

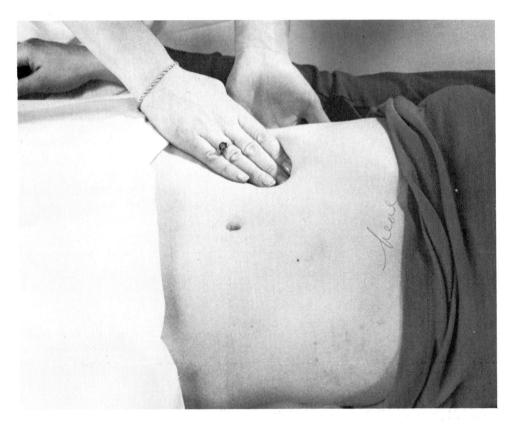

FIGURE 11.16
Palpation of the liver with the examiner's left hand on the posterior thorax.

right hand is then placed below the left costal margin. Sliding the fingertips under the rib cage is the easiest way to reach the spleen. Short fingernails are a must! The patient should again be asked to inspire; the spleen will descend as did the liver edge. If the spleen can be felt at all, it will be during inspiration.

If the examiner suspects splenic enlargement and is unable to confirm her suspicion, she may ask the patient to roll completely on

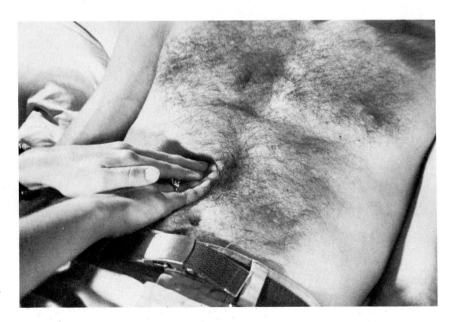

FIGURE 11.17
Palpation of the liver with super-imposition of the hands.

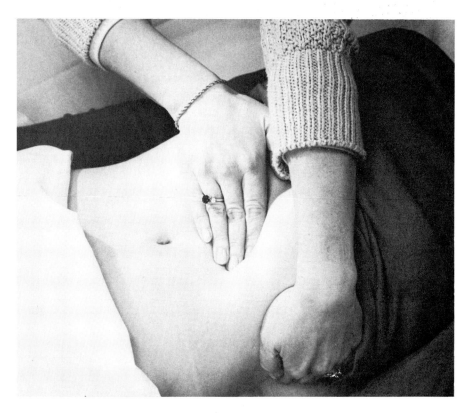

FIGURE 11.18
Palpation of the spleen.

his right side. The principles of gravity will be evidenced as the spleen becomes more anterior and easier to feel, if it is enlarged. Another point to keep in mind is that if the spleen is significantly enlarged and the examiner places her hand under the rib cage, she may be above the edge of the spleen. Therefore, it is appropriate to check (by palpation) below the costal margin to see if the spleen can be felt.

PANCREAS

The pancreas is not normally palpable in the healthy adult. If the examiner elicits tenderness, rebound tenderness, or a soft area when palpating the epigastrium, pancreatitis is suspected. Pancreatic masses are almost impossible to palpate.

THE KIDNEYS

It is very difficult to palpate the normal kidneys except in a child or a very thin adult. However, the right kidney is more likely to be felt. Picturing the kidneys anatomically

helps to understand the approach to palpation. The kidneys lie along the midaxillary line lateral to the rectus muscle. The goal of palpation is for the examiner to feel the lower pole of the kidney between her palpating hands (Fig. 11.19).

The right-handed examiner places her right hand along the inferior edge of the costal margin on the right anterior abdominal area. The other hand is placed on the posterior thorax at about the same place. The patient is asked to inspire, and the examiner pushes her hands together. The kidney will descend with inspiration, and the pole will be felt between the hands. The procedure is repeated for the other kidney. The examiner reaches across the patient, placing her right hand along the inferior edge of the costal margin and the other hand on the posterior thorax.

COSTOVERTEBRAL ANGLE TENDERNESS

Costovertebral angle (CVA) tenderness occurs when there is inflammation of the kidney(s). The palm of the examiner's hand is placed

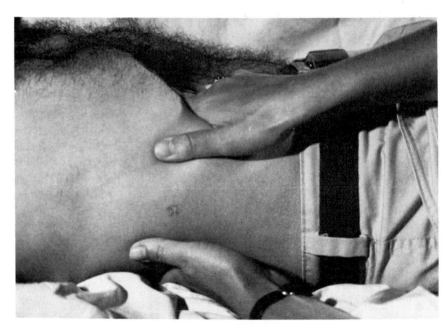

FIGURE 11.19
Palpation of the right kidney.

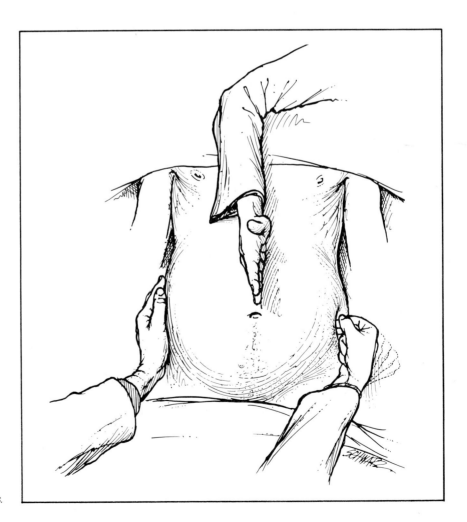

FIGURE 11.20
Palpation for ascites.

over the posterior lower flank area, better known as the costovertebral angle. A light blow is delivered in the posterior flank area over each kidney. If pain is elicited, then it is likely that inflammation exists. (See the recorded example at the end of this chapter to note how this finding is transcribed.) The same is repeated on the right side. Occasionally, the first time the patient feels the examiner's tapping, a startle reaction occurs. If this happens, the examiner should deliver the light blow again to confirm this response.

THE AORTA

This tube-like structure is palpated to the left of the umbilicus in the epigastric area. The examiner rolls her fingertips horizontally over this area while applying pressure. The aortic pulsation will be felt slightly to the left once the aorta is located. Palpating a strong pulse in a lateral movement may indicate the presence of an aortic aneurysm.

PALPATION OF ASCITIC FLUID

This test is not often reliable and may be positive only when advanced ascites already exists. The test requires an additional pair of hands that can be those of an assistant or the patient's. The patient, already in a supine position, is asked to place the ulnar surface of his hand (or the assistant places her hands) firmly down the midline of the abdomen. The examiner places one hand, palm surface, against the lateral flank area on one side. She then taps the other lateral flank area with her other hand (Fig. 11.20). A sensation to the examiner's palmar hand will be transmitted if ascites exists.

It is important to remember that the accuracy of these findings depends on the patient's relaxation, cooperation, and trust in the examiner. Therefore, as with any procedure, a thorough explanation of the procedure as well as telling the patient when he may experience discomfort are essential.

Screening Examination of the Abdomen

1. Inspection of the abdomen
2. Auscultation of the abdomen with the diaphragm for bowel sounds
3. Auscultation of the aorta, renal and femoral arteries with the bell*
4. General percussion of the abdomen
5. Percussion and measurement of the liver span and splenic dullness
6. General light palpation of the abdomen
7. General deep palpation of the abdomen
8. Palpation of the liver, spleen, and kidneys
9. Palpation of the inguinal and femoral nodes
10. Assessment for costovertebral angle tenderness

In adults only.

EXAMPLE OF A RECORDED HISTORY AND PHYSICAL

SUBJECTIVE:

Chief Complaint: "I've had a stomach ache for 4 days."

HPH: This 54-year-old female considers herself to be in "basically good health except for the usual flus, colds, etc." In the last few months, she has had intermittent episodes of "burning, gnawing" epigastric and left-upper quadrant pain. This happened the first time 4 months ago, shortly after her mother passed away. She had "waves of this pain for a couple of days at a time." It would appear between meals and get worse over a period of 15 minutes, "then I'd take a Rolaid and it would go away. Eating doesn't seem to make it worse or better. I wouldn't be bothered again for several days. It seems to be happening weekly now for the last 6 weeks. This week the pain lasted 4 days instead of the usual 2."

She notices some mild nausea associated with the pain but not enough to have a decreased appetite. There is no radiation of the pain, vomiting, change in bowel habits, diarrhea, constipation, heart burn, belching, flatulence, food allergies, fever, rectal bleeding, or mucus in stools.

She has a large amount of formed brown stool every other day. Her bowel habits have not changed in frequency or character. She has no food intolerances but cannot "eat a lot at one time or I get the pain." She tries to eat "a balanced diet—a lot of fruit and vegetables. I never fry or eat greasy foods." She drinks a mixed drink or two on a weekend night on an irregular basis. She smokes 1 ppd of True filters and has been smoking for 15 years.

Patient considers herself under some stress presently. Since her mother died, there is "a lot of business I must attend to. We were very close, and I miss her a lot." Patient is a secretary for a project that will end next month, "and then I'll be out of work." She feels she gets a lot of support from her family and "my husband tells me not to worry about finding another job."

She is taking no medicines other than an occasional aspirin (10 grains 1 or 2 times/month) and a Rolaid or two when the pain is "bad." She has not found changing positions helpful. She has not tried eating dairy products when she has the pain.

She has never had any abdominal pain prior to the onset of this and has not sought treatment until today. Her mother died of "cancer of the colon." She was 80. No other family history of abdominal disorders. Patient can still go to work with the pain, but is "frightened, as my mother had the same symptoms 2 years ago."

OBJECTIVE:

T. 98.4°F orally; P. 86 radial; R. 18; B.P. 146/86 sitting.

Abdomen: Round abdomen, loose muscle tone, symmetrical. No scars, lesions, moles, rashes. Peristalsis not visible. Bowel sounds audible in all quadrants. Abdomen soft and nontender throughout, except in the epigastric area. Some guarding with deep palpation. No rebound tenderness or masses. LIVER: 8 cm. span at MCL. Nontender. SPLEEN: Not palpable. Nontender. AORTA: pulsations palpable. No tenderness. No bruits. CVA: No tenderness.

REFERENCE

Judge, R., & Zuidema, G. (1982). Methods of Clinical Examination: A Physiological Approach (4th ed.). Boston: Little, Brown.

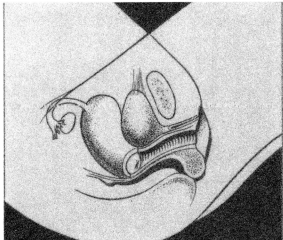

12

The Female Genitalia

E xamination of the genital area is viewed with hesitation by many women. The adolescent girl may approach her first examination with anxiety or a fear of the unknown. The same may be true for the pregnant woman who has heard unpleasant stories from friends or relatives about their experiences with childbirth. Commonly, once a woman is past her childbearing years, she will stop coming for routine pelvic examinations.

Although the male child is routinely examined for testicular problems, hernia, and placement of the urethra, there is still some taboo about examining the genitalia of the female child (Driscoll, 1982). The first female examination should be done in the delivery room or birthing room. From then on, an examination of the external genital area should be a part of all well-child exams. By examining the genital area early and regularly, the female child will learn to view it as normal, and the examination will not be new or terrifying to her when she reaches adolescence.

The complete adult female genitalia exam includes an examination of the *external genitalia*, a *speculum examination*, a *Papanicolaou smear* (Pap smear) which is a simple, painless test for cervical cancer, a *bimanual examination* and a *rectovaginal examination*. A young woman's first complete pelvic should be done just prior to beginning sexual activity or by the age of 18 or 20 years, if she is not sexually active. An initial examination is performed between the ages of 14 and 16 if menarche has not yet occurred. A young female known or suspected of being exposed to *diethylstilbestrol* (DES) in utero should be examined after menarche or by the age of 14 years if menarche has not occurred (Prenatal diethylstilbestrol, 1983). There is an increased incidence of vaginal and cervical adenocarcinoma in daughters of women who took DES while pregnant and the mothers may be at increased risk for breast cancer. Both mothers and daughters require additional medical check-ups and medical consultations as necessary.

The American Cancer Society recommends the following guidelines for obtaining a complete pelvic examination, a Pap smear, a rectal examination, a blood stool slide test, and *proctosigmoidoscopy* or procto (an inspection of the rectum and lower colon with a hollow, lighted tube) (American Cancer Society, 1985):

1. All asymptomatic women age 20 and over, and those under 20 who are sexually active, should have a Pap smear annually for two negative examinations and then at least every three years.
2. Women who are at high risk of developing cervical cancer due to early age at first intercourse, multiple sexual partners, or other risk factors may need to have more frequent Pap smears.
3. A pelvic examination should be done as part of a general physical examination every three years from age 20 to 40 and annually thereafter in asymptomatic women.
4. At menopause, women at high risk of developing endometrial cancer (cancer of the uterine lining) should have a Pap smear, pelvic examination, and endometrial tissue sample. Women are at high risk if they have a history of infertility, obesity, failure of ovulation, or have been on prolonged estrogen therapy.
5. A digital rectal examination should be done yearly starting at age 40.
6. After 50 years of age, a blood stool test should be done every year and a procto exam every 3 to 4 years after two initial negative tests one year apart. Blood stool tests should begin earlier in women at risk for rectal cancer. Risk factors include a family history of rectal or colon cancer, a history of polyps or prior cancer surgery, and ulcerative colitis.

Most clinics develop their own approach to the female examination based on the above guidelines. For example, if a woman is using a diaphragm, oral contraceptives, or an intrauterine device, check-ups more regular than every 3 years are indicated.

Unfortunately most women of today did not have the benefit of having an annual genital examination starting in infancy. For these and other reasons, many concerns for privacy and modesty remain. Very modest women (e.g., many of Mexican-American and Indian descent) may hesitate to have a pelvic examination. If great concern for modesty is apparent, efforts should be made for a female to conduct the examination. Many of the concerns felt by women can be identified during the gynecology history taken prior to the physical examination. The nurse's attitude can make a great deal of difference in how the woman views the pelvic exam. The best approach is to have a calm, reassuring, and attentive manner. Once rapport is established, the nurse may be able to dispel much of the anxiety.

DEVELOPMENTAL CHANGES OF THE FEMALE GENITOURINARY SYSTEM THROUGHOUT THE LIFESPAN

Sexuality begins at the moment of birth for both boys and girls. The female infant often has vaginal discharge (*leukorrhea*) at the time of birth. This is a natural phenomenon secondary to estrogen stimulation in the mother and disappears in a few weeks.

Urinary tract infections in infancy are more common in males than females. However, during the toddler and preschooler stage of development, girls are more susceptible to *urinary tract infection* than boys. Estimates indicate that from 5 to 10 percent of girls will have at least one urinary tract infection before 18 years of age (Chow, et al., 1984). In a large number of these cases, the child is asymptomatic and infection is identified on a routine screening of the urine. The short female urethra and the milestone of becoming potty-trained puts a little girl at risk if personal hygiene is not properly monitored by the child's caretaker. Complete neuromuscular control of urination should be achieved by the age of 4 or 5 in girls. Little girls need to be taught the importance of wiping from front to back at the onset of potty training to prevent introducing bacteria from the rectum into the urethra. This will lower the risk for developing urinary tract infections.

Puberty is defined as that period during adolescence when maximal growth of the body occurs as well as the acquisition of secondary sexual characteristics (Robie, 1983). The first sign of puberty is usually a rapid increase in stature followed by the onset and growth of the breast tissue. The appearance of pubic hair occurs about 6 months after the onset of breast budding between the ages of 11 and 12. The adult pattern is established at about 14 years.

Menarche or the onset of menstruation occurs toward the end of puberty. The average time from initial breast development to menarche is approximately 28 months. The mean time from menarche until the establishment of regular cyclic menstrual period is 14 months, and usually there are about 24 months between the time of menarche and the establishment of ovulatory cycles (Robie, 1983). The average age at which menarche occurs is 12 years 9 months with a range from 9 to 18 years. Generally blacks and Asians tend to reach pubertal maturity more rapidly than do Caucasians (Eveleth & Tanner, 1976).

The adult woman has increased susceptibility to urinary tract infections at several points in her development. Many women develop urinary tract symptoms when they first become sexually active or when they resume frequent intercourse after a period of infrequent or no activity. Symptoms are caused by trauma to the anterior urethra during prolonged or very active intercourse (Fogel, 1981). Some women first develop symptoms when they are pregnant or during the postpartum period. During postpartum some women have difficulty voiding resulting in urinary retention and infection (Fogel, 1981).

The *climacteric* is the transition time between the reproductive and nonreproductive ability of a woman. This period of time is divided into three phases including the *premenopausal, menopausal, postmenopausal.* During the premenopausal phase the woman is still menstruating, but she may have irregular cycles due to occasional ovulatory failure. This phase occurs 4 to 5 years prior to menopause which is the actual cessation of menstruation for 1 year. However, a woman is not considered infertile until 2 years after her last period

and needs to be counseled about birth control when appropriate. The average age of menopause is 52 with a range from 40 to 60 years (McKinlay, et al., 1972). The decrease in estrogen which occurs during this phase is responsible for the *night sweats* and *hot flashes* that are experienced by the majority of women (McKinlay & Jeffreys, 1974; Jaszmann, et al., 1969). Postmenopause is the phase when all traces of ovarian activity are lost. Approximately 5 to 10 years into the postmenopausal phase, some women experience the late effects of decreased estrogen including *vaginal atrophy* and *osteoporosis.*

A woman again becomes susceptible to urinary problems during the postmenopausal phase of her development. The decreased levels of estrogen and relaxed musculature associated with pregnancy may cause the urethral orifice to *prolapse* and become displaced into the vaginal outlet. This exposes the urethra to trauma and allows the flora of the vagina to enter the urethra with resultant infection. *Atrophic distal urethritis* and stricture formation affect bladder function by causing obstruction, residual urine, and ascending infection (Fogel, 1981). Another problem common among elderly women who have had children is relaxation of the muscles of the pelvic floor. This results in the development of *stress incontinence* which is involuntary loss of urine when laughing, sneezing or coughing.

ANATOMY

The External Female Genitalia

The external female genitalia consist of the *mons pubis, labia majora, labia minora, clitoris,* and *vestibule* (Fig. 12.1). In front of the symphysis pubis lies a rounded pad of fat called the mons pubis. At puberty this becomes covered with hair. The labia majora are two folds of skin and fat that extend backward from the mons pubis toward the rectum. The skin of the labia majora contains hair follicles, sweat glands, and sebaceous glands. The labia minora are reddish folds of stratified squamous epithelium located between the labia majora. These folds are soft and devoid of hair follicles and sweat glands. Anteriorly, the labia minora meet to form the *prepuce*

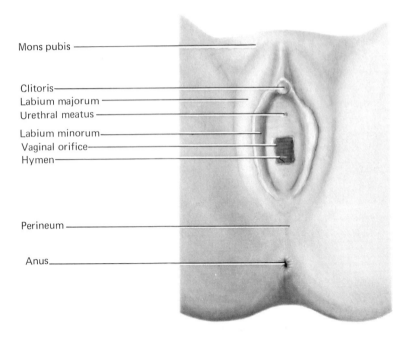

Mons pubis

Clitoris
Labium majorum
Urethral meatus

Labium minorum
Vaginal orifice
Hymen

Perineum

Anus

FIGURE 12.1
*External female genitalia. (From Heagarty,
M., et al. Child Health: Basics for Primary
Care. New York: Appleton-Century-Crofts,
1980, p. 162, with permission.)*

that partially covers the *clitoris*. The clitoris
is composed of erectile tissue similar to that
of the penis. Posteriorly, the labia minora are
connected by a slight transverse fold called
the *fourchette*. The *perineum* extends from the
introitus (vaginal orifice) to the *anus* (Fig.
12.1).

The vestibule is the cleft between the labia
minora and behind the clitoris. The vagina
and the *urethra* open into this area. The
urethra is located on the anterior surface of
the vagina about 2.54 centimeters behind the

clitoris. The *Skene's glands* are located just
posterior and to either side of the urethral
opening. The *Bartholin's glands* are situated
in the floor of the vestibule, one on either side
of the vaginal orifice.

The Internal Female Genitalia

The internal female genitalia consist of the
vagina, cervix, uterus, ovaries, and *uterine
tubes* (Fig. 12.2). The vagina is a muscular

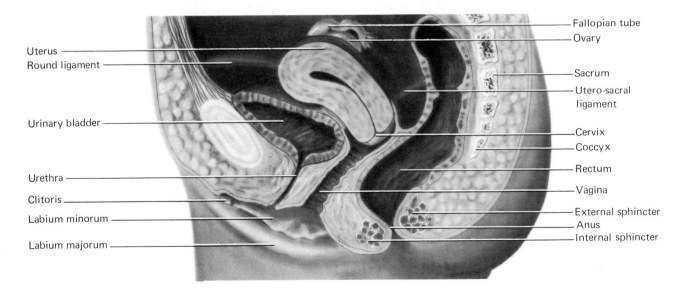

Uterus
Round ligament

Urinary bladder

Urethra
Clitoris
Labium minorum
Labium majorum

Fallopian tube
Ovary

Sacrum
Utero-sacral
ligament

Cervix
Coccyx

Rectum

Vagina

External sphincter
Anus
Internal sphincter

FIGURE 12.2
*Internal structure of the female genitalia. (From Heagarty, M., et al. Child Health: Basics for
Primary Care. New York: Appleton-Century-Crofts, 1980, p. 162, with permission.)*

tube measuring 8 to 10 centimeters in length. The vagina is covered by a mucous membrane which lies in transverse folds called *rugae.* The upper end of the vagina is attached to the cervix. There are recesses of the vagina behind, at both sides of, and in front of the cervix. These are called the *posterior fornix,* the *lateral fornices,* and the *anterior fornix.*

The uterus is a muscular organ that communicates with the vagina below and the uterine tubes above. The upper portion of the uterus is called the *body* and the lower portion the cervix. The upper portion of the uterus between the uterine tubes is referred to as the *fundus.* The cervix projects into the vagina, where it forms lips that surround the *os.* The uterine cavity reaches into the vagina through the cervical os.

The *ovaries* are almond-shaped structures about 3 centimeters in length. They are located on either side of the uterus, below the uterine tubes. The two uterine tubes (*fallopian tubes*) are approximately 10 centimeters long. They each penetrate the uterine wall and open into the uterine cavity. The free end is in intimate contact with the ovary. This is called the *fimbriated end* due to finger-like projections, or *fimbriae.*

The *levator ani* and the *coccygeus* are the muscles of the pelvic floor that support the uterus. The levator ani is a paired muscle arising from the pubis and extending backward toward the midline. The urethra, vagina, and anal canal pass through this muscle. On contraction it raises the pelvic floor. The coccygei are two small muscles that extend from the spines of the ischium and insert on the sacrum and coccyx. When contracted they pull the coccyx forward.

The Anus and Rectum

The anal canal extends from the anus to the rectum and is about 4 centimeters in length. Strong sphincter muscles guard the anal opening. The voluntary external sphincter is a cylinder of skeletal muscle that helps close the anus. In the upper part of the anal canal is the involuntary internal sphincter. The rectum extends from the *anal canal* to the *sigmoid colon.* It ascends from the tip of the coccyx along the coccyx to the hollow of the sacrum. In the lumen of the rectum are three folds called *valves of Houston.* These folds support the fecal mass held in the rectum. The lowest one, which projects posteriorly, can sometimes be felt. Through the anterior wall of the rectum it is possible to palpate the male prostate, the female cervix, and, in some instances, the female uterus.

HISTORY

The gynecologic history of a patient needs to be adjusted for age. The pediatric history differs significantly from the history obtained from an adult, therefore, it will be discussed separately.

The Pediatric History

The infant's history is geared toward identifying signs of urinary or vaginal infection, congenital abnormalities and parental concerns. The nurse should keep in mind that the clinical presentation of urinary tract infection in the infant is nonspecific.

The parent or guardian of the female infant should be asked the following questions:

1. Has she had any unexplained fevers, unsatisfactory weight gain, vomiting, diarrhea, lethargy or irritability?
2. How many times do you have to change wet diapers?
3. What is the strength of her urine stream?
4. Have you noticed any change in the color of her urine?
5. Have you noticed any discharge from the vagina? (If yes, describe.)
6. Have you noticed any rashes or lesions in the diaper area?
7. How do you clean her genital and rectal area?
8. Did her mother take any drugs or experience any infections during her pregnancy?
9. Is there a family history of genital or gonadal abnormalities, nephritis, nephrosis, or kidney masses?
10. Do you have any questions or concerns regarding the development of her genital organs?

The health history of the toddler and pre-schooler is obtained from the parent with increasingly more input from the child. As the child grows older, symptoms of urinary tract infection become more specific, so these are included along with questions regarding potty training. Additional information to be obtained includes:

1. Does she complain of urgency, frequency, burning, flank pain, blood in the urine, anorexia, vomiting, abdominal pain or diarrhea?
2. What is the color and odor of her urine?
3. When was potty training started and what techniques were used?
4. At what age did she achieve bladder and bowel control?
5. Does she ever wet the bed?
6. Does she ever have daytime incontinence?
7. What are her personal hygiene skills and techniques?
8. Have you noticed any vaginal discharge, odor or irritation?
9. Has she had a past history of urinary or genital infections?

The school-age history is similar to the preschool history. The exception is the history of potty training. This is obtained only if indicated by the rest of the history. As the young girl approaches the preteenage years (9 to 12 years of age), historical developmental milestones are added. These include the age at first appearance of breast budding, axillary hair and pubic hair, and age of menarche. Once menstruation has begun, the format for the adult health history is followed.

The sexual history is a part of every pediatric gynecologic history. See Chapter 1 for the age-appropriate questions.

The Adult History

The essentials of the adult history include *demographic data*, the *menstrual history*, the *obstetric history*, the *contraceptive* and *hormonal history*, the *genitourinary history*, and the *sexual history*.

DEMOGRAPHIC DATA

Demographic data relevant to the genitourinary system include the patient's age, marital status, and number and ages of any children.

These data, which can usually be obtained from the patient record prior to beginning the interview, help to direct questions appropriate to the patient's place in the life cycle.

MENSTRUAL HISTORY

To put the patient at ease during the interview, the nurse should begin with questions that provoke minimal to no anxiety. The menstrual history is nonthreatening to most women, so this is a good place to begin the interview. With the exception of the very young female, most women will answer the questions directly without embarrassment. The menstrual history includes age at menarche and a description of the woman's menstrual pattern.

Menarche. As mentioned earlier, the mean age of menarche is 12 years 9 months with a range from 9 years to 18 years. A young girl and her mother may become concerned if menarche does not occur within this normal range. In this case the examiner should gain information about the presence of other secondary sex characteristics, the presence of menstrual symptoms (e.g., breast tenderness or bloating), and the mother's and sisters' ages at menarche. There may be an inherited tendency for late onset of menstruation, but this has not been established. Physician consultation should be sought if there is any question of a hormonal problem or if the girl has not experienced menarche before 16 years of age. In every patient with established menses, the examiner should inquire into the circumstances of the onset of menses. For example, the patient is asked how she was prepared for its occurrence and how she reacted to the onset. This may give clues regarding how the patient views herself as a woman.

Menstrual Pattern. Information necessary for determining a woman's menstrual pattern includes:

1. What was the date of your last normal menstrual period?
2. What was the date of your last menstrual period? (This may be the same as 1.)
3. What is the average number of days between the first day of one period and the first day of the next period?
4. Have you skipped any periods?
5. What is the amount and duration of flow?
6. Do you notice any symptoms prior to the

onset of your menses (i.e., breast tenderness, bloating, irritability)?

7. Do you have *dysmenorrhea* (painful menstruation)?

8. Have you experienced any spotting between periods?

When a woman between the ages of 40 and 55 has had no menstrual period for one year or longer, she is commonly considered to have gone through menopause. Immediately premenopausal and postmenopausal women should be asked if they are experiencing any symptoms related to hormonal changes. The main symptoms experienced around the time of menopause include night sweats and hot flashes. In addition, inquiry should be made about her attitude toward menopause and her use of treatment to alleviate symptoms (e.g., estrogens and Vitamin E).

The young woman of child-bearing age usually has a regular menstrual cycle occurring approximately every 29.5 days and lasting 2 to 5 days. However, there is a wide variation among women. The interval between cycles is considered normal if the variation of the interval does not exceed 5 days. Irregularity is frequently found in the young woman beginning her cycle and again as she approaches menopause. However, the examiner should not overlook the possibility of pregnancy. The duration of flow is relatively constant for most women.

Premenstrual symptoms usually occur just prior to menstruation and subside once the flow begins. A wide variety of symptoms have been considered to be premenstrual, including breast tenderness, low abdominal pain, headache, bloating, diarrhea, constipation, and irritability.

Symptoms of *dysmenorrhea* begin with the onset of menstrual flow. *Primary dysmenorrhea* usually develops once the menstrual cycles become ovulatory and improves after pregnancy or once the woman is into her late twenties. Many women will experience mild cramping or lower abdominal pain, but the pain of dysmenorrhea is usually colicky and cyclic. *Secondary dysmenorrhea* occurs after an established period of time with relatively painless periods (Fogel, 1981). Further investigation is required to identify the causative factor.

Intermenstrual spotting is commonly encountered with women taking low dose oral contraceptives. When pregnancy is suspected, it could indicate a threatened abortion. Spotting in a woman who is postmenopausal requires further evaluation for the presence of endometrial cancer.

THE OBSTETRIC HISTORY

The obstetric history includes the following information:

1. How many times have you been pregnant (*gravity*)?

2. How many live births (*parity* or number of births with a fetal size compatible with extrauterine life)?

3. How many *miscarriages?*

4. How many *abortions?*

5. Have you, as a couple, ever experienced a problem with infertility?

Each pregnancy is explored in relation to the type of delivery, duration of the pregnancy, birth weight, condition of the infant, and complications of the pregnancy or postpartum period. Miscarriages and abortions are explored regarding the time in pregnancy they occurred. When a woman has had a miscarriage she should be asked if she had any follow-up care. If the woman had an abortion, then inquiry is made regarding the type of procedure performed. Most important, women who give a history of a past miscarriage or abortion should be given the opportunity to express the feelings they had then or have presently about the event.

THE CONTRACEPTIVE AND HORMONAL HISTORY

The current and past contraceptive practices of every woman of childbearing age should be elicited. The young adolescent and premenopausal woman should be included, because ironically, it is during these time periods that women are often most lax and pregnancy is least desired. Questions to be asked about the use of contraceptives and hormones include:

1. Do you presently use birth control?

2. (If yes) What type of birth control are you presently using? How long have you used that method? Are you experiencing any problems with your present form of birth control? Are you and your partner happy with your present method?

3. (If no) Are you in need of birth control?

4. What methods have you used in the past? (For each method, determine the duration of use, side effects, and reason for discontinuing the method.)
5. What are your and your partner's plans for future pregnancies?
6. Did your mother take any hormones while she was pregnant with you or did you take any hormones while pregnant?

The patient should be evaluated for risk factors that may make the method of birth control she is using or is requesting inappropriate for her. Also, the patient is questioned regarding any side effects she may be experiencing with her present method of birth control. You are referred to *Contraceptive Technology* by Hatcher, et al. (1984) for historic questions specific to each method.

Inquiry should be made of menopausal and postmenopausal women about the present or past use of estrogen replacement therapy. Women presently on therapy require ongoing follow-up.

THE GENITOURINARY HISTORY
The patient is asked if she is presently experiencing or has experienced in the past any of the following problems:

1. Vaginal itching, discharge, or odor
2. Painful vaginal intercourse (*dysparunia*)
3. Urinary frequency, urgency, dysuria, hematuria, or stress incontinence
4. A past history of any sexually transmitted disease including *syphillis, gonorrhea, herpes progenitalis, trichomoniasis, candida albicans, gardnerella,* or *chlamydia trachomatis*
5. A past history of urinary tract infections
6. A family history of nephritis, nephrosis, or kidney masses

If the patient has a positive past history of any of these she should then be asked when she was diagnosed, what the symptoms were, the treatment she received, and the follow-up care.

THE SEXUAL HISTORY
Once the woman has discussed the previously given information, she may be at ease and comfortable enough to discuss her sexual history. The goal of this portion of the history is to identify her feelings about her sexuality and detect any problems (see the section on "Sexual History" in Chapter 1). Use of the developmental approach will help facilitate the discussion and gather data appropriate to her stage in the life cycle.

PHYSICAL ASSESSMENT

Preparing the Room

All necessary equipment should be set up in the examining room. It is very inconsiderate of the examiner to have to leave the patient for forgotten equipment in the middle of the examination. The following equipment is needed (Fig. 12.3):

1. A good *light source* such as a goose neck lamp or a head set with a light
2. *Drapes*
3. Two to three glass slides, 10 percent *potassium hydroxide solution, saline solution,* and 2 to 3 *sterile swabs* to be used in preparing vaginal smears for the identification of the causative organism of vaginitis
4. One to three *slides,* 1 *swab, Ayre spatula,* and *cytology fixative* for the Pap smear
5. One swab and *chocolate agar media* for the gonorrhea culture
6. *Lubricant* for the bimanual examination
7. *Tissue* to clean the perineum
8. *Vaginal specula* in at least 3 different sizes. Specula come in either metal or plastic. The metal specula can be stored on a comfortably warm heating pad
9. A *pencil* to mark the specimens and the appropriate laboratory slips
10. A waste paper basket should be placed handy to the examining table
11. A small, transparent, sagital plastic *model of the female pelvis*
12. A microscope to examine vaginal smears.
13. A stool guaiac slide to test the stool for blood

Prior to having the patient enter the examining room, the nurse should survey the room

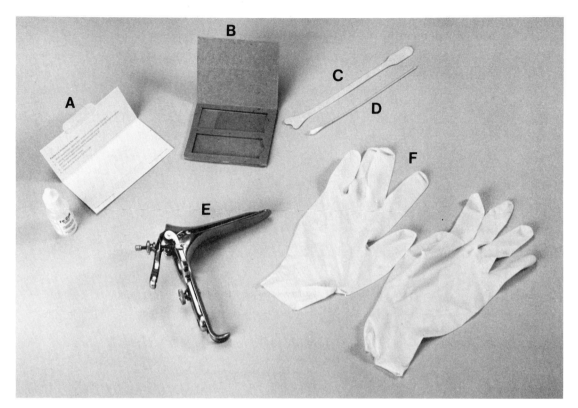

FIGURE 12.3
Equipment for the pelvic and rectal examination. **A.** *Stool guaiac slide test.* **B.** *Pap slide.* **C.**
Ayre spatula. **D.** *Swab.* **E.** *Speculum.* **F.** *Gloves. (Not pictured: Pap fixative, lubricant, and chocolate
agar media.)*

for all the necessary equipment. She should then test the light source to see if it is working. Finally, she should always open and close the speculum several times so she knows how it operates and she is sure it is functioning. It is uncomfortable for both the patient and the examiner if the examiner does not know how to remove the blades once inserted. The placement of mobiles, clever signs or pictures over the examination table can promote relaxation.

The genital area is not devoid of bacteria, so it is not necessary to use sterile technique for a routine pelvic examination. The goal is to have a working area with a minimal number of microorganisms and to prevent spread of infection to other patients or to the examiner. This is achieved by the use of *clean technique.* The examiner is using clean technique when she washes her hands with warm, soapy water between examinations and uses clean rubber gloves. Each patient should be draped with a freshly laundered sheet. Metal specula are washed in a disinfectant solution and plas-

tic specula are discarded at the completion of the examination.

Preparing the Patient

At the time the adult patient calls in to make an appointment for a screening pelvic examination, she is reminded that she should not douche or insert chemicals into her vagina for 24 hours prior to her examination and that she should not be menstruating. Douching can interfere with accurate evaluation of vaginal secretions, smears, and cultures. Chemicals such as contraceptive creams and jellies do not allow for adequate visualization of the vagina and cervix, and menstruation may result in an inaccurate Pap smear.

Prior to the examination, the patient should empty her bladder. This will facilitate palpation of the uterus and adnexa as well as make the woman more comfortable during the examination.

The female nurse can perform the examination unassisted. It is good practice for the male examiner to have a female attendant present during the examination as a chaperone. A young girl is usually examined with her parent or guardian in the room. As she approaches adolescence she may or may not want the parental support. The adult female may wish to have her partner accompany her. This should be done only at the patient's request and not be due to any pressure from her partner.

Patient explanation before beginning the pelvic examination is important to allay fears and to obtain the patient's cooperation. The instruments should be shown to the patient while explaining the procedure. The use of a small, transparent, sagital plastic model of the female pelvis is helpful in demonstrating to the patient what is going to be done. The woman can be asked if she would like to view the examination with the use of a mirror. Many women are interested in knowing what their internal anatomy looks like.

Usually a child is left undraped so she can see what is happening. The adult patient should be asked whether or not she would like a drape to be used. Some women object to the use of a drape because they feel that it makes the examination something to be embarrassed about. Others feel that the examiner is hiding behind the drape and is detached from them (the patient) as a person. A drape is placed over the abdomen of the patient who wishes it. It preserves modesty and still allows the examiner to assess the patient's face during the examination. The head of the examining table is elevated to about 30 to 45 degrees. This provides the examiner with a better view of the woman's face and promotes relaxation of the abdominal muscles (Beckmann, et al., 1986).

The young girl is placed in a *frog-leg position* up to the age of 10 years (Driscoll, 1982) (Fig. 12.4). The adult is asked to put her heels into the stirrups. Shortening the stirrup brackets helps the patient to bend her knees more and brings the cervix down. She then is asked to bring her buttocks just beyond the end of the examining table. For the elderly woman this position may need to be modified due to physical limitations.

At this time the mirror is positioned for those patients who are interested. First the head of the examining table should always be elevated to 45 degrees. The patient holds the mirror above her body just over her pubic and perineal area at about a 30- to 45-degree angle. Then the examiner should come around to the head of the table so her eyes are parallel to those of the patient. By doing this the examiner will know whether the mirror, light, speculum, and eyes are in the right position for adequate visualization (Wallis, 1982).

Once the examination begins the patient should have her hands on her chest (if she is not using the mirror) to relax her abdominal muscles. The tense patient is encouraged to take slow breaths in and out through her mouth while fixing her stare on something on the ceiling. The examination proceeds from the external examination of the genitalia, to the speculum examination and finally to the bimanual examination, which includes the rectovaginal exam. The nurse should explain each phase as she moves along.

If the examination proves very anxiety-producing for the woman and the examination is not urgent, she can be asked to return in another 2 or 3 weeks. During that time she should be encouraged to introduce 2 clean fingers into her vagina once a day and to practice tightening and relaxing her perineal muscles (Wallis, 1982).

External Examination

Gloving for the examination of the infant and child is not always necessary, because rarely does the exam involve any more than inspec-

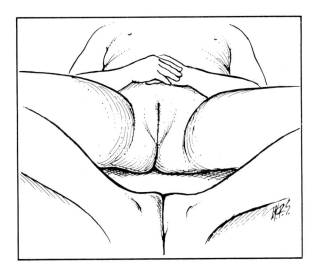

FIGURE 12.4
Positioning the young female in the frog-leg position.

tion. However, it is recommended that the nurse glove both hands for the examination of the adult female. This will allow her to completely assess the genitalia and prevent the spread of infection to herself and to other patients.

INSPECTION

The examiner should be seated at the foot of the table with the light positioned between the patient and herself, a few inches below her chin. The examiner views the external genitalia over the light. To begin the examination, the nurse tells the woman she is going to touch her and places one hand on the woman's inner thigh at about the level of the knee and moves her hand toward the perineum. This eliminates the startle reaction usually obtained when the perineum is touched directly and signals to the woman that the exam is about to begin. The external genitalia are then systematically inspected, beginning with the *pubic hair, labia majora* and *labia minora, skin, clitoris, hymen, urethra, perineum* and *rectal area.*

The Pubic Hair. The pubic hair is assessed for presence, distribution and quantity. The growth and distribution of pubic hair has been classified by Tanner (1962) into the following five developmental stages (Fig. 12.5):

Stage 1. Preadolescent—no pubic hair
Stage 2. Sparse, lightly pigmented, straight, over the medial border of the labia

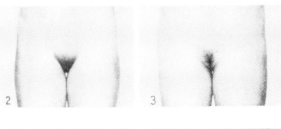
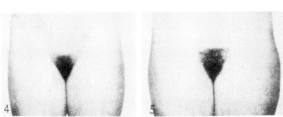

FIGURE 12.5
Developmental stages for pubic hair rating in girls. (Reprinted with permission from Tanner, J. Growth at Adolescence. Oxford, England: Blackwell Scientific Publications, Plate 6, p. 36, 1962.)

Stage 3. Darker, beginning to curl, increased amount
Stage 4. Coarse, curly, abundant but amount less than in the adult
Stage 5. Adult feminine triangle, spread to the medial surfaces of the thighs.

When a girl has onset of pubic or axillary hair before the age of 9 or has pubic or axillary hair growth, but is without any breast development there is concern about virilization or total lack of estrogen (Robie, 1983). Absence of pubic hair after 16 is considered abnormal. After menopause the pubic hair becomes sparse, straightens, and grays.

The Labia. The labia majora differ with age and parity. In the full-term infant the labia minora are often more prominent than the labia majora. This is always the case in the premature infant (Oehler, 1981). They are scaphoid and smooth in a child, plump and well formed in the menstruating woman, and atrophied in the postmenopausal woman. In the nulligravida, the labia majora cover the labia minora. After childbirth the labia minora become more prominent between the now-separated labia majora. The surfaces of the labia are covered by uniformly pink epithelium in the young woman. The skin surfaces in older women will appear thinner, less elastic and shiny due to hormonal changes.

The Skin. The skin is generally inspected for lesions or interruptions in skin integrity, abnormal exudate, erythema, and cleanliness. Among the most common abnormal genital findings are pubic lice (*Pediculosis pubis*), genital herpes (*Herpes progenitalis*), and anogenital warts (*Condylomata acuminata*). The nits or adult lice adhere to the base of the pubic hair or hair around the anus, abdomen, and thighs (Campbell & Herten, 1981). The lesions of herpes usually appear in the form of vesicles which eventually rupture, draining clear fluid and leaving a single or multiple painful ulcers. Condylomata acuminata are genital warts that are small to begin with, but eventually coalesce to form large warty growths. These warts are white-pink in color and often look like cauliflower.

A milky white, blood-tinged mucoid vaginal discharge is normal in the neonate until 2 to 3 weeks of age. The presence of vaginal discharge in the older infant and child needs further exploration. This can be due to poor hygiene practices, but occasionally, specific pathogens are isolated which may prove to be a clue for abnormal sexual relationships. You are referred to Robie (1983) for techniques used in obtaining vaginal smears on young girls. Normal versus common abnormal vaginal discharges observed in the menstruating and postmenopausal woman are discussed in the section on the speculum examination (p. 316).

At this point the labia are separated with the thumbs to adequately view the vestibule. The child may be asked to assist in this portion of the examination to help allay her anxiety.

Labial adhesions of the labia minora are not uncommon in children. The predisposing factors are a relatively atrophic genital tract and the close anatomical position of the labia combined with a vulvar inflammation. After adequately exposing the vestibule, the *clitoris*, *hymen*, and *urethra* are inspected.

The Clitoris. The clitoris is examined for size and lesions. It is difficult to measure the clitoris in any accurate way with a child and is not necessary. True enlargement of the clitoris is usually obvious. In the adult female the clitoris may vary from 2 millimeters to 1 centimeter, and is estimated at 4 to 5 millimeters both in the transverse and longitudinal planes (Woods, 1981). When there is any question about enlargement, the patient should be referred. In the adult female it may need to be retracted for clear visualization. The clitoris is a common location for the *chancre* of *syphilis* in a young woman and a cancerous lesion in the older woman. The chancre of syphilis is usually singular, nontender, beefy red, has a smooth appearance, and has raised borders. A cancerous lesion may appear raised, red, and ulcerated.

The Hymen and Urethra. The presence of a *hymenal tag* protruding from the vagina is a normal finding in the neonate (Oehler, 1981). This is a redundant segment of the hymen which disappears in a few weeks. The hymen in the child is usually red and shows no evidence of estrogen stimulation. The urethral meatus of the child is inspected for location. Children with ambiguous genitalia or with other congenital anomalies frequently do not have a urethra in the normal location

(Capraro, 1972). The urethral meatus of both children and adults is observed for signs of inflammation. It is normally pink without any exudate. The inner deep red lining of the urethra may be observed in some postmenopausal women. This is due to pelvic relaxation associated with decreased estrogen levels.

The Perineum and Rectal Area. The buttocks may need to be spread to adequately inspect the perineum and the rectal area. If an *episiotomy* was done during a vaginal delivery a scar will be present on the perineum. The rectal area is inspected for the presence of external *hemorrhoids, lesions,* and *worms.*

This concludes the examination of the young female genitalia. The only time the examiner goes further with a young girl is when there is bleeding, discharge, or itching. You are referred to Robie (1983) for discussion of the speculum and bimanual examination of the child.

PALPATION

Palpation of the external genitalia includes palpation of the *Skene's* and *Bartholin's* glands and assessment of the *support of the vaginal outlet.* The Skene's glands are palpated by inserting the gloved index finger of the dominant hand palm side up into the introitus approximately 2 to 3 centimeters (Fig. 12.6). The urethra is then milked from the bladder neck down. If any discharge is present it should be cultured for gonorrhea (see "Vaginal Smears and Cultures," page 316).

The Bartholin's glands are not palpable except in infection. The index finger is now moved to the posterior introitus and the thumb is placed outside the posterior part of the labia majora (Fig. 12.7). The examiner palpates between the index finger and the thumb for swelling and tenderness of the Bartholin's gland. The hand is rotated to examine the other side.

To assess the support of the vaginal outlet the patient is asked to bear down. Bulging observed on the anterior wall of the vaginal outlet indicates the presence of a *cystocele.* A cystocele is a prolapse of the anterior wall of the vagina and the bladder into the vagina. A *rectocele* is a prolapse of the posterior wall of the vagina and the rectum into the vagina. This is identified by noting bulging on the posterior

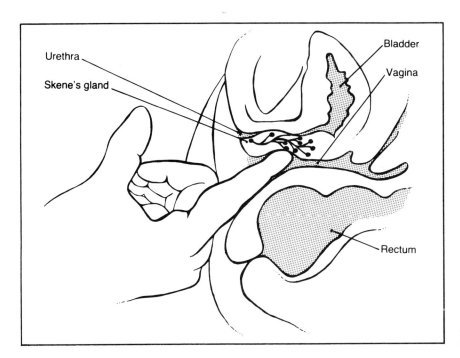

FIGURE 12.6
Palpation of Skene's glands.

wall of the vagina. Another sign of weak vaginal support is the observation of *stress incontinence* as the woman bears down.

Next, two fingers are inserted into the vagina and the fourchette is depressed to check resistance. Strong resistance indicates that the perineal body is intact. The patient is then asked to contract her pelvic muscles around the examiner's fingers. If she has difficulty knowing which muscles to contract she should be asked to pretend she is holding her urine back. The examiner should feel pressure or

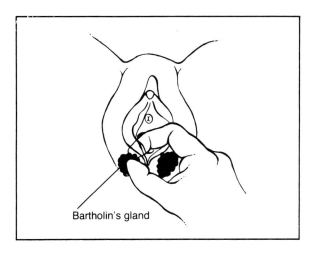

FIGURE 12.7
Palpation of Bartholin's glands.

tightening around her fingers within the vagina if the muscles are intact.

Speculum Examination

The examiner should be sure that the speculum is the correct size (Fig. 12.8). This involves a rather rough estimate, based primarily on the patient's sexual and obstetrical history. If the woman is virginal, the smallest size speculum is used. A medium speculum can be used comfortably with most sexually active women. A medium to large speculum is used with women who have had children.

As mentioned previously, the metal speculum can be warmed on a heating pad or it can be warmed by running lukewarm water over it just prior to insertion. Lubricant should not be used on the blades if any smears or cultures are to be taken, as this will contaminate the results.

If the woman is having difficulty relaxing, it often helps to have her practice tightening her perineal muscles as if she were trying to hold back her urine and then relaxing. By repeating this several times prior to beginning the examination, she will learn which muscles to relax. Several deep breaths also aid in relaxation.

If the woman has never had a vaginal ex-

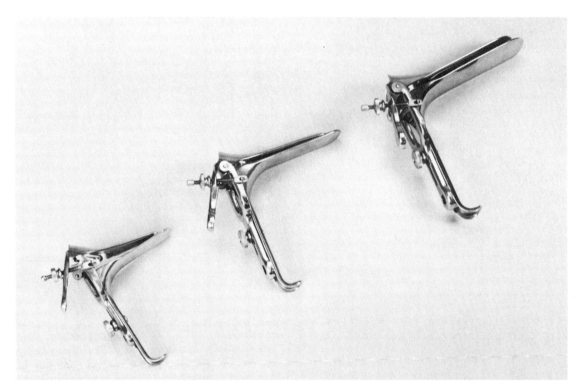

FIGURE 12.8
Vaginal speculi. **Left.** *Small.* **Center.** *Medium.* **Right.** *Large.*

amination, it is recommended that the examiner insert two fingers into the vagina and explore the introitus prior to insertion of the speculum. This is to make sure that there are no abnormalities in the vagina. This is also a good practice in general to help locate the cervix and give a clue as to where to direct the speculum.

Prior to introduction of the instrument, the patient is asked to bear down. The examiner then admits the index and middle fingers of her non-dominant hand into the vagina approximately 2 centimeters and spreads open the vagina with pressure on the posterior wall (Fig. 12.9A). The speculum, with the blades firmly together is held in the free dominant hand and inserted obliquely over the two vaginal fingers (Fig. 12.9A). This is to avoid contact with the sensitive urethra on the anterior vaginal wall. The fingers are then removed. Once in the vagina, the blades are turned parallel to the table for 2 to 3 centimeters and then directed at a 45-degree angle into the vagina (Fig. 12.9B and C). The speculum is inserted into the vagina as far as it will go. This is usually the entire length of the blades (Fig. 12.9C). When a firm structure is reached, the

instrument is opened and the cervix should be observable between the blades of the speculum (Fig. 12.9D). If the cervix cannot be seen, the speculum should be withdrawn slightly. If the cervix does not come into view the speculum is reinserted. It is better to begin the insertion over completely rather than to get involved in a lot of upward and downward movement of the speculum in search of the cervix. Once the cervix is identified, the speculum is secured in place by turning the upper thumb screw of the metal speculum (Fig. 12.10). The speculum will now remain in place without being held. If this does not provide adequate visualization, the lower thumb screw on the handle of the speculum is turned gently to expand. The *cervix* is inspected for *shape* and *size, color, lesions,* and *discharge.* Next, the *vaginal cultures* and *smears* are obtained. Finally, the *vaginal walls* are closely inspected as the blades of the speculum are removed.

SHAPE, SIZE, AND COLOR OF THE CERVIX
The cervix is usually round and symmetrical. The presence of a *cervical collar* is associated with exposure to DES prior to birth. The nulliparous *os* is small and either round or oval

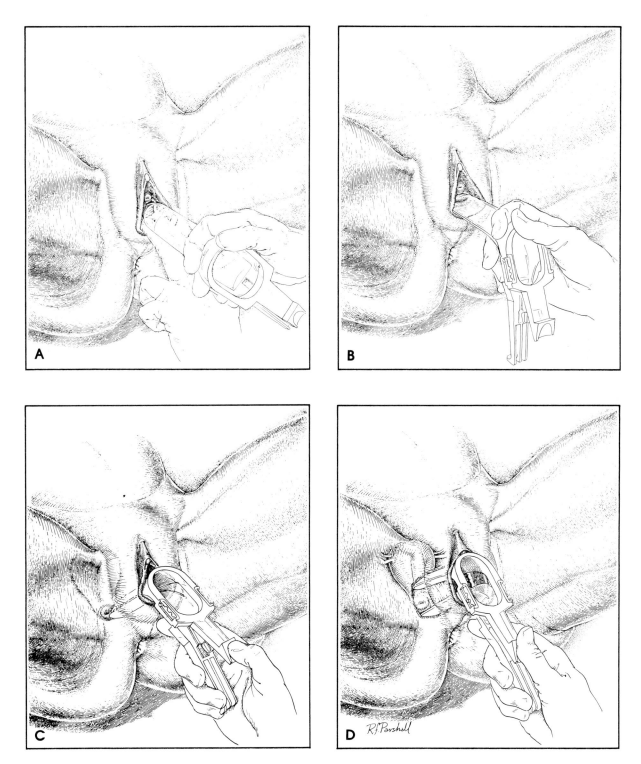

FIGURE 12.9
Procedure for insertion of the vaginal speculum. **A.** Opening the introitus and oblique insertion of the speculum blades. **B.** Speculum blades parallel to the table. **C.** Speculum blades directed at a 45-degree angle into the vagina. **D.** Opening the speculum blades.

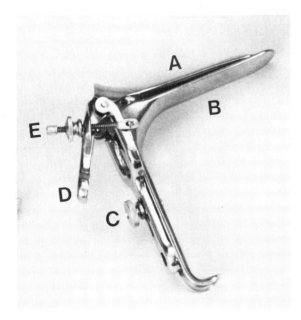

FIGURE 12.10
The parts of the vaginal speculum. **A.** Upper blade. **B.** Lower blade. **C.** Lower thumb screw. **D.** Thumb hinge. **E.** Upper thumb screw.

(Fig. 12.11A). After childbirth, the cervical os presents with a slit-like appearance (Fig. 12.11B). The cervix is usually pink in color, but after menopause is normally pale, glistening, and thick in appearance. The cervix has a bluish appearance in early pregnancy called *Chadwick's sign* (see Chapter 16 for further discussion of changes related to pregnancy).

CERVICAL LESIONS

The three most common changes on the surface of the cervix are *eversions, erosions, nabothian cysts,* and *polyps.* An eversion is present when the lining of the cervical canal pouts out. It appears red, symmetrical, and smooth (Fig. 12.11C). An eversion can be due to a previous childbirth laceration or can be a variation within normal limits. An erosion presents as a beefy red, irregular area around the cervical os that bleeds easily on touch (Fig. 12.11D). This is not easily distinguished from a cancerous lesion and requires further assessment. Nabothian cysts are typically small, round, smooth, yellow elevations on the cervix (Fig. 12.11E). They are due to obstruction or occlusion of the mucosal folds of the cervix and can be associated with chronic cervicitis. Polyps are usually seen protruding through the cervical os. They are usually light red and soft

appearing. Cysts and polyps require additional evaluation.

CERVICAL DISCHARGE

The characteristics of the cervical discharge are observed. Normal cervical discharge varies with the menstrual cycle. Following menstruation, estrogen levels are low, so there is little discharge. Several days before ovulation the discharge becomes a cloudy yellow and is sticky. The discharge at ovulation is highly lubricative, with the consistency of egg white. This discharge, which can be heavy, persists for 1 to 3 days after ovulation. As the progesterone levels increase, the discharge becomes cloudy and sticky. Then immediately prior to menstruation the discharge may become clear and watery. Following menopause when the estrogen levels are low, there is minimal cervical discharge.

Discharge that is colored, appears purulent or has a foul odor is abnormal. The most common vaginal infections are *Trichomoniasis vaginalis, Candida albicans, Gardnerella, Neisseria gonorrhea,* and *Chlamydia trachomatis.* Trichomoniasis is associated with profuse, purulent, malodorous discharge. The classic greenish yellow, bubbly discharge is present in only about one third of women (Eschenbach, 1983). Small hemorrhages may be observed on the cervix and vaginal walls. Discharge from Candida albicans may be thin but is characteristically thick, white, and curdy. This discharge may cling to the walls of the vagina, giving the appearance of cottage cheese. The most common characteristic of Gardnerella is a foul fishy amine vaginal odor. The discharge has a nonviscous appearance. Both Neisseria gonorrhea and Chlamydia trachomatis cause a yellow purulent discharge. Correct identification of the specific type of discharge is not possible by observation alone. When there is suspicion of a vaginal infection vaginal cultures and smears should be obtained.

VAGINAL CULTURES AND SMEARS

Gonorrheal Culture. Discharge for a Neisseria gonorrhea culture is obtained prior to any other specimens so that the necessary discharge is not removed resulting in a false negative culture. To obtain the gonorrhea culture, a swab is placed in the cervical canal and rotated 360 degrees. It should remain in the os for approximately 15 to 20 seconds. If the his-

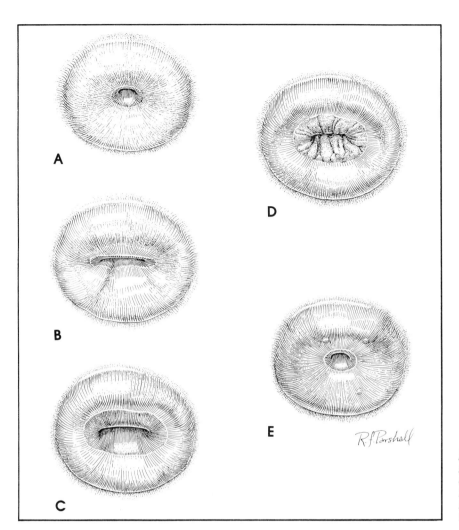

FIGURE 12.11
*Normal and common abnormal
appearances of the cervix.* **A.**
Healthy nulliparous. **B.** *Healthy
multigravida.* **C.** *Everted.* **D.**
Eroded. **E.** *Nabothian cysts.*

tory indicates exposure to gonorrhea through oral or rectal intercourse, the specimen is obtained from the appropriate location. The discharge is placed on a *Thayer Martin Plate* or *Transgrow bottle* in a Z pattern. The Thayer Martin culture is placed upside down in a large jar with a candle. The candle is lit and the cover secured in place. The Transgrow bottle requires the placement of a CO_2 tablet in the plate. Both types of medium are placed in an incubator.

Chlamydial Culture. Until recently the diagnosis of Chlamydia trachomatis was one of exclusion. Because the signs and symptoms of a chlamydial genital tract infection often resembled those of gonorrhea a chlamydial infection was not suspected until the culture report came back negative for Neisseria gonorrhea. Cell culture of chlamydia was available primarily through state health de-

partments, research, or reference laboratories. Now there is an easy-to-perform test available called a *direct fluorescent antibody stain test* (Schachter, 1984). This rapid slide test is specific for Chlamydia trachomatis. The test comes in a kit including a slide, swab, and fixative.

The procedure for collecting the specimen is as follows:

1. Because the chlamydial organism appears to live in the columnar epithelium, it is important to first wipe the cervix with a cotton or dacron swab (not provided in the kit) to remove excess mucus.
2. The swab provided is inserted into the endocervical canal until most of the tip is not visible.
3. The swab is then rotated for 5 to 10 seconds inside the endocervical canal using sufficient pressure to dislodge the cells.

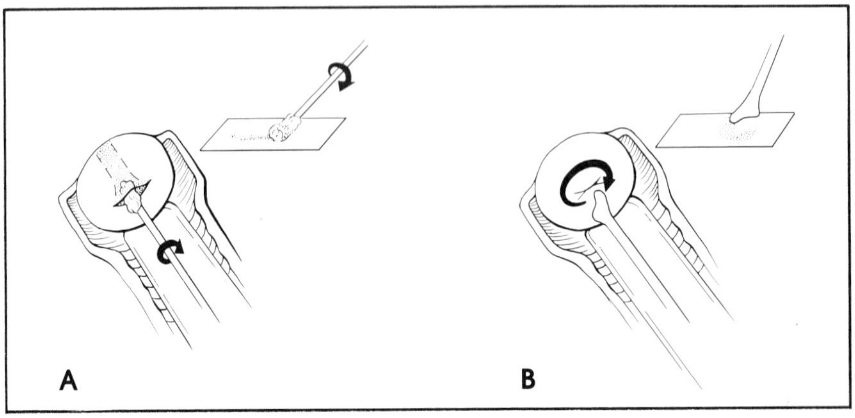

FIGURE 12.12
Procedure for obtaining a Pap smear. **A.** *Endocervical smear.* **B.** *Exocervical smear.*

4. The swab is withdrawn without touching any vaginal surfaces and rolled on the slide where indicated.
5. The slide is allowed to completely air dry prior to flooding with the acetone fixative.
6. After the fixative has evaporated, it is packaged and transported or refrigerated and stained within 7 days of collection.

In the laboratory, the specimen is stained with an antibody stain and read with a fluorescent microscope. Frequently, gonorrhea and chlamydia vaginal infections coexist so when available, this rapid staining test should be done along with a gonorrhea culture as symptoms and examination findings indicate. At present, this test is not used for routine screening in the asymptomatic patient.

Papanicolaou Smear. Discharge is obtained from two or three different locations for the Pap smear. These include the *endocervix, exocervix,* and *vagina.* A saline swab is inserted into the os of the cervix and rotated 360 degrees several times (Fig. 12.12A). This discharge is rolled onto the slide in the location marked E. The longer end of the Ayre spatula is placed at the *squamocolumnar junction* (the junction between the endocervix and the cervix) and is rotated a full 360 degrees (Fig. 12.12B). This discharge is smeared thinly onto the slide in the location marked C. If a vaginal lesion is present or the woman has been exposed to DES, a direct scrape is obtained from the lesion or wall. This specimen is obtained with the handle of the Ayre spatula and is smeared onto the slide in the location marked V. The slides are sprayed immediately with a fixative or placed in a Pap smear specimen bottle filled with 95 percent ethanol and sent to the laboratory for analysis.

Smears for Vaginal Infections. Secretions that look suspicious of a vaginal infection should be obtained from the vaginal pool, os, or walls of the vagina and placed on a glass slide. The nurse can readily learn to identify the causative organism by the use of a microscope. To test for Trichomonas vaginalis and Gardnerella, the secretions are mixed with a drop of normal saline, and a cover slip is applied. The specimen should be observed immediately under the microscope to identify the spindle-shaped, highly mobile trichomonads (Fig. 12.13). They are slightly larger than a white blood cell and have a characteristic undulating swimming motion. If Gardnerella is the causative organism, *"clue cells"* will be seen. These are epithelial cells to which a large number of organisms attach, obscuring the entire cell border (Eschenbach, 1983). The borders of clue cells are granulated, unlike the clear cell border of the normal epithelial cell.

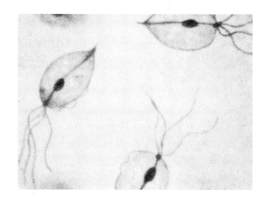

FIGURE 12.13
Trichomoniasis. (Reprinted with permission from Campbell, C. and Herten, R. VD to STD: Redefining venereal disease. American Journal of Nursing, 81, p. 1632, 1981.

A large amount of vaginal fluid is mixed with a drop of 10 percent potassium hydroxide (KOH), and the odor is noted. A fishy, amine odor is characteristic of Gardnerella. The solution is then placed on a slide and a cover slip is applied. The specimen is observed under a microscope to identify the characteristic buds and mycelia of Candida albicans (Fig. 12.14). Because of the uncertainty as to which type of vaginal infection may be present, it is best to prepare both a KOH slide and a saline slide and to examine both under the microscope.

EXAMINATION OF THE VAGINAL WALLS AND REMOVAL OF THE SPECULUM

The upper thumb screw is loosened and slight pressure is put on the thumb hinge to open the blades further. This avoids catching the cervix between the blades as the speculum is withdrawn. After clearing the cervix, pressure on the thumb hinge is gradually released. As the speculum is withdrawn the walls of the vagina are inspected. The vaginal walls of the woman of childbearing age are deep pink and rugations are observed. The vaginal walls of the postmenopausal woman are light pink, thin, and without rugations. By the time the end of the blades are at the introitus there should be no pressure on the thumb hinge and the blades should be in the closed position.

Bimanual Examination

The bimanual examination includes palpation of the *vagina, cervix, uterus,* and the *adnexae* (including the ovaries and fallopian tubes).

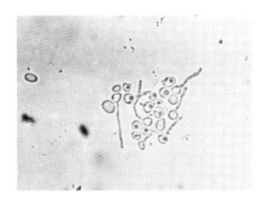

FIGURE 12.14
Candida albicans (moniliasis). (Reprinted with permission from Campbell, C., and Herten, R. VD to STD: Redefining venereal disease. American Journal of Nursing, 81, 1981, p. 1632.)

This examination is to be done in a systematic fashion, working from the exterior to the interior. The examiner should be standing between the legs of the woman for this examination. Lubricant is applied to the index and the middle finger of the gloved examining hand. These two fingers are inserted into the vagina. At the same time the thumb is hyperextended, and the ring and little fingers are flexed into the palm (Fig. 12.15). The surfaces of the hand should remain perpendicular to the floor.

VAGINAL WALL AND CERVIX

The vaginal wall is palpated for any nodularity or tenderness. The *cervix* is located and described in terms of position, consistency, mobility, and patency of the os. The position of the cervix is determined by the direction in which the os is pointing. If the os is directed toward the anterior wall of the vagina, the cervix is in the *anterior position.* The cervix is in a *midline position* when the os is pointed toward the vaginal outlet. The os is directed toward the posterior wall of the vagina when the cervix is in the *posterior position.* The consistency of the cervix is normally firm, like the tip of the nose. During pregnancy the cervix softens and feels like the lips of the mouth (*Goodell's sign*) (see Chapter 16 for further discussion of pregnancy-related changes). In the presence of a tumor the cervix becomes very hard. As the index finger is swept around the cervix, the cervix normally feels smooth, but if *nabothian cysts* are present they may be palpated as small, round elevations.

Mobility of the cervix is determined by holding the cervix between the index and middle finger and moving it laterally and medially. Normally the cervix is freely movable, and this movement causes no discomfort. If there is malignancy or scarring due to chronic pelvic inflammatory disease, the cervix will be fixed in one position. In the presence of acute pelvic inflammatory disease, the patient will experience great discomfort. The examination may have to be discontinued at this point because the woman will be too uncomfortable to allow adequate palpation of the pelvic organs.

The index finger is placed at the cervical os to check for *patency.* Normally, the os is 3 to 5 millimeters in diameter. If the examiner is able to admit the tip of her finger, something may have recently passed through the os, such as the contents of an abortion.

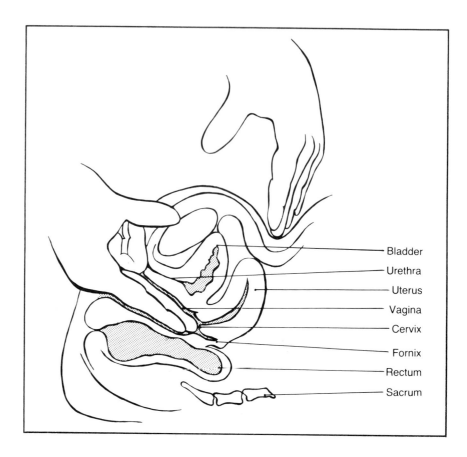

Bladder
Urethra
Uterus
Vagina
Cervix
Fornix
Rectum
Sacrum

FIGURE 12.15
Bimanual palpation of the uterus.

UTERUS

The *uterus* is palpated by placing the free ungloved hand on the abdomen halfway between the umbilicus and the symphysis pubis (Fig. 12.15). The examiner decides whether the dominant hand should be used as the vaginal or abdominal hand after trying both approaches. The examiner simultaneously locates the vaginal fingers in the anterior vaginal fornix. Starting at the umbilicus the abdominal hand is moved slowly toward the pubis until the uterus is trapped between the two hands. If the uterus is not felt, the vaginal fingers are placed in the posterior fornix, and the uterus is lifted upward as the examiner again attempts to trap it between the two hands. When neither of these two methods is successful, the middle finger is placed in the rectum, leaving the index finger in the vagina. The uterus may then be palpated in the posterior position through the rectal wall. However, this maneuver should be delayed until the adnexae are examined.

The five positions of the uterus are *anteverted, anteflexed, midposition, retroverted,* and *retroflexed* (Fig. 12.16A–E). When the os

of the cervix is pointed posteriorly and the uterus is palpated between the abdominal hand and the vaginal hand located in the anterior vaginal fornix, the uterus is anteverted. If the cervix is pointed anteriorly and the uterus is palpated between the abdominal hand and the vaginal hand located in the anterior vaginal fornix, the uterus is anteflexed. The uterus is in a midline position when the cervix is midline and the uterus is palpated by the abdominal and vaginal hands deep in the abdomen. The uterus is retroverted when the cervical os is pointed anteriorly and the uterus is palpated either in the posterior vaginal fornix or through the rectum. The uterus is retroflexed when the cervix is directed posteriorly and the uterus is palpated either in the posterior vaginal fornix or through the rectum.

The size of the uterus varies normally in relation to childbearing and the production of estrogen. The uterus is usually about the size of a fist and is located within the pelvic cavity. True enlargement of the uterus (above the level at the symphysis pubis) in a young woman should make one suspicious of preg-

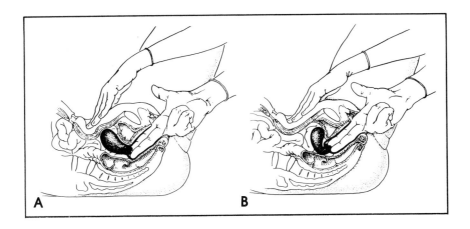

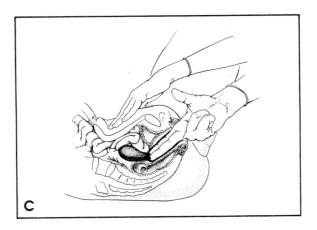

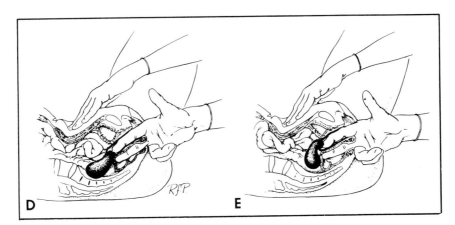

FIGURE 12.16
Positions of the uterus palpated on vaginal and rectovaginal examination. **A.** *Anteverted.* **B.**
Anteflexed. **C.** *Midposition.* **D.** *Retroverted.* **E.** *Retroflexed.*

nancy or tumor. The regularity and consistency of the uterus are determined by walking the fingers of the abdominal hand down the sides of the uterus. The surfaces of the uterus are normally smooth. Irregularities may indicate the presence of fibroids. The normal consistency of the nonpregnant uterus is firm. The

uterus softens in pregnancy due to hormonal influence and increased circulation. As early as the fifth week of pregnancy, softness will be noted on the anterior side of the uterus just above the uterocervical junction. This is known as *Ladin's sign.* Around the sixth week of pregnancy the lower uterine segment becomes very compressible. This is *Hegar's sign* (see Chapter 16 for further discussion of pregnancy-related changes). The uterus is normally freely movable but may become fixed due to the adhesions of malignancy, pelvic surgery, chronic pelvic inflammatory disease or endometriosis.

ADNEXAE

The *adnexae* are examined one at a time. First the abdominal hand is placed on the right-lower quadrant and the vaginal hand is placed in the right-lateral fornix. The abdominal hand is maneuvered downward along the iliac crest to trap the right ovary. This procedure is repeated on the left side. The *ovaries* are assessed for *size, consistency, mobility,* and *tenderness.* If the ovary is palpable, it should be less than 3 to 4 centimeters long. Ovaries are palpable in about half of normal menstruating women (Beckmann, et al., 1986). They are smaller in the postmenopausal woman, and if one is palpable, a tumor should be suspected. Ovaries are usually smooth and quite mobile. Irregularities on the surface of the ovary may suggest malignancy. Anything that may cause adhesions in the pelvic cavity, such as endometriosis, may cause the ovary to become fixed. There is some discomfort normally when the ovary is compressed between the fingertips. The *fallopian tubes* are rarely palpable and if they are palpable, an abnormality is suggested. Excessive discomfort in the adnexa indicates inflammation or the possibility of an ectopic pregnancy.

Rectovaginal Examination

The last part of the pelvic examination involves assessment of the rectovaginal area. A new glove is placed on the examining hand and the fingers are well-lubricated to ease insertion. The middle finger is slowly moved into the rectum following the natural curve of the rectal canal. This is upward at a 45-degree angle for 1 to 2 centimeters, then down-

ward (Beckmann, et al., 1986). Once the rectal finger has reached the bend where the angle turns downward, the index finger is inserted into the vagina. The vaginal finger is placed in the posterior fornix and the rectal finger is inserted as far as it will go.

The lateral, anterior, and posterior walls of the rectum are systematically palpated for the presence of tumors and polyps. The anterior wall is called the rectovaginal septum and is normally thin, smooth, and pliable. The vaginal finger is kept on the cervix to prevent confusion when palpating through the anterior wall (Fig. 12.16 D and E). Here the posterior surface of the uterus may be palpated in the retroverted or retroflexed position. The uterosacral ligaments may not be palpable or may be felt as resilient, band-like structures. Any mass not identified as an ovary or the uterus is abnormal.

BLOOD STOOL TEST

After completing the examination, the nurse should inspect the stool left on the glove. If it is tarry black, it indicates the possible presence of blood in the upper gastrointestinal tract. A *stool guaiac* slide test for occult blood should be done on all women age 50 and over. To perform this procedure, a small stool sample is collected on one end of an applicator and thinly smeared on a piece of filter paper. Two drops of solution containing hydrogen peroxide and denatured alcohol are applied directly over the slide. Results are read after 60 seconds. Any trace of blue at the edge of the smear indicates a positive test for occult blood.

Completion of the Examination

Upon completion of the female genitalia examination, the patient is asked to move upward on the table and then sit up. If she attempts to sit prior to moving upward she may fall. The woman should then be given some tissue to clean herself.

Screening Examination of the Female Genitalia

The screening examination of the female genitalia includes:

1. Inspection of the external genitalia and rectum
   a. Pubis
   b. Labia majora and labia minora
   c. Introitus

        1) Hymen
        2) Vagina
        3) Clitoris
        4) Urethra
     d. Rectum
  2. Palpation of the Bartholin and Skenes glands*
  3. Assessment of vagina support*
  4. Speculum examination*
  5. Bimanual examination*
     a. Palpation of the vagina, cervix, uterus, and adnexae
  6. Palpation of the rectum*

Adolescents and adults only

EXAMPLE OF A RECORDED HISTORY AND PHYSICAL

SUBJECTIVE:

Chief Complaint: Vaginal itching for 3 days.

HPH: This 30-year-old white female considers herself to be in good health. Three days ago she first noticed vaginal itching which has become increasingly worse. It is accompanied by a thick, white, odorless discharge. Her LMP was 10 days ago on March 10th. This was a normal 5 day menses with a moderate flow. She has been on oral contraceptives (Ortho Novum 1/50) for the past 8 years without any known side effects. She is para 0, gravida 0. She has a satisfying sexual relationship with her husband. She feels that they are both monogamous. She denies urinary frequency, burning, urgency, hematuria, fever, or abdominal pain. No past history of urinary tract infection, venereal disease, or vaginal infections. She is not taking antibiotics. The family history is negative for diabetes. She finds this problem to be a "nuisance."

OBJECTIVE:

External Genitalia: Normal female hair distribution, no lesions or rashes. Bartholin's and Skene's glands not palpable.

Urethra: No discharge.

Vaginal: Reddened; thick, white discharge clinging to the walls; no odor.

Cervix: Dark pink to red, no lesions, whitish discharge at os, nulliparous, posterior position, firm, movable, nontender.

Uterus: Small, smooth, freely movable, anteverted. No tenderness.

Adnexae: Not palpable. No tenderness.

Rectovaginal: No masses.

REFERENCES

American Cancer Society (1985). 1985 Cancer Facts and Figures. New York: American Cancer Society.

Beckmann, C., Ellis, J., Ling, F., Barzansky, B., et al. (1986). The woman's health evaluation. In C. Beckmann, F. Ling, and J. Ellis, (Eds.), A Clinical Manual of Gynecology (2nd ed.). Norwalk, Conn.: Appleton-Century-Crofts.

Campbell, C., & Herten, R. (1981). VD to STD: Redefining venereal disease. American Journal of Nursing, 81, 1629–34.

Capraro, V. (1972). Gynecologic examination in children and adolescents. Pediatric Clinics of North America, 19(3), 511–28.

Chow, M., Durand, B., Feldman, M., & Mills, M. (1984). Handbook of Pediatric Primary Care. New York: John Wiley & Sons.

Driscoll, C. (1982). Pediatric gynecology. The Female Patient, 7, 4–12.

Eschenbach, D. (1983). Vaginal discharge. In J. Duenhoelter, (Ed.), Greenhill's Office Gynecology (10th ed.). Chicago: Year Book, pp. 84–101.

Eveleth, P., & Tanner, J. (1976). World Wide Variation in Human Growth. New York: Cambridge University Press.

Fogel, C. (1981). The gynecologic triad: Discharge, pain, and bleeding. In C. Fogel, and N. Woods, (Eds.), Health Care of Women—A Nursing Perspective. St. Louis: C. V. Mosby, pp. 220–50.

Hatcher, R., Guest, F., Stewart, F., Stewart, G., et al. (1984). Contraceptive Technology 1984–1985 (12th ed.). New York: Irvington Publishers.

Jaszmann, L., Van Lith, N., & Zaat, J. (1969). The perimenopausal symptoms: The statistical analysis of a survey (Parts A and B). Medical Gynecology and Sociology, 4, 268–77.

McKinlay, S., & Jeffreys, M. (1974). The menopausal syndrome. British Journal of Preventive and Social Medicine. 28, 108–15.

McKinlay, S., Jeffreys, M., & Thompson, B. (1972). An investigation of the age of menopause. Journal of Biosocial Science, 4, 161–73.

Oehler, J. (1981). Family-centered Neonatal Nursing Care. Philadelphia: J. B. Lippincott.

Prenatal diethylstibestrol exposure. (1983). Clinical Pediatrics, 22(2), 139–43.

Robie, G. (1983). Pediatric gynecology. In J. Duenhoelter, (Ed.), Greenhill's Office Gynecology (10th ed.). Chicago: Year Book, pp. 238–322.

Schachter, J. (1984). Chlamydia trachomatis: An overview. Syva Monitor, 2(1), 1–8.

Tanner, J. (1962). Growth at Adolescence (2nd ed.). Oxford, England: Blackwell Scientific Publications.

Wallis, L. (1982). The patient as partner in the pelvic exam. The Female Patient, 7, 28/4–28/7.

Woods, N. (1981). Woman's body. In C. Fogel, and N. Woods, (Eds.), Health Care of Women—A Nursing Perspective. St. Louis: C. V. Mosby, pp. 68–100.

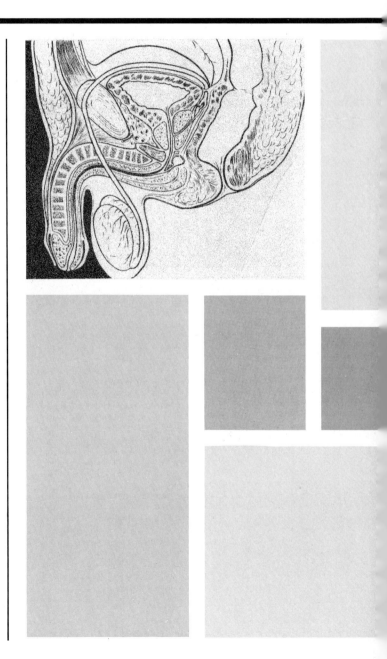

13

The Male Genitalia and Hernia Areas

Examination of the genitalia of the young male should be done in the delivery or birthing room and thereafter at all well-baby, preschool and school physicals. Many parents of newborn boys have been raising questions regarding whether or not to have their child circumcised. These questions arose because of the 1971 Committee on Fetus and Newborn of the American Academy of Pediatrics statement that there were no valid medical indications for circumcisions in the neonatal period (Gracely-Kilgore, 1984). Parents of infants and young boys have questions about the development of their child's genitals which they may be hesitant to mention. The nurse can anticipate these questions by offering reassurance of normal findings while examining the child.

Preadolescent (10–12 years) and adolescent (13–20 years) boys wonder about their own physical development and often compare themselves to peers. During this stage of development the boy may be embarrassed to have his genitals examined, particularly by a woman. Throughout the examination the nurse should stress to the adolescent that his genitals are normal. As young men approach the age of 20, most have established their sexual identity, and this embarrassment generally decreases (Haggerty, 1983).

Scrotal cancer is the most common neoplasm in men between the ages of 20 and 34 years, affecting approximately 3.1 men per 100,000 (Haggerty, 1983). The prognosis is good if the diagnosis is made early. This problem can easily be detected by the man if a systematic monthly self-examination is performed. Ideally the male should be instructed in the performance of *testicular self-examination* in midadolescence (16–20 years). He should be encouraged to perform the examination at the same time each month so that it becomes a habit. There are no set guidelines regarding frequency of professional examination of the male genitalia, but it has been suggested that professional examination be performed every third year after age 20 (Lindberg, 1980). A history of undescended testicles, whether surgically corrected or not, increases the risk of testicular cancer and may require more frequent examinations.

As men age, the incidence of *prostatic disease* and *cancer of the colon* and *rectum* increases. In men 55 to 74 years of age cancer of the colon and rectum is the second most common cause of cancer death and cancer of the prostate is the third (Cancer Statistics, 1985). After the age of 75, cancer of the prostate ranks second and cancer of the colon and rectum third as the most common cause of cancer death in men. Cancer of the prostate is more common in Caucasians than other racial groups (Rhodes, et al., 1974). A national study done by the American Cancer Society indicated that most people had their colon and rectum checked infrequently by health care providers and most thought disease was usually found in advanced stages when survival chances were minimal (American Cancer Society, 1985).

Examination of the prostate and rectum remains one of the best means for detecting cancer of these organs. This examination should be performed yearly on every man over the age of 40. A biannual examination of the prostate should be performed if the patient has a family history of cancer of the prostate or a positive history for *benign prostatic hyperplasia* (Shortridge & McLain, 1979). The American Cancer Society recommends two tests for the early detection of cancer of the rectum and colon. Starting at age 50 a *stool test* for blood should be done on an annual basis and a *proctosigmoidoscopy* should be done every 2 to 3 years, following two annual examinations with negative results (American Cancer Society, 1985). Those persons at high risk for developing rectal cancer should begin to have a blood slide test prior to the age of 50. High risk factors include a family history of cancer of the colon or rectum, a history of polyps or prior colon cancer and ulcerative colitis. In addition, there is some evidence that a diet high in beef or deficient in fiber may be a causitive factor (American Cancer Society, 1985).

DEVELOPMENTAL CHANGES OF THE MALE GENITOURINARY SYSTEM THROUGHOUT THE LIFESPAN

Sexuality exists at the moment of birth. The boy infant has an erection shortly after his first lung-filling cry. Infants soon discover that touching the genitalia gives pleasurable sensations and masturbation often occurs before the first birthday. In the child, testes are nonfunctional, but after 6 years of age the seminiferous tubules show the first signs of developing.

Complete neuromuscular control of urination should be achieved by the age of 5 or 6 in boys. *Enuresis* is involuntary bedwetting during sleep in a child whose age and development indicate that he should have control. It is *primary enuresis* if the child has never established bladder control and *secondary enuresis* if the child has previously established control and later loses it.

Boys are at significantly greater risk than girls for *urinary tract* infection in the first year of life. Studies indicate that fewer than 1 percent of infants have a urinary tract infection and that two-thirds of these are boys. The reasons for this susceptibility are not fully understood, but it is presumed that these infections are blood borne (Cunningham, 1984). After the age of 1 the incidence of infections in females exceeds that in males by a factor of 5 or 10 to 1. It has been estimated that less than 1 percent of boys will have even one urinary tract infection before the age of 18 (Chow, et al., 1984).

Boys begin sexual maturation 6 months to 2 years later than girls. The first sign of pubertal change in a boy is enlargement of the testes between the ages of 10 and 13½ years. However, it is hard to detect this earliest change. The complete development of the testes takes 5 to 6 years, with the fastest growth occurring between 13 and 14 years of age (Tudor, 1981). As the testicles grow in size so does the scrotum. Enlargement and lengthening of the penis begins about 1 year after the onset of testicular growth and takes about 2½ years to reach adult size. Associated with beginning penile enlargement there is a slight growth of long straight, slightly pigmented hair laterally at the base of the penis. This is usually the first visible sign of puberty occurring at approximately age 13. Hair growth on the medial thigh areas between 14 and 18 years of age signals the end of pubertal development. The time between onset and completion of puberty for the male is approximately 4 years.

Ejaculation usually occurs in boys 1 to 2 years after the first appearance of pubic hair, and may occur earlier. Spermatozoa are frequently present in the ejaculate of males 1 year after the visible onset of puberty and after 2 years most are able to father children. Spontaneous *nocturnal emissions* occur about 1 year after ejaculatory ability has been achieved through masturbation. Spermatogenesis does diminish with advancing age. Beginning with the fifth decade of life there are fewer sperm and fewer viable sperm (Markley, 1982). Sperm production, however, has been found to persist into the ninth decade of life and beyond.

An older man can take up to twice as long to achieve an erection as a young man. There may be a decrease in firmness of an erection in the male over 60 years of age (Markley, 1982). With advancing age a man can maintain an erection longer before ejaculation and the refractory period, the time between ejaculations, tends to be longer.

Urinary tract infections increase in frequency in the elderly male. This is related to the use of instrumentation such as cystoscopy or catheterization, the presence of bladder outlet changes, the presence of diabetes or neurologic disease, the presence of benign prostatic hypertrophy, and the use of medications (Yurick, et al., 1980).

ANATOMY

The anatomy of the male genitalia, hernia areas, and prostate will be covered in this section (see Chapter 12 for anatomy of the rectum).

The Male Genitalia

The male genitalia include the penis and the scrotum (Fig. 13.1). The penis consists of the *shaft, glans, foreskin,* and *urethra.* The shaft of the penis is formed dorsally by two lateral columns, the *corpora cavernosa,* and ventrally by one column, the *corpus spongiosum,* which contains the urethra (Fig. 13.2). These three columns are bound together by heavy fibrous tissue. At the end of the shaft is the glans penis. The urethra traverses through the glans to its termination point at the tip of the glans. The point where the glans and the shaft meet is called the corona. The prepuce or foreskin is a flap of skin that covers the glans. This is the piece of skin that is removed at the time of circumcision.

The scrotum is a pouch-like sac that is internally separated by a septal fold. Each half contains a *testis* with its *epididymis* and *spermatic cord.* The testis is an oval body about 1.5 inches in length. The testes should be descended by birth. Of those that are undescended, one half descend by the first month and one fourth by the end of the first year. The epididymis is a comma-shaped structure attached to the posterolateral surface of the testis. In approximately 7 percent of men, it is on the anterior surface of the testis. The spermatic cord consists of the *vas deferens, blood vessels, lymphatic vessels,* and *nerves.*

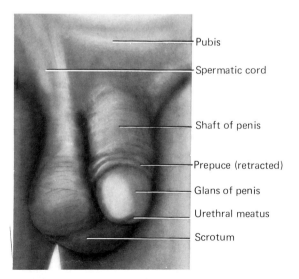

FIGURE 13.1
External male genitalia. (From Heagarty, M., et al. Child Health: Basics for Primary Care. New York: Appleton-Century-Crofts, 1980, p. 164, with permission.)

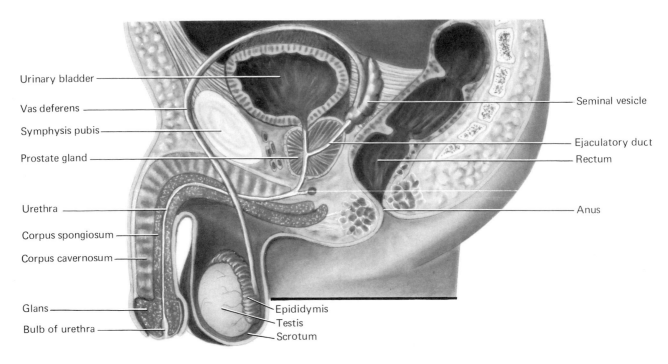

Urinary bladder

Vas deferens

Symphysis pubis

Prostate gland

Urethra

Corpus spongiosum

Corpus cavernosum

Glans

Bulb of urethra

Seminal vesicle

Ejaculatory duct

Rectum

Anus

Epididymis

Testis

Scrotum

FIGURE 13.2
Internal structure of the male genitalia. (From Heagarty, M., et al. Child Health: Basics for Primary Care. New York: Appleton-Century-Crofts, 1980, p. 164, with permission.)

The vas deferens passes from the epididymis through the inguinal canal and enters the abdominal cavity, eventually descending into the pelvic cavity.

Hernia Areas

The inguinal ligament goes from the anterior superior iliac spine to the pubic tubercle. Just above and lateral to the pubic tubercle is the *external inguinal ring* of the *inguinal canal* (Fig. 13.3). The inguinal canal, a flattened tunnel between superficial and deep layers of abdominal muscle, extends to the internal ring, which is 1 to 2 centimeters above the midpoint of the inguinal ligament.

The *femoral canal* is a potential space below the inguinal ligament. It is located medial to the femoral artery and lateral to the pubic tubercle.

There are two types of hernias: *inguinal* and *femoral* (Fig. 13.3). An inguinal hernia can be either *direct* or *indirect*. The direct hernia originates above the inguinal ligament, close to the pubic tubercle and near the external inguinal ring. It emerges directly from behind and through the external ring. The indirect hernia originates above and near the midpoint of the inguinal ligament at the internal inguinal ring. It comes down the canal. A femoral hernia presents on the anterior surface of the thigh just below the inguinal ligament.

The Prostate Gland

The *prostate gland* is a solid, heart-shaped structure about 2.5 centimeters in length (Fig. 13.2). It lies in the pelvis 2 centimeters posterior to the symphysis pubis. The posterior surface is in close contact with the anterior rectal wall and is the only portion accessible to palpation. Three lobes comprise the prostate: the *median lobe* and the *right* and *left lateral lobes.* The two lateral lobes are on the posterior surface of the gland and are divided by a *shallow median furrow.* The seminal vesicles lie above and along the lower posterior surface of the bladder (Fig. 13.2).

HISTORY

The genitourinary history of the male patient differs with the age of the patient.

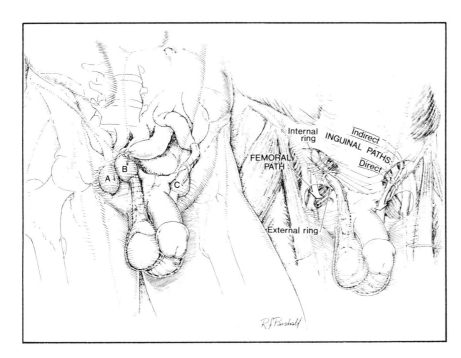

FIGURE 13.3
*Common hernia areas. **A.** Femoral hernia. **B.** Direct inguinal hernia. **C.** Indirect inguinal hernia.*

The Pediatric History

The infant's history should be geared toward identifying signs of urinary tract infection, hygiene practices, genital anomalies, and parental concerns. The nurse should keep in mind that the clinical presentation of urinary tract infection in an infant is non-specific. Answers to the following questions should be obtained from the parent or guardian of the male infant:

1. Has the child had unexplained fevers, poor feeding, failure to gain weight, vomiting, diarrhea, or irritability?
2. How often do you have to change wet diapers?
3. What is the strength of his urine stream?
4. Have you noticed any rashes or lesions in the diaper area?
5. Have you noticed a change in the color or odor of his urine?
6. Was the child circumcised?
7. How do you clean his genital area?
8. Have you noticed any scrotal swelling or masses?
9. Have the testes been felt in the scrotum?
10. Did his mother take any drugs during her pregnancy?
11. Is there a family history of genital or gonadal abnormalities, nephritis, nephrosis, or kidney masses?

12. Do you have any questions about the development of his sexual organs?

The history of the toddler and preschooler can be obtained from the parent with input from the child. As the child grows older the symptoms for a urinary tract infection become more specific, and questions relative to potty training should be included. Additional questions for the parent of the toddler and preschooler include:

1. When was potty training initiated and what techniques were used?
2. When did he attain bladder and bowel control?
3. Does he wet the bed at night?
4. Does he ever have daytime incontinence?
5. Has he experienced any urgency, frequency, burning, flank pain, blood in his urine, anorexia, vomiting, abdominal pain, or diarrhea?
6. Have you noticed a change in the color or odor of his urine?
7. Has he ever had a urinary tract infection in the past?

The history from a school-age child is similar to the preschool history. As the young boy enters the preteenage years (10–12 years), signs of development should be obtained, including the age at first appearance of pubic hair, axillary hair and voice change. He should also be asked if he has any concerns about his genitals.

The sexual history is part of every pediatric genitourinary history. See Chapter 1 for the age-appropriate questions.

The Adult History

Obtaining the genitourinary history of an adolescent or adult male can be sensitive for the female examiner and patient alike. The examiner should be comfortable with her own sexuality and view exploration of this system as necessary to holistically understand the patient. Questions should be presented in a matter-of-fact way using precise terms that are familiar to the patient. Included in the review of the male genitourinary system are questions that may uncover the presence of urinary tract disease, venereal disease, hernias, testicular and prostate disease, cancer risk factors, and a family history of kidney disease. A sexual history should also be obtained.

Symptoms of *urinary tract infection* in the adult are usually specific. Every patient should be asked if he is experiencing painful urination, urgency, hematuria, decreased output or no urine output, backache, lethargy, abdominal pain or incontinence. In addition, the examiner should go over the course and treatment of any past urinary tract infection.

Each patient should be asked about symptoms that may indicate the presence of sexually transmitted diseases (STD). These include lesions or rashes in the genital area or rectum, discharge from the urethra, and painful urination. The examiner should ask about any past history of STD and how it was treated. Finally, she should determine the man's knowledge of STDs, including symptoms, prevention, and treatment.

To explore for the presence of *testicular disease*, the nurse should ask the patient if he has noticed any lumps, soreness, or heaviness in his testicles. To determine if the patient is at risk for testicular cancer he should be asked if he has a history of undescended testicles and if his mother took hormones during pregnancy. Even if surgical correction for undescended testicles was performed before age 5 there is an increased risk for cancer. There may be some increased risk for testicular cancer in males whose mothers took oral contraceptives or *diethylstilbesterol* (DES) during pregnancy. The patient should be asked if he practices a monthly testicular self-examination and if not be instructed on the necessity of doing so.

Middle-aged and elderly patients should be asked about symptoms related to *prostatic disease* including hesitancy, slow stream, a change in stream, urinary frequency, and dribbling. There is increased risk for prostatic cancer when there is family history of prostatic cancer in the father or grandfathers.

The examiner should ask every adolescent and adult male if he has noticed any swelling in the groin or scrotum that is accentuated with straining, lifting, or coughing. If his occupation requires heavy lifting, he may be at risk for the development of a hernia. In addition, the nurse should obtain a family history of kidney problems on all males. Important information includes a family history of nephritis, nephrosis, and kidney masses.

The sexual history is often integrated with the genitourinary history. The goal is to identify any of the patient's concerns or problems. The sexual history often helps to direct questions related to the genitourinary system. See Chapter 1 for the age-appropriate questions.

PHYSICAL ASSESSMENT

Equipment

The equipment necessary for the male genital examination includes:

1. *Gloves*
2. Gonorrhea *culture plate* and *swabs*
3. A *penlight* to transilluminate a *hydrocele* or *spermatocele* (see "Transillumination," page 336)
4. *Lubricant* for the rectal and prostate examination
5. A stool guaiac slide to test the stool for blood

Preparation of the Patient

The examination of school-age boys should be performed with a parent present. Siblings, however, should be removed from the examining room in the interest of privacy. Examination of an adolescent can be performed without the parent; this assures confidentiality. Patient or parent explanation prior to beginning the male genital examination is important. A systematic, quick approach should be used in consideration of the patient's modesty. If the examiner has further questions during the exam, it is best to delay them until the examination is completed and the patient is clothed. These measures help to prevent a potentially embarrassing or uncomfortable situation for the examiner and patient. Findings should be communicated to the patient or his parents. Parents of both young children and adolescents need reassurance that there are no problems.

In a complete physical examination, the genitalia examination logically follows that of the abdomen. The examination of the infant and toddler can be done with the child in a supine position. The preschooler and early school-age child may be easier to examine with the child standing on the examining table. The adult patient should be standing at the foot of the examining table with the examiner sitting in front of him. The patient's underwear should be removed to allow a complete view of the genitalia and groin.

Examination of the Male Genitalia

The examination includes general inspection of the genitalia and groin, followed by inspection and palpation of the penis and scrotum. Abnormalities of the scrotum are evaluated by transillumination. Next the hernia areas are inspected and palpated. Finally, the prostate and rectum are examined in patients over 40 years of age.

GENERAL INSPECTION

General inspection includes examination of the *pubic hair, skin,* and *groin.* The pubic hair is assessed for presence, distribution, and quantity. The growth and distribution of pubic hair has been classified by Tanner (1962) into the following *developmental stages* (Fig. 13.4).

Stage 1. None
Stage 2. Scanty, long, slightly pigmented
Stage 3. Darker, starts to curl, small amount

Stage 4. Resembles adult type, but less in quantity; coarse, curly
Stage 5. Adult distribution (diamond shaped), spread to medial surface of the thighs

Onset of pubic hair before the age of 9½ years may be indicative of precocious adolescent sexual development. The elderly male will have less pubic hair, and it will become gray with age. The skin over the genital area is inspected for lesions. Nits seen at the base of the pubic, genital, abdominal, or rectal hair are caused by *Phthirus pubis.* This condition requires treatment. Finally, the groin is inspected for any signs of swelling which may be due to enlarged lymph nodes or hernias.

THE PENIS

Inspection. The penis is inspected for size, lesions, placement of the urethral opening, and discharge. In infancy, the nonerect penis is 2 to 3 centimeters, increasing in size between the ages of 11 and 14½ years. A mature flaccid size of approximately 8 to 10 centimeters is reached by 13½ to 17 years of age. An infantile penis at adolescence suggests a hormonal problem. The penis decreases in size in the elderly male, but it does not change in general appearance.

Inspect the shaft, prepuce, and glans of

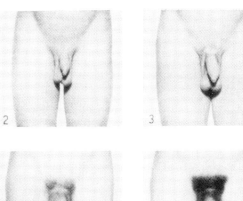

FIGURE 13.4
Developmental stages for pubic hair ratings in boys. (Reprinted with permission from Tanner, J. Growth at Adolescence. Oxford, England: Blackwell Scientific Publications, Plate 6, 1962, p. 36.)

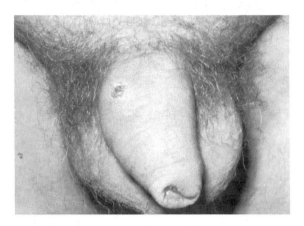

FIGURE 13.5
Syphilitic chancre. (Reprinted with permission from Felman, Y., et al. Wellcome Atlas of Sexually Transmitted Diseases. New York: Park Row Publishers, 1984, p. 21.)

the penis for lesions and nodules. The most common lesions are due to *syphilis, condylomata accuminata* and *herpes progenitalis.* The *syphilitic chancre* is the primary lesion of syphilis (Fig. 13.5). It appears as an oval, dark red erosion with a smooth, rounded border. It is typically painless and singular. Venereal warts, called condylomata accuminata, are small, elongated projections which may be either moist or dry (Fig. 13.6). Herpes lesions

often first appear as tiny, painful blisters which break open after a few days and become ulcerous (Fig. 13.7). The red sores eventually form scabs and heal. The lesion associated with carcinoma of the penis may be dry and scaly or ulcerated. This occurs most frequently in men who were not circumcised in childhood, and may be masked by the prepuce.

If the prepuce is present, it is retracted by the examiner or the patient so that the glans can be observed. It should be easily retractable. A normal exception is in the first 2 to 3 months of life, when the foreskin is normally tight and should not be forceably retracted. After 1 year of age, 50 percent of males will have a fully retractable foreskin, but it is not until 3 years of age that it is retractable in most males (Chow, et al., 1984). *Phimosis* is a condition in which the prepuce cannot be retracted. *Paraphimosis* exists when the prepuce is partially retracted and cannot return to normal position. At the time of retraction the external meatus is examined for position and discharge. The meatus is normally positioned centrally in the glans. *Hypospadias* is the congenital displacement of the urethral meatus to the inferior (ventral) surface of the penis. *Epispadias* is malpositioning of the meatus on the dorsal surface of the penis (Fig. 13.8).

To observe for discharge from the urethra, have the patient hold the penis with his thumb and index finger at the base and then milk it downward. Any urethral discharge is

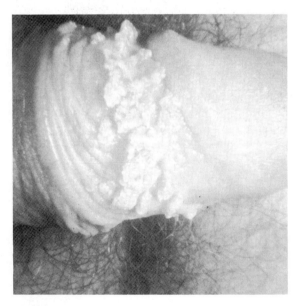

FIGURE 13.6
Condylomata accuminata. (Reprinted with permission from Felman, Y., et al. Wellcome Atlas of Sexually Transmitted Diseases. New York: Park Row Publishers, 1984, p. 11.)

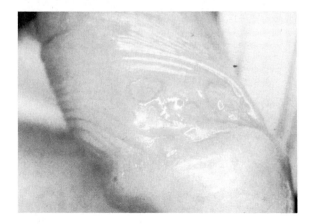

FIGURE 13.7
Genital herpes lesions. (Reprinted with permission from Felman, Y., et al. Wellcome Atlas of Sexually Transmitted Diseases. New York: Park Row Publishers, 1984, p. 11.)

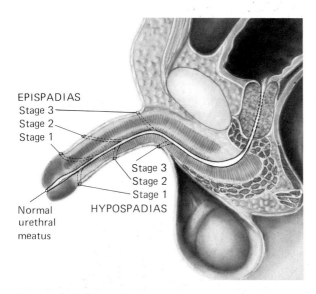

FIGURE 13.8
Abnormalities of the urethral meatus. (From Heagarty, M., et al. Child Health Care: Basics for Primary Care. New York: Appleton-Century-Crofts, 1980, p. 164.)

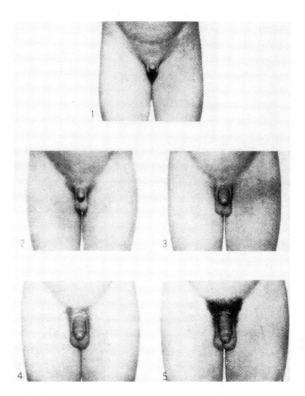

FIGURE 13.9
Developmental stages for genitalia maturity rating in boys. (Reprinted with permission from Tanner, J. Growth at Adolescence. Oxford, England: Blackwell Scientific Publications, Plate 5, 1962, p. 32.)

abnormal and should be cultured for Neisseria gonorrhea.

Palpation. Gloves should be worn while palpating the genitalia. Hold the penis between the thumb and first two fingers and gently palpate. Note any tenderness of lesions and the size of nodules that were observed or inspected. Some patients have non-tender hard plaques just beneath the skin, usually along the dorsum of the penis. These patients often complain of crooked, painful erections. This is known as *Peyronie's disease,* a chronic disease of unknown cause.

THE SCROTUM

Inspection. When inspecting the scrotum, it is important to lift the sac up to observe the undersurface. The scrotum should be inspected for size and color, symmetry, lesions, and swelling. Tanner (1962) has identified five stages of *scrotal development* (Fig. 13.9). The first is the preadolescent stage when the scrotum is small, smooth, and pink. The second stage occurs at approximately 12 to 13 years of age. At this time the scrotum enlarges, becomes reddened and rugae begin to appear. During the third stage the scrotum further enlarges, and at the fourth stage it darkens. The fifth stage is when the genitalia reach adult

size and shape. When physical signs of puberty have not appeared by age 16, puberty is considered delayed. In the aging man, there is significant loss in elasticity of the scrotal skin which leads to increased relaxation, folding, and sagging of the scrotal tissue (Yurick, et al., 1980).

The *dartos muscle* of the scrotum contracts when the scrotum is cold and relaxes when it is warm. In the adult, the left scrotum is lower than the right because of a longer spermatic cord on that side. *Sebaceous cysts* are common benign cutaneous skin lesions found on the scrotum. They are yellow-white in appearance and on palpation are firm and non-tender. A taut swelling of the scrotum with pitting *edema* may be associated with the generalized edema of cardiac or nephrotic disease.

Palpation. Gently palpate the scrotum between the thumb and first two fingers on both sides. The contents of the scrotum, including the testes, epididymis, vas deferens, and spermatic cord should be palpated separately. First, determine the presence of each testis. The incidence of *undescended testis* in full-term infants is approximately 4 percent (Marshall & Elder, 1982). The incidence of undescended testis drops rapidly over the first few months and at 1 year appears to be just under 1 percent. If the testicles are not in the scrotum, the examiner should search for them in the inguinal canal or in the abdomen just proximal to the internal ring. This is done by placing the index finger (the little finger is used for the young child) at the bottom of the scrotum to allow enough skin to invaginate as the finger is brought up to the inguinal ring. Be aware of the cremasteric reflex in boys (see Chapter 15), which causes the testes to ascend into the superficial inguinal pouch when the boy is cold or embarrassed. This reflex becomes active after the age of 3 months and may cause a normal testicle to appear undescended. The reflex can be eliminated by having the child sit *cross-legged* on the table. Any child with undescended testes should receive further evaluation and treatment.

Compression of the testis is painful, so palpate them gently. The testis is smooth, egg shaped, and of a rubbery consistency. A very hard testicle or lump in a portion of the testicle should make the examiner suspect cancer.

The epididymis is normally resilient and slightly tender. A hard, enlarged, non-tender epididymis may be due to tuberculosis. Tenderness and swelling are signs of acute epididymitis, perhaps secondary to trauma or infection. Palpate each spermatic cord with its vas deferens between the thumb and index finger from the epididymis to the external inguinal ring. Note any swelling or nodules. A *varicocele* consists of varicose veins of the spermatic cord (Fig. 13.10A). It is more common on the left side, because the left spermatic vein empties into the left renal vein and is competing for blood from the kidney. The right spermatic vein empties directly into the vena cava. A varicocele feels like a bag of worms and disappears when the patient is in the supine position. It is frequently associated with infertility. If the varicocele does not disappear in the supine position, obstruction from a malignancy should be suspected.

Transillumination. Transillumination is used to evaluate any swelling or mass in the scrotum. This is done in a darkened room by pulling the scrotal wall tightly over the mass and putting a flashlight against the posterior side of the scrotum. A beam of light shines through the mass. If the mass transilluminates, a red glow is produced. Serous fluid will transilluminate; tissue and blood will not. Two masses that transilluminate are a hydrocele and a spermatocele.

A *hydrocele* is the most common mass in the scrotum (Fig. 13.10B). It is a soft or tense fluid filled sac in front of the testis and epididymis or it is located in the spermatic cord above the testis. A non-communicating hydrocele in an infant results from residual peritoneal fluid that may remain after the closure of the processus vaginalis, a sac of peritoneal tissue that preceded the descent of the male

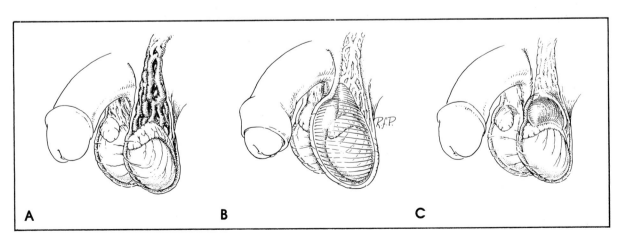

FIGURE 13.10
Scrotal abnormalities. **A.** *Varicocele.* **B.** *Spermatocele.* **C.** *Hydrocele.*

testis into the scrotum. This usually resorbs during the first year of life. When the processus vaginalis remains open, a communicating hydrocele exists. This is associated with an undescended testis and an inguinal hernia. Such a finding requires referral for further evaluation and treatment. A hydrocele in an adult may be due to infection or trauma.

A *spermatocele* is a cyst of the epididymis resulting from a partial obstruction of the spermatic tubules. It is located just above or behind the testis (Fig. 13.10C). This cyst contains a milky mass with or without spermatozoa and feels like a third testis.

In general, any scrotal mass needs additional evaluation.

EXAMINATION OF THE HERNIA AREAS

A hernia is the protrusion of a part of an organ or tissue through the structures that normally contain it. There are three main types of pelvic area hernias. *Indirect inguinal* hernias are the most common type, occurring more frequently in males than females. They result when the processus vaginalis remains open. This type of hernia is generally present in the majority of patients with undescended testis. The hernia can be limited to the inguinal canal or emerge from the external ring into the scrotum. *Direct inguinal* hernias usually result from congenital weakness combined with an additional factor such as heavy lifting or obesity. They most frequently occur in men over 40 years of age. They rarely enter the scrotum and are easily reduced when the patient reclines. *Femoral hernias* are less common than inguinal hernias and are more frequently found in women than men. They emerge through the femoral ring, femoral canal and the fossa ovalis. Femoral hernias are acquired. They can occur with loss of muscle substance and frequent stooping. The incidence of strangulation is high, therefore, immediate referral for treatment is required.

When the patient is relaxed, the inguinal and femoral areas are inspected for any obvious bulges that may indicate the presence of a hernia. This is followed by palpation for the presence of *inguinal* and *femoral hernias.*

Inguinal Hernias. Inguinal hernias are palpated by having the patient stand with his ipsilateral leg slightly flexed and the examiner seated in front of him. Using the right index finger for

examining the patient's right side (the little finger is used with children) and the left index finger for the left side, the examiner invaginates the loose scrotal skin, starting at a low point on the scrotum (Fig. 13.11). The spermatic cord is followed upward to the external ring. With the finger either at the external ring or within the canal, the patient is asked to turn his face to one side, strain down, and cough. The examiner notes any palpable herniating mass as it touches the finger. Inguinal hernias can be either indirect or direct. An indirect inguinal hernia comes down the inguinal canal and will strike the side of the examiner's finger. In the female, a small indirect hernia may produce a bulge at the midpoint of the inguinal canal at the internal inguinal ring. Palpation of the canal is usually unsatisfactory in females. However, it may enter the labia majora as a labial hernia. In the presence of a direct inguinal hernia, a bulge will strike the top of the examiner's finger when the patient is straining, since it comes directly through the abdominal wall instead of down the inguinal canal.

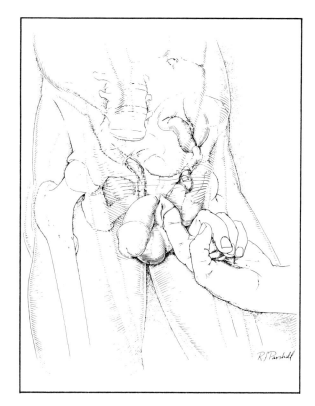

FIGURE 13.11
Examination of a male patient for an indirect inguinal hernia.

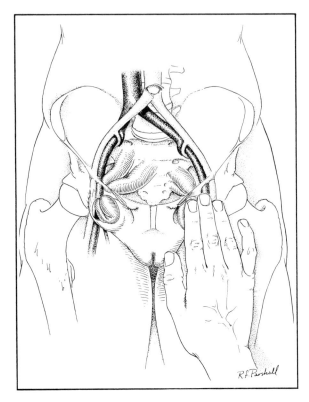

FIGURE 13.12
Examination of a female patient for a femoral hernia.

Femoral Hernias. The location of the femoral canal can be approximated by placing the right index finger on the patient's right femoral artery. The middle finger will then lie over the femoral vein and the ring finger will be over the femoral canal (Fig. 13.12). If a femoral hernia is present, a soft mass will be felt which becomes larger as the patient strains or coughs.

EXAMINATION OF THE RECTUM AND PROSTATE

Positioning of the patient for the rectal examination varies according to age and physical health. To begin the examination of the rectal area, the young child should be in the supine position with his knees and hips flexed toward the abdomen. The adult patient is given instructions to empty his bladder before beginning examination, because a full bladder causes loss of definition at the base of the prostate gland. Then he is asked to turn around and lean on the examination table with his toes pointed toward each other (Fig. 13.13A and B). If the patient is debilitated, a lateral Sims position is used (Fig. 13.14). The rectal area is then inspected followed by palpation

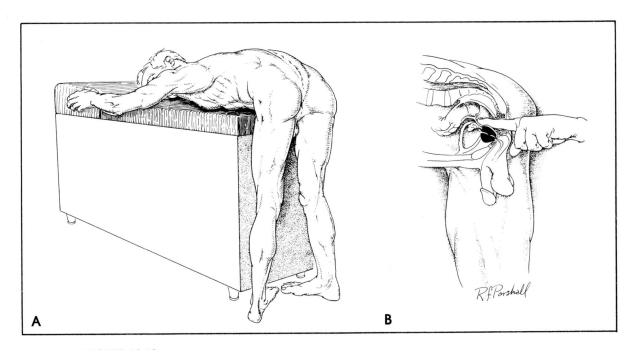

A   B

FIGURE 13.13
*A. Positioning of the male patient for a prostate examination. **B.** Palpation of the prostate gland and seminal vesicles.*

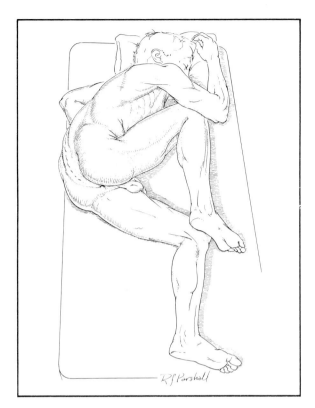

FIGURE 13.14
The lateral Sims' position.

The examiner places the index finger (the fifth finger may be used with children) at the anus and waits a few seconds to relax the sphincter. She then gently inserts her finger noting sphincter tone, muscle tone, and tenderness (Fig. 13.13B). The lateral and posterior walls are systematically palpated for *tumors, polyps,* and *stool.* The *prostate gland* is felt through the anterior wall of the rectum. Palpate each lobe, starting from the median furrow and moving out to the lateral aspects. Every portion of the gland is covered. Note its *symmetry, consistency, size,* and *tenderness.*

A normal prostate is symmetric and has a smooth, firm, rubbery consistency. The three main causes for an abnormal prostate are infection, benign enlargement and cancer. In an infectious process the prostate is boggy, tender and somewhat asymmetrical. *Benign prostatic hypertrophy* is extremely common in men older than 50 years of age. The prostate may bulge more than 1 centimeter into the rectal lumen, and the hypertrophied tissue tends to obliterate the median furrow. It is smooth, symmetrical and non-tender. Any stony, hard nodule or asymmetry should make the examiner strongly suspect cancer. The initial cancerous lesion usually involves the posterior portion of the prostate, which is readily palpable. As the cancer grows in size it can eventually obliterate the median furrow. Cancerous lesions are usually non-tender.

Finally, an attempt is made to palpate the *seminal vesicles* above the prostate (Fig. 13.13B). They are normally not palpable, but if they are involved in an inflammatory reaction, they may be dilated and extremely tender. At the completion of the examination the examiner should inspect the stool left on the glove for the presence of blood. A stool guaiac slide test is done on all men age 50 and over (see Chapter 12, page 332).

of the rectum and prostate in all patients 40 years of age and older. Palpation is not routinely done in children or young males, unless the history indicates a problem.

Inspection. In children, the examiner observes for *fissures, skin tags,* a *pilonidal dimple* (an opening leading to a hair containing sinus or cyst), *bleeding,* and signs of scratching (possibly due to the presence of *pinworms*). Inspect the anus of the adult for fissures, hemorrhoids, signs of scratching and bleeding.

Palpation. The examining hand should be gloved and the index finger well lubricated.

Screening Examination of the Male Genitalia

The screening examination of the male genitalia includes:

1. Inspection of the pubis
2. Inspection of the penis
   a. Shaft
   b. Prepuce

  c. Glans
  d. Urethra
3. Palpation of the penis
4. Inspection of the scrotum
5. Palpation of the scrotum
  a. Testis
  b. Epididymis
  c. Spermatic cord
6. Palpation for inguinal and femoral hernias
7. Inspection of the rectum
8. Palpation of the rectum and the prostate (40 years of age and over)

EXAMPLE OF A RECORDED HISTORY AND PHYSICAL

SUBJECTIVE:

Chief Complaint: "I have had pain when urinating since yesterday."

HPH: This 19-year-old white college male considers himself to be in good health. Last night he had a sudden onset of urgency and painful urination. This morning he noticed a small amount of yellowish discharge from his penis. He has casual sexual relationships with three women. His last sexual contact was 3 days ago. He is not aware of having been exposed to venereal disease. He has never experienced these symptoms in the past. He denies hematuria, backache, lethargy, chills, fever, rashes in the genital area, genital lesions, past history of urinary tract infection, and past history of venereal disease. There is no family history of kidney disease. He is very concerned that he may have the "clap."

OBJECTIVE:

Abdomen: No tenderness over general abdomen or suprapubic or costovertebral junction. No masses palpated.

Penis: Circumcized. No lesions or rash; normal size; no masses; small amount of yellow discharge from the urethra with milking.

Scrotum: No rash, lesions, masses, or swelling; testes descended. No tenderness of epididymis or spermatic cord.

Prostate: Firm, no masses or tenderness.

Lymph nodes: Inguinal and femoral nodes not palpable or tender.

REFERENCES

American Cancer Society (1985). 1985 Cancer facts and figures. New York: American Cancer Society.

Cancer Statistics (1985). Ca-A Cancer Journal for Clinicians, 35(1), 19–35.

Chow, M., Durand, B., Feldman, M., & Mills, M. (1984). Handbook of Pediatric Primary Care (2nd ed.). New York: John Wiley & Sons.

Cunningham, R. (1984). Urinary tract infection in infants and children. Postgraduate Medicine, 75(1), 59–64.

Haggerty, B. (1983). Prevention and differential of scrotal cancer. Nurse Practitioner, 8(10), 45–52.

Gracely-Kilgore, K. (1984). Penile adhesion: The hidden complication of circumcision. Nurse Practitioner, 9(5), 22–24.

Lindberg, S. (1980). Periodic preventive health screening for adult men and women. Nurse Practitioner, 5(5), 9–21.

Markley, V. (1982). Sexuality and aging. In E. Lion, (Ed.), Human Sexuality in Nursing Process. New York: John Wiley & Sons, pp. 143–66.

Marshall, F., & Elder, J. (1982). Cryptorchidism and Related Anomalies. New York: Praeger Publishers.

Rhodes, G., Glober., & Stemmermann, G. (1974). A review of some tumors of interest for demographic study in Hawaii. Hawaii Medical Journal, 33, 283–84.

Shortridge, L. & McLain, B. (1979). Primary care and prostate cancer. Nurse Practitioner, 25–30.

Tanner, J. (1962). Growth at Adolescence (2nd ed.). Oxford, England: Blackwell Scientific Publications.

Tudor, M. (1981). Child Development. New York: McGraw-Hill.

Yurick, A., Robb, S., Spier, B. & Eber, N., (Eds.). (1980). The Aged Person and the Nursing Process. New York: Appleton-Century-Crofts.

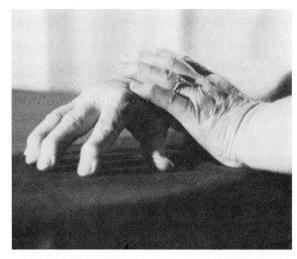

14

The Musculoskeletal System

The musculoskeletal system is highly complex and rarely evaluated independently. Because of the interrelationship of this system to the neurologic system, these systems would ordinarily be assessed together. This is particularly true of the extremities. For the purposes of this chapter, however, the specifics of history taking and examination of the musculoskeletal system will be dealt with separately.

The musculoskeletal system in children is usually thoroughly assessed at each well-child check. Adults, however, rarely need as complete an assessment as is described in this chapter, unless specific complaints are presented. Then the importance of being thorough cannot be overemphasized. An adult screening examination of the musculoskeletal system would consist primarily of joint inspection and determination of active range of motion and strength on resistance. Any difficulties would then be investigated more thoroughly, including assessment of the degrees of range of motion.

The examiner should develop the habit of establishing baseline data for each patient. This will allow for comparison of data, especially important for older patients so that true changes in function can be established quickly.

DEVELOPMENTAL CHANGES OF THE MUSCULOSKELETAL SYSTEM THROUGHOUT THE LIFESPAN

The musculoskeletal system changes in structure and ability to function throughout one's life. Because this system works so interdependently with other systems, it is difficult to isolate developmental changes that relate only to this system. Obviously, the ability of an infant to walk is as dependent on intact neurologic function as it is on a normally developing musculoskeletal system. The interconnectedness of these systems is always present. There are, however, some musculoskeletal changes throughout the lifespan that are unique to this system.

Moments after birth, the musculoskeletal system is evaluated for the first time. It comprises a major portion of the Apgar score.* Muscle tone is one of the first features assessed in a newborn. All extremities should move actively immediately after birth. Babies who have inadequate muscle tone are called "floppy." Poor muscle tone can come from asphyxiation, central nervous system disease, or excessive drugs given to the mother during labor and delivery.

Significant musculoskeletal development takes place during infancy. Most infants walk by 12 to 14 months of age, some earlier. In order to accomplish this milestone, normal development of the bones, joints, and muscles must take place. At all well-child exams until 1 year of age, the hips are assessed for congenital dislocation or instability. (See discussion of "Ortolani click" page 368.) This problem does not commonly occur, but it can. If hip dislocation or instability is suspected, then referral is indicated. The infant's spine is also assessed at birth for alignment. It should be straight from the cervical area to the sacrum. A malaligned spine can severely hamper the infant's ability to walk normally.

The feet are another potential source of developmental problems in the infancy period. Many of the foot deformities can be attributed to positioning in utero from hip flexion and abduction, (see definition of terms, Chart 14.1, page 347) and external rotation. In utero, the ankles are in an equinus position (pointed down) and the heels are in a *varus* position (bent medially). The forefoot is adducted (see definition of terms, Chart 14.1, page 347) (DeAngelis, 1984). The patella point out and the feet point forward. Therefore, when the infant is born, the lower extremities are in a frog-like position (DeAngelis, 1984). During the first year of life this changes dramatically. The psoas muscle lengthens, thus the patella move to a more midline position. The feet also become more normally positioned. There are, however, a certain percentage of infants and children who develop problems of the lower extremities that need correction in the early years.

Most children toe in when they first walk. They also have a wide stance and gait until toddlerhood, when they develop more confidence in walking. A condition called *metatarsus adductus*, (Fig. 14.69, p. 376) which is toeing in of the forefoot, can occur. This is usually the result of in utero positioning. In many instances, the examiner can easily straighten out the foot using passive range of motion. If the foot cannot be straightened out with manipulation, the child should be referred for further evaluation. Another cause of toeing in is *inward tibial torsion* (DcAngelis, 1984). In this condition the tibia is somewhat rotated (DeAngelis, 1984). For most children this condition will resolve itself by 18 months of age. Toeing out can also occur, but is much less common.

Most infants are *bow-legged* (*genu varum*). This term is used if there is a gap between the knees when the medial malleoli are touching at midline. Most of the time this will resolve itself by 18 months of age, too. In fact, many children go from being bow-legged to becoming slightly knock-kneed (*genu valgum*). In this condition, if the knees are touching the medial malleoli cannot be brought together. Boys are more likely to get this than girls (DeAngelis, 1984).

Infants are flat-footed due to the fat pads on the feet and an undeveloped arch of the foot. Arches in the feet normally develop around 3 years of age. Therefore, until 3 years of age, most children have flat feet (DeAngelis, 1984). If after 3 years, these arches do not develop, then the child is considered flat-footed (*pes planus*). Most flat feet are the result of lax joints and thus the body weight is being placed over the medial support of the foot. In a normally arched foot, the body weight is transmitted to the os calcis or calcaneus metatarsal heads (McMillan, et al., 1982).

The school-aged child is evaluated carefully for *scoliosis* (lateral curvature of the spine). Scoliosis occurs more commonly in girls. It can be found easily on routine screen-

---

* *A method to assess a newborn's health status immediately after birth.*

ing exams and should be evaluated at regular intervals. Generally speaking, any scoliotic curve should be x-rayed. If more than a slight degree of curvature is present (i.e., 10 degrees) or the scoliosis is progressing, than referral is in order.

Injuries are common to adolescents. Most commonly occurring are fractures, sprains, strains, dislocations and tears in muscles, ligaments and menisci. These injuries are the result of direct trauma.

Other than trauma, there is one musculoskeletal problem that occurs in this age group. It is called *Osgood-Schlatter disease* and is described as tenderness and swelling at the site of the infrapatellar tendon insertion into the tibial tubercle (Fig. 14.53, p. 371) (Hoppenfeld, 1976). Osgood-Schlatter disease occurs more often in boys than in girls and can be bilateral. There seems to be an increased incidence in athletes and during growth spurts (DeAngelis, 1984). Diagnosis is made by noting the bulge and pinpoint tenderness over the tibial tubercle. X-rays confirm the physical findings.

Athletics and competitive sports become very important in the school-age child and adolescent. If a child is involved in regular sporting activities, not only is it important that he be evaluated for physical problems, but also that equipment (i.e., shoes, boots, skis, etc.) is appropriate. Growth spurts and pubescent changes cause rather rapid alterations in the height, weight, and shape of these young people. One of the quickest ways to promote injury to the bones, muscles and joints is to be using ill-fitting equipment. Therefore, equipment should be checked and refit regularly by appropriate individuals.

As with adolescents, young adults do not usually have musculoskeletal problems that are not related to injury. However, jogging and competitive running have become common in the world of adult exercise. In fact, many adults have built this fairly seriously into their world. The long term effects of running on the musculoskeletal system will not be established for some time. It will be interesting to note if any problems arise for runners in 10 to 20 years that may not be encountered by their non-running, middle-aged counterparts. Within the next decade, data should begin to emerge regarding the long-term effects of running.

Most of the musculoskeletal changes during adulthood are due to the wear, tear, and degeneration of the bones, muscles and joints. Back pain, back injuries and generalized pain in the extremities are common in the middle adult and elderly years. Much of the etiology of these problems is related to *degenerative joint disease, osteoporosis* and *rheumatoid arthritis.* Degenerative joint disease is a non-inflammatory disorder that affects joint cartilage, and to some degree synovial membrane, causing degeneration of the bone. Most often, the weight-bearing joints such as the spine, hips, knees, shoulders, the cervical spine and the distal interphalangeal and proximal interphalangeal joints of the hands are affected (Harvey, et al., 1984). Osteoporosis, which occurs after menopause in women (also occurs in men), is a disorder that results in loss of bone mass, creating the potential for easily encountered fractures. Common fracture sites are the distal radius, vertebrae and upper end of the femur. These fractures can also occur spontaneously as a result of weight bearing (Harvey, et al., 1984). Rheumatoid arthritis is a systemic disease which involves chronic inflammation of the synovial membrane ultimately causing erosion and destruction of the joint cartilage and support structures. Rheumatoid arthritis most commonly occurs in women and involves the joints of the hands (the proximal interphalangeal joints and the metacarpal joints), wrist, feet, shoulders, hips, toes, ankles, and knees (Yurick, et al., 1984). Immobility enhances all these conditions. Most believe that immobilization often makes these diseases worse.

These diseases, as well as other physiologic changes related to aging, make up much of the musculoskeletal alterations among the elderly. The profile of the person at highest risk for osteoporosis is the thin, fair complected, postmenopausal woman. Other factors that play a role in the development of osteoporosis include cigarette smoking, calcium deficiency and immobilization. Adequate calcium intake and regular exercise through the lifespan hold promise as a means of preventing osteoporosis (Beuchamp & Held, 1984). Along with alterations in bone structure are changes in the muscle mass. Often this can be the result of disease and atrophy, as well as a decrease in the number and diameter of the muscle fibers (Yurick, et al.,

1984). Hormonal factors influence this, but even more important is that there does not seem to be any regeneration of muscle tissue in the elderly (Yurick, et al., 1984). Muscle atrophy is usually obvious in the dorsal side of the hands, the upper arms, legs and buttocks. One further change that correlates with these others is a change in gait. Elderly people may have a widened stance and gait, but more commonly, one can observe deliberate small, shuffling steps with feet barely lifted from the floor (Yurick, et al., 1984). Some of this is due to a lack of confidence and a fear of falling. Falling is a fear many elderly have, and justifiably so. The prevalence of cardiovascular disease and cerebrovascular disease, and decreased visual acuity combined with the decreased bone mass of osteoporosis are contributing factors to hip fractures in the elderly. Annually, in the United States, more than 120,000 fractures of the hip occur resulting in 50,000 deaths (Beuchamp & Held, 1984). Often, when an elderly person is recovering from an injury such as a fracture, the family and health care team come to a conclusion that changes must take place in the degree of independence this person has. Needless to say, this has multiple implications. For this reason, and others, the elderly see falling as a terrible threat to their sense of well-being.

ANATOMY

The skeletal system provides structure and support for the body and its 206 bones. This system is also involved in blood cell formation and acts as a protective structure for underlying organs (i.e., the brain and lungs). Individual bones are generally classified in four categories:

1. Irregular (i.e., vertebra)
2. Short (i.e., hand)
3. Long (i.e., leg)
4. Flat (i.e., pelvis)

Groups of bones are classified into two categories:

1. The axial skeleton (bones of the head, vertebral column, and ribs).
2. The appendicular skeleton (shoulder, pelvis, and extremities).

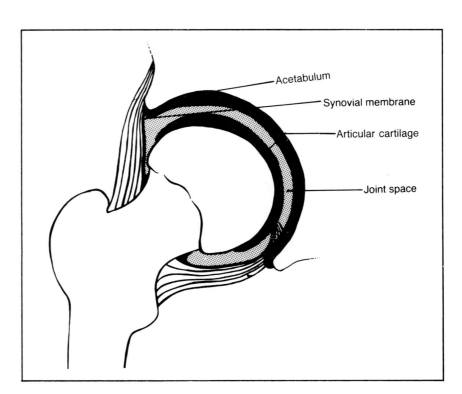

FIGURE 14.1
The anatomic structure of the joint capsule.

CHART 14.1
SYNOVIAL JOINT MOTION

Flexion	Bending of a joint as to approximate its connective parts. Flexion decreases the angle between two bones
Extension	Extension increases the angle between two bones
Abduction	Moving away from the midline of the body
Adduction	Moving toward the midline of the body
Rotation	Movement of a part around its long axis
Circumduction	Movement of a part in a circular motion
Supination	Movement toward the supine position—i.e., hand facing palm side up
Pronation	Movement toward the prone position—i.e., palm facing down
Eversion	Movement turning outward—i.e., toes facing out, heel more in
Inversion	Movement turning inward—i.e., foot pointing in

Voluntary or striated muscles, of which there are over 600, comprise approximately 40 percent of the body's muscle mass and attach themselves to various points on the bony skeleton. Involuntary or smooth muscles are found in parts of the body which act automatically or without effort on the part of the individual (i.e., blood vessels and the stomach). The heart is usually listed separately, for though it consists of striated muscle, it is not under voluntary control.

The articular system consists of various joints throughout the body and is generally broken down into three functional categories:

1. *Synovial joints*
2. *Fibrous joints*
3. *Cartilaginous joints*

The synovial joint consists of a *joint space,* a *joint capsule,* a *synovial membrane,* and an *articular cartilage* which forms over the ends of two adjoining bones (Fig. 14.1).

The *articular cartilage* acts as a nearly friction-free cushion between two joint bones. The loose synovial membrane surrounds the joint space and secretes synovial fluid; both the membrane and the fluid allow for freedom of movement within the joint capsule. The

knee and hip are examples of synovial joints. These joints can move in ten directions (Chart 14.1). During physical examination, these joints should be evaluated for the appropriate kind and degree of movement.

Fibrous joints consist of two bones bound by fibrous material and are found where little, if any, movement is needed—i.e., the suture lines of the skull.

Cartilaginous joints allow for only limited motion. The *hyaline* type of cartilage is found where the first rib joins the sternum. The *fibrocartilaginous* type is found in the vertebral column.

Tendons are tough fibers which are part of the muscle and join muscle to bone. *Ligaments* are fibers which join bone to bone. These are connective tissues which are also assessed in the physical examination.

Various joints of the body will be discussed at length in terms of their anatomy and range of motion. There are many differences in these joints among individuals due to age, general health, and amount of exercise undertaken. Degrees of motion given are averages. Chart 14.2 can act as a guide during the nurse's assessment. Only major bony and muscle structures will be discussed. (For further information see the reference section at the end of this chapter.)

The Temporomandibular Joint

This joint is the point of articulation of the mandible with the skull and is the only movable joint in this portion of the axial skeleton (Fig. 14.2). It is also one of the most used joints in the body and is subject to great stress in the course of a lifetime. The hinge and glide motion is usually symmetrical and can be felt by placing an index finger in the anterior external auditory canal, or directly over the joint, while the patient opens and closes his mouth.

The Shoulder

Many of the structures of the shoulder can be easily identified (Fig. 14.3):

1. The *clavicle* articulates with the *manubrium sternum* at the *sternoclavicular*

CHART 14.2
RANGE OF MOTION[a]

Joint	Motion	Approximate Measurement
Temporomandibular	Open wide (active)	Able to insert three fingers
	Mandible forward	Top teeth behind lower teeth
Neck	Flexion	45°
	Extension	55°
	Rotation	70°
Trunk	Flexion	70–90°
	Extension	30° standing/20° prone
		30–45°
	Rotation	35°
	Lateral bending	
Shoulder	Forward flexion (arm straight)	180°
	Backward extension (arm straight)	50–60°
	Internal rotation (toward shoulder)	55°
	External rotation (arm back)	45°
	Abduction (arm straight)	180°
	Adduction (arm straight)	45–50°
Elbow	Flexion	150°
	Extension	0°
	Hyperextension	0–15°
	Supination[b]	90°
	Pronation[b]	90°
Wrist	Flexion	80–90°
	Extension	70° ±
	Radial deviation	20°
	Ulnar deviation	30–50°
Fingers		
Metacarpophalangeal joints	Flexion	90°
	Extension	0°
	Hyperextension	30°
	Abduction	20° between fingers
	Adduction	Fingers should touch
Proximal interphalangeal joints	Flexion	100–200°
	Extension	0°
Distal interphalangeal joints	Flexion	80–90°
	Extension	0°
Thumb	Flexion	Transpalmar adduction
	Extension	Able to touch tip of thumb to base of little finger and then extend away from the palm 50° between thumb and index finger
Metacarpophalangeal joint	Flexion	50°
	Extension	0°
Interphalangeal joint	Flexion	90°
	Extension	0°
Palmar	Abduction	70°
	Adduction	70°
Opposition	Able to touch each fingertip with tip of thumb	
Hip	Flexion	
	Knee flexed	10–120°
	Knee straight	90° or less
	Extension (prone)	0°
	Abduction	45–50°
	Adduction	20–30°
	Internal rotation	35–40°
	External rotation	45°
Knee	Flexion	120–130°
	Extension (hyper)	10–15°
	Internal rotation	10°
	External rotation	10°

CHART 14.2—Continued.

Joint	Motion	Approximate Measurement
Ankle and foot	Extension (dorsiflexion)	20°
	Flexion (plantar flexion)	45–50°
	Inversion (passive), hind foot	5–20°
	Eversion (passive), hind foot	5–20°
	Abduction, forefoot	10°
	Adduction, forefoot	20°
Toes		
First metatarsophalangeal joint	Flexion (active)	45°
	Extension (active)	70–90°
Interphalangeal joints	Distal	
	Flexion	60°
	Extension	30°
	Proximal	
	Flexion	35°
	Extension	0°
Metatarsophalangeal joints	Flexion	40°
	Extension	40°
Toe spread	Abduction/adduction	Degrees vary

[a] Active unless otherwise stated.
[b] Elbow held at side and flexed.

joint and with the *scapula* at the *acromioclavicular joint* in the shoulder. This is the only bone joining the shoulder girdle to the axial skeleton.

2. The *greater* and *lesser tuberosities* of the *humerus* on the anterior aspect of the shoulder.
3. The *groove* for the biceps tendon.
4. The *deltoid muscle* which overlies the shoulder.
5. The *scapula*.
6. The *glenohumeral joint* between the scapula and the humerus.
7. The *biceps* muscle.
8. The *triceps* muscle.

The subacromial bursa, which lies between the deltoid and supraspinatus muscles, is not normally identifiable.

The Spine

From the posterior view the spinal column is normally straight from the base of the skull (Fig. 14.4). There are 7 *cervical*, 12 *thoracic*, 5 *lumbar*, 5 *sacral*, and 4 *coccygeal vertebrae*. The spinous processes may be seen easily if the patient is not obese, particularly the prominent processes of C_7 and T_1 on a plane with the superior tip of the scapula. L_4 can be identified by drawing a line between the right and left iliac crests.

Major muscle bodies which can be identified in the neck include the *sternocleidomastoid*, which extends from behind the ear to the sternoclavicular junction, and the *trape-*

zius, which extends posteriorly from the base of the skull to the shoulder and to the midthoracic region in a triangle. Motions of both the neck and the rest of the spine include flexion, extension, rotation, and lateral bending.

The Elbow

The bony structures of the elbow are readily identified, as follows (Fig. 14.5):

1. The *olecranon* (the most visible point posteriorly).
2. The *olecranon fossa* (just anterior to the olecranon).

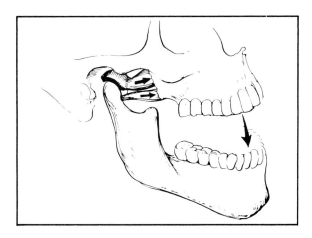

FIGURE 14.2
The external pterygoid muscle's two heads act asynchronously to open the temporomandibular joint. (From Hoppenfeld, S. Physical Examination of the Spine and Extremities. New York: Appleton-Century-Crofts, 1976, p. 129.)

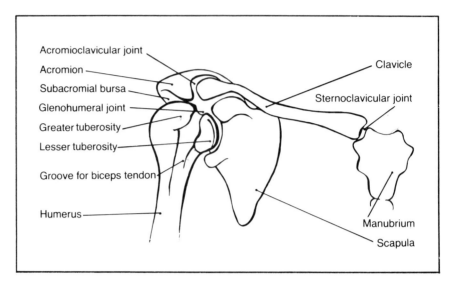

FIGURE 14.3
Bony structures of the shoulder.

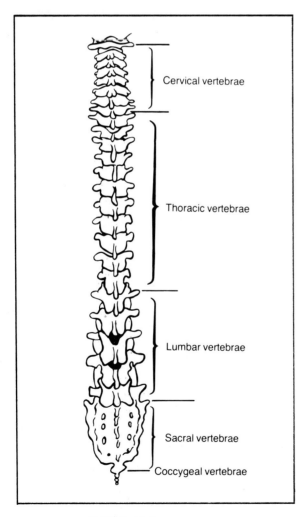

FIGURE 14.4
Posterior view of the spine.

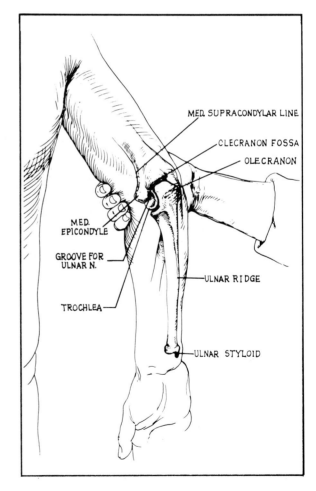

FIGURE 14.5
Anatomy of the elbow (posterior view). (From Hoppenfeld, S. Physical Examination of the Spine and Extremities. New York: Appleton-Century-Crofts, 1976, p. 38.).

3. The *medial* (closest to the body) and *lateral epicondyles* of the humerus.

4. The groove for the ulnar nerve just postero-lateral to the medial epicondyle (frequently referred to by the patient as the "funny bone"); the *medial collateral ligament* overlies this groove and is not normally palpable. The wrist flexors are palpable along the antero-medial portion of the forearm and the extensors are palpable on the anterior aspect. The motions of the elbow include flexion, extension, hyperextension, supination, and pronation.

The Wrist, Hand, and Fingers

The bones of the forearm, the *radius,* and *ulna* meet at the *distal radioulnar* joint. In the hand there are 8 *carpal bones,* 5 *metacarpals,* and 14 *phalanges* (Fig. 14.6). The first joints of the hand distal to the wrist are called the *carpal–metacarpal joints.* With the exception of the thumb, which lacks the middle phalanx, the next joint is called the *metacarpophalangeal joint* followed by the *proximal interphalangeal*

joint, and finally the *distal interphalangeal joint.* The thumb is considered the first finger, the index the second finger, and so on. Each of the bones and joints, with the exception of several of the carpal bones, can be easily identified.

Prominent landmarks include the *ulnar styloid process* and the *radial styloid.* The *anatomic snuff box* just distal and dorsal to the radial styloid can be seen when the thumb is extended. It is bordered by the *extensor pollicis longus* and *abductor pollicis longus.* The size of the *palmaris longus muscle,* the tendon of which lies superficially near the center of the flexor surface of the wrist, is variable among populations. It cannot be detected in 15 to 25 percent of patients of European descent, but is generally observable in Oriental and black patients (Barnicot, 1977). Many muscles and tendons are involved in performing the complex actions of the fingers, hands, and wrist.

The motions of the wrist include flexion, extension, radial deviation, and ulnar deviation. At the metacarpophalangeal joints, motion includes flexion, extension, abduction,

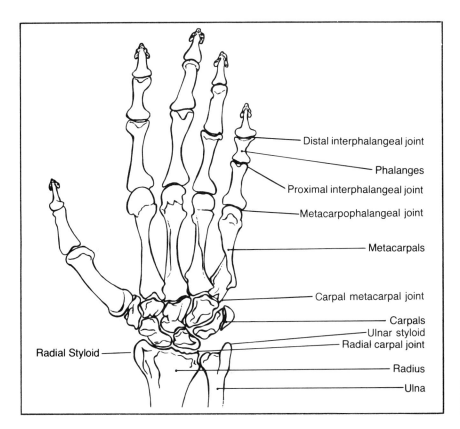

Distal interphalangeal joint

Phalanges

Proximal interphalangeal joint

Metacarpophalangeal joint

Metacarpals

Carpal metacarpal joint

Carpals
Ulnar styloid
Radial carpal joint

Radius

Ulna

Radial Styloid

FIGURE 14.6
The anatomic structure of the wrist, hand, and finger.

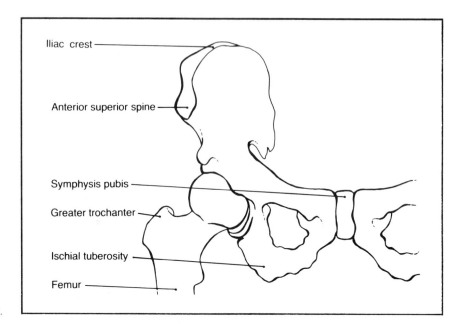

FIGURE 14.7
The hip joint (anterior view).

and adduction. At the proximal and distal interphalangeal joints, motion includes flexion and extension. Motions of the thumb include flexion, extension (radial abduction, palmar abduction/adduction), and opposition.

The Hip

Only a small portion of the hip and pelvis can be directly identified. Palpable landmarks include the *iliac crests*, the *anterior–superior spines*, the *symphysis pubis*, and the *ischial tuberosities* (Fig. 14.7). If the examiner places her fingertips on the lateral aspects of the iliac crest and has her hand resting laterally, her palm will rest on the *greater trochanter* of the *femur*. There are three joints within the pelvic girdle: (1) the *symphysis pubis*, (2) the *sacroiliac*, and (3) the *hip joint*. The first two are nearly immobile, with the hip joint providing nearly all mobility needed.

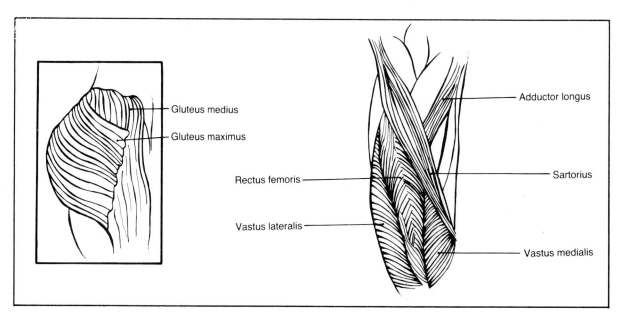

FIGURE 14.8
Muscles of the hip and thigh.

The major muscle groups that assist in movement of the hip are identifiable. They include the *sartorius,* the *adductor longus,* the *gluteus medius,* the *gluteus maximus,* the *iliopsoas,* and the *rectus femoris* (Fig. 14.8). The *sartorius* is a long thin muscle that lies obliquely along the anterior medial portion of the thigh. The *adductor longus* extends from the symphysis pubis toward the middle of the thigh. The *gluteus medius* inserts into the upper lateral portion of the trochanter. The *gluteus maximus* is the primary hip extensor and extends from the ischial tuberosity to the coccyx across to the area of the greater trochanter. The *iliopsoas* is the primary hip flexor and is not accessible to exam. It lies under other muscles and fascia from the iliac spine down to the inferior medial aspect of the femur. The rectus femoris is one of the quadricep muscles that crosses the hip and knee joint. It acts as a flexor for the hip and extensor for the knee (Spuhler, 1950). Motions of the hip include flexion, extension, abduction, adduction, internal rotation, and external rotation.

The Knee

The knee areas in Figure 14.9 are easily identifiable. Ordinarily the *synovium,* the *medial* and *lateral collateral ligaments,* and the

menisci are not palpable. The *anterior* and *posterior cruciate ligaments* are located behind the *patella* near the center of the knee joint. They provide stability to the knee and prevent dislocation of the *tibia* and *femur* anteriorly and posteriorly. The motions of the knee include flexion, occasionally hyperextension, and internal and external rotation.

The Ankle and Foot

The ankle is composed of more than one joint, but the major one is called the *tibiotalar joint.* The major landmarks are the *Achilles tendon,* the *medial malleolus* of the *tibia,* and the *lateral melleolus* of the *fibula* (Fig. 14.10). There are many muscles, ligaments and tendons in the ankle and foot. The major muscles supplying the ankles are the *soleus* and *gastrocnemius,* the so-called calf muscles. The peroneus tertius muscle assists in dorsiflexion of the foot at the ankle and in elevation of the lateral border of the foot. Its tendon can be felt running from the region of the lateral malleolus at the ankle to the base of the fifth metatarsal. This muscle may be reduced or absent in some populations; absence is more frequent in black and American Indian populations than in European or Oriental patients. Interestingly, this muscle may be present asymmetrically (in one

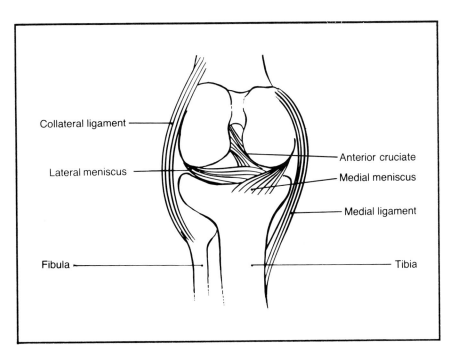

FIGURE 14.9
Anterior view of the knee.

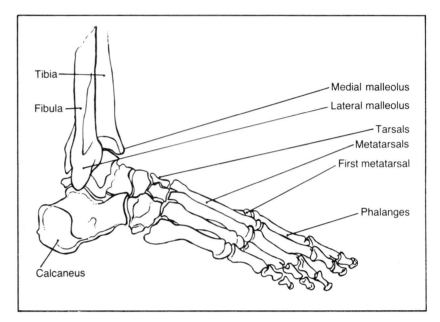

FIGURE 14.10
Lateral view of the ankle and foot.

leg only) (Hoppenfeld, 1976). The motions of the ankle and foot include extension (dorsiflexion), flexion (plantar flexion), inversion, eversion, abduction, and adduction.

The *calcaneus* is the most posterior bone of the foot and is referred to as the heel. The *talus* prominent bony landmark lies just distal to the medial malleolus. There are 5 *tarsal bones*, 5 *metatarsals*, 14 *phalanges* and 2 *sesamoid* bones. The great toe lacks a middle phalange and so the foot corresponds approximately in composition to the hand. The motions of the toes include flexion, extension, abduction, and adduction.

HISTORY

A careful history of the musculoskeletal system is absolutely vital. Frequently, what may appear superficially to be a musculoskeletal disorder can be, in fact, the result of changes in the cardiovascular, respiratory, neurologic, or other systems.

A general review of the system for the child and adult includes a history or presence of joint pain, joint swelling, or limitation of motion; pain or swelling in the extremities or muscles; hip or feet deformities or problems; back pain; postural irregularities, change in stature; injuries or fractures; and a known deficiency of vitamin D and calcium. If the history reveals any of the above, inquiry should be made regarding dates the problem existed, diagnostic studies done, and treatments implemented.

All patients should be asked what type of exercise they engage in and how often they do exercise. The purpose is to screen for age-appropriate exercise (or lack of), the appropriateness of the exercise for maintaining bone mass, and the extent to which patients guard themselves against injury.

Historic data should also be obtained on factors in the patient's environment that may put him at risk for musculoskeletal injury. For example, the mother of the infant and toddler should be asked if safety gates are installed at stairwells in the home. The elderly patient should be asked if stair railings and night lights are in place and whether or not there are loose rugs on the floor.

A birth history relevant to the musculoskeletal system is obtained on all children from birth to 5 years of age. This information includes the occurrence of a breech presentation, congenital abnormalities and birth injuries, and at what age walking took place and whether there were problems in achieving this developmental task.

Family history is obtained about the presence of back problems, painful joints, curved spine and congenital or other abnormalities of the hip or feet. The patient should be asked if anyone in his family was diagnosed with rheumatoid arthritis, osteoarthritis, or osteoporosis.

PHYSICAL ASSESSMENT

The examination should proceed in an orderly fashion, with a general inspection first and then a separate examination for each part, from the temporomandibular joint down. Inspection should always come first; palpation and measurement should come later. A flexible protractor or a measuring tool called a *goniometer* is helpful in accurately assessing range of motion in degrees. A comfortably warm room is a must because the patient must be undressed to do an adequate examination. The standing, sitting, supine, and prone positions are used throughout the examination.

General Inspection

The assessment actually begins when the patient first walks into the examining room, because he is then least apt to be aware that the examiner has already begun an early assessment. In addition, the examiner should have the patient walk away from her in a straight line and then return to assess his gait. Assessing gait is very important in infancy, early childhood, and in the elderly. As soon as a child is able to walk, his gait should be assessed. This should be included in all well-child examinations. The child is asked to walk across a room (adequate distance is necessary). If the child is too young to understand instructions or slightly afraid, ask the parent to stand on the other side of the room or down a hall. The child is likely to go to the parent when called. While the child is walking, the examiner assesses his gait. The examiner also looks at the shape of the child's legs and the position of the child's feet when he places them on the floor. Remember that almost all children are bow-legged until about 18 months

and many will become slightly knock-kneed following that. Additionally, children toe in when they begin walking. These are considered normal findings.

In the elderly patient, the quality of the gait may have direct bearing on his independence. If a patient's gait becomes hazardous, that may reflect his ability to manage independently. Posture can be observed. If the patient stands tall with shoulders back and head up, that can also reveal significant information about mood and self image. Elderly people tend to be more round shouldered and may have trouble standing straight. This is a normal degenerative change of aging. Further assessment of posture can be done when the back is inspected and palpated.

Gait assessment is broken into the *stance* phase and *swing* phase. The stance phase has three parts: (1) the *heel strike*, (2) *midstance*, and (3) *push-off*. The swing phase also has three parts: (1) *acceleration*, (2) *swing-through*, and (3) *deceleration*. There should be minimal shifting of the pelvis and trunk during the gait, and the normal distance between the heels while walking is 2 to 4 inches. A wider gait is indicative of pathology. The examiner should watch for foot dragging, shuffling, or limping and record abnormalities in relation to the phase of the gait. While the patient is walking the examiner should also note the position of the trunk in relation to the gait. Active range of motion of the trunk should be within the following range (Figs. 14.11–14.14; Chart 14.2):

- Flexion: 70–90°
- Extension: 30° standing; 20° prone
- Rotation: 30–45°
- Lateral bending: 35°

A person with *acute low back pain* due to strain or disc problems will favor the side of greatest pain, the trunk will be tilted forward slightly or over the painful side, the lumbar curve will be absent or nearly absent, the gait will be hesitant and more widely spaced, and occasionally a marked pelvic tilt will be present. If an *unstable hip* or weak musculature is present, the pelvis will fall on the side of the uninvolved hip rather than staying level as it usually does during normal gait or weight-bearing. As a general rule, gait is an

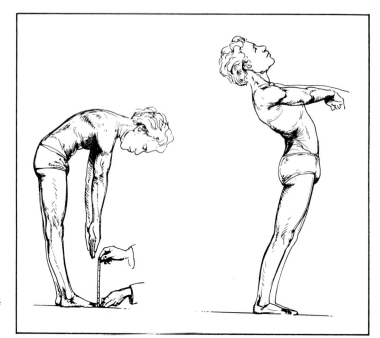

FIGURE 14.11
Left: *Range of flexion in the lumbar spine.*
Right: *Range of extension in the lumbar spine.*
(From Hoppenfeld, S. Physical Examination of the Spine and Extremities. New York: Appleton-Century-Crofts, 1976, p. 248.)

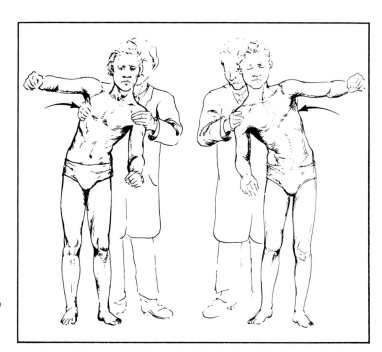

FIGURE 14.12
The range of lateral bending in the lumbar spine should be equal on both sides. (From Hoppenfeld, S. Physical Examination of the Spine and Extremities. New York: Appleton-Century-Crofts, 1976, p. 248.)

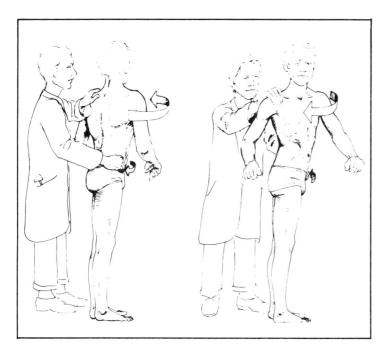

FIGURE 14.13
Range of rotation in the lumbar spine. (From Hoppenfeld, S. Physical Examination of the Spine and Extremities. New York: Appleton-Century-Crofts, 1976, p. 249.)

excellent indicator of problems within the musculoskeletal and neurologic systems. The examiner should look at the patient's posture from the anterior and posterior views. She should check the spinal curves looking for any displacement—i.e., *scoliosis* (Figs. 14.15 and 14.16), which is a lateral curve seen on the posterior view, usually of the thoracic spine. *Kyphosis,* an increased convexity of the thoracic spine (Fig. 14.15) on the lateral view is seen frequently in older persons. *Lordosis* is an increased concavity of the lumbar spine (Fig. 14.15). *Lumbar lordosis* is normally present in small children who have protuberant abdomens. This normal curvature is more pronounced in black children. In the elderly patient, loss of lordosis may indicate the collapse of one or more vertebrae. The examiner should also look for any gross deformities or asymmetry. She should observe how the patient gets onto the examining table and record any difficulties or need for assistance.

The Spinal Column

While the patient is still standing, the examiner should have him bend over as far as he can. The spinal column should then have a smooth convex curve. A *functional scoliotic curve* due to poor posture will disappear. True scoliosis will be accentuated when the patient bends over. This quick and easy test is frequently skipped in children. The importance of checking for scoliosis in children cannot be too highly stressed. This is a critical exam for the school nurse and other nurses that work with children. Early referral of even borderline scoliosis may prevent a worsened curvature, extensive surgery, and emotional trauma for the child. The spinal column will spread up to 4 inches in length and depending on the patient's age and general condition, the examiner should be able to record forward flexion of between 70 and 90 degrees. Next,

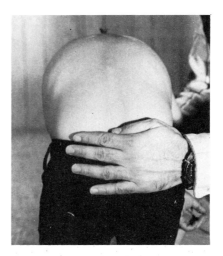

FIGURE 14.14
Testing forward flexion of the trunk and checking for curvature of the spine.

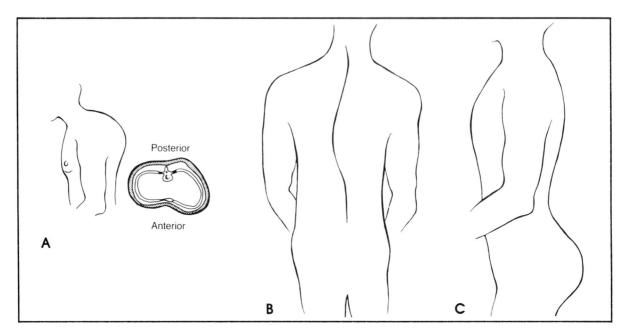

FIGURE 14.15
Abnormal curvatures of the spine. **A.** *Kyphosis.* **B.** *Scoliosis.*
C. *Lordosis.*

the examiner should palpate the spinal processes and paravertebral muscles to assess for points of tenderness or swelling and record the level where pain occurs.

The Temporomandibular Joint

The examiner should observe the patient's face and note any asymmetry, swelling, or evidence of trauma. She should have the patient open his mouth and note the smoothness of motion and any hesitancy of that movement. There should not be any shift of the mandible to the right or left and the examiner should be able to insert three fingers vertically into the patient's fully opened mouth.

To check the ease of joint function, the examiner should place the tips of the little fingers in both ear canals and press gently on the anterior portion of the canals. She should have the patient open his mouth, noting any marked click (possibly a *damaged meniscus*) or a grating sensation (*arthritis*). Poor dentition or poor occlusion may also cause trauma to the temporomandibular (TM) joint, in which case external palpation will elicit tenderness. If there is *spasm of the external ptery-goid muscles,* pressure on the maxillary buccal mucosa posterior to the molars will cause ten-

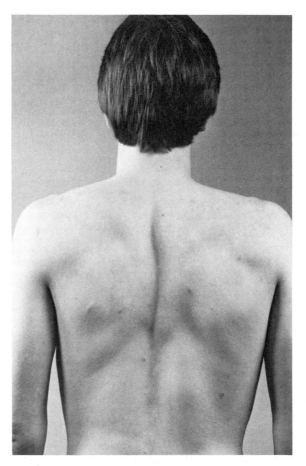

FIGURE 14.16
Scoliotic curvature of the spine.

derness. If there is *spasm of the external ptery-goid muscles,* pressure on the maxillary buccal mucosa posterior to the molars will cause tenderness. Occasionally opening the mouth wide into hyperextension, as in a big yawn, will cause the mandibular condyles to slip out of the glenoid fossa, creating an inability to close the mouth. The *dislocation* may be unilateral or bilateral. The displacement might occur as a result of a blow, traumatic injury to the chin, or with chronic disease of the temporomandibular joint. In either case immediate referral to a physician for reduction of the dislocation is imperative.

The Cervical Spine

The examiner should observe the neck in the anterior, lateral, and posterior positions. She should check the cervical curvature for any abnormalities. Loss of curvature may result from severe muscle spasm after a *whiplash* accident. The examiner should compare the size and symmetry of the neck muscles, particularly the sternocleidomastoid and trapezius, and note any deviations or masses. She should palpate along the spinous processes and also along the supraclavicular fossa for any points of tenderness, swelling, or nodules. Active range of motion (ROM) should be within the following range from the 0 degree position (Figs. 14.17–14.19, Chart 14.2):

- Flexion: 45°
- Extension: 55°
- Rotation: 70° or chin in line with the shoulder
- Lateral bending: 40–45°

The nurse should attempt to find a passive range of motion if the patient has difficulty with ROM on his own. She should test the strength of the neck muscles by providing resistance during active range of motion and compare sides. It is important to note that passive range of motion in an acute injury of the cervical spine is contraindicated and dangerous. If there is a complaint of neck, shoulder, or arm pain, the *Adson test* should be performed to determine whether pressure is being exerted on the subclavian artery by the scalenus anticus muscle or a cervical rib (Fig.

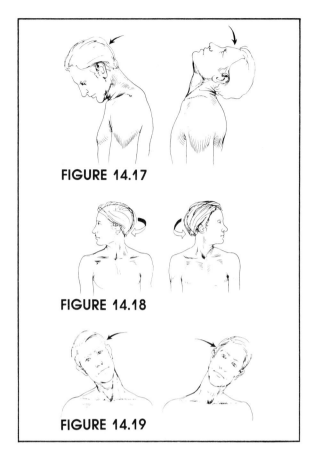

FIGURE 14.17

FIGURE 14.18

FIGURE 14.19

FIGURES 14.17–14.19
(*14.17*) *Left. Normal range of neck flexion. **Right.** Normal range of neck extension.* (*14.18*) *Normal range of neck rotation.* (*14.19*) *Normal range of lateral bending.* (*From Hoppenfeld, S. Physical Examination of the Spine and Extremities. New York: Appleton-Century-Crofts, 1976, p. 115.*)

14.20). To perform this test the examiner should palpate the left radial artery and then have the patient extend his chin upward slightly, rotate his head to the left, and take a deep breath. If the pulse diminishes or disappears, the test is positive. This should be repeated on the opposite side for comparison.

The Shoulder

The examiner should inspect and compare both shoulders in terms of bony and muscular symmetry. She should note the presence of atrophy of the muscles, deformity, or masses involving elevation or depression of the shoulder. She should identify the bony landmarks as indicated in the anatomy section and note

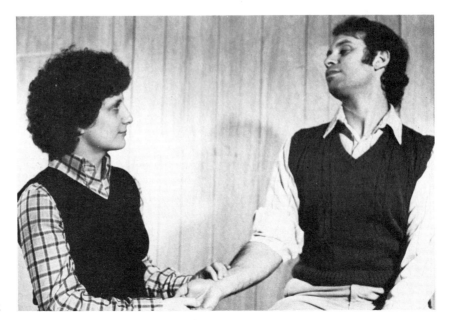

FIGURE 14.20
The Adson test.

any point tenderness or crepitation and its location. She should palpate the muscular structure and note any tenderness or spasm. The patient should be asked to attempt active range of motion, as follows (Figs. 14.21–14.28, Chart 14.2):

- Forward flexion: 180°
- Backward extension: 50–60°
- Abduction: 180°
- Adduction: 45–50°

The examiner should note crepitation or any motions which elicit pain and record at what angle the pain or loss of function occurred. If difficulty is encountered, the examiner should do passive ROM to see if shoulder mobility can be increased. She should also note the angle at which the scapula begins to move or elevate as the extended arm is abducted from the body. She should test muscle strength bilaterally by providing resistance against the arm in each motion. She should also have the patient shrug his shoulders against resistance. The stability of the scapula should be tested by having the patient face a wall and push his hands against it. If there is weakness in the serratus anterior muscle, the scapula will become mobile and prominent, giving a "winged" effect.

TEARS IN THE ROTATOR CUFF

The four muscles that guard and stabilize the shoulder joint can be assessed by passively abducting the extended arm to a 90-degree angle. The patient should be asked to slowly lower his arm. If a tear is present, he will be unable to do so; the arm will fall abruptly. Any suspicion of a tear should be referred for further follow-up as soon as possible.

A common sports injury, aside from dislocation, is *subluxation* of the acromioclavicular joint. The patient will support his arm with the opposite hand and be reluctant to flex or abduct the shoulder. The nurse should have him place the hand of the affected side on the opposite shoulder and lean forward. Pressure on the distal end of the clavicle will cause pain and the clavicle will be mobile. Subluxation may also be encountered in the stroke patient when the paralyzed shoulder and arm are inadequately supported.

If *fracture* of the upper arm, particularly of the neck of the humerus, is suspected, the examiner should be sure to determine if pulses are present in the lower arm. In addition, the neurologic status, particularly of the radial nerve, should be assessed to see if it is intact. Radial nerve damage can be diagnosed if there is wrist drop of the involved arm or numbness on the dorsum of the hand.

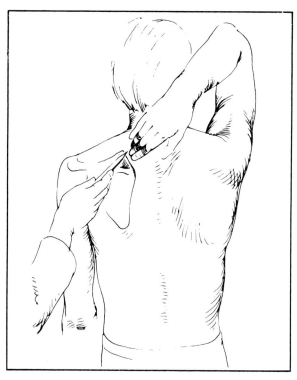

FIGURE 14.21
Example of the Apley scratch test: external rotation and abduction. (From Hoppenfeld, S. Physical Examination of the Spine and Extremities. New York: Appleton-Century-Crofts, 1976, p 21.)

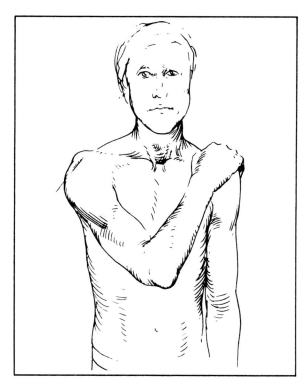

FIGURE 14.22
Test for internal rotation and adduction. (From Hoppenfeld, S. Physical Examination of the Spine and Extremities. New York: Appleton-Century-Crofts, 1976, p. 21.)

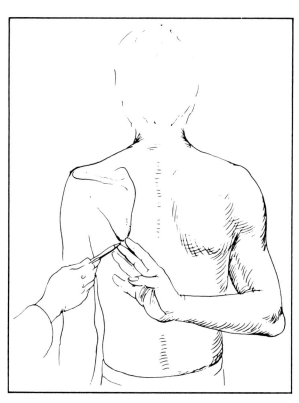

FIGURE 14.23
Internal rotation and adduction. (From Hoppenfeld, S. Physical Examination of the Spine and Extremities. New York: Appleton-Century-Crofts, 1976, p. 21.)

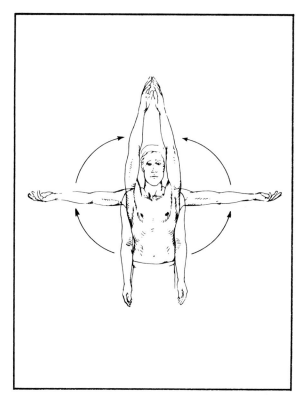

FIGURE 14.24
Range of motion. (From Hoppenfeld, S. Physical Examination of the Spine and Extremities. New York: Appleton-Century-Crofts, 1976, p. 22.)

362

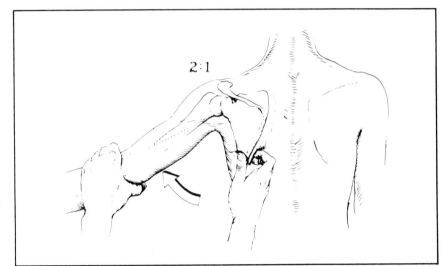

FIGURE 14.25
Test for abduction: motion occurs at the glenohumeral and scapulothoracic articulation in a 2:1 ratio. (From Hoppenfeld, S. Physical Examination of the Spine and Extremities. New York: Appleton-Century-Crofts, 1976, p. 23.)

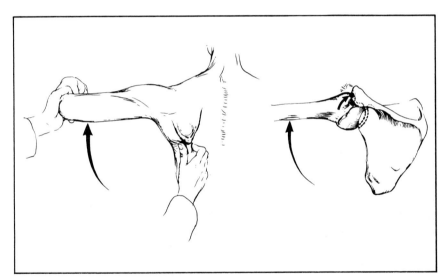

FIGURE 14.26
Abduction continues to approximately 120°, where the surgical neck of the humerus strikes the acromion. (From Hoppenfeld, S. Physical Examination of the Spine and Extremities. New York: Appleton-Century-Crofts, 1976, p. 24.)

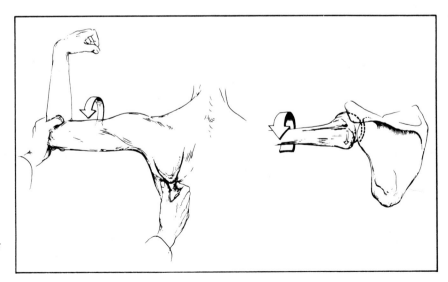

FIGURE 14.27
Full abduction is possible only when the humerus is externally rotated. (From Hoppenfeld, S. Physical Examination of the Spine and Extremities. New York: Appleton-Century-Crofts, 1976, p. 24.)

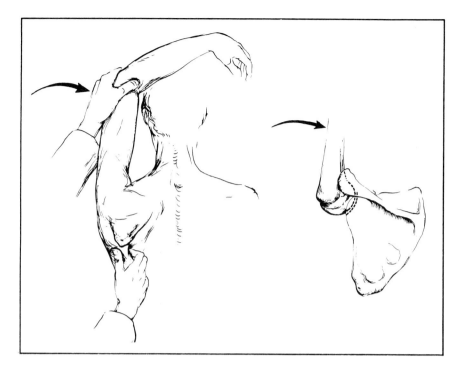

FIGURE 14.28
External rotation increases the articulating surface of the humeral head and turns the surgical neck away from the tip of the acromiom. (From Hoppenfeld, S. Physical Examination of the Spine and Extremities. New York: Appleton-Century-Crofts, 1976, p. 24.)

The Elbow

The examiner should inspect the elbow while it is in 90 degrees of flexion, noting any redness, swelling, nodules, or deformities. A soft swelling over the olecranon process may be indicative of *olecranon bursitis.* The examiner should note the muscle structure in the forearm and upper arm and compare it with that of the opposite arm. She should palpate the elbow in a position of flexion and extension, determine the bony landmarks, and note any point tenderness, bogginess, or crepitation around the joint itself. The muscle bodies should be palpated to determine if tenderness or spasm is present. The examiner should then have the patient put his elbow through active range of motion (Figs. 14.29 and 14.30; Chart 14.2). During supination and pronation, the arm must be tested with the arm adducted against the lateral chest wall; otherwise the shoulder motion may falsely increase the forearm motion:

- Flexion: 150°
- Extension: 0°
- Hyperextension: 0–15°
- Supination: 90°
- Pronation: 90°

Lateral epicondylitis of the humerus (tennis elbow) is a condition caused by excessive strain of the extensor muscles of the wrist. On exam, one will find tenderness along the lateral epicondyle and along the *extensor aponeurosis* muscle. Referred pain may go to the shoulder. It is possible to replicate the pain of tennis elbow. The patient extends his forearm while the examiner stabilizes it. The patient makes a fist and then extends his wrist. With the other hand, the examiner applies pressure to the dorsum of the fist trying to flex the wrist. If the patient has tennis elbow, there will be pain at the lateral epicondyle (Hoppenfeld, 1976).

The Wrist

The examiner should inspect the wrist for shape, deformity, swelling, lumps, or redness. She should palpate the prominent bony landmarks, the muscles, and the tendons, comparing the two wrists and determining whether any point tenderness exists. This part of the body is susceptible to dysfunction in *rheumatoid arthritis* and the *migratory arthritis* of rheumatic fever in children.

The examiner should have the patient

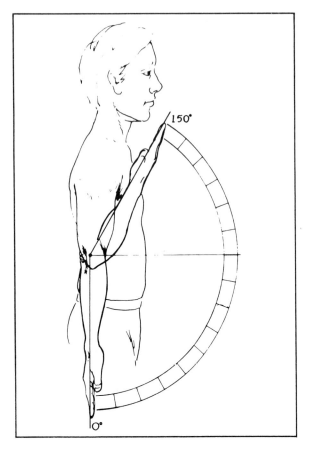

FIGURE 14.29
The elbow range of motion in flexion and extension. (From Hoppenfeld, S. Physical Examination of the Spine and Extremities. New York: Appleton-Century-Crofts, 1976, p. 50.)

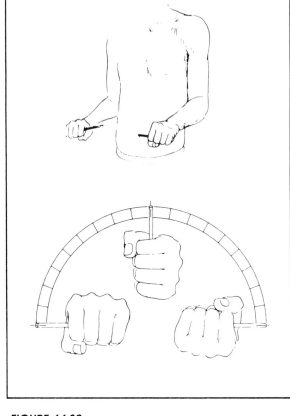

FIGURE 14.30
The elbow range of motion in supination and pronation. (From Hoppenfeld, S. Physical Examination of the Spine and Extremities. New York: Appleton-Century-Crofts, 1976, p. 51.)

move the wrist through active range of motion (Figs. 14.31 and 14.32; Chart 14.2):

- Flexion: 80–90°
- Extension: 70°
- Radial deviation: 20°
- Ulnar deviation: 30–50°

If the patient has complained of difficulty flexing and extending his thumb and if tenderness is present in the tendons bordering the anatomic snuffbox, he may have *de Quervain's disease,* or *chronic stenosing tenosynovitis.* To test for this, the patient is asked to clench his fingers over his thumb and then put his wrist sharply into ulnar deviation. This is called the *Finkelstein test* and is positive if the patient experiences sudden pain from the snuffbox into his thumb. *Ganglions* are not uncommon

on the posterior or dorsal surface of the wrist. These are soft, round, discrete cysts that arise from the joint capsule or tendon sheaths and are therefore fixed at their origins. They rarely cause pain or inhibit function in the wrist. If the patient has complained of pain, numbness or weakness in his thumb, index or middle fingers, there may be *compression of the median nerve* by the *volar carpal* ligament. Tapping the wrist on a ligament over the median nerve will cause pain in the fingers supplied by this nerve. This is called a positive *Tinel's sign.* A positive Tinel's sign is an indication of *carpal tunnel syndrome.* Carpal tunnel syndrome is the entrapment of the median nerve as it passes through the carpal tunnel. It causes numbness of the fingers that are innervated by the median nerve (the median nerve innervates the radial portion of the palm and the palmar surfaces of the thumb, index and middle fingers; may also supply the dorsum of the terminal phalanges of these fingers). The syndrome can also cause pain and weakness of the hand.

The most common deformity in the wrist due to fracture is the silver fork deformity of a *Colles' fracture.* This is a fracture within 2 to 3 centimeters of the distal end of the radius with dorsal displacement including a fracture of the ulnar styloid process. When the wrist and hand are placed on a flat surface, the displacement looks like a fork turned with the tines pointing down on the surface. This is usually caused by a fall on an outstretched hand.

The Hand and Fingers

The examiner should inspect and compare the hands in terms of bony and muscular structure, looking for signs of swelling, redness, nodules, deformities, extra fingers (*polydactyly*), very short fingers (*brachydactyly*), or webbing between the fingers (*syndactyly*). The thenar eminence (the muscle body proximal to the thumb) should be compared with the hypothenar eminence (the heel of the hand or palm). The examiner may be able to delight the patient by telling him which hand he uses for the majority of activities simply by noting that the muscles are more prominent in the thenar and hypothenar areas in the dominant hand. In addition, the hand creases are deeper and more noticeable in that hand. In darkskinned individuals, the palmar surfaces of the hands and plantar surfaces of the feet may normally show darkly pigmented creases. The presence of *palmar muscle atrophy* should also be noted. If pronounced, the palm (or volar surface) will have a hollowed out appearance.

The examiner should palpate the body landmarks of the hand, paying particular attention to the joints. She should note the presence of tenderness, bogginess, or nodules. *Heberden's nodes,* which occur in osteoarthritis, may be present at the distal interphalangeal joints (Fig. 14.33).

The patient should be asked to perform active range of motion of the thumb and fingers. Independent movement of the distal phalanges is usually not possible without the examiner stabilizing the proximal interphalangeal joints in zero position—i.e., with

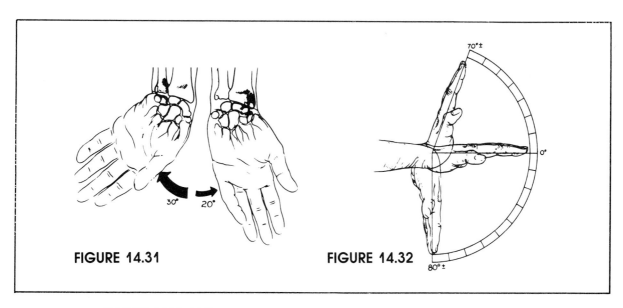

FIGURE 14.31

FIGURE 14.32

FIGURES 14.31–14.32
(**14.31**) *Ulnar and radial deviation of the wrist.* (**14.32**) *Wrist flexion and extension range of motion. (From Hoppenfeld, S. Physical Examination of the Spine and Extremities. New York: Appleton-Century-Crofts, 1976, p. 89.)*

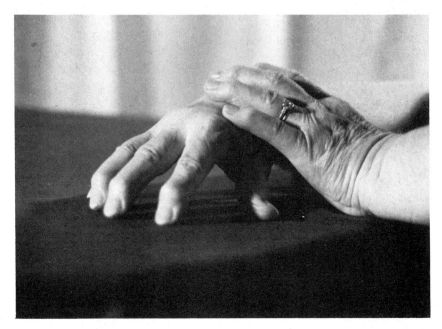

FIGURE 14.33
Example of Heberden's nodes.

the fingers extended in straight line position from the palm.

Further ranges of motion are listed as follows (Figs. 14.34–14.41, Chart 14.2):

1. Fingers*
   a. Metecarpophalangeal joints
      1) Flexion: 90°
      2) Hyperextension: 30°
      3) Extension: 0°
      4) Abduction: 20° between fingers
      5) Adduction: Fingers should touch
   b. Proximal interphalangeal joints
      1) Flexion: 100–120°
      2) Extension: 0°
   c. Distal interphalangeal joints
      1) Flexion: 80–90°
      2) Extension: 0°
2. Thumb*
   a. Flexion and extension: transpalmar adduction; able to touch tip of thumb to base of little finger and then extend

away from palm 50° between thumb and index finger
   b. Metacarpophalangeal joint
      1) Flexion: 50°
      2) Extension: 0°
   c. Interphalangeal joint
      1) Flexion: 90°
      2) Extension: 0°
   d. Palmar
      1) Abduction: 70°
      2) Adduction: 70°
   e. Opposition: Able to touch each fingertip with tip of thumb
   f. Radial deviation: 20°

The examiner should observe any difficulty performing active or passive range of motion and note where the problem occurs. A *contracture* of one of the fingers due to adherence of the tendon to the tendon sheath may prevent full extension of the fingers away from the palm. This is called *Dupuytren's contracture.* This flexion deformity is caused by the myofibrillar elements of the palmar fascia.

Because *rheumatoid arthritis* most commonly affects the proximal interphalangeal and metacarpophalangeal joints, the examiner may note tenderness and swelling of those joints. With advanced disease, a *swan's neck*

---

* *Metacarpophalangeal and interphalangeal motion is extremely variable from individual to individual, but should be symmetrical from left to right within the individual patient.*

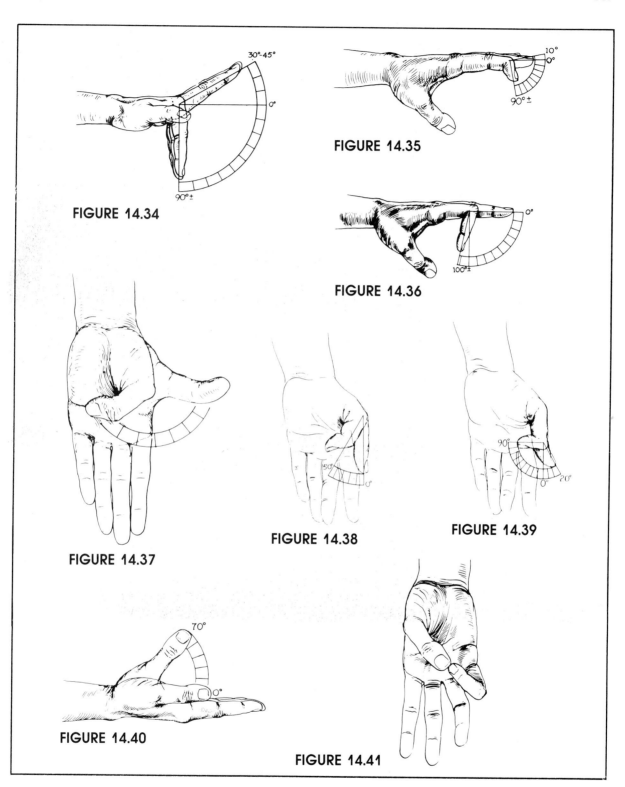

FIGURE 14.34

FIGURE 14.35

FIGURE 14.36

FIGURE 14.37

FIGURE 14.38

FIGURE 14.39

FIGURE 14.40

FIGURE 14.41

FIGURES 14.34–14.41
(14.34) *Metacarpophalangeal joint range of motion: flexion–extension.* **(14.35)** *Proximal interphalangeal joint range of motion: flexion–extension.* **(14.36)** *Distal interphalangeal joint range of motion: flexion–extension.* **(14.37)** *Thumb flexion and extension.* **(14.38)** *Thumb flexion and extension: metacarpophalangeal joint.* **(14.39)** *Thumb flexion and extension: interphalangeal joint.* **(14.40)** *Palmar abduction/adduction of the thumb.* **(14.41)** *Opposition of the thumb and fingertips. (From Hoppenfeld, S. Physical Examination of the Spine and Extremities. New York: Appleton-Century-Crofts, 1976, p. 89–91.)*

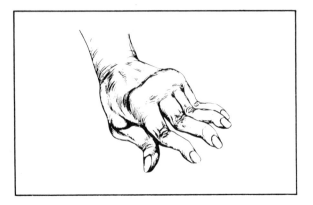

FIGURE 14.42
Swan's neck deformity. (From Hoppenfeld, S. Physical Examination of the Spine and Extremities. New York: Appleton-Century-Crofts, 1976, p. 87.)

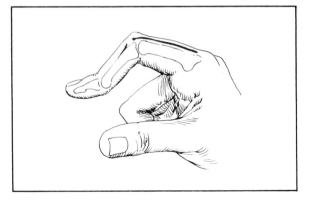

FIGURE 14.43
A boutonniere deformity. (From Hoppenfeld, S. Physical Examination of the Spine and Extremities. New York: Appleton-Century-Crofts, 1976, p. 87.)

or *boutonniere* deformity may be present (Figs. 14.42 and 14.43).

The Hip and Pelvis

The pelvis should be inspected with the patient in the sitting position. The level of the iliac crests should be level or parallel to the floor. The examiner should look for signs of trauma—i.e., bruising, abrasion, or swelling. She should palpate the crests, the anterior spines, and, when the patient is lying down, the symphysis, and the ischial tuberosities. If pressure exerted on any of these areas elicits a pain response from the patient and there is a history of body or pelvic trauma, *pelvic fracture* must be considered. The examiner should palpate along the spine for tenderness, swelling, or nodules.

With the patient in the supine position, the fingertips are placed over the iliac crest and the palm over the lateral hip. The greater trochanter of the femur will lie just under the palm. The area is palpated for tenderness and deformity. The muscles of the hip, thigh, and buttocks are palpated for tenderness. The examiner should have the patient perform active range of motion. He may need passive assistance to complete ROM (Figs. 14.44–14.49; Chart 14.2):

- Flexion: knee flexed, 110–120°; knee straight, 90°
- Extension (prone): 0°
- Abduction: 45–50°

- Adduction: 20–30°
- Internal rotation: 35–40°
- External rotation: 45°

The examiner should test for strength of the muscles by providing resistance during active range of motion. A *flexion contracture* of the hip may be demonstrated by having the patient, while in supine position, flex his leg against his chest. Ordinarily, the opposite leg barely rises during this motion. If contracture is present, the straight leg will begin to flex and this is measured in degrees. This is considered a positive *Thomas test* for hip flexion contracture. Pain precipitated in the lumbar spine by straight leg raising is called a positive *Lasègue's sign*. The degree at which pain occurs is then recorded. The sacroiliac joint is tested by the *Patrick's test* in which the heel of the tested leg is placed on the opposite knee and the hip is abducted. Back pain implies sacroiliac joint pathology.

In infants an *Ortolani click* may be heard in congenital dislocation of the hip(s) (Figs. 14.50 and 14.51). The knees of the infant are flexed to 90° and the hips are abducted and externally rotated so that the legs are flat on the table. If dislocation is present, a click will be heard and felt as the head of the femur slips back into the acetabulum. A positive *Allis' sign* in congenital hip dislocation is present if one leg appears shorter than the other when the knees are flexed in the supine position and viewed anteriorly.

At this point the examiner should measure the leg lengths. This is done in two ways:

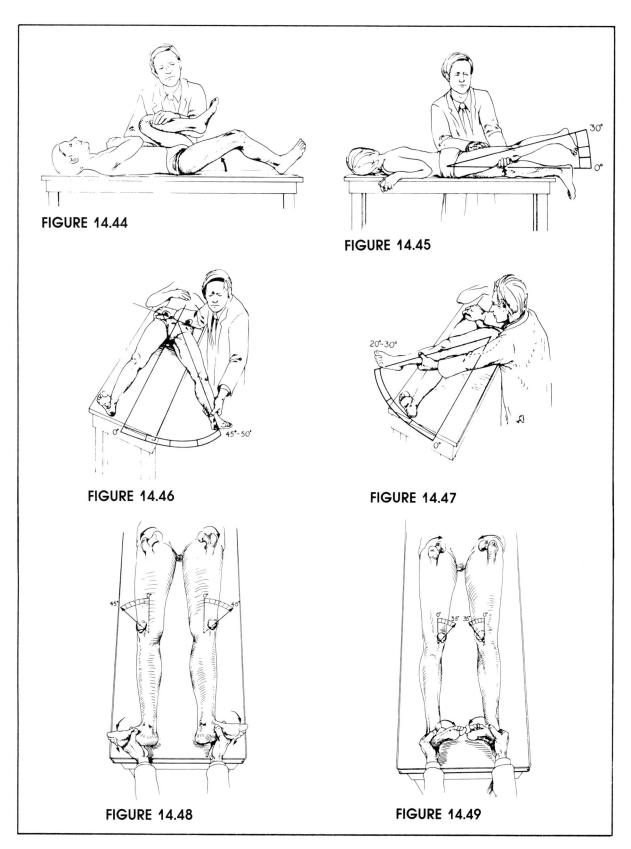

FIGURE 14.44

FIGURE 14.45

FIGURE 14.46

FIGURE 14.47

FIGURE 14.48

FIGURE 14.49

FIGURES 14.44–14.49
(14.44) *The normal limit for hip flexion is approximately 135°.* **(14.45)** *Test for hip extension.* **(14.46)** *The normal limits for hip abduction are 45° to 50°.* **(14.47)** *The normal limits for hip adduction are 20° to 30°.* **(14.48)** *The normal limit for internal rotation is 35°.* **(14.49)** *The normal limit for external rotation is 45°. (From Hoppenfeld, S. Physical Examination of the Spine and Extremities. New York: Appleton-Century-Crofts, 1976, pp. 156–8.)*

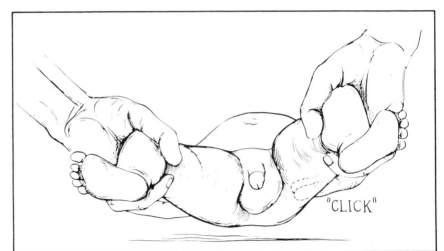

FIGURE 14.50

A diagnosis of a congenital dislocation of the hip. This may be confirmed by the Ortolani "click" test. The involved hip is not able to be abducted as far as the opposite one, and there is a "click" as the hip reduces. (From Hoppenfeld, S. Physical Examination of the Spine and Extremities. New York: Appleton-Century-Crofts, 1976, p. 168.)

1. **Apparent leg length:** The examiner picks a nonfixed point, such as the umbilicus, and measures from that point to the medial malleolus. This is repeated on the opposite side.
2. **True leg length:** The examiner measures from the anterior–superior spine of the pelvis to the medial malleolus. This is repeated on the opposite side.

These maneuvers determine if one leg is actually shorter than the other or if the pelvis is tilted.

Since the low back and hip are sites for referred pain from disease in the pelvis, the examiner may want to perform a pelvic exam on a female or a prostate exam on a male.

The Knee

The knees should be inspected while the patient is in the sitting position. Any deformities, redness, swelling, or nodules should be noted. All children should be screened for *tibial torsion*. Tibial torsion is an abnormal rotation of the tibia along its axis. Tibial torsion exists if an imaginary line is drawn from the center of the patella and does not intersect the toes of the foot. The examiner should have the child stand and note the position of the legs. Bow-leggedness, or *genu varum* (Fig. 14.52) may be present if the medial malleoli are touching and the knees are more than 1 inch apart. Conversely, *genu valgum* (Fig. 14.52) may be present if the knees are touching and

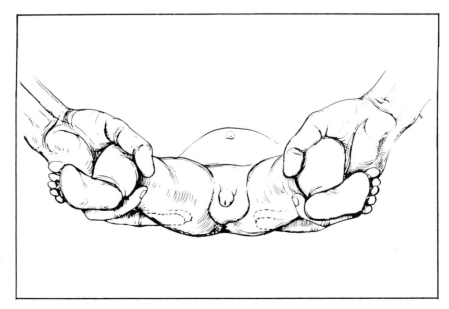

FIGURE 14.51

In the newborn, both hips can be equally flexed, abducted, and externally rotated without producing a "click." (From Hoppenfeld, S. Physical Examination of the Spine and Extremities. New York: Appleton-Century-Crofts, 1976, p. 168.)

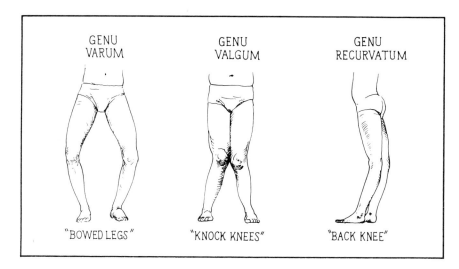

FIGURE 14.52
Common types of knee deform-
ity. (From Hoppenfeld, S. Physi-
cal Examination of the Spine
and Extremities. New York: Ap-
pleton-Century-Crofts, 1976, p.
172.)

the medial malleoli are more than 2 to 3 centimeters apart. Another way to describe the difference between the valgus and varus is to think in terms of the angle along the medial aspect of the joint. If that angle is less than 180 degrees, the deformity is *varus*. If the angle is greater than 180 degrees, it is *valgus*. Hyperextension of the knees that cannot be straightened voluntarily is considered abnormal. This hyperextension is known as *genu recurvatum* (Fig. 14.52).

The examiner should palpate the bony and muscular structures and note any points of tenderness in the joint, muscles, or tendons and compare sides. The patella should move freely without discomfort. In adolescents, *Osgood–Schlatter* disease may be present if tenderness and swelling are found at the insertion of the infrapatellar tendon onto the tibial tubercle (Fig. 14.53). *Chondromalacia* may be present if pain is produced as the patella is moved while pressing it against the femur.

Next, the examiner should have the patient move the knee through active range of motion and assist as necessary (Fig. 14.54; Chart 14.2).

Tibial tuberosity is
tender and
enlarged

FIGURE 14.53
Osgood–Schlatter syndrome.

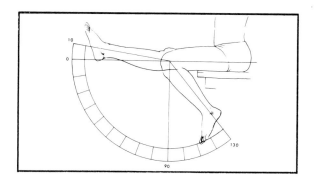

FIGURE 14.54
The range of knee motion in flexion and extension. (From
Hoppenfeld, S. Physical Examination of the Spine and Ex-
tremities. New York: Appleton-Century-Crofts, 1976, p.
187.)

372

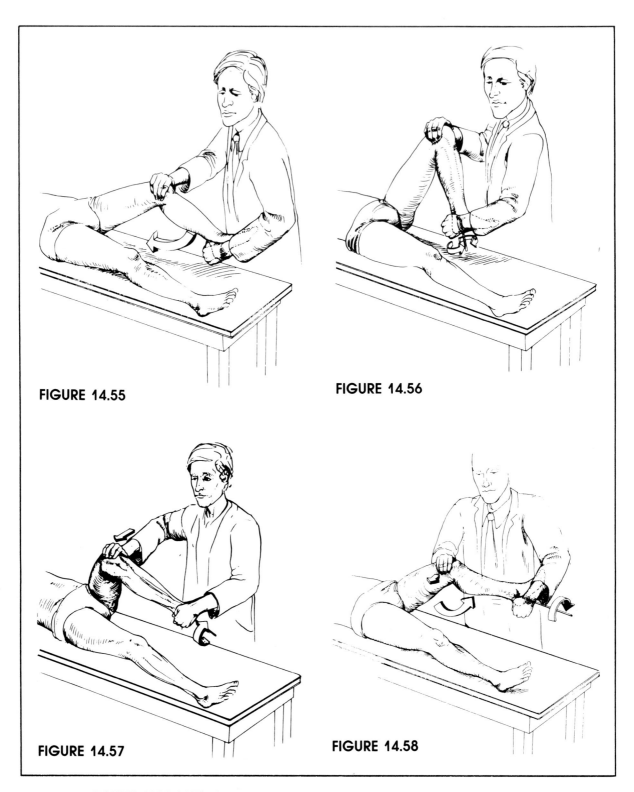

FIGURE 14.55

FIGURE 14.56

FIGURE 14.57

FIGURE 14.58

FIGURES 14.55–14.58
(14.55) *McMurray's text for meniscal tears. The knee is flexed.* **(14.56)** *While the knee is being flexed, the examiner internally and externally rotates the tibia on the femur.* **(14.57)** *With the leg externally rotated, the examiner places a valgus stress on the knee.* **(14.58)** *With the leg externally rotated and in valgus, the examiner slowly extends the knee. If a click is palpable or audible, the test is considered positive for a torn medial meniscus, usually in the posterior position.* (From Hoppenfeld, S. Physical Examination of the Spine and Extremities. *New York: Appleton-Century-Crofts, 1976, p. 192.*)

- Flexion: 120–130°
- Extension (hyper): 10–15°
- Internal rotation: 10°
- External rotation: 10°

The nurse should test the strength of the muscles by providing resistance during active range of motion and perform a neurologic check of the lower extremities (see Chapter 15).

There are a number of tests the examiner can perform to check for stability and obstruction in the knee. The following are among the major tests.

McMURRAY'S TEST (FOR MENISCAL TEARS)
With the patient in a sitting position with the knee flexed, the examiner places her fingers over the joint line and *passively* extends the knee while the foot is rotated inward and out-

ward. A palpable click in either the medial or lateral joint line suggests a torn meniscus (Figs. 14.55–14.58).

TEST FOR INTEGRITY OF THE COLLATERAL LIGAMENTS
The patient can be sitting or in the supine position for this test. If he is sitting, the knee is slightly flexed (approximately 15–30°). To test the *lateral collateral ligament,* the examiner places her hand on the medial aspect of the leg, just below the knee joint and stabilizes the lower leg with her other hand on the lateral side above the ankle. The hand on the medial side applies pressure laterally in an attempt to open the knee joint on the lateral side. The lateral aspect of the knee will open if the lateral collateral ligament is not intact. The examiner should remember that some play in the knee joint is normal and one knee must be compared to the other. To test the *medial collateral ligament,* hand positions are

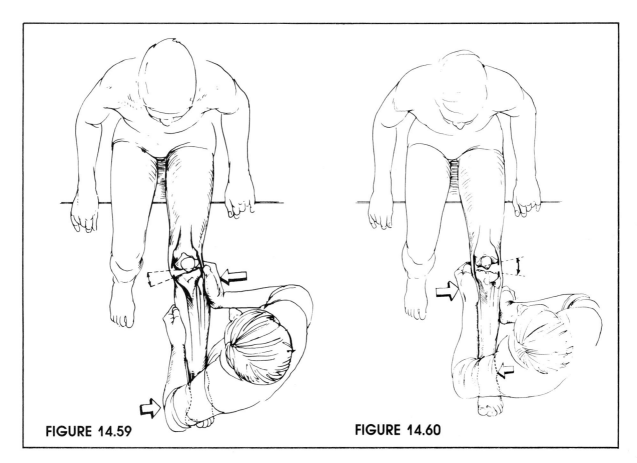

FIGURE 14.59   **FIGURE 14.60**

FIGURES 14.59–14.60
(14.59) To test the medial collateral ligament, the examiner applies valgus stress to open the knee joint on the medial side. **(14.60)** To test the lateral knee for stability, the examiner applies varus stress to open the knee joint on the lateral side. (From Hoppenfeld, S. Physical Examination of the Spine and Extremities. New York: Appleton-Century-Crofts, 1976, p. 185.)

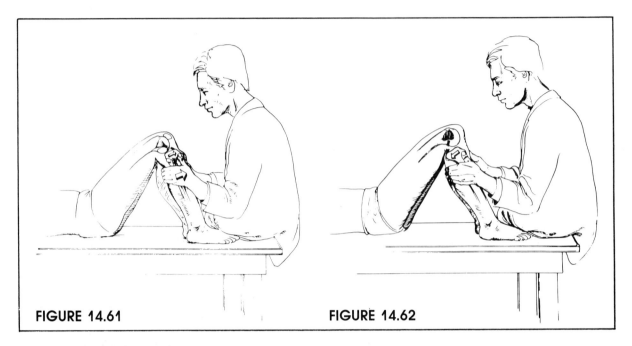

FIGURE 14.61

FIGURE 14.62

FIGURES 14.61–14.62
(14.61) A positive anterior draw sign: torn anterior cruciate ligament. **(14.62)** A positive posterior draw sign: torn posterior cruciate ligament. (From Hoppenfeld, S. Physical Examination of the Spine and Extremities. New York: Appleton-Century-Crofts, 1976, p. 186.)

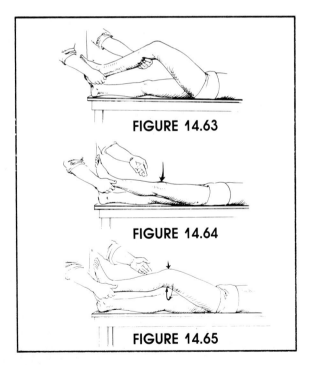

FIGURE 14.63

FIGURE 14.64

FIGURE 14.65

FIGURES 14.63–14.65
(14.63) The "bounce-home" test. The examiner flexes the knee. **(14.64)** The knee is allowed to passively extend. It should fully "bounce home" into extension. **(14.65)** Fluid in the knee joint prevents the knee from "bouncing home"; instead it may rebound. (From Hoppenfeld, S. Physical Examination of the Spine and Extremities. New York: Appleton-Century-Crofts, 1976, p. 194.)

reversed and medial pressure is applied with the proximal hand (Figs. 14.59 and 14.60).

TEST FOR INTEGRITY OF THE ANTERIOR AND POSTERIOR CRUCIATE LIGAMENTS (DRAW SIGN)

The examiner has the patient assume the supine position with his knees flexed to 90 degrees. She then sits on the patient's foot, fixing it to the table and applies pressure to the tibia with her hands, pushing toward the patient. If a tear or weakness of the posterior cruciate ligament is present, the tibia will slide posteriorly. The examiner then pulls the tibia toward her. If there is a tear or weakness of the anterior cruciate ligament, the tibia will slide forward (Figs. 14.61 and 14.62).

TEST FOR TORN CARTILAGE OR A FOREIGN BODY IN THE KNEE JOINT

With the patient in a supine position, the examiner flexes the patient's knee and raises the leg off the table. She then holds the ankle in her hand and passively lowers the leg. The leg should extend fully. If it does not, some type of tear or foreign body exists in the joint (Figs. 14.63–14.65). The acutely injured patient will resist this motion due to pain.

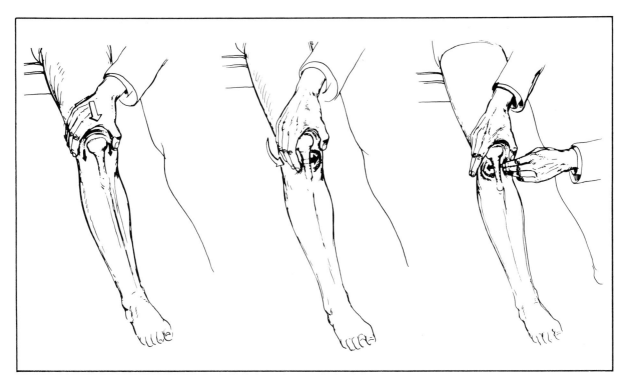

FIGURE 14.66
Test for minor effusion. (From Hoppenfeld, S. Physical Examination of the Spine and Extremities. *New York: Appleton-Century-Crofts, 1976, p. 196.)*

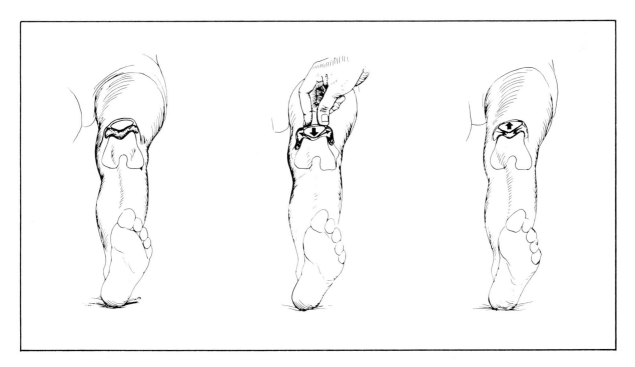

FIGURE 14.67
Test for major effusion: a ballottable patella. (From Hoppenfeld, S. Physical Examination of the Spine and Extremities. *New York: Appleton-Century-Crofts, 1976, p. 195.)*

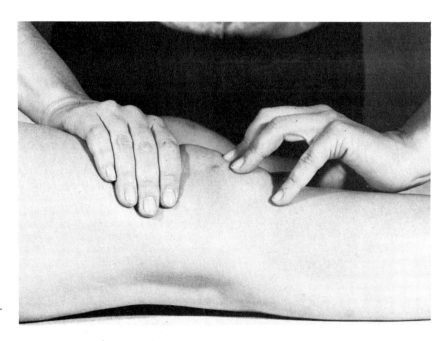

FIGURE 14.68
Testing for ballottement of the pa-
tella.

TEST FOR MINOR SWELLING BENEATH THE PATELLA

The examiner applies pressure or milks the
patella downward and then applies pressure
to the medial or lateral side. A bulge will appear on the side opposite the pressure if fluid
is present (Fig. 14.66).

TEST FOR MAJOR SWELLING BENEATH THE PATELLA

The examiner presses the patella sharply
against the femur. If fluid is present, the patella will rebound or bounce back quickly. Another name for this test is *ballottement of the*
patella (Figs. 14.67 and 14.68).

The Ankle, Foot, and Toes

The ankle is inspected for swelling, redness,
nodules, and deformity. Swelling, redness,

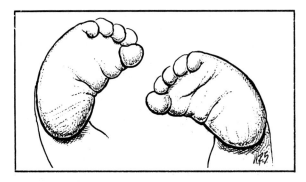

FIGURE 14.69
Metatarsus adductus.

and marked tenderness to the lightest of palpation in either of the first metatarsal phalangeal
joints may be indicative of *gout.* The examiner
should note the presence or absence of the
longitudinal arch of the foot, as well as any
deformities of the toes (such as a *hammer toe*
or flexion contracture) and any calluses or
warts. She should look for the presence of *hal-
lux valgus*, which occurs when the great toe
is laterally deviated toward the second toe and
occasionally overlaps it. Continuous trauma
due in part to ill-fitting shoes may result in
a bursa over the first metatarsophalangeal
joint, resulting in the so called painful *bunion.*
The nurse should note the position of the ankle: the position is valgus if the medial malleolus angulates inward and varus if the lateral
malleolus angulates outward. Inspecting the
shoes for points of wear is often helpful in
determining ankle and foot stress points.

In children it is important to note whether
the entire foot toes out (*pes valgus*) or toes
in (*pes varus*). *Metatarsus adductus* (Fig.
14.69) describes the condition in which only
the forefoot turns in. If attempts to passively
correct these conditions fail, then referral for
correction is necessary.

The sole of the foot should be inspected
for any abnormalities—i.e., excessive callus
formation, flattened arches, or warts. The
nurse should palpate the bony and muscular
structures of the foot for any points of tenderness and record any findings. The patient

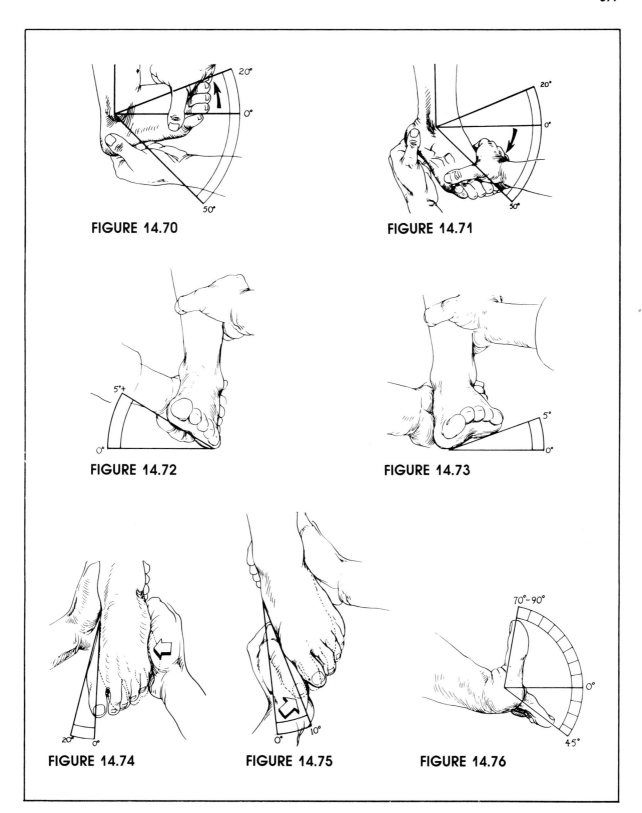

FIGURE 14.70

FIGURE 14.71

FIGURE 14.72

FIGURE 14.73

FIGURE 14.74

FIGURE 14.75

FIGURE 14.76

FIGURES 14.70–14.76

(14.70) *Range of ankle dorsiflexion.* **(14.71)** *Range of ankle plantar flexion.* **(14.72)** *Foot inversion test.* **(14.73)** *Foot eversion test.* **(14.74)** *Forefoot adduction test.* **(14.75)** *Forefoot abduction test.* **(14.76)** *The normal flexion/extension range of the first metatarsophalangeal joint.* (From Hoppenfeld, S. Physical Examination of the Spine and Extremities. *New York: Appleton-Century-Crofts, 1976, p. 223, 225, 226.*)

should be asked to perform active range of motion of the ankle, foot, and toes. Several of the maneuvers will have to be done passively, as listed below (Figs. 14.70–14.76; Chart 14.2).

1. Ankle and foot
   a. Extension (dorsiflexion): 20°
   b. Flexion (plantar flexion): 45°–50°
   c. Inversion (passive), hind foot: 5°–20°
   d. Eversion (passive), hind foot: 5°–20°
   e. Abduction, forefoot: 10°
   f. Adduction, forefoot: 20°
2. Toes
   a. First metatarsophalangeal joint
      1) Flexion (active): 45°
      2) Extension (active): 70°–90°
   b. Interphalangeal joints
      1) Distal
         a) Flexion: 60°
         b) Extension: 30°
      2) Proximal
         a) Flexion: 35°
         b) Extension: 0°
   c. Metatarsophalangeal joints
      1) Flexion: 40°
      2) Extension: 40°
   d. Toe spread (abduction/adduction): degrees vary

CHART 14.3
MUSCLE GRADING CHART

Muscle Gradations	Description
5—Normal	Complete ROM against gravity, with full resistance
4—Good	Complete ROM against gravity, with some resistance
3—Fair	Complete ROM against gravity
2—Poor	Complete ROM, with gravity eliminated
1—Trace	Evidence of slight contractility; no joint motion
0—None	No evidence of contractility

Strength of muscle groups is tested by providing resistance during active range of motion (Chart 14.3). A test for strength of the gastrocnemius and soleus muscles in the posterior lower leg can be conducted by having the patient hop on the ball of his foot. If the muscles are weak the foot will land flat on the floor. He will not be able to hold himself on the ball of his foot. This test should be done in accordance with the age and general condition of the patient.

Screening Examination of the Musculoskeletal System

1. Assessment of stance and gait.
2. Assessment for strength and symmetry of the temporomandibular joint.
3. Assessment for range of motion of the cervical spine (neck).
4. Assessment for strength, range of motion, and symmetry of the upper extremities including:
   a) The shoulders
   b) The elbows
   c) The wrists
   d) The fingers
5. Assessment for strength, range of motion, and symmetry of the lower extremities including:
   a) The hips
   b) The knees
   c) The ankles
   d) The feet
6. Assessment for strength, range of motion and symmetry of the spine.

EXAMPLE OF A RECORDED HISTORY AND PHYSICAL

SUBJECTIVE:

Chief Complaint: ". . . pain in my hip for 10 hours."

HPH: This 54-year-old truck driver was admitted to Memorial Hospital for "control of my diabetes." He considered himself to be in "pretty good" health prior to admission. Because of extreme lethargy he was placed on bedrest for the first 24 hours after admission. On the second day he began to complain of "rheumatism in my right hip. I knew this was going to happen if I stayed in bed too long. I do O.K. if I keep moving—even when I drive my truck, I have to stop every 2 hours or so and walk around. My doctor told me I had rheumatism—I guess he called it arthritis—about 5 years ago." He describes the pain as "a steady deep aching in my right hip" that started about 10 hours ago. He stated it "feels real stiff, too; I can hardly move my leg." He denies low back pain or radiation to his (R) leg; aching increases with initial activity and eases if he continues the activity—i.e., walking. He usually takes 2 or 3 plain aspirin tablets "when I feel the aching begin" and gets "good" relief. There is no regular pattern of medication use. No known allergies. Denies fever, redness, or swelling in (R) hip. Denies history of trauma to either hip, pelvis, or lower extremities. Both parents had "rheumatism real bad when they got older."

States "I usually just keep right on truckin' as they say; can't let it get me down. I just try not to do a whole lot of stair climbing or lifting heavy boxes any more."

OBJECTIVE:

T.98.4°F orally; P. 88 (radial); R. 18; B.P. 160/88 (sitting)

General: Patient presents as an alert, cooperative, 54-year-old man sitting on the edge of his bed. He grimaces occasionally when he tries to change his position. Needs assistance to ambulate three steps. Avoids putting full weight on (R) leg.

Face: Temporomandibular joint → crepitations felt bilaterally; able to open mouth 3 cm.

Neck: Full active ROM without complaints of pain or stiffness. No muscle atrophy, deformities, or masses noted.

Shoulders: Symmetrical; full active ROM without complaints of pain or stiffness. No muscle atrophy, deformities, masses, redness, or swelling noted.

Elbows: As for shoulders above.

Wrists: As for shoulders above.

Fingers: Deformities noted in distal interphalangeal joints of the second and third fingers, bilateral—flexion limited to 45° in these joints and 0° extension. All other joints have full active and passive ROM. No redness, swelling, or muscle atrophy seen.

Some 2 to 3 mm. nodules noted below nailbed; one on second finger, one on third finger of right hand.

Spine: In sitting position appears straight in posterior view. Accentuated curve at cervical/thoracic junction in lateral view. No redness, swelling, tenderness or deformities seen.

Pelvis: In sitting position → iliac crests appear level. No tenderness to palpation or pressure.

Hips: Tender to pressure over (R) hip joint. No redness or swelling seen; no visible deformity. In lying position: full active/passive ROM in (L) hip.

- With knee straight < 45° before ↑ pain.
- With knee flexed < 60° before ↑ pain.
- Extension: Unable to extend right leg in prone position; 10° on left.
- Abduction: 25–30°
- Adduction: < 10°
- Internal rotation: < 20°
- External rotation: < 20°

Knees/Ankles/Toes: Full active/passive ROM without complaints of pain or stiffness. No redness, swelling, tenderness, muscle atrophy, or masses found.

REFERENCES

Barnicot, N. (1977). Biological variation in modern populations. In G. Hanson, et al. (Eds.), Human Biology: Introduction to Human Variation Growth and Ecology (2nd ed.). New York: Oxford Press, pp. 181–300.

Beuchamp, P., & Held, B. (1984). Estrogen replacement therapy. Universal remedy for the post menopausal woman? Post Graduate Medicine, 75 (7), 42–53.

DeAngelis, C. (1984). Pediatric Primary Care (3rd ed.). Boston: Little, Brown.

Harvey, A., Johns, R., McKusick, V., et al. (Eds.) (1984). The Principles and Practice of Medicine (21st ed.). Norwalk, Conn: Appleton-Century-Crofts.

Hoppenfeld, S. (1976). Physical Examination of the Spine and Extremities. New York: Appleton-Century-Crofts.

McMillan, J., Neiburg, P., Stout, C., & Oski, F. (1984). The Best of the Whole Pediatrician Catalogue Volumes I–III. Philadelphia: Saunders.

Spuhler, J. (1950). Genetics of three morphological variations. Patterns of superficial veins of the anterior thorax, peroneus tertius muscle and number of vallate papillae. Cold Spring Harbor Symposium on Quantitative Biology, 15, 175–89.

Yurick, A., Spier, B., Robb, S., Ebert, N. (1984). The Aged Person and the Nursing Process (2nd ed.). Norwalk, Conn.: Appleton-Century-Crofts.

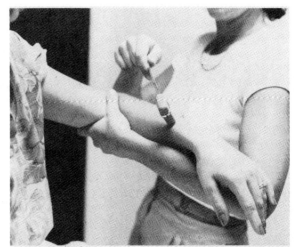

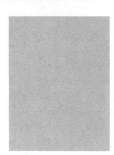

15

The Neurologic System

The nervous system is the "integrator" of all the other systems in the body. Without its "intactness," many homeostatic controls will not function. The nervous system, which begins to develop in early embryonic life, starts its role as integrator even then.

By the time a baby is born, this system has already been very active. Because of the nervous system's major role in growth and development, it is vital that accurate assessments be made from birth. Throughout life the nervous system needs to be evaluated routinely. A detailed neurological assessment can take up to 45 minutes, however, this is neither feasible nor necessary for a routine screening of a well-child or adult. There are simple tests that check the functioning of the patient's *mental status, cranial nerves, motor system, sensory system* and *reflexes.* If the results of any screening tests are questionable, a more detailed evaluation can be made. When choosing an appropriate level of depth for this exam, there are other considerations. The condition of the patient makes a great deal of difference—not only in his level of consciousness, but also in his ability to ambulate. Many portions of the exam require the patient's ability to move and coordinate his extremities. Another factor in determining how much detail is required in the exam is the chief complaint of the patient. If his chief complaint relates to the neurologic system, as with "headaches," a most thorough assessment is essential. However, if the reason for the visit is routine health maintenance, a screening level will be more appropriate. The last, but none the less important, consideration is the cooperation and participation of the patient.

DEVELOPMENTAL CHANGES OF THE NERVOUS SYSTEM THROUGHOUT THE LIFESPAN

During the neonatal and infancy periods, frequent and precise neurological assessment is warranted. In these months, so much neurological development goes on, that detailed examinations must be done. Almost immediately after a baby is born, after breathing has been established, and a quick inspection of body parts reveals that all is intact, the neurological assessment is begun. The presence of certain reflexes, the character of a baby's cry and the tone of his body are some of the indicators used to assess whether or not the neonate is neurologically intact. Other responses like the blinking of the eyes when a bright light is shone in his eyes, or a startle when a loud noise is made, reinforce that the crucial senses of vision and hearing are present.

There are certain reflexes present during the neonatal and infancy periods that are important for evaluating neurological development. The major reflexes are: *rooting, sucking, Moro's, palmar grasp, dancing, tonic neck,* and *Babinski's.* The intensity of these responses, however, may vary considerably among population groups. The reflexes are described in detail in the "Physical Assessment" section of this chapter.

As the reflexes diminish in the course of normal development, there are new milestones that are watched for that indicate normal neurological function. Neurological development is evaluated in 5 categories: *mental status* (which includes *speech, language* and *intellectual* functioning), the *cranial nerves,* the *motor system,* the *sensory system,* and the *reflexes.* At different intervals in a person's life, one area of assessment may be a more valuable indicator than another. For instance, some cranial nerve function, like taste or sensation in the face, might be important to assess in an elderly patient to determine if there is neurological degeneration or a malignant lesion. It is not usually necessary to assess these areas in a toddler. In a toddler, however, motor and intellectual skills need careful evaluation, but in a young, healthy, adult, these categories might not reveal much valuable data about the patient.

For the infant and toddler, neurological assessments are done at well-baby exams by taking a thorough history, doing a complete physical (including an appropriate neurologic exam), and administering a Denver Developmental Screening Test. With these three tools, most developmental abnormalities can be picked up.

The Denver Developmental Screening Test (DDST) is a test constructed to assess four areas: *gross motor,* which involves the musculoskeletal as well as the nervous system; *communication skills,* including speech, hearing and comprehension; *fine motor skills* and *interactional* (social) skills. This test is both valid and reliable (Frankenberg, 1984). It can be administered until 6 years of age. Although there are other tests similar to the Denver that are used to assess these areas, the DDST is considered a classic that is fairly easy to administer and score.

A shorter version of the DDST has recently been developed. It is called the DDST-R. The discussion regarding which test to implement is provided in detail later in this chapter under the heading "Developmental Assessment is Children," page 416.

There are many milestones to be evaluated during the infant and toddler years. Some of these include rolling over, sitting, crawling, walking, talking, etc. Each of the expected tasks of development needs to be carefully evaluated at each well-child visit.

As with infancy and toddlerhood, the preschool years have an important neurological focus, as well. Toilet training may have begun for some children in late infancy, but for most, it is a task to be accomplished in the early preschool period. Socialization, interest in others, longer attention spans and improved motor skills are other important developmental features of this period. The child may be in preschool, or if not, is about to enter school. It is necessary for a child to accomplish these tasks in order to be at an appropriate developmental level when he enters school.

Not many neurological problems typically occur in the school-age and adolescent years. However, school is a good screening facility for many such problems in this age group. Health care for this age group deals mostly with acute treatment and periodic physicals. It is important, therefore, that thorough neurological screening be done during the annual physical exam. Accidents are a major cause of morbidity and mortality among this population. Often when these tragedies occur, much neurological damage can be seen.

In the young and middle adult, again, neurologic problems are not common. There are some degenerative neurological diseases that have a high incidence during these years. Two of the more common diseases are multiple sclerosis and amyotrophic lateral sclerosis. These diseases usually begin with very vague complaints, like weakness or numbness, and are often hard to diagnose until the disease process is much more advanced. Therefore, it is important for all health care providers to evaluate all vague complaints as thoroughly as the more obvious ones. Sometimes vague complaints are assumed to have a psychogenic origin only. Although in some instances this may be true, in many instances, it is not. For this reason, it is important to always indicate to the patient that if a problem does not completely resolve or improve significantly, follow-up is necessary. For some degenerative neurological diseases, early diagnosis and intervention can help prevent rapid or further degeneration.

In the geriatric patient, special concerns exist. Many elderly people have decreasing motor skills, unexplained fears, depression, confusion and phobia, decreased sensory abilities, and disruption of memory. These people may have difficulty walking or walk more slowly. Vision and hearing decreases. Often these changes go unnoticed by the patient; for others, these changes create great anxiety and fear. Many disease processes, like diabetes or cerebral vascular disease, create neurologic or other related problems. Diabetic neuropathies can cause constant pain and can destroy many organs in the body. Patients who have strokes (cerebral vascular accidents) are often left with some residual paralysis or limitation. Therefore, it is easy to see that the health care provider must always be concerned about the neurologic system even if the disease process seems to stem from other systems like the vascular or endocrine system.

Depression is a common emotional disorder in the elderly, possibly due to the multiple losses experienced with advanced age. However, it should be considered a part of the normal aging process. Research indicates that successful suicide attempts in persons over the age of 65 years is well above the national average for suicide attempts (Kahn, et al., 1960). Therefore, it is important that the nurse pursue a complaint of depression with a thorough history, physical and, appropriate referral, if needed.

Confusion, an altered mental state, is more often associated with the elderly client than any other age group. The term confusion is used to describe a variety of patient behaviors such as decreased concentration and attention span, inappropriate response to questioning, recent or remote memory loss, disruptive or bizzare behavior, and a general inability to carry out activities of daily living. Confusion is also related to such terms as senility, organic brain syndrome, and dementia. Until recently, an assessment of confusion from the mildest to the most severe form, was thought to be irreversible. However, as research has begun to identify pathology as a possible cause of altered behavior patterns, confusion is now more often thought to be reversible. Wolanin and Phillips suggest that reversible confusion is of the acute or rapid-onset type. This is due to a variety of pathological states such as compromised brain support, sensoriperceptual problems, altered environmental factors and altered physiologic states. Irreversible confusion, on the other hand, is of the chronic or slow-onset type such as arteriosclerotic cerebral disease or true dementia, Alzheimer's disease, Pick's disease, or Jakob–Creutzfeldt disease (Wolanin & Phillips, 1981). Confusion should not be assessed as part of the normal aging process. Normal elderly, as in all age groups, can be expected to demonstrate a variety of emotional patterns to give evidence of accurate memory recall, and to be able to perform tests that involve comprehension and abstraction (Mezey, et al., 1980).

When a patient notices decreasing mobility, loss of memory, and other similar problems, it can be frightening to him. With a gradual decrease in neurological functioning, his whole independent existence is threatened, and this has many implications. Not only is independence an issue, but the patient's self-image may be threatened as well. If the nurse is astute and includes anticipatory guidance in her care, the potential for a situational crisis may be decreased.

ANATOMY

The study of the anatomy and physiology of the nervous system is difficult for two reasons. First, the nervous system's structure, function, and effect on the human body is very complex. Second, there are many varied and contradictory theories and explanations for the structure, function, and effect of this system.

For all practical purposes, the nervous system can be separated into the *central nervous system* and the *peripheral nervous system*. The *brain* and *spinal cord* make up the central nervous system. The *spinal nerves* and the *cranial nerves* compose the peripheral nervous system.

The Central Nervous System

THE BRAIN

The brain can be divided up in several different ways. The simplest division includes the *forebrain*, the *brainstem*, and the *cerebellum* (Fig. 15.1). The forebrain includes the cerebrum (telencephalon) and diencephalon (thalamus and hypothalamus) and the brainstem includes the midbrain, pons, and medulla.

The Forebrain. The *cerebrum* is the largest portion of the brain center. In addition to its sensory and motor functions, it is said to be the place of the highest mental function. It stores

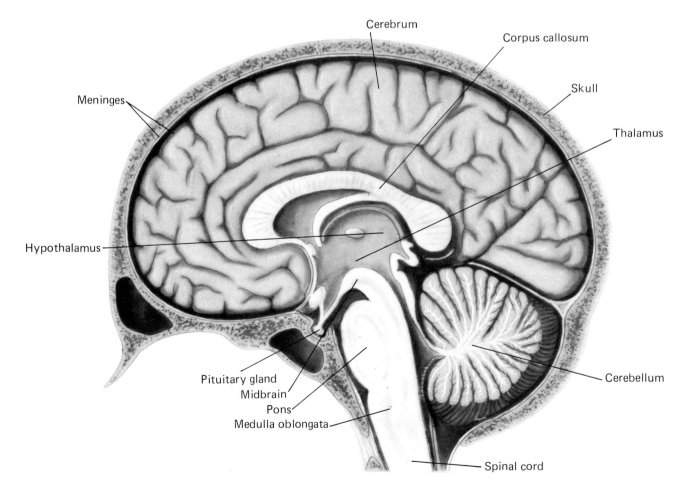

FIGURE 15.1
The brain: major structures. (From Heagarty, M., et al. Child Health: Basics for Primary Care. New York: Appleton-Century-Crofts, 1980, p. 169.)

all knowledge. The cerebrum is divided into lobes, totaling four on each side, which have the same anatomical construction, but very different functions. Anteriorly are the *frontal lobes,* followed by the *parietal lobes.* The posterior lobes are called the *occipital lobes.* The remaining lobes are called *temporal* and they lie above each ear (Zuidema, 1977).

The *diencephalon* is composed of the *thalamus* and the *hypothalamus.* The thalamus is the largest part of the diencephalon and is considered a very important relay center and information processor. It works along with the hypothalamus to affect hormones, smooth muscles, and glands. The hypothalamus is known as the regulator of the internal environment. It integrates and correlates autonomic, somatic, and hormonal operations. The hypothalamus also plays a part in emotion and satiation.

The Brainstem. All the *afferent and efferent tracks* between the spinal cord and the brain go through the brainstem. Many cranial nerves come from there and all the cell bodies of the efferent section of the cranial nerves are in the brainstem. The overall function includes the control of subconscious and reflex activity. The *midbrain* is involved in motor coordination. The *medulla* contains the autonomic control centers for breathing, arterial blood pressure, and vomiting. Not much is known about the pons and its separate function. It contains many fiber tracks between the spinal cord and the brain. It does seem to be a "relay center," with most messages going to the *cerebellum.*

The Cerebellum. The cerebellum is located in the occipital region of the head. It attaches to both the cerebrum and the brainstem. Functionally, the cerebellum deals with balance, posture, and equilibrium. The cerebellum also has a major role in reflex skeletal muscle tone and in the coordination and regulation of all voluntary muscular activities (Jensen, 1980).

The Peripheral Nervous System

THE SPINAL NERVES

There are 31 pairs of spinal nerves: 8 cervical, 12 thoracic, 5 lumbar, 5 sacral, and 1 coccygeal. Each spinal nerve has an afferent and efferent component as well as a *dorsal* and *ventral branch* (Fig. 15.2). The ventral portion

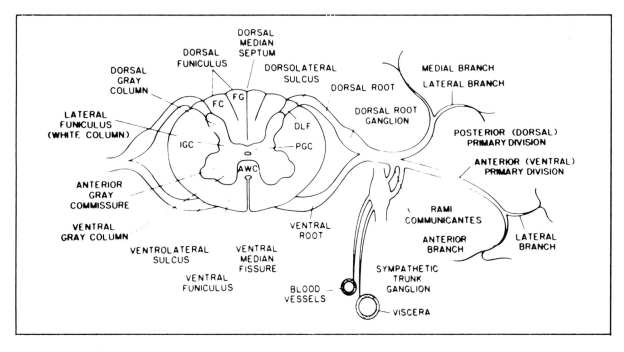

FIGURE 15.2
The spinal nerve: dorsal and ventral branches. (From Jensen, D. The Human Nervous System. New York: Appleton-Century-Crofts, 1980, p. 41.)

serves the limbs as well as the front and lateral aspects of the trunk. The area of skin supplied with afferent innervation from a single dorsal root is called a dermatome (Fig. 15.3). It is important to note that each spinal nerve may have a very large dermatome to serve.

THE CRANIAL NERVES

There are 12 pairs of cranial nerves. In this case, each pair does not necessarily have an afferent and efferent component. Some have both and others have only an efferent or afferent component. These 12 cranial nerves are: *olfactory* (CN I), *optic* (CN II), *oculomotor* (CN III), *trochlear* (CN IV), *trigeminal* (CN V), *abducens* (CN VI), *facial* (CN VII), *acoustic* (CN VIII), *glossopharyngeal* (CN IX), *vagus* (CN X), *spinal accessory* (CN XI), and *hypoglossal* (CN XII). Each nerve has specific functions and is either sensory, motor, or both (Chart 15.1).

The peripheral nervous system can be further divided into afferent and efferent sections because most of the cranial nerves and all of the spinal nerves have both components.

The efferent segment is divided again into the *somatic* and *autonomic systems.* The somatic efferent motor nerves innervate skeletal

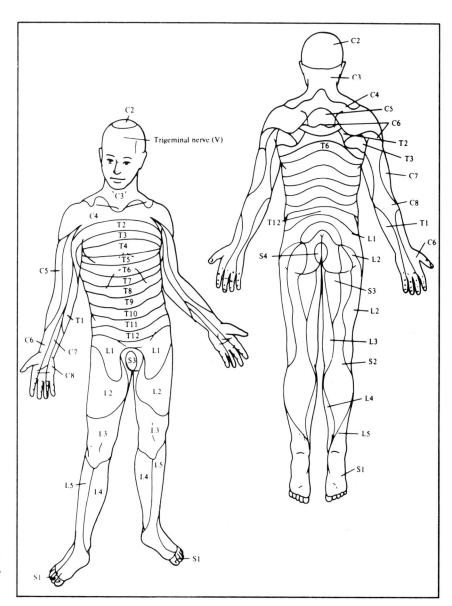

FIGURE 15.3
Dermatomes. (From Brill, E. and Kilts, D. Foundations for Nursing. New York: Appleton-Century-Crofts, 1980, p. 225.)

CHART 15.1
THE CRANIAL NERVES

Cranial Nerve	Motor (M) or Sensory (S) Origin	Function
CN I (olfactory)	S	Smell
CN II (optic)	S	Vision
CN III (oculomotor)	M	
	Autonomic	Pupillary constriction
	Somatic	Extraocular muscles: superior rectus, medial rectus, inferior rectus, inferior oblique
CN IV (trochlear)	M	Extraocular muscles: superior oblique
CN V (trigeminal)	S	Face and scalp; three divisions: ophthalmic, maxillary, mandibular
	M	Mandibular muscles: masseter, temporal, pterygoid
CN VI (abducens)	M	Lateral deviation of eye
CN VII (facial)	S	Taste: anterior ⅔ of the tongue; external ear; soft palate; anterior pharynx
	M	Facial muscles: face, scalp, outer ear, forehead, mouth Submandibular, sublingual, and salivary, lacrimal glands, and glands of nasal and palatine mucosa
CN VIII (acoustic)	S	Hearing, balance
CN IX (glossopharyngeal)	S	Taste: posterior ⅓ of the tongue
	M	Pharynx: swallowing, gagging, parotid gland
CN X (vagus)	S	Larynx; pharynx; esophagus; heart, abdominal organs
	M	Pharynx; larynx; heart; esophagus; abdominal organs; trachea and bronchi
CN XI (spinal accessory)	M	Muscles: sternocleidomastoid, trapezius
CN XII (hypoglossal)	M	Tongue

muscle and the autonomic nerves stimulate smooth muscle, cardiac muscle, and the glands.

AUTONOMIC NERVOUS SYSTEM
The autonomic nervous system is not simply another nervous system. The autonomic nervous system functions very interdependently and is not as major a unit as the central nervous system and peripheral nervous system. This unit functions involuntarily and is a division of the peripheral nervous system. It is, in fact, one of the efferent portions of the peripheral nervous system. This innervation further breaks down into the *sympathetic and parasympathetic sections.*

The feature unit of this system involves the *ganglia,* which are groups of cells that lie outside the central nervous system (Fig. 15.4). The synapse of neural transmission occurs along this pathway. One difference in the sympathetic and parasympathetic divisions depends on the location of these ganglia. For the most part the ganglia in the sympathetic

system lie close to the spinal cord. In the parasympathetic system the ganglia lie closer to the organ receiving the stimulation. The fibers on either side of the ganglia are called either *preganglionic* or *postganglionic.*

At the junction of the preganglionic and postganglionic neurons, where the synapse occurs, a chemical transmitter is released. This must happen prior to the synapse. The type of chemical released depends on the site of the ganglia. *Acetylcholine* is released between *preganglionic* and *postganglionic fibers* in both the sympathetic and parasympathetic systems. The nerve fibers that release acetylcholine are *cholinergic* fibers. Acetylcholine is also released between the parasympathetic postganglionic fiber and the effector cell (Fig. 15.4). At the synapse of the sympathetic postganglionic fiber and effector cell, *adrenergic* (adrenalin) fibers release *norepinephrine.* Whereas, in the parasympathetic response acetylcholine is again released between the postganglionic fiber and the effector cell.

The function of the autonomic nervous

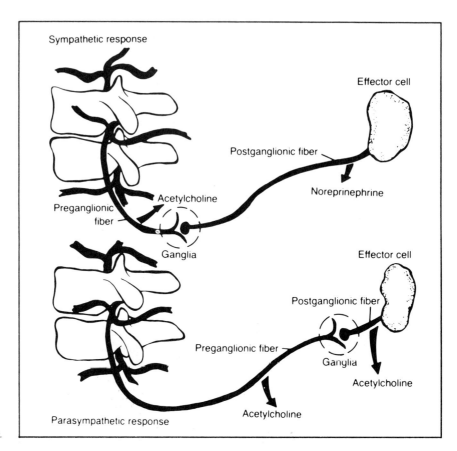

FIGURE 15.4
Autonomic nervous system.

system is to provide a homeostatic environment for the body by controlling the activities of specific organs—primarily the smooth muscles, cardiac muscles, and glands. For the most part, this function is accomplished by involuntary controls.

Most organs that the autonomic nervous system affects receive dual innervation. This means that the organs have both sympathetic and parasympathetic stimulation. These systems work antagonistically against one another. The sympathetic deals with "fight or flight"; the parasympathetic effect is most easily evidenced at rest or recovery from sympathetic stimulation.

THE MOTOR SYSTEM

In order for the motor system to function appropriately, the following organs must be intact: the *cerebral cortex,* the *basal ganglia,* the *cerebellum,* the *brainstem,* and the *spinal cord nuclei.*

The cerebral cortex has an important role in motor function. The area of the cortex most involved is the posterior portion of the frontal lobe. This is known as the *motor cortex.*

The basal ganglia act as relays in the motor system. They receive messages from the cortex to stimulate purposeful control of fine, coordinated, rapid and slow movement. The mechanism of postural control lies here also. The brainstem, spinal cord nuclei, and *reticular formation* are portions of the descending tract that act in conjunction with the basal ganglia. The reticular formation is an area of the upper spinal cord that contains a group of interconnected nerve fibers and cells. This important regulatory system is a polysynaptic pathway for afferent and efferent impulses (Jensen, 1980).

The cerebellum houses both afferent and efferent nerve fibers. Every motor stimulus must pass through the cerebellum. Motor stimulation is not initiated here, but all the integration of information from the basal ganglia and motor cortex takes place in the cerebellum.

If damage occurs in the cerebellum, not only does movement become uncontrolled and uncoordinated, but vestibular function is affected. Thus balance and posture are involved in the function of the cerebellar region.

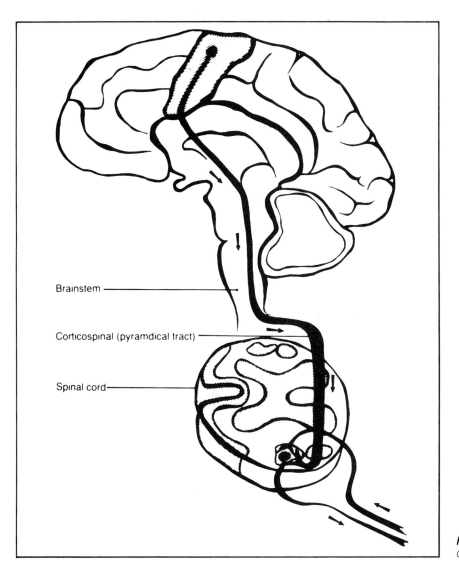

FIGURE 15.5
Corticospinal pathways.

Brainstem

Corticospinal (pyramdical tract)

Spinal cord

The descending pathways which influence motor function and are an intricate part of this system are the *corticospinal* (pyramidal tract) and the *multineuronal* pathways (Fig. 15.5). Two-thirds of the nerve fibers in the corticospinal pathways cross over in the medulla before reaching the spinal cord. Thus if right-sided symptoms appear, damage will have most likely occurred on the left side of the brain.

The multineuronal pathway is not a separate descending pathway. It is the first connecting point for some motor neurons that synapse in the nuclei of the brainstem and cerebrum. Although the synapse occurs outside the motor cortex, the integration of all this electric activity is what allows for coordinated movement of the skeletal muscles.

The Reflex Arc. The reflex arc is a homeostatic mechanism of the motor system. This is the basis for the *muscle stretch reflex.* The muscle stretch reflex is a *monosynaptic reflex.* This means that there is only one synapse between the receptor and the effector.

Deep tendon reflexes are examples of the monosynaptic reflex arc. This simple reflex arc can be described most easily by imagining what occurs between the moment a tendon is tapped by a reflex hammer and the concentration of the muscle (Fig. 15.6). Reflexes are involuntary.

The *tendon* is tapped. The *muscle spindle* is activated, and the impulse travels along an afferent nerve fiber along the peripheral nerve to the spinal nerve. Further along the pathway and just outside the spinal cord is the *posterior*

THE REFLEX ARC

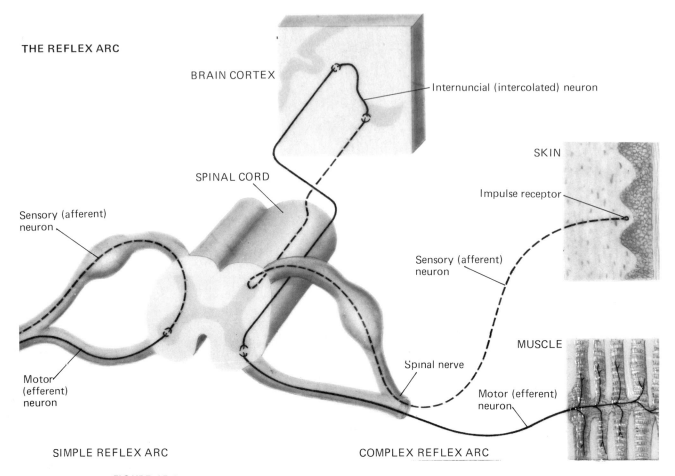

BRAIN CORTEX

Internuncial (intercolated) neuron

SKIN

Impulse receptor

SPINAL CORD

Sensory (afferent)
neuron

Sensory (afferent)
neuron

MUSCLE

Motor
(efferent)
neuron

Spinal nerve

Motor (efferent)
neuron

SIMPLE REFLEX ARC

COMPLEX REFLEX ARC

FIGURE 15.6
*Nervous reflex: the reflex arc. (From Heagarty, M., et al. Child Health: Basics for Primary Care.
New York: Appleton-Century-Crofts, 1980, p. 170.)*

root. When the stimulus enters the cord, the synapse takes place. The *anterior root* picks up the stimulus, and it travels along efferent pathways, including the spinal nerve and the peripheral nerve. Ultimately, the impulse reaches the muscle and the contraction occurs. This illustrates *lower motor neuron function.*

THE SENSORY SYSTEM

The *sensory system* is made up of *sensory receptors, afferent neurons, ascending pathways,* and the *primary sensory areas* of the cerebral cortex.

There are many different kinds of sensory receptors. These vary according to the types of stimuli they receive. The receptors are classified according to position, movement, and

the sensations of heat, cold, pain, and touch. There are other types for muscle, joint, and tendon stimulation. There are also receptors in the viscera and blood vessels. These are not necessarily conscious receptors.

Two ascending pathways known to scientists at present are the *lateral spinothalamic* and the *posterior* columns. The lateral spinothalamic is responsible for pain and temperature. The posterior column is the tract that deals with position and movement.

Like all the other divisions within the nervous system, all the units must be intact and functioning for an appropriate response to occur, regardless of the orientation of the stimulus. If there is any interruption along the way, symptoms will appear. The history and physical assessment of the nervous system will help pinpoint the location of that interruption.

HISTORY

The neurological history is important for two reasons: (1) to get the patient's description of the functioning or malfunctioning of his nervous system and (2) to establish the mental status of the patient. Although assessment of mental status is part of the physical, much can be checked while eliciting the history, including the patient's orientation, intellectual abilities, language, and speech. If the nurse senses some confusion or inaccuracy while taking a neurological history on an elderly patient, she may find the use of Kahn's Mental Status Questionnaire (Wang, 1980) to be a concise and efficient tool in assessing the presence and degree of chronic brain syndrome in the elderly client. It will also serve as a future guide to changes in mental status of the patient (see Chart 15.3, page 396).

To say that there is one method or one format for the neurological history would be incorrect. It has already been stated that the level of consciousness, the chief complaint, and the cooperation of the patient must be considered. Additional criteria include the developmental age and stage of the patient. Obviously, there are certain questions relevant to infant development that are not pertinent to the adolescent. However, there are some questions that are important to ask at any age. These concern any history of loss of consciousness, fainting, convulsions, trauma, tingling or numbness, tremors or tics, limping, paralysis, speech disorders, loss of memory, disorientation, mood swings, anxiety, depression, or phobias.

If the answer to any of these questions is yes, further inquiry regarding circumstances is necessary—when they occurred, the cause(s), treatment(s), and course of recovery. Essentially, exploring the eight areas of investigation or eliciting a brief HPH will provide necessary details of past problems.

A complaint of pain does not typically arise in relation to this system. If pain from a neurological disorder is mentioned, it will probably come up during the system review for the head, back, or extremities.

Other complaints that may arise in this discussion are anxiety, nervousness, moodiness, and clumsiness. The patient should be queried about all these complaints, which should then be listed as pertinent negatives if the patient denies their occurrence.

Discussion concerning problems with smell, vision, taste, etc. is not necessarily included here. Although these senses are related to the cranial nerves, they are more appropriately covered under the system review of the eyes, nose, and oral cavity. (See history within the appropriate chapters.)

To approach the specific developmental areas of the system review, it is easiest to begin with infancy and work through the various stages of life.

In *infancy*, special attention is paid to the presence of the reflexes mentioned earlier. Not only can the nurse elicit the reflex response during the physical, but she can also question the parents about certain movements they should notice. This also gives the nurse information on the parent's observation of their child. Do they notice that if they touch the baby's cheek, he turns his head toward the side touched (*rooting reflex*)? Does the baby have difficulty with sucking or swallowing? Does he gag? When a loud noise is made or the crib is jarred, does the baby seem to be startled (*Moro reflex*)? When an object or finger is placed in the baby's palm, does he grasp it (*palmar grasp reflex*)? When they hold the baby in a "standing" position with his feet on a flat surface, does he appear to be dancing (*dancing reflex*)? All these reflexes and others can be assessed as part of the DDST during the physical. There are certain times specific reflexes are expected to disappear. The disappearance is as important as their presence. (See the section on description of infant reflexes.) However, even these reflexes may vary among population groups. In reporting on ethnic differences in infants, Freedman found that American Indian and Chinese babies showed a reduced Moro reflex and "defense reaction" (turning away or swiping at a cloth held over the nose) when compared with Caucasian and black babies (Freedman, 1979).

As the neonate progresses through infancy, additional growth and developmental tasks must be accomplished, such as rolling over, sitting, pulling himself up, and walking. All of these are milestones. Approximate dates of occurrence can be elicited during the history, and documentation can be done during the physical and the DDST. Although racial variation has been reported in the rate of motor development (black infants reportedly sit, stand, and walk at earlier ages than their Caucasian counterparts), no standardized developmental scales have used cross-racial subjects. Consequently, the examiner must also rely on family reports when assessing the developmental level of ethnic children of color (Freedman & DeBoer, 1979).

Parents of children in this age group should also be questioned about inappropriate movement or obvious problems with balance that may have been observed in the child. A balance problem may not be noticeable until late infancy, when the baby begins to walk. If there is a concern, most parents will observe inappropriate falling. It is important for the nurse to remember that normalcy in growth and development depends on the accomplishment of developmental tasks appropriate to that age and stage. If any discrepancies are found, evaluation of past accomplishment is necessary.

The last area of investigation in the neurologic review concerns any history of seizures. Seizures in this age group occur for one of two reasons: high fever or a neurologic disease. If elevated temperature is suspected as the reason, it is important to record the description of the seizure, including body temperature, body movement, loss of consciousness (for how long?), loss of urine or feces, number of occurrences within that illness, length of time they lasted, previous history of seizures, other members of the family who have had a seizure, and treatments implemented. If neurologic dysfunction is suspected, the same types of questions should be asked.

The *toddler* has many developmental milestones, too. Most of these were reviewed in Chapter 1 (see Chart 1.2). Again, questioning the parents about the approximate dates of accomplishment of these milestones is worthwhile. Any inappropriate movements, falling, tics, tremors, head nodding, or head banging should be recorded. Seizing with an elevated temperature is not atypical in this age group. In fact, this response to a high fever may exist late into the school-age years. The nurse should always inquire if this has occurred at other times in the past. It is also important to assess exposure to lead, particularly with children from poor families. The greatest incidence of lead poisoning occurs in children living in old houses in the inner city. Frequent exposure to lead may produce symptoms of "dullness." The child may thus be viewed as developmentally retarded when he is actually the victim of a poverty-perpetuated disease (Branch & Paxton, 1976).

During the preschool, school-age, adolescent, and young adult years, the nurse should inquire about the completion of developmental tasks (see Chapter 1, Chart 1.2). Successful accomplishment of these and a negative general history (see general review of neurologic system) will take care of this system review. However, if any of the general questions asked get a positive response, further investigation is necessary. The developmental milestones of infancy and toddlerhood are reviewed in all children under the age of 5 years. This past developmental data is reviewed with the older child only if a developmental problem presents itself.

Generally, the middle-aged patient has few neurologic complaints. He may notice some gradual changes, such as problems with presbyopia. Other neurologic changes are minimal during these years if the person is in reasonably good health.

With the patient in the later years, the nurse must pay special attention to neurological changes. Obtaining a past history regarding the elderly patient's personality and self concept is often helpful in determining if present characteristics are exaggerated effects of past behavior or are age-related. The nurse can ask the patient what kinds of things are particularly bothersome to him and if these issues are life-long feelings or have just recently developed. The answer(s) to this question might provide some insight about his personality. Obtaining a past history of any psychiatric treatment or central nervous system injuries is also helpful in developing an accurate neurological assessment. The past and present cardiac, respiratory, and nutritional status of the elderly client, in addition to an accurate medication history are also important factors that directly affect the aged client's neurological state. Changes in cardiac and respiratory status may decrease the amount of oxygen available to the brain and thus, affect mental status. Lack of appropriate food and fluids can also cause behavioral changes. It is also extremely important to remember that drugs used in the elderly may affect them very differently than they affect a healthy, younger adult. Any renal or hepatic failure will completely alter the drug's half-life, and this can result in significant changes in the patient's ability to function.

The elderly person may not always be aware of gradual neurological changes or losses. There may be a gradual impairment in recent memory with good remote memory. For example, the elderly patient may fail to notice any general overall muscle weakness. Therefore, he should be questioned about any weakening or paralysis of the extremities, any vision or hearing changes, any sensory symptoms such as paresthesias, numbness and tingling. In terms of motor function, any problems with falling, dizziness, uncontrolled muscle movements, tics, tremors, or speech disturbances, should be elicited from the patient and recorded.

When the client complains of frequent falls, a detailed history and physical exam should be completed. The elderly person should be asked about the frequency of falling, precipitating factors, and whether there was any loss of consciousness. Falls can lead to serious injury in the elderly and frequently accompany acute illness.

In the history of the older adult, the nurse may find she must use more direct questioning to elicit specific concrete information. Sometimes an older person will have trouble remembering details. Direct questioning will help the patient focus his answer. It is important to develop a warm and trusting relationship prior to examining these sensitive areas. It is often difficult to get the patient to be specific about complaints. The more concrete the data, the more helpful they will be. For this reason, the nurse may find herself using direct questioning and guiding the patient to specific points.

PHYSICAL ASSESSMENT

The physical assessment of the neurologic system involves two different approaches, depending on the reason for the examination. If the patient is undergoing a routine health assessment, a screening level exam is appropriate. If the chief complaint relates to the neurologic system, as with headaches, numbness,

or weakness of an extremity, then a more detailed assessment is required.

The screening examination includes a brief assessment of mental status; developmental level in children; assessment of specific cranial nerves II, III, IV, V (motor), VI, VII (motor), VIII, IX (motor), X (motor), XI, and XII—most of these are unavoidably tested in the examination of the head, ears, eyes, nose, and throat; assessment of motor function, including walking, knee bends, hopping, balance (Romberg), walking on heels, toes, and tandem gait (the examiner should test only those tasks appropriate to age and ability); evaluation of sensory function, including pain and vibration in the hands and feet; coordination; assessment of deep tendon reflexes; and developmental status at appropriate ages.

The equipment needed for the neurologic screening exam includes a Snellen chart, an ophthalmoscope, a tuning fork, a tongue depressor, a safety pin (sharp and blunt ends needed), and a reflex hammer. For a more detailed exam the examiner needs two test tubes (one filled with warm water and one with cold), a wisp of cotton, a quarter, a paper clip, two distinct substances with odors (alcohol swab, coffee grounds, or a peppermint), and four food items to represent the four areas of taste on the tongue (i.e., sugar, lemon, salt, and aspirin).

Mental Status

Much of the mental status exam can be done during the interview. This is especially true for testing orientation to time, person, and place, and is also true for testing recall. The patient's responses to questions about his past health history reflect his memory for events that occurred earlier in his life. Elicitation of data about a recent complaint illustrates his recall for more recent events. The patient's orientation to person, place, and time are intact if he knows who he is, where he is, and the time of day. Although the nurse elicits subjective data, her observation of the patient's responses are objective data.

The additional components of the mental status examination include:

1. *General appearance:* It is important to notice not only hygiene and grooming,

but also whether the patient's clothing is appropriate for the place and weather.

2. *Posture:* The patient's sitting or standing position may be either upright or slouched. This can point out a mechanical problem or reflect his self-image.

3. *Facial expression.*

4. *Mood:* This is often evidenced in the posture and facial expression. The nurse should be careful to document this with her observational skills and not just give her opinion.

5. *Speech:* This includes tone and verbalization as well as the quality of what is being stated. The nurse must be sure that there are no educational or language barriers while making this observation.

6. *Level of awareness and state of consciousness:* This includes orientation to time, person, and place; ability to concentrate; and the level of consciousness (Chart 15.2).

7. *Intellectual functioning:* This includes memory (both recent and remote), basic knowledge (understanding and ability to learn), abstract thinking (the ability to explain abstract statements, such as "A rolling stone gathers no moss."), similarity association (the ability to take similar concepts and make an association—i.e., a chair is to a table as a pencil is to paper), and judgment (the ability to make decisions with common sense and appropriate thought processes).

Using a tool like Kahn's Mental Status Questionnaire (Chart 15.3) may prove to be a valid indicator of the elderly patient's mental status and tests his recent, as well as, remote memory. All these observations are invalid if the nurse is testing at a level at which the patient cannot understand or participate. Therefore, the nurse should be subtle in her approach in gathering this information and scatter the tests throughout the interview (Chart 15.2).

The Cranial Nerves

The decision as to whether or not to test all or some of the cranial nerves for screening purposes is a moot point. It takes so little time to test their intactness because so many of

CHART 15.2
ALTERED STATES OF CONSCIOUSNESS

Term	Characteristics
Conscious	Alert, awake Aware of one's self and environment
Confusion	Disorientation in time Irritability and/or drowsiness Misjudgment of sensory input Shortened attention span Decrease in memory
Delirium	Disorientation, fear Misperception of sensory stimuli Visual and auditory hallucinations Loss of contact with environment
Stupor	Unresponsive, but can be aroused back to a near normal state
Coma	Unresponsive to external stimuli
Akinetic mutism	Alert-appearing Immobile Mental activity absent
Locked-in syndrome	No effective verbal or motor communication Consciousness may be intact EEG indicates a preservation of cerebral activity Secondary to bilateral supranuclear paralysis at the level of the brain stem
Chronic vegetative state	Secondary to severe brain damage Often follows a period of coma Vital functions preserved with no evidence of active mental processes EEG indicates absence of cerebral activity

(*From Plum, F. and Posner, J. B. The Diagnosis of Stupor and Coma (3rd ed.). Philadelphia, Davis, 1981, with permission.*)

them are tested within the head, ear, eye, nose, and throat exams. Some providers prefer to test them all. However, for screening purposes, the following cranial nerves are tested: CN II (optic); CN III (oculomotor); CN IV (trochlear); CN V (trigeminal-motor); CN VI (abducens); CN VII (facial-motor component); CN VIII (acoustic); CN IX (glossopharyngeal—motor only); CN X (vagus); CN XI (spinal accessory); and CN XII (hypoglossal). Remember that many of the following are tested during other parts of the physical. For instance, CN II, III, IV, and VI are included in the eye exam. The first cranial nerve (CN I—olfactory) is only tested if a problem is suspected. This is also true regarding the sensory components of CN VII and CN IX.

CRANIAL NERVE I (OLFACTORY)

This nerve controls the sense of olfaction. The patient is told that he will be asked to smell

CHART 15.3
THE KAHN TEST

1. Where are we now?
2. Where is this place (located)?
3. What is today's date—day of month?
4. What month is it?
5. What year is it?
6. How old are you?
7. What is your birthday (the day and the month)?
8. What year were you born?
9. Who is the president of the United States?
10. Who was the president before him?

RATING OF MENTAL STATUS QUESTIONNAIRE

Number of Errors	Presumed Mental Status
0–2	Mild Organic Impairment
3–8	Moderate Organic Impairment
9–10	Severe Organic Impairment

a particular substance and identify it. For this he will have to close his eyes. After he closes his eyes, he is asked to place a finger over one nostril so he can only smell through one side at a time. The examiner should make sure the patient's nose is not obstructed from sinus drainage. She then places an odorous substance at the open nares—i.e., alcohol, coffee grounds, an orange, or a mint (especially good for children). The patient is asked to identify the scent, after which the other nostril is tested with a different substance. This is not done on the screening level.

CRANIAL NERVE II (OPTIC)
The optic nerve is tested by evaluating visual acuity (with the Snellen chart and a funduscopic exam) and visual fields (with confrontation testing) (see Chapter 5, page 130).

CRANIAL NERVES III (OCULOMOTOR), IV (TROCHLEAR), AND VI (ABDUCENS)
These are all tested together because of their related functions (see Chapter 5, page 123–137). These nerves are tested for appropriate extraocular movements, direct and indirect pupillary constriction, ptosis, lid lag, and nystagmus.

CRANIAL NERVE V (TRIGEMINAL)
This nerve has both a sensory and a motor component. The motor portion deals with the strength and symmetry of the masseter and

temporal muscles. The patient is asked to clench his teeth. The examiner palpates the temporomandibular area and asks the patient to swallow. She feels the strength of these muscles during the contraction. Unequal muscle contraction is significant and worthy of documentation and should be referred. The *sensory* division has three areas that need evaluation. The *ophthalmic area* is assessed by testing for the presence of the *corneal reflex* (see Chapter 5, page 136). The *maxillary* and *mandibular* divisions are tested for the sensations of pain or light touch. The nurse explains to the patient that he will be feeling a sharp or dull sensation scattered around his face. He is to identify which sensation he feels. It is helpful to demonstrate the sensations he will feel by placing the sharp end, then the blunt end of a safety pin on the patient's hand. The patient is then asked to close his eyes. The nurse places either the blunt or sharp end of the pin along the lateral aspect of the face, the forehead, the cheek, and chin. If there is any doubt after this test, the nurse asks the patient to identify the difference between hot and cold temperatures. For this the nurse has two test tubes filled with water—one hot, one cold. She applies the base of either tube in the same general area as she did the safety pin. The patient is asked to identify which is hot and which is cold. The nurse must remember to scatter the stimuli and alter the temperatures. The nurse can also stroke the patient's face at these selected areas with a wisp of cotton. The patient should be able to tell when the cotton is touching his face.

CRANIAL NERVE VII (FACIAL)
The motor component of CN VII is included in the routine screening exam. The nurse initially observes the face for any tics, unusual movement, or asymmetry. The muscles of the face are tested by asking the patient to clench his teeth forcefully and smile, (Fig. 15.7) blow out his cheeks and with his mouth closed, frown or wrinkle his forehead, raise his eyebrows, and close his eyes tightly, not letting the examiner open them.

The taste buds on the anterior two-thirds of the tongue are tested to evaluate the sensory component of CN VII. The tongue can pick up the sensations of sweet (sugar), salty, sour (lemon), and bitter (aspirin). The patient should be able to differentiate among the

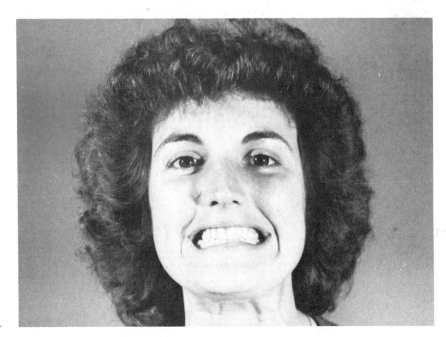

FIGURE 15.7
Testing cranial nerve VII.

tastes. The nurse should be sure to have him rinse his mouth between tastes to avoid overlap. The taste test is not done at the screening level.

CRANIAL NERVE VIII (ACOUSTIC)

Auditory acuity can be tested by audiometry, the Weber and Rinné tests. These tests are easily included in a screening examination (see Chapter 6, pages 160 and 163). Testing vestibular function also assesses cranial nerve VIII. This testing is not performed by nurses as a rule. The test involves injecting ice water into the external ear and observing for nystagmus, vertigo, or falling. Anyone with intact vestibular function will have nystagmus. Patients find this test most uncomfortable; it therefore, is only done when symptoms of vertigo exist.

CRANIAL NERVES IX (GLOSSOPHARYNGEAL) AND X (VAGUS)

These two nerves are tested together. To test the glossopharyngeal nerve, the patient is asked to open his mouth and say "ah." The nurse should note the soft palate rising as well as the uvula. The nurse touches the uvula with a tongue depressor and elicits a gag reflex. This gag reflex tests the motor function of the vagus nerve. The nurse listens for any hoarseness of the voice. All this can be observed in taking the history and while examining the mouth.

CRANIAL NERVE XI (SPINAL ACCESSORY)

The strength of the sternocleidomastoid and trapezius muscles is tested. The nurse places her hands on the patient's shoulders. The patient shrugs his shoulders, and the nurse pushes down on them. The patient is asked to resist this pressure (Fig. 15.8). For the other portion of this test, the examiner puts her hand on the side of the patient's face (Fig. 15.8). She asks him to push against her hand while she applies pressure toward his face. The patient should be able to resist this pressure with the strength in his facial muscles. The other side of the face is then tested.

CRANIAL NERVE XII (HYPOGLOSSAL)

The patient's tongue is inspected. The nurse notes the size of the mouth and any irregular movement or asymmetry. The patient is then asked to stick out his tongue and move it from side to side, while the nurse looks for irregularities in the medial and lateral movements of the tongue.

This completes the tests for the twelve cranial nerves.

The Motor System

Consistent with the other components of the neurological examination, the testing of the motor system has a screening level and a more

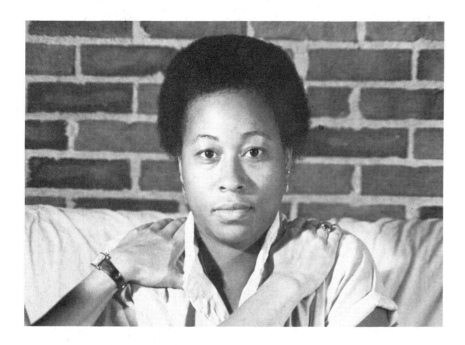

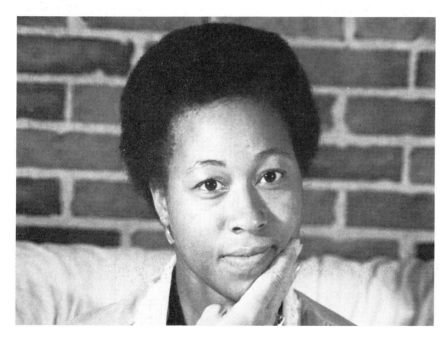

FIGURE 15.8
Testing cranial nerve XI.

detailed approach. Some parts of the screening exam can be completed by watching the patient as he walks into the room and while he is sitting during the interview. The screening exam includes the objective assessment of posture and muscle tone (especially in children and older people), as well as muscle strength and coordination.

The more detailed version of the examination of motor system function is the same for both children and adults. The objective information obtained depends on the patient's ability and cooperation. This portion of the exam becomes necessary when abnormalities are suspected from the results of the screening exam. The evaluation at this point involves a further assessment of muscle tone, muscle strength, and coordination.

POSTURE AND MUSCLE TONE

Posture can be evaluated by observing the patient's walk, his sitting position, and obvious deviation along the spinous process, back, or shoulders. Most people when they sit will have some degree of rounding of the shoulders. However, if this is exaggerated or corresponds with a portion of the chief complaint, further evaluation is necessary.

The posture and muscle tone of the newborn should be evaluated as well. In normal resting posture, the baby's legs are partially flexed and there is a slight abduction of the hips. Thorough inspection and palpation of muscle tone is essential, especially in infants and children (see Chapter 14, page 344). In the older patient, muscle mass may atrophy and will appear to have less "substance."

Swinging of the arms in conjunction with movement of the legs can be observed easily when the patient walks into the room. Abnormalities in this movement are obvious. Elderly patients may take shorter steps and have a wider gait between their feet as part of the normal aging process.

BALANCE

Observing the patient's overall balance is the first step. Again, obvious abnormalities can be detected when he walks into the room.

The Romberg test, a test for cerebellar function, is a quick screening test for balance that should be done with all age groups, from toddlers to the elderly. For this test the patient is asked to stand up with his feet together. He is then asked to close his eyes. He is observed for swaying. The nurse should be close to the patient with her arms extended around him in case the patient starts to fall (Fig. 15.9). Some swaying is normal, especially in older patients.

Other cerebellar tests for balance, for the ambulatory patient who is able, include a shallow deep-knee bend, hopping in place (one foot at a time), heel-to-toe walking, walking on tip-toes and then on heels, and standing on one foot at a time with the eyes closed.

INSPECTION OF THE GENERAL MUSCLE MASS

The muscles of the body are inspected for atrophy, asymmetry, fasciculations (twitching) and involuntary movement. Further discussion of this examination can be found in Chapter 14.

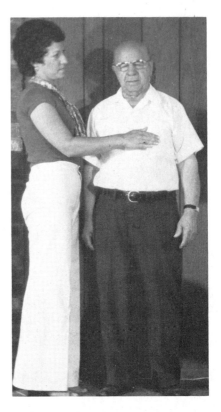

FIGURE 15.9
The Romberg test.

A more detailed exam, when necessary, includes the following.

Muscle Tone. The patient should be lying in a supine position. The nurse should explain to him that the extremities of his body will be flexed and extended to test for pain, resistance, and flaccidity. Testing each side separately, the examiner supports the extremity being tested and takes it through a *passive range of motion.* On the upper half of the body, the fingers, wrists, elbows, and shoulders are assessed. Then the toes, ankles, and knees are flexed, extended, abducted, adducted, and rotated for the same purpose.

Muscle Strength. Muscle strength is tested against the resistance of the examiner. Symmetrical responses are significant and permit the examiner to use the patient as his own control. Considerations should be given to the age and health of the patient as well as to the integrity of the skeletal muscles. The specific tests should be applied quickly and systematically, without fatiguing the patient. These include:

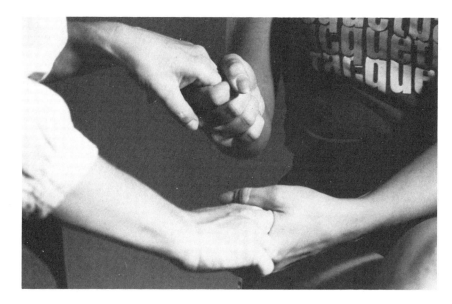

FIGURE 15.10
Symmetrical finger-grip strength.

1. *The finger-grip:* The patient is asked to squeeze the examiner's first two fingers. The grip should be reasonably strong, but most important, it should be equal in both hands (Fig. 15.10). It may also be noted that hand grip strength does not appreciably diminish with age, but there is less strength difference between the dominant and non-dominant hands after 70 years of age.

2. *Finger abduction:* The patient is asked to separate his fingers. The examiner explains to him that she will try to push them together. The patient is to resist this pressure. The examiner notes any weakness or asymmetry in strength (Fig. 15.11).

3. *Wrist dorsiflexion:* The patient is asked to make a fist with both hands. The examiner tries to push them down while the patient resists. Any weakness is noted (Fig. 15.12).

4. *Flexion and extension of the elbow:* The patient is asked to push against the examiner's hands with his forearm (extension) (Fig. 15.13A). He is then asked to

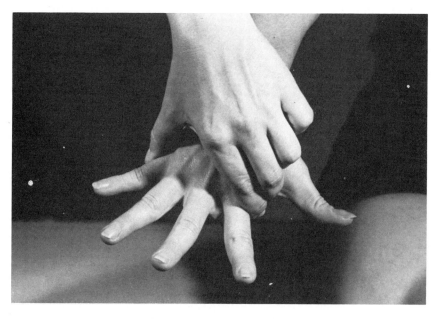

FIGURE 15.11
Finger abduction.

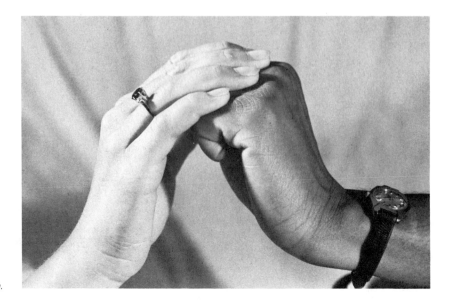

FIGURE 15.12
Wrist dorsiflexion.

pull against the resistance of the examiner's hand at the forearm (flexion). Any pain or resistance is noted (Fig. 15.13B).

5. *Shoulder and scapulae resistance:* The patient is asked to extend both arms out in front of him for 20 seconds. He is told to resist the push about to be applied. The nurse then tries to push the arms down (Fig. 15.14). Any pain or weakness with this maneuver is noted. This is a common site for sports injuries, arthritis, and bursitis. Next the patient is asked to raise both arms above his shoulders. The nurse tries to push his arms down to his sides. The patient is once again instructed to resist this maneuver.

6. *Lateral bending, flexion, and extension of the trunk:* The lower half of the body is assessed in a manner similar to that used for the upper half, with the patient lying down. (See Chapter 14, page 355.)

7. *Hip flexion:* The patient is asked to raise his leg against the examiner's hand, which is applying pressure on the thigh, trying to flatten the leg. Any pain with this movement is noted, especially in the geriatric patient.

8. *Hip abduction:* The patient is asked to flex his knees so that his feet are flat on the table (or bed). The nurse places her hands over the lateral collateral ligaments. The patient then tries to push against the examiner's hands with his

knees. The nurse resists the push (Fig. 15.15). There should be no pain or asymmetry in strength.

9. *Hip adduction:* The patient's legs are in the same position used with hip abduction, except that they are slightly spread apart. This time the nurse places her hands over the medial collateral ligaments. The patient is asked to bring his knees together against the nurse's resistance.

10. *Knee extension and flexion:* Again the patient's legs are flexed at the knees with his feet flat on the bed. To test extension of the knee, the nurse places one of her hands behind the patient's knee and the other on the ankle. The patient is asked to straighten his leg against the nurse's hand, which is on his ankle (Fig. 15.16A). Then the nurse's hand at the knee is taken from behind and placed on top of the knee. The patient is asked to keep his foot flat on the bed as the nurse tries to extend his leg and straighten it. (Fig. 15.16B)

11. *Plantar flexion and dorsiflexion of the ankle:* This test is commonly used to help locate the origin of back and leg pain. The patient is still supine with his legs flat on the bed. The nurse puts her hand on the ball of the patient's foot. The patient is asked to push against the nurse's hand while the nurse applies resistance to the patient's push (plantar

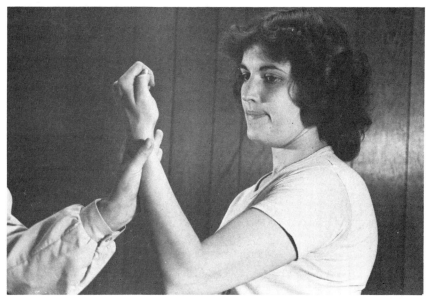

A

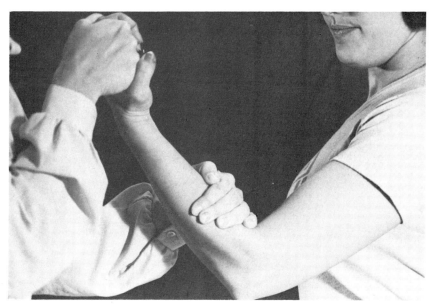

B

FIGURE 15.13
A. Extension of the elbow. B. Flexion of the elbow.

flexion) (Fig. 15.17A). Then the patient is asked to pull against the nurse's hand, which is cupped around the superior aspect of each foot (dorsiflexion) (Fig. 15.17B). In specific back injuries, pain will be elicited with this test.

12. *Abdominal muscle strength:* While the patient is in the supine position, he is asked to raise himself at the waist or sit up. A child is asked to look at his "belly button." Pain with this maneu-ver may be indicative of meningeal irritation.

COORDINATION

This portion of motor system function, which in fact tests for intact cerebellar function, evaluates fine, purposeful movement and coordination of the upper and lower extremities. The tests are not complicated, but the instructions may be confusing. In order to be sure that the patient understands the directions, it is

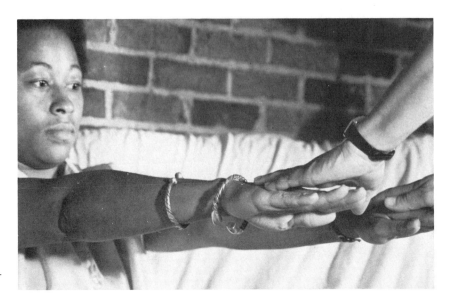

FIGURE 15.14
Shoulder and scapulae resistance.

wise for the nurse to demonstrate to the patient what she expects him to do. Assessing rapid rhythm movement is the first test. There are two phases in this evaluation. One phase tests upper extremity coordination and the other phase assesses the lower extremities. First the patient, who is sitting up, is asked to pat the superior aspects of his thighs with the palms of his hands as rapidly as possible. He is then asked to turn his hands back and forth with the same rapid motion (palm to dorsum of hand) (Fig. 15.18). This is observed

for 30 seconds. Speed and symmetry are noted.

For the second test, the patient is asked to take his thumb and touch all his fingers consecutively, repeating this several times. Each hand is tested separately. The examiner notes problems with consecutive touching or missing the fingers completely.

Next, the nurse asks the patient to touch his nose with his index finger and then put that finger on the examiner's finger. The nurse holds her finger 2 feet in front of the patient's

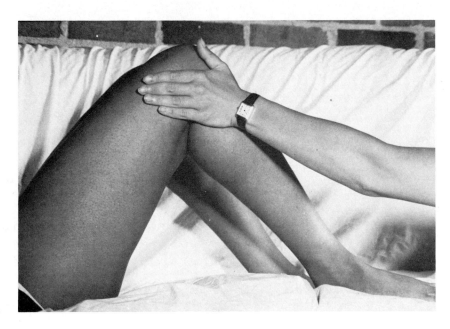

FIGURE 15.15
Hip abduction.

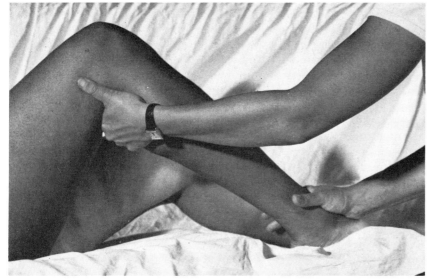

A

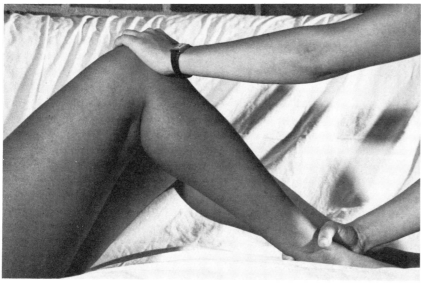

B

FIGURE 15.16
A. Knee extension. B. Knee flexion.

face. The patient is asked to touch the examiner's finger with his index finger and then touch his nose with his index finger. He must move his finger back and forth several times from the nurse's finger to his nose. The patient is then asked to close his eyes, after noting the location of the nurse's finger. Again he is to touch his nose and then her finger—this time with the eyes closed. The nurse should not move her finger during this part of the test.

Testing fine coordination of the lower ex-

tremities is simple. The patient should be in a supine position. He is instructed to close his eyes and place the heel of his foot on the opposite knee. Next he is asked to slide his heel down his shin to his foot. He is asked to do this a few times in a row. The nurse observes the smoothness of this maneuver. This test is repeated on the other extremity.

Another test of the lower extremities can be done with the patient in a sitting position and the nurse kneeling in front of him. The

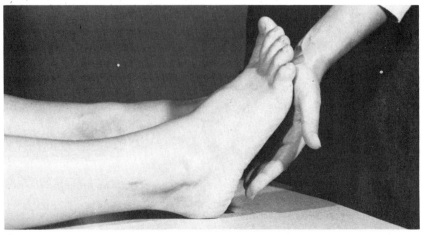

A

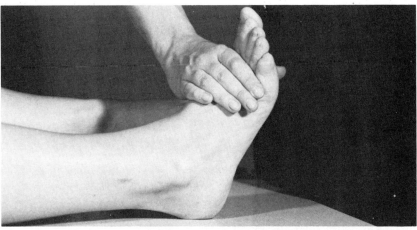

FIGURE 15.17
A. Plantar flexion of the ankle. **B.**
Dorsiflexion of the ankle.

B

nurse holds her index finger approximately 2 feet from the patient's foot. The patient is asked to touch her finger with his great toe as rapidly as possible. The nurse then moves her finger in several different locations as the patient repeats the process. Any problem with missing the moving or stable target is noted. The test is repeated with the other foot.

For screening purposes, one test is selected to test the cerebellar function in the upper extremities and one test is selected for the lower extremities. In testing the elderly patient, his increased reaction time to verbal suggestions must be taken into account. The nurse should also be alert for patient fatigue during this extensive testing. Accuracy and validity are essential.

With children, many of these tests are made into games. It is important to remember that geriatric patients tire more easily and that some decrease in their motor abilities is within normal limits.

The Sensory System

The screening examination for the sensory system includes assessment of pain, vibration, and light touch. Where a more detailed evaluation is required, the nurse adds *temperature sensation, position sense, discriminative sensation* (*stereognosis* and *two-point discrimination*), *point localization,* and *extinction.*

The sensory examination can be done quickly and efficiently, without fatiguing the patient if an organized approach is used. There are certain rules that should be applied consistently throughout the exam. First, stimuli

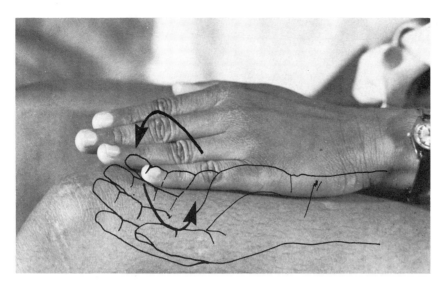

FIGURE 15.18
Hand coordination.

should be scattered and applied symmetrically wherever possible, so that all the dermatomes and peripheral areas are covered. Second, the more distal areas should always be tested first. If they are undamaged, the more proximal areas will be intact. Third, if any areas are suspect, the boundaries of the sensory changes need to be clearly mapped out.

The equipment used is a wisp of cotton, a safety pin, two straight pins, and a tuning fork. If the pain or light touch sensations are questionable, two test tubes with hot and cold water should be available.

The patient needs a careful explanation of the procedure because he will be asked to keep his eyes closed during the testing. Reassuring him that nothing will hurt him will help to gain his trust. In fact, it is helpful to demonstrate to the patient what will be done, while his eyes are still open, so that he knows what to expect.

SCREENING FOR THE SENSORY SYSTEM

Pain. A response to painful stimuli can be easily elicited with a safety pin. The patient is asked to close his eyes. Either the sharp or the dull end of the pin is placed at specific points on the body. The patient should be able to distinguish between sharp and dull. The nurse should start with the more distal areas (face, feet, and hands) and apply the pin in symmetrical positions, going from right to left or left to right. For screening purposes, the pin is applied to sites around the patient's an-

kles and wrists. If the distal locations are intact so are the proximal locations. The sharp and dull stimuli should be varied irregularly so that the patient does not come to rely on a pattern.

Vibration. This testing is carried out in a manner similar to that used for sharp and dull testing. The patient is again asked to close his eyes. The nurse places the vibrating tuning fork on bony prominences, such as the wrist, ankles, and forehead. The patient should be able to say when he feels the vibration on his body. A low-pitched (large) tuning fork will give stronger sensations. An alternate method involves placing the vibrating fork on a bony prominence and stopping the vibrations suddenly. The patient is asked to say when the sensation stops. If there is any doubt after testing the distal areas, little time is needed to evaluate the elbows, shoulders, knees, iliac crests, and spine. If these are found to be normal, the distal places should be retested to confirm findings.

Light Touch. Using the wisp of cotton, the nurse strokes the patient, while his eyes are closed, on different parts of his body. He is asked to state where he is being touched. Symmetrical testing is important here.

Detailed Examination of the Sensory System. These tests are used when there are complaints of numbness, tingling or loss of sensation, loss of motor function, areas of tissue breakdown, or muscle atrophy. Obviously, these tests can also be used to expand on information elicited during the screening test.

Temperature. This is applied when the patient is unable to distinguish between sharp and dull stimuli. The two test tubes, filled with hot and cold water, are placed on various parts of the body. The patient is asked to distinguish between hot and cold.

Position. The patient is asked to close his eyes. He is told that his big toe will be moved either up or down. He is to say when the toe is up and when it is down. The toe is held on the lateral aspects. When the nailbed is held, it is too easy for the patient to determine the position of the toe. This is repeated with the other foot and then with each hand.

DISCRIMINATIVE SENSATION

Stereognosis. For this test, a familiar object, such as a key, coin, or paper clip, is used. The patient is asked to open his hand and close his eyes. The nurse places the object in one hand and the patient is allowed to feel it with that hand. He is asked to identify the object. Another variation of this test is to write a number familiar to the patient in his palm. The blunt end of the reflex hammer or the nurse's finger will do. The patient should be able to identify the number. Both hands are tested.

Two-point Discrimination. The heads of two straight pins are placed on the patient's fingertip about 3 centimeters apart. The points are brought closer and closer together until he can only distinguish one point. The pins should not be more than 2 or 3 millimeters apart. One finger is tested on each hand (Fig. 15.19).

Point Localization. This test is relatively simple. The patient, with his eyes closed, is touched by the nurse somewhere on his body. She removes her hand. After that he opens his eyes and points to where he has been touched. This test is repeated on various parts of the patient's body.

Extinction. The patient's eyes are closed, and the nurse touches him on corresponding parts of his body at the same time (upper arms, knees, etc.). He is asked to state where he has been touched.

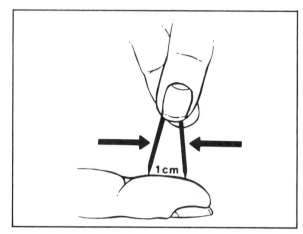

FIGURE 15.19
Two-point discrimination.

If discrepancies are found after completing the above tests, a referral is usually necessary. However, several factors may skew the results: fatigue on the part of the patient, poor instructions, or common skin abnormalities, such as callouses. Evaluating test results in children may be difficult. Making games out of all these tests will add to a child's cooperation. While evaluating the elderly patient, it must be remembered that during the normal aging process, perception of intense pain and temperature variations are decreased. However, normal aging does not affect the perception of light touch and mild pain. In assessing the sensory system and discriminative sensations of the elderly patient, the nurse must also be aware of the additional time needed for the patient to respond to the stimuli.

If there is a degree of uncertainty, evaluation on a different day, in a different setting, or at a different time may prove worthwhile. It should be remembered that documenting the specific boundaries of areas under suspicion is essential. To record the information, it may be easier to draw an outline of a person on the chart and label the involved areas. If there is any question, prompt referral is in order.

Reflexes

The discussion of assessment of the reflexes will include *infant reflexes, superficial reflexes,* and *deep tendon reflexes.* In all three cases, a reflex is a "reaction" to a provocation within the nervous system. It is not voluntary, learned, or conscious. However, with infant reflexes it is important to remember that the disappearance of specific reflexes at certain ages is appropriate and normal.

The quality of a reflex response to a stimuli will vary among individuals. In certain pathologic conditions (i.e., thyroid disorders), an abnormal reflex response may be a sign of the problem. Since the nervous system of the aging person may deteriorate gradually, it is possible that a patient's reflex responses will become less intense through the years.

REFLEX ACTIVITY IN THE NEWBORN AND INFANT

The major reflexes in the newborn and infant are the *rooting, sucking, Moro's, palmar grasp, dancing, tonic neck,* and *Babinski's.* As previously discussed, the intensity of these responses may vary considerably among population groups.

The Rooting Reflex. When the baby's cheek is stroked, he will turn his head toward the side being stroked. This response should be present from birth to about 4 months. If the upper lip on either side of the face is stroked, the baby will tip his head back, turn toward the stimulus, and open his mouth.

The Sucking Reflex. This reflex is also present at birth and can last to about 7 months. Putting something (a finger, nipple, etc.) in the baby's mouth will cause vigorous sucking. This is the action of the sucking reflex.

Moro Reflex. This is also known as the startle reflex. It can be elicited by creating a sudden noise, shaking the bed, or changing the baby's position suddenly. The first two of these stimuli will give a more accurate response. The loud noise can be supplied easily by clapping loudly over the baby's head. An alternate method of eliciting this response is to lift the baby by his hands from a supine position about 30 degrees. He is then lowered slowly to the table. As soon as his head touches the table the nurse lets go of his hands (Fig. 15.20A). The response is an abduction of the arms at the shoulder and an extension of the forearms at the elbow (Fig. 15.20A). The hands open, too. The next portion of this response is the baby's bringing all the extended extremities closer to his body. The legs follow an elongating movement like the upper torso response, but not as exaggerated. This reflex is present at birth and lasts up to 3 months.

The Palmar Grasp Reflex. When a finger or another object is placed in the palmar aspect of the baby's hand (usually the object is slid in on the ulnar side), the baby will surround the object with a strong grip for an extended period of time (Fig. 15.20B). After the infant grasps the examiner's hand and she draws her fingers upward, the baby's grip tightens as the muscle contraction spreads to the flexor muscles of his arm. The grip is so strong that the infant can be lifted from the bed (Rudolph & Hoffman, 1983). This reflex is present at birth and lasts for 6 months.

The Dancing (Stepping) Reflex. The baby is held in a standing position with support under the arms. When the baby's feet touch a flat surface, he will make dancing or stepping movements (Fig. 15.20C). The times this appears and disappears can vary. However, in most babies it can be elicited by the time the infant is 1 month old and can last for 12 months.

The Tonic Neck Reflex. This reflex does not usually develop until 2 months and only lasts until 6 months. The tonic neck reflex resembles the fencing position. When the baby is in the supine position and his head is turned in one direction, the arm and leg on the side he is facing will extend. The other arm and leg will flex. Special attention should be paid to the disappearance of this reflex.

Babinski's Reflex. There is some controversy over the validity of this reflex in an infant. Because there are reflexes which cause extension and flexion of the toes, some authorities hesitate to trust its validity. To elicit the Babinski, the bottom of the baby's foot is stroked from the heel, along the lateral aspect of the foot to the big toe and across the ball of the foot. A finger or an object, like the bottom of the reflex hammer, can be used. The great toe will dorsiflex and the four little toes will fan out, then extend (Fig. 15.21A). The final stage is the relaxation of the toes which gives the impression of curling around the examiner's finger (Fig. 15.21B). The reaction remains in babies until approximately 18 months.

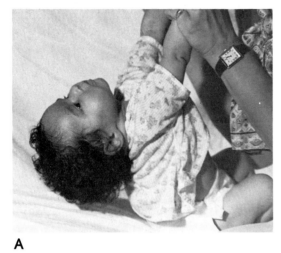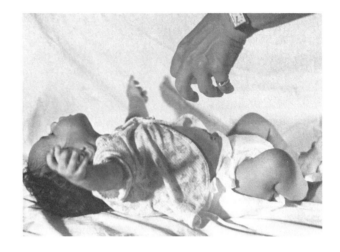

A

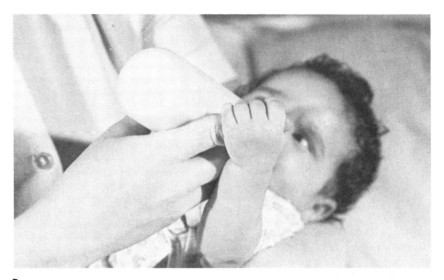

B

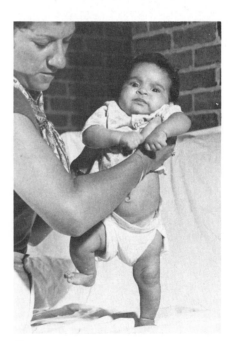

C

FIGURE 15.20
A. Moro reflex. **B.** Finger grasp reflex. **C.** Dancing reflex.

410

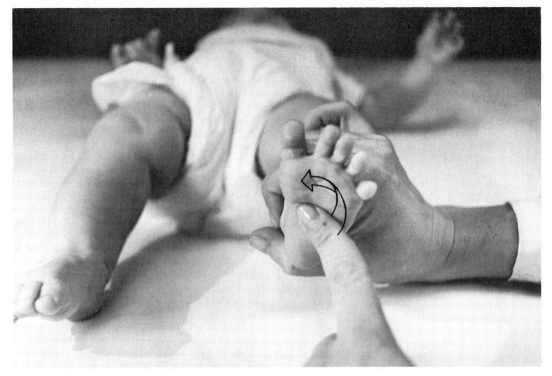

A

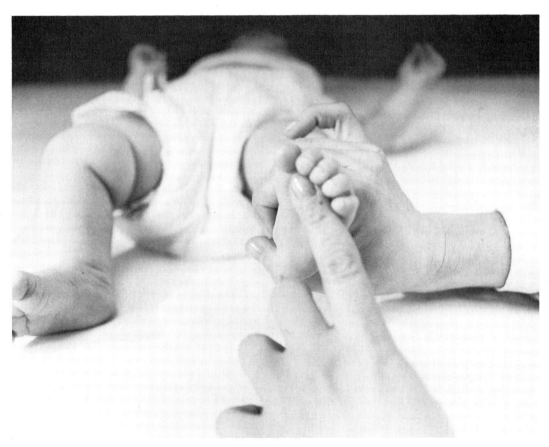

B

FIGURE 15.21
Babinski response. **A.** *Dorsiflexion motion.* **B.** *End response.*

Ankle Clonus. Ankle clonus can be elicited in infants. The thumb of the examiner is placed on the ball of the infant's foot. The foot is then dorsiflexed abruptly and held in that position. The response is rhythmic contractions and relaxation of the gastrocnemius muscle. There may be several contractions after each stimulus.

This is not actually a reflex. However, it is an involuntary oscillation of a specific area which may be indicative of upper motor neuron disease in adults. Most healthy adults have no oscillation with this maneuver. Ankle clonus is most frequently tested if the Achille's response (the contraction of the gastrocnemius when it is tapped with a reflex hammer, also known as "the ankle jerk") is hyperactive.

Deep Tendon Reflexes. Proper technique in eliciting deep tendon reflexes is essential for two reasons. First, it has already been stated that everyone will have a different quality of response to the stimulus. For example, in advanced age, deep tendon reflexes are diminished and may even be absent. The nurse must know how to evaluate the boundaries of different ranges of "normal." Second, if technique is faulty, there is likely to be an asymmetrical response, which will result in false findings. A bilateral symmetrical reflex response is probably the most valid tool for ascertaining absence of disease. Thus, good dexterity with and knowledge of this skill is a must.

A reflex hammer is used to elicit a deep tendon reflex. The hammer is held loosely between the thumb and index finger. The wrist must also be very loose and the hammer is swung up and down. The loose wrist motion is similar to the wrist motion used with percussion. Further detail on how to elicit each deep tenson reflex is presented below.

Appropriate elicitation of reflexes involves more than the dexterity of the nurse. The patient must be relaxed, or no response will occur. Therefore, the nurse must be sure that the patient understands the procedure, so that he can relax.

For measurement of the reflex response, a scale is available with a gradation from 0 to +4 (Chart 15.4). Because there is so much room for subjective interpretation of this scale, it is most reliable to evaluate the response in terms of symmetry. For this reason, the nurse should test each reflex bilaterally before moving down the body. This allows for immediate comparison of the response.

The deep tendon reflexes to be elicited are: the *biceps,* the *triceps,* the *brachioradialis* (supinator), *patellar,* and *Achilles tendon* reflexes. All of these are tested with a reflex hammer.

The Biceps Reflex (Spinal Cord Level: C_5, C_6). The patient's arm is flexed at the elbow and held by the nurse. The nurse places her thumb horizontally over the biceps tendon. A blow is delivered with the hammer to her thumb (Fig. 15.22). There will be slight flexion of the elbow, and the nurse will be able to feel the biceps contraction through her thumb.

The Triceps Reflex (Spinal Cord Level: C_6, C_7, C_8). The patient's arm is again flexed at the elbow. The nurse palpates for the triceps tendon about 2 to 5 centimeters (1 or 2 inches) above the elbow. She then delivers the blow with the hammer directly to the tendon (Fig. 15.23). The patient is observed for contraction of the tricep tendon and slight extension of the elbow.

The Brachioradialis Reflex (Spinal Cord Level: C_5, C_6). The patient's forearm can rest on the nurse's forearm or his own leg. The hammer strikes the tendon over the radius 2 to 5 centimeters (1 or 2 inches) above the wrist. The patient is observed for flexion and supination of the forearm (Fig. 15.24). The fingers of the patient's hand may also extend slightly in this response.

The Patellar Knee Jerk (Spinal Cord Level: L_2, L_3, L_4). This can be more difficult to elicit if the patient is not relaxed completely. The patient should be sitting up if possible with his legs dangling over the side of the bed or table. If he is unable to sit up, the examiner slides her arm under the patient's knees as he flexes them. The patellar tendon is tapped with the

CHART 15.4
GRADATION OF REFLEX RESPONSES

0 = No reflex response
+1 = Below normal
+2 = Average
+3 = Stronger than average
+4 = Very intense response (may resemble clonus)

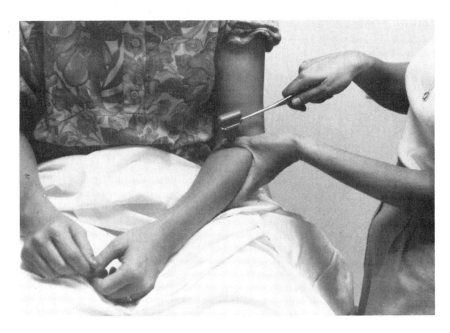

FIGURE 15.22
The biceps reflex.

hammer (Fig. 15.25). The tendon is usually found directly below the patella itself. When no response can be obtained, often the patient's legs are not relaxed enough. In this case he is asked to interlock his fingers and pull while the examiner taps the tendon. This allows him to loosen up his legs so that the accuracy of the brisk response is not distorted.

The Achilles Tendon Reflex (Spinal Cord Level: L₅, S₁, S₂). This should follow the patella reflex so that the patient can remain in the same position. To tap this reflex, the patient's ankle is dorsiflexed. With the foot held in this position, the examiner delivers the blow to the Achilles tendon just above the heel (Fig. 15.26). This reaction will be plantar flexion of the heel. The nurse will feel this in her hand as well as see it. If the patient is unable to sit up, the nurse can take the foot and place it on the opposite shin. This forces dorsiflexion as well. Another method to use if the patient is ambulatory is to ask him to kneel on the seat of the chair with his feet dangling over

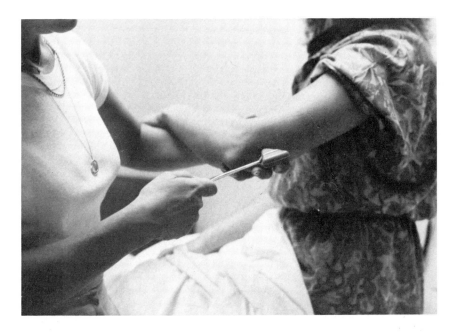

FIGURE 15.23
The triceps reflex.

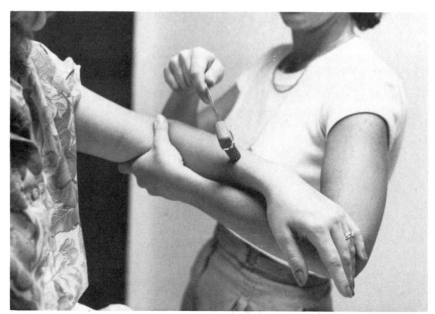

FIGURE 15.24
The brachioradialis reflex.

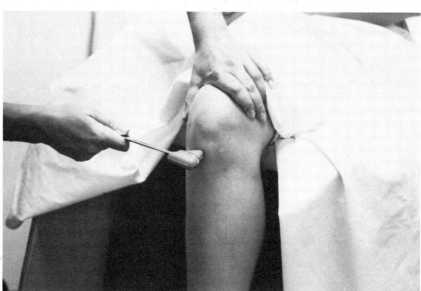

FIGURE 15.25
The knee-jerk reflex.

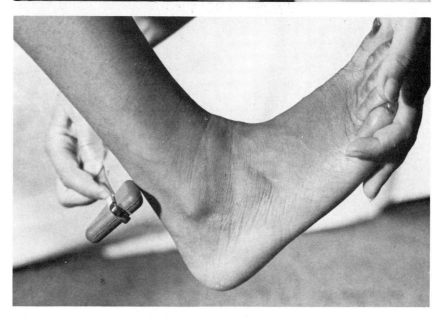

FIGURE 15.26
The Achilles tendon reflex (patient sitting).

414

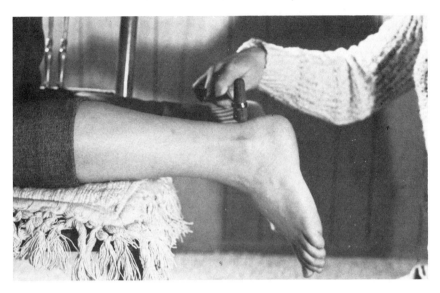

FIGURE 15.27
The Achilles tendon reflex (patient kneeling over a chair).

the edge (Fig. 15.27). This, too, forces dorsiflexion of the foot.

SUPERFICIAL REFLEXES
The superficial reflexes include the *abdominal reflex,* the *cremasteric reflex,* the *corneal reflex,* and *Babinski's reflex.*

The Abdominal Reflex (T_6–T_{12}). The abdominal reflex is elicited by stroking each quadrant of the abdomen toward the umbilicus with a blunt firm object (a key, the handle of the reflex hammer) (Fig. 15.28).

The response will be a contraction of the subadjacent abdominal muscles and the movement of the umbilicus toward the stimulus. This superficial reflex may be absent in abdomens with poor muscle tone as in multiparity, obesity, or the elderly.

The Cremasteric Reflex (Spinal Cord Level: L_1, L_2). This can only be elicited in males. It is

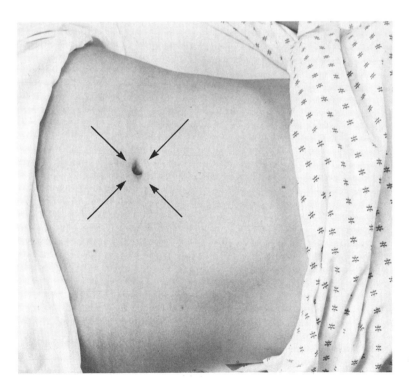

FIGURE 15.28
The abdominal reflex.

present by the age of 6 months. The inside of the patient's upper thigh is stroked upward with an object (a finger will do). The response to note is the rising of the testicle on the side being stroked.

The Corneal Reflex. See the section on "The Cranial Nerves" in this chapter; also see Chapter 5, page 136.

Babinski's Reflex (Spinal Cord Level: L_4, L_5, S_1, S_2). As stated earlier, this should not be positive in an adult. Performance of this test is the same for both infants and adults. In an adult, if upper motor neuron disease is present, there will often be a positive Babinski's response (Fig. 15.29).

Tests for Meningeal Inflammation

Meningeal inflammation is not assessed for screening purposes. However, any time a child presents with symptoms of an upper respiratory infection, these tests should be done. In an adult, any suspicion of intracranial dysfunction (due to infection, for instance), systemic problems, or trauma, is an indication for this evaluation. Any positive findings justify immediate referral and further investigation. The signs tested for the presence of meningeal inflammation include Brudzinski's sign, Kernig's sign, and nuchal rigidity.

BRUDZINSKI'S SIGN

The patient should be lying flat on his back. The nurse places her hand under the patient's head (on the occiput) and raises his head toward his chest. A child may comply more readily if asked to look at his "belly button." The patient with a positive sign will resist this or have pain. Hip and knee flexion may also occur.

KERNIG'S SIGN

The patient is still supine. One leg is flexed at the hip and then the knee at about 90 degrees. The nurse attempts to straighten the knee (Fig. 15.30). Resistance or pain in the hamstrings is a postive sign for meningeal irritation.

NUCHAL RIGIDITY

Any pain or resistance with flexion or rotation of the neck can be indicative of meningeal irritation. However, this may be the result of muscular problems. The nurse should be sure the history and other symptoms correlate with a neurologic problem as opposed to muscular injury or tension.

Developmental Assessment in Children

Assessment of the developmental level of a child is not only important in the neurologic examination, but also serves as major screening for all children. The developmental level is measured by testing certain abilities, including motor, communicative, and interactive skills. Special emphasis is placed on the population between birth and 6 years of age. After 6 years, one assumes that the school will take over the testing regarding learning ability. Even so, the examiner performing the annual health assessment should ask certain questions pertinent to the developmental tasks and test certain motor skills that are appropriate to each age group.

There are several standardized tests available to measure the accomplishment of these tasks. In selecting a particular test, it is important to consider its reliability, validity, standardization, simplicity of administration, expense, ease in scoring, and interpretation. As

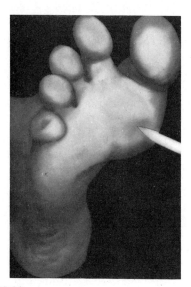

FIGURE 15.29
Babinski's reflex. Pathologic response in an adult. (From Heagarty, M., et al. Child Health: Basics for Primary Care. New York: Appleton-Century-Crofts, 1980, p. 170.)

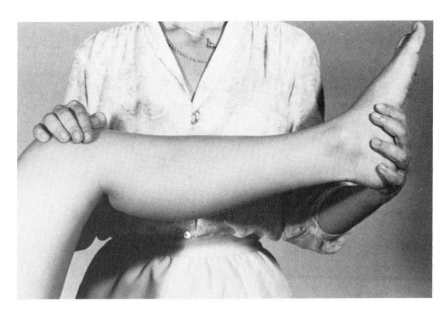

FIGURE 15.30
Kernig's sign.

previously discussed, while racial developmental differences have been reported, no cross-racial standardized tests are yet available.

To exemplify the screening process, the most universally accepted test will be described: The Denver Developmental Screening Test (DDST). This test was developed at the University of Colorado in the late 1960s. Its widespread use is due to its high rate of reliability and validity in testing as well as its ease in administration.

The DDST evaluates four areas of development:

1. Gross motor, which involves an emphasis on the musculoskeletal and nervous systems.
2. Communication skills, including comprehension, expression, hearing, and speech.
3. Fine motor skills, which involve eye–hand coordination.
4. Personal, including social behavior, which relates to self-care and interaction with others.

The DDST is *not* a diagnostic test. It does test the developmental level in children from birth to age 6. Lack of achievement in certain areas warrants further investigation but does not label a child as retarded, handicapped, or slow.

There are two ways to approach the DDST: the indirect and the direct methods. In the indirect method, the examiner asks the parent about specific abilities and behaviors. In the direct approach the examiner observes the child performing a task.

The direct method is much more valid. However, there are some tasks the child may refuse to perform, but which he is capable of doing. In this instance, the examiner should check with the parents and accept their word.

There are several factors to consider before testing the child:

1. *The facility:* The setting should be non-threatening, well lit, and quiet.
2. *Health of the child:* The test should be deferred if the child has been ill or under stress or has experienced recent trauma.
3. *Attention span:* If the child is at a stage where his attention span is short, this should be taken into account.
4. *Fatigue:* If the child has spent a long day in school or it is late in the day, another time should be scheduled.
5. *Eating:* If an infant has just been fed, he is likely to want to sleep. In addition, some spitting up may occur just after feeding, especially during motor skill testing. A hungry child may not be cooperative either.
6. *Painful or frightening procedures:* All testing should be done before any painful

or frightening procedures are administered.

7. *Explanation to parents:* An explanation to the parents is essential. The nurse should emphasize that this is *not* an intelligence test, that the child will be asked to do certain things on levels he will not be expected to have achieved yet. Whether or not the parent should be present depends on the interaction between the parent, child, and examiner. If the child is more comfortable with the parent(s) present, then the parent(s) should be allowed to stay.

8. *Rapport:* This may be the most important uncontrollable item on this list. A sense of trust must exist between the examiner and the child or all the information elicited may be invalid.

THE TWO STAGE SCREENING PROCESS

Although the DDST is considered extremely valuable and important in assessing developmental level in children, there has been considerable reluctance among health care providers to use it. Research studies have indicated that physicians tend to rely on their own clinical judgment to assess developmental problems. (Carr, 1964; Bierman, et al., 1964; Smith, 1978). For this reason, as well as the need to update the format of the test, a two-stage screening process has been devised.

A further change in the testing concept has been made, as well. There is now a questionnaire used to include parental opinion, and in certain cases, information about the child's home environment. The questionnaire chosen depends on the educational level of the parents. There has been recent documentation that socioeconomic level can have an effect on a child's development (Sameroff, 1975; Werner, et al., 1971). Therefore, one questionnaire was developed to be used for parents in whom one or both has less than a high school education. The other is used when both parents have at least a high school education.

The tool used when one or both parents have less than a high school education is called the *Home Screening Questionnaire (HSQ)* (Coons, et al., 1978). It has been shown that one of the main correlations with lack of school achievement is a home environment that is not conducive to a child's development

(Coons, et al., 1978). This test, therefore, is designed to quickly evaluate the home environment. The test takes 5 to 8 minutes to score and can be done so by a non-professional.

The questionnaire used when both parents have at least a high school education is a parent-answered form. This tool can be administered easily in a waiting room setting. It has been shown that parents of this educational level are able to report accurately their child's developmental status (Frankenberg, 1984). Both questionnaires help to confirm the objective findings of the DDST.

The screening process has two stages. The first step includes a quick or abbreviated version of the full DDST. When the quick screening is used, if any items are missed, a full test is administered. In order to better understand the principles and process of administering the test, the full version will be explained in detail prior to the abbreviated form.

The equipment needed for this test is available in an inexpensive kit. The kit's contents include red wool, raisins, a rattle with a narrow handle, eight 1-inch square colored blocks (red, blue, yellow, green), a small glass bottle with an opening no bigger than ⅝ inch, a small bell, a tennis ball, and a pencil. Also needed are the test sheet and the instructions on its reverse side (Figs. 15.31 and 15.32).

How to Administer the Test

1. The chronologic age of the child must be established. This is done by subtracting the birthdate from the date of the test.

DATE	YEAR	MONTH	DAY
Date of test	86	7	15
Birthdate	81	3	10
Chronologic age	5	4	3

2. The nurse takes the test form and draws a line from the top to the bottom of the page at the corresponding age. The line should be drawn through all four areas of development. If the child was premature, the number of weeks premature should be subtracted from the chronologic age (Fig. 15.32). The line is drawn at the adjusted age.
3. The date the test is administered is written at the top of the age line. If an adjust-

DATE
NAME
DIRECTIONS
BIRTHDATE
HOSP. NO.

1. Try to get child to smile by smiling, talking or waving to him. Do not touch him.
2. When child is playing with toy, pull it away from him. Pass if he resists.
3. Child does not have to be able to tie shoes or button in the back.
4. Move yarn slowly in an arc from one side to the other, about 6" above child's face.
   Pass if eyes follow 90° to midline. (Past midline; 180°)
5. Pass if child grasps rattle when it is touched to the backs or tips of fingers.
6. Pass if child continues to look where yarn disappeared or tries to see where it went. Yarn
   should be dropped quickly from sight from tester's hand without arm movement.
7. Pass if child picks up raisin with any part of thumb and a finger.
8. Pass if child picks up raisin with the ends of thumb and index finger using an over hand
   approach.

 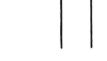

9. Pass any en-   10. Which line is longer?   11. Pass any   12. Have child copy
    closed form.   (Not bigger.) Turn   crossing   first. If failed,
    Fail continuous   paper upside down and   lines.   demonstrate
    round motions.   repeat. (3/3 or 5/6)

When giving items 9, 11 and 12, do not name the forms. Do not demonstrate 9 and 11.

13. When scoring, each pair (2 arms, 2 legs, etc.) counts as one part.
14. Point to picture and have child name it. (No credit is given for sounds only.)

 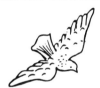 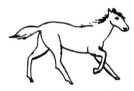 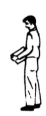

15. Tell child to: Give block to Mommie; put block on table; put block on floor. Pass 2 of 3.
    (Do not help child by pointing, moving head or eyes.)
16. Ask child: What do you do when you are cold? ..hungry? ..tired? Pass 2 of 3.
17. Tell child to: Put block on table; under table; in front of chair, behind chair.
    Pass 3 of 4. (Do not help child by pointing, moving head or eyes.)
18. Ask child: If fire is hot, ice is ?; Mother is a woman, Dad is a ?; a horse is big, a
    mouse is ?. Pass 2 of 3.
19. Ask child: What is a ball? ..lake? ..desk? ..house? ..banana? ..curtain? ..ceiling?
    ..hedge? ..pavement? Pass if defined in terms of use, shape, what it is made of or general
    category (such as banana is fruit, not just yellow). Pass 6 of 9.
20. Ask child: What is a spoon made of? ..a shoe made of? ..a door made of? (No other objects
    may be substituted.) Pass 3 of 3.
21. When placed on stomach, child lifts chest off table with support of forearms and/or hands.
22. When child is on back, grasp his hands and pull him to sitting. Pass if head does not hang back
23. Child may use wall or rail only, not person. May not crawl.
24. Child must throw ball overhand 3 feet to within arm's reach of tester.
25. Child must perform standing broad jump over width of test sheet. (8-1/2 inches)
26. Tell child to walk forward, ⚯⚯⚯⚯ heel within 1 inch of toe.
    Tester may demonstrate. Child must walk 4 consecutive steps, 2 out of 3 trials.
27. Bounce ball to child who should stand 3 feet away from tester. Child must catch ball with
    hands, not arms, 2 out of 3 trials.
28. Tell child to walk backward, ←⚯⚯⚯⚯ toe within 1 inch of heel.
    Tester may demonstrate. Child must walk 4 consecutive steps, 2 out of 3 trials.

DATE AND BEHAVIORAL OBSERVATIONS (how child feels at time of test, relation to tester, attention
span, verbal behavior, self-confidence, etc,):

FIGURE 15.31
*Directions for Denver Developmental Screening Test. (From Frankenburg, W. K. and Dodds,
J. B., University of Colorado Medical Center, 1969.)*

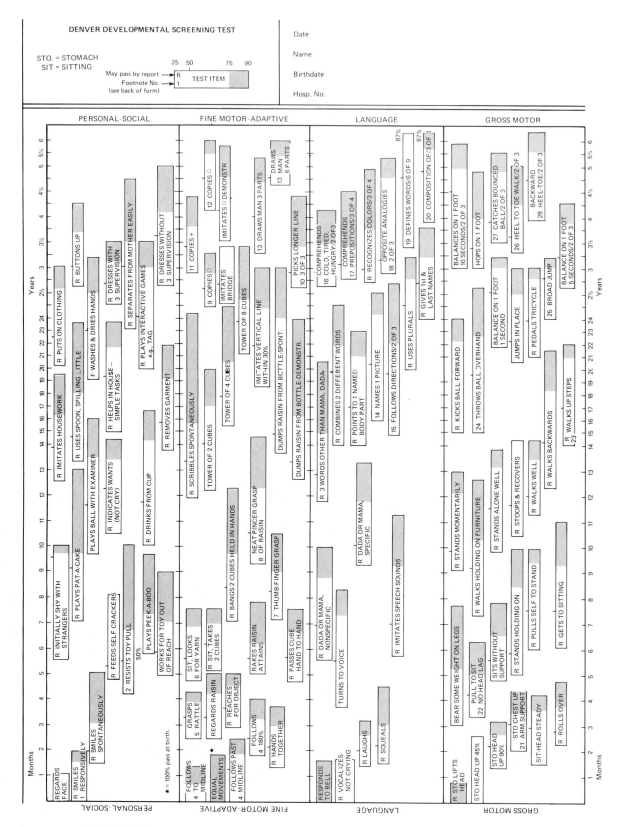

FIGURE 15.32
Form for Denver Development Screening Test. (From Frankenburg, W. K. and Dodds, J. B., University of Colorado Medical Center, 1969.)

ment was made for prematurity, this should be indicated under the date.

4. Full instructions are on the back of the sheet.

5. At this point the child is tested. The tasks he should be asked to do are listed along the drawn line.

6. Each item is represented by a bar. The bar is placed on paper to show that 25, 50, 75, or 90 percent of all children (standardized population) can perform that task at that age. The short slash shows the 50 percent cut-off, the left end of the shaded area represents the 75 percent group, and the right end of the shaded area shows the 90 percent performance level.

7. There is also a standardized method of scoring. If a child refuses to perform a particular item, the nurse should let the parent try. If still unsuccessful, *R* (refusal) should be recorded, as opposed to *F* (failure). *P* is the letter used to indicate a "pass." The last score option is *N.O.* (no opportunity). In some cases, a child may not have had the opportunity to learn certain skills, such as riding a tricycle. In other instances, cultural differences may interfere with performance. If this is the case, it is certainly not fair to fail the child in that area. Thus, the score "N.O." should not be used in the interpretation.

Before designating the score *F*, it is important to give the child at least three chances to perform the test. Administering the test on another day should be considered, too.

A "delay" is any item failed by the child which is completely to the left of the age line. In other words, the child may have failed an item which 90 percent of children normally pass at a younger age. This is documented on the form by coloring the right end of the bar of the delayed item. If the bar touches the age line, it should not be considered a delay.

The child should be tested on all items which pass through the age line. In addition, the child should be tested within each section for at least three expected failures and three expected passes. It helps build up the child's confidence to start with three items well below his age level.

At the completion of the test, the parents should be asked if the child's performance was typical of his activities at other times.

The results are classified within each sector as *normal, abnormal,* or *questionable.* The term *normal* is accepted when there is no doubt about the results. The term *abnormal* can be used under the following circumstances: (1) there are two or more delays in two or more sectors or (2) there are two or more delays in one sector, one delay in one or more sectors, and no passes intersecting the age line in the latter sector(s). The term *questionable* can be used when there are (1) two or more delays in one sector or (2) one delay in one or more sectors and no passes intersecting the age line in that (those) sector(s).

Children whose test scores are *abnormal* or *questionable* should be reevaluated within 2 or 3 weeks. If another *abnormal* score is obtained and the parent indicates that this is a typical performance level for the child, further evaluation is warranted.

There is an alternative form to the DDST, called the DDST-R (Fig. 15.33). It is not considered a replacement form, but an alternative to the original form. The DDST-R was designed to look more like the standardized growth forms that health care providers use to chart a child's physical growth and development. Some providers may find the revised form easier to use from a visual standpoint. Either is acceptable.

How to Administer the Abbreviated or First Stage DDST

The complete DDST can take 15 to 20 minutes to administer. Some health care providers feel they cannot justify this time (Smith, 1978). For this reason, the more brief version of the DDST has been developed and proven valid.

To administer this test, the examiner tests only 12 total items. She tests any three items in each sector that are immediately to the left, but not touching, the age line. The child must successfully complete all 12 items, or the complete DDST must be given. (Frankenberg, 1984). Statistics gathered recently demonstrated that only 25 percent of all children will fail this first-stage screening (Frankenberg, 1984).

422

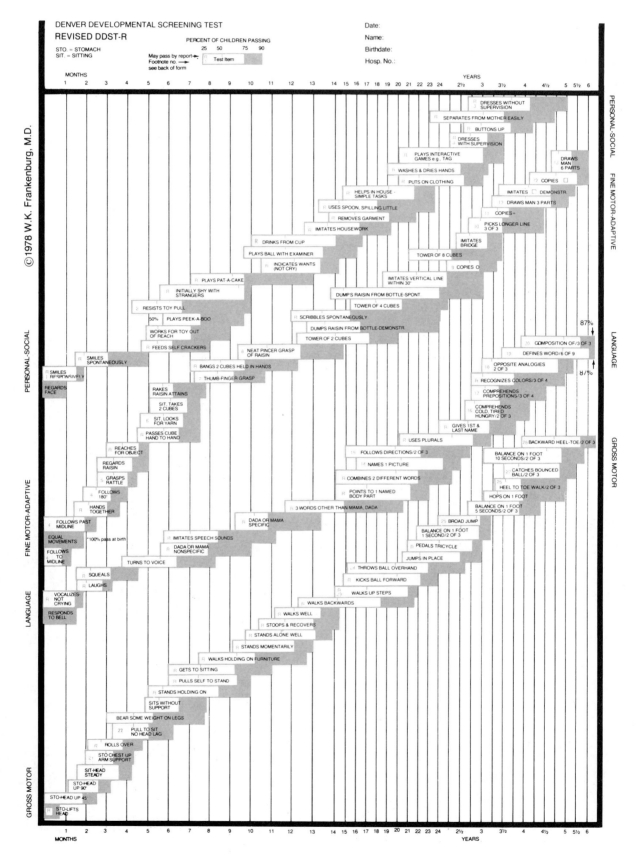

FIGURE 15.33
DDST-R Screening Test. (From Frankenburg, W. K. and Dodds, J. B., University of Colorado Medical Center, 1969.)

The reliability of the test results depends a great deal on the sensitivity of the examiner to the child and the environment. Illness, fear, or the atmosphere of the testing area may distort the results. For this reason, it is important for the nurse to write down her observations of the child's behavior. The behavior observed includes attention span, nonverbal communication, and the relationship with the nurse or parent.

Observation of the parent–child interaction during the test may prove valuable to the nurse. Any signs of overdependency or hostility may manifest here. The nurse can also assess problems of emotional development during this entire process—for instance, lack of interest, lack of eye contact, preoccupation, withdrawal, or excessive shyness.

Above all, it is important to remember that this is a screening test, *not* a diagnostic tool. Its basic purpose is to alert the examiner to any need for further evaluation.

Screening Examination of the Neurologic System

1. Assessment of mental status.
2. Evaluation of Cranial Nerves II, III, IV, V (motor), VI, VII (motor), VIII, IX (motor), X (motor), XI, and XII. (Remember most of these tests are done within the exam of the head, face, eye, ear, and mouth.
3. Assessment for motor function includes:
   a. Walking
   b. Kneebends (if the patient is able)
   c. Hopping
   d. Balance (Romberg)
   e. Heel-toe walking
4. Evaluation of sensory function includes:
   a. Vibratory sensation in the hand and feet; or
   b. Sharp and dull testing in the hands and feet
5. Assessment of coordination
   a. Hand coordination—See Figure 15.18 (to test upper extremities)
   b. Position sense (to the test lower extremities)
6. Assessment of deep tendon reflexes.
7. Developmental status at appropriate ages.

EXAMPLE OF A RECORDED HISTORY AND PHYSICAL

SUBJECTIVE:

Chief Complaint: "Headache and dizziness twice today."

HPH: This 75-year-old male considers himself to be in "fair" health. He has "severe arthritis" which has been a problem for "years." His day began as usual with no problems until 10:00 A.M, when he suddenly noticed he had a dull ache behind his forehead. About 15 minutes later he felt dizzy, too. "The room began spinning around." He took two aspirin, laid down for an hour and "felt fine." About 2 hours ago, the same pain in his head began again, but was more "intense." About 1 hour ago his wife told him that his words were slurring. Half an hour ago his vision became blurry—only out of his left eye. He has no previous history of this type of episode, loss of consciousness, fainting, convulsions, trauma, tingling or numbness, tremors or tics, paralysis, or speech disorders. He takes Motrin 400 mg. t.i.d. for his arthritis. Does not take any other medications except an occasional aspirin. There is a family history of heart disease. Both parents died in their "mid-seventies" of a "stroke." His wife called their family doctor, and he instructed her to take her husband to the emergency room. Patient feels he is "losing control of the situation."

OBJECTIVE:

T. 98.8°F axillary; P. 96 radial; R. 24; B.P. (R) 180/100 (lying), (L) 182/106.

MENTAL STATUS. Patient, when sitting in wheelchair, was somewhat slouched. He is frowning and his face reflects tension. His speech is slurred, but words can be understood. He is oriented to time, person, and place. He recalls recent and remote events. Abstract thinking and similarity association testing deferred.

CRANIAL NERVES

I: Deferred at present.

II: Right—able to read paper 1 foot away. Left—not able to distinguish letters or words. *Visual fields:* right—within normal limits; Left—(?) < on periphery. *Funduscopic:* Right—unremarkable; Left—A–V ratio approximately 2:4, disc unremarkable; no A–V nicking, exudates, or hemorrhages.

III, IV, VI: Right—no ptosis, lid lag, PERRLA; no nystagmus; extraocular movements intact. Left—ptosis present, unable to hold glance at upper-left outer quadrant; no nystagmus, lid lag; consensual reaction to light slow.

V: *Sensory*—corneal reflexes present in both eyes. Able to distinguish light touch and sharp from dull on right side of face, chin, and right temporal area. Unable to feel stimulus from wisp of cotton on left temporal or left side of face. Can distinguish sharp from dull all over left side of face. Can also distinguish between hot and cold in the area where light touch is decreased. *Motor*—unable to clench teeth firmly. Temporomandibular contractions weaker on left side.

VII: No tics, tremors, unusual movement, or asymmetry. When asked to clench teeth, smile, unable to hold this position. Difficulty blowing out cheeks with mouth closed, more pronounced on left. Taste testing deferred at present.

VIII: Deferred at present.

IX, X: Uvula rises. No asymmetry of soft palate. Gag response elicited. No hoarseness.

XI: Left—weakness of shoulder when push applied to shrugged shoulders. Weakness also noted when patient pushes face against hand. Right—can resist shoulder shrug and push face against hand.

XII: No asymmetry, unusual movement or deviation of tongue.

MOTOR SYSTEM. Dragging left foot when walking from wheel chair to stretcher. Romberg—could not stand without falling with eyes closed.

	RIGHT	LEFT
Finger grip	Strong	Very weak
Finger abduction	Unremarkable	Weaker than right
Wrist dorsiflexion	Unremarkable	Weaker than right
Flexion and extension of elbow	Unremarkable	Weaker than right
Shoulder and scapulae resistance	Unremarkable	Weaker than right
Hip flexion	Unremarkable	Weaker than right
Hip abduction	Unremarkable	Weaker than right
Hip adduction	Unremarkable	Weaker than right
Knee extension and flexion	Unremarkable	Weaker than right
Plantar flexion and dorsiflexion of ankle (no pain with testing)		

Sensory: Able to distinguish sharp from dull along the right side from shoulder to foot. On left side not able to do this on foot or shin, hand or forearm. Thigh, hip, abdomen, chest, and upper arm intact. Able to distinguish vibratory sensation along right side, wrist, knee, elbow, shoulder, hip, and foot. Unable to feel vibratory sensation on left wrist and left hip. Other areas distinguishable. Unable to distinguish position (up or down) of left big toe. Other areas intact. Rest of sensory exam deferred at present due to fatigue of patient.

Deep Tendon Reflexes: All intact; +2 and symmetrical. No right or left ankle clonus.

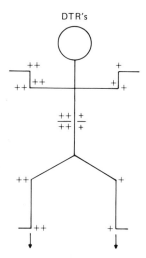

DTR's

Chest: Respirations regular. Chest expansion symmetrical. Clear to auscultation. No adventitious breath sounds.

Heart: Regular rate. No murmurs heard. Left carotid bruit present. Right carotid, no bruit.

Pulses:

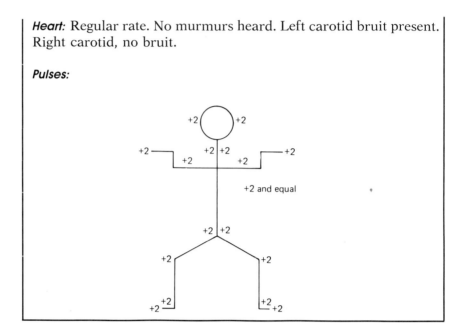

REFERENCES

Bierman, J., Connor, A., Veage, M., et al. (1964). Pediatrician's assessment of intelligence of two-year olds and their mental test scores. Pediatrics, 34, 680.

Branch, M., & Paxton, P. (1976). Providing Safe Nursing Care for Ethnic People of Color. New York: Appleton-Century-Crofts.

Carr, J. (1964). Pediatricians and developmental tests. Developmental medicine. Child Neurology, 6, 614.

Coons, C., Frankenberg, W., Garrett, E., et al. (1978). Proceedings Second International Conference and Developmental Screening. Denver: University of Colorado Press.

Frankenberg, W. (1984). Routine, periodic developmental screening: Practical approaches for primary health care providers. Ross Timesaver–Public Health Currents. Columbus, Ohio: Ross Laboratories.

Freedman, D. (1979). Ethnic differences in babies. Human Nature, 2, 36–44.

Freedman, D., & DeBoer, M. (1979). Biological and cultural differences in early child development. Annual Review of Anthropology, 8, 379–600.

Jensen, D. (1980). The Principles of Physiology (2nd ed). New York: Appleton-Century-Crofts.

Kahn, R., Goldfarb, A., Pollack, M., & Peck, A. (1960). Brief objective measures for the determination of mental status in the aged. American Journal of Psychiatry, 117, 326–28.

Mezey, M., Rauckhorst, L., & Stokes, S. (1980). Health Assessment of the Older Individual. New York: Springer Publishing.

Rudolph, A., & Hoffman, J. (Eds.). (1983) Pediatrics (17th ed.). Norwalk, Conn.: Appleton-Century-Crofts.

Sameroff, A. (1975). Early influences on development: Fact or fancy? Merrill-Palmer Q, 21, 267–94.

Smith, R. (1978). The use of developmental screening tests by primary care physicians. Journal of Pediatrics, 93, 524.

Wang, H. (1980). Diagnostic procedures. In C. Busse and D. Blazer, (Eds.),

Handbook of Geriatric Psychiatry. New York: Van Nostrand Reinhold, p. 294.

Werner, E., Bierman, J., & Franch, F. (1971). The Children of Kauai. Honolulu: University of Hawaii Press.

Wolanin, M., & Phillips, L. (1981). Confusion: Prevention and Care. St. Louis: C. V. Mosby.

Zuidema, G. (1977). The Johns Hopkins Atlas of Human Anatomy. Baltimore: Johns Hopkins University Press.

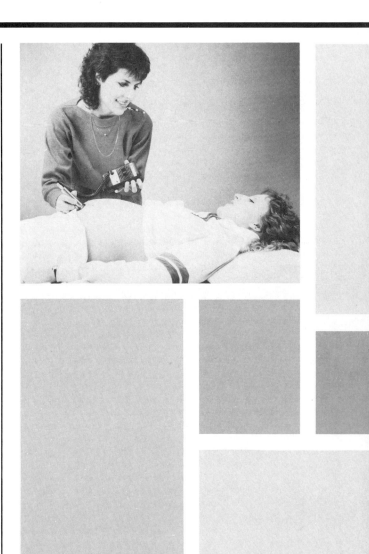

16

The Prenatal Patient

As nursing expands its horizons, and its practice accepts new challenges, the question arises: What is the role of nursing in prenatal assessment? There are a variety of opinions on this subject. However, one point of view is maintained. Pregnancy is a state of wellness, not illness. If a major portion of nursing care is wellness-oriented, then nurses have an important place in the care of the pregnant patient and her family.

For nurses to be able to assess the pregnant patient, some fundamental knowledge needs to be obtained. Not only is it important to be able to locate and count the fetal heart rate, it is also essential to know the physiological changes that are occurring in the mother and the fetus at the time the heart rate is heard. Of equal importance are the psychological changes experienced by the pregnant woman. Knowledge of these changes will help the nurse to identify variations from normal. A nurse with a firm grounding in both the physiological and psychological changes of pregnancy will be able to obtain accurate and relevant historical and physical data.

To facilitate the discussion of the changes of pregnancy and the prenatal assessment, some basic terminology will be covered. First, there are different terms used to describe fetal age and some are confusing. The *gestational age or menstrual age* (Chart 16.1) is the age calculated by referring back to the date of the last menstrual period before conception. Therefore, the date for fetal age is calculated to be 2 weeks prior to ovulation and fertilization, which is almost 3 weeks before implantation. Birth should occur 40 weeks or 280 days from the date of the last menstrual period

432

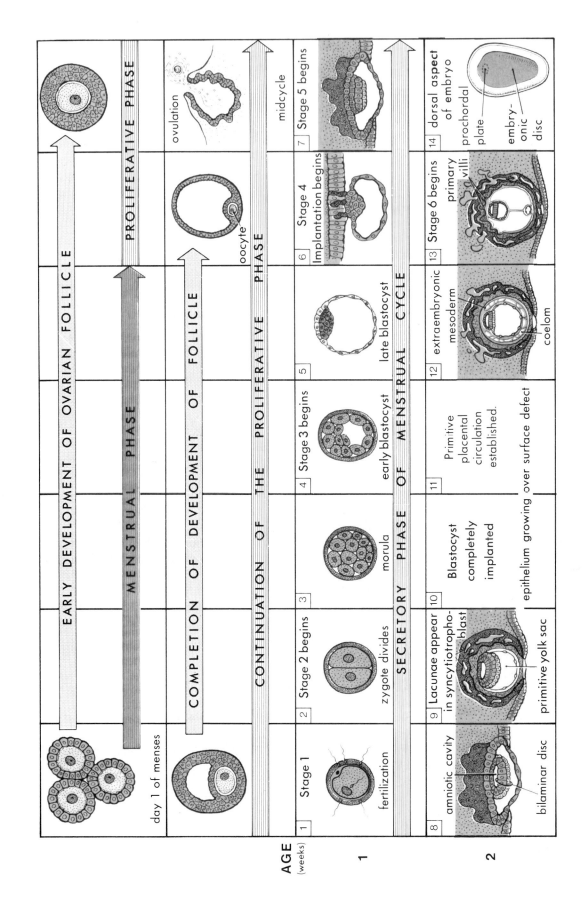

433

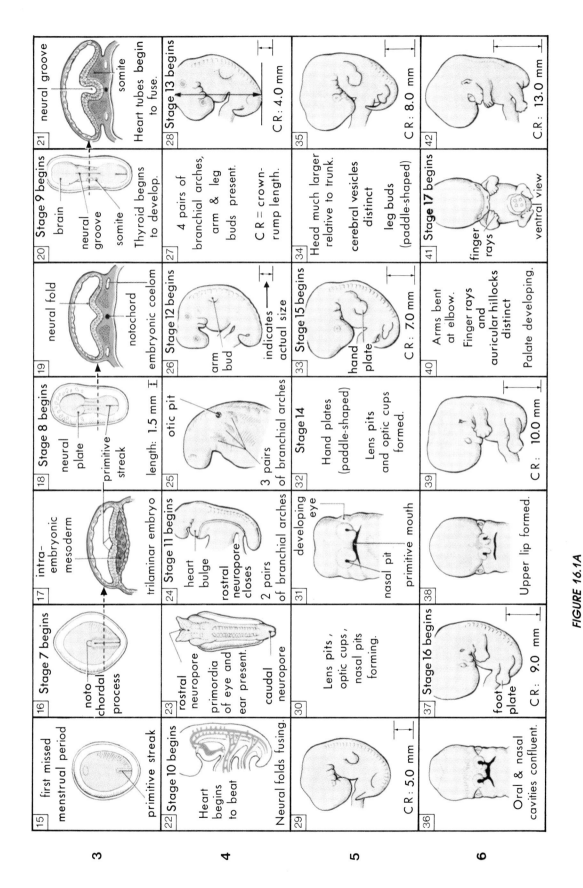

FIGURE 16.1A
Timetable of human prenatal development, 1 to 6 weeks. (Continued.)

434

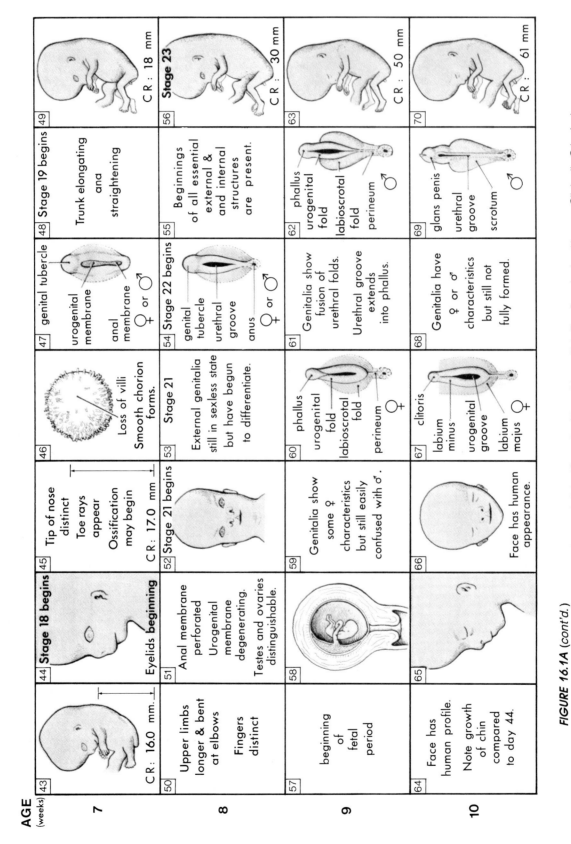

AGE (weeks)

7	43 CR: 16.0 mm.	44 **Stage 18 begins** Eyelids beginning	45 Tip of nose distinct Toe rays appear Ossification may begin	46 Loss of villi Smooth chorion forms.	47 genital tubercle urogenital membrane anal membrane ♀ or ♂	48 **Stage 19 begins** Trunk elongating and straightening	49 CR: 18 mm

Row 7: 43 CR: 16.0 mm.; 44 Stage 18 begins — Eyelids beginning; 45 Tip of nose distinct, Toe rays appear, Ossification may begin; 46 Loss of villi, Smooth chorion forms.; 47 genital tubercle, urogenital membrane, anal membrane ♀ or ♂; 48 Stage 19 begins, Trunk elongating and straightening; 49 CR: 18 mm

Row 8: 50 Upper limbs longer & bent at elbows, Fingers distinct, CR: 17.0 mm; 51 Anal membrane perforated, Urogenital membrane degenerating. Testes and ovaries distinguishable.; 52 Stage 21 begins; 53 Stage 21 External genitalia still in sexless state but have begun to differentiate.; 54 Stage 22 begins, genital tubercle, urethral groove, anus ♀ or ♂; 55 Beginnings of all essential external and internal structures are present.; 56 Stage 23 CR: 30 mm

Row 9: 57 beginning of fetal period; 58; 59 Genitalia show some ♀ characteristics but still easily confused with ♂.; 60 phallus, urogenital fold, labioscrotal fold, perineum ♀; 61 Genitalia show fusion of urethral folds. Urethral groove extends into phallus.; 62 phallus, urogenital fold, labioscrotal fold, perineum ♂; 63 CR: 50 mm

Row 10: 64 Face has human profile. Note growth of chin compared to day 44.; 65; 66 Face has human appearance.; 67 clitoris, labium minus, urogenital groove, labium majus ♀; 68 Genitalia have ♀ or ♂ characteristics but still not fully formed.; 69 glans penis, urethral groove, scrotum ♂; 70 CR: 61 mm

FIGURE 16.1A (cont'd.)
Timetable of human prenatal development, 7 to 10 weeks. (From Moore K. L. The Developing Human: Clinically Oriented Embryology (3rd ed.). Philadelphia: W. B. Saunders, 1982, with permission.)

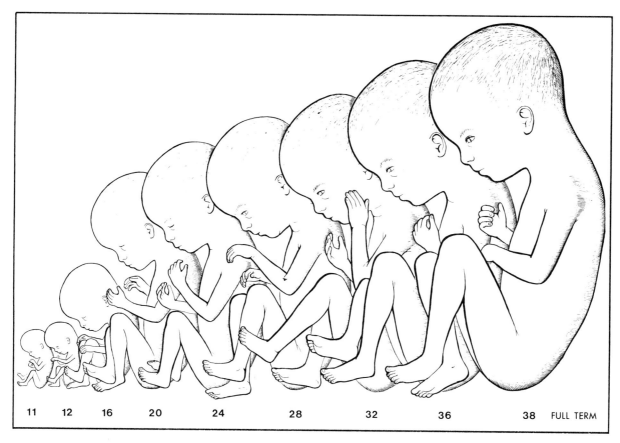

FIGURE 16.1B
*Timetable of human prenatal development, 11 to 38 weeks. (From Moore, K. L. The Developing
Human: Clinically Oriented Embryology (3rd ed.). Philadelphia: W. B. Saunders, 1982, with permis-
sion.)*

and legs, and cries weakly. This infant may
survive with the technology of neonatal intensive care.

Eighth Lunar Month. At the end of 32 weeks, the
length of the fetus is 40 to 42 centimeters (approximately 16″) and weighs 1,700 to 1,800
grams (approximately 4 lbs.) (Bobak & Benson, 1984). The skin is pinker and smoother
(Fig. 16.1B). His awareness goes beyond the
uterus as he responds to sounds outside his
mother's body. This baby has the ability to
survive if born.

Ninth Lunar Month. By 36 weeks, the fetus
weighs 2,000 to 2,500 grams (approximately
5 lbs.) and is 45 to 47 centimeters (approximately 18″) long (Bobak & Benson, 1984). The
body is plump and the lanugo is disappearing.
This baby, if born now has a fine chance for
survival (Fig. 16.1B).

Tenth Lunar Month. At 40 weeks or at term, the
fetus is 45 to 55 centimeters (approximately
18–22″) long and weighs 3,400 grams (approximately 7½ lbs.) (Bobak & Benson, 1984). The
skin is pink and his body is round. The lanugo
continues to decrease and will be present on
the upper torso and shoulders at birth. The
vernix caseosa is also decreasing.

Maternal Physiology

There are multiple physiological changes going on in the mother's body during pregnancy.
These changes extend beyond the reproductive system, and in fact all body systems are
affected. Some physiological changes are
more dominant in one trimester than another,
while some occur consistently throughout the
pregnancy. While one tries to assess the progression of the pregnancy in terms of growth

of the fetus, it is also helpful to look at maternal changes in relationship to fetal development.

The following sections present a discussion of maternal physiology in pregnancy. Included are all relevant body systems in which the mother will notice differences, and the health care provider should expect changes.

FIRST TRIMESTER

The Uterus. For the first few weeks of the pregnancy, the pear shape of the pre-pregnant uterus is maintained. Around the 6th week of pregnancy, the isthmus of the uterus softens significantly. This is known as *Hegar's sign.* Shortly after, the uterus begins to become more globular in shape. As the shape changes, the initial increase is more in the length than in width. Eventually the uterus takes on an ovoid shape and begins to grow out of the pelvis. By the 12th week of pregnancy, the uterus can be palpated at the level of the symphysis pubis (Fig. 16.2).

Cervical Changes. Throughout pregnancy, the cervix undergoes many changes. Some of the cervical variations are due to the increased vascularity and edema of the cervix. Additionally, a mucus plug is formed in the cervix soon after conception to block the cervical canal. This plug remains in the cervix until the baby is ready to be born.

About the 8th week of pregnancy, the cervix begins to soften (*Goodell's sign*) and often gets a blue cyanotic appearance (*Chadwick's sign*). The softening of the cervix continues throughout pregnancy to help prepare for the ultimate *dilatation* (enlargement) and *effacement* (thinning and shortening) necessary for the birthing process.

Cervical erosions are rather common during pregnancy. They represent an extension of the proliferating endocervical glands and the columnar epithelium. These eversions have a red-velvety appearance and are considered to be a normal variant (Pritchard, et al., 1985). The cervical mucus also changes during pregnancy. It increases in quantity and patients notice this particularly in the first trimester. When looked at under a microscope, this mucus does not fern, as it would if it were the thickened estrogenic discharge of ovula-

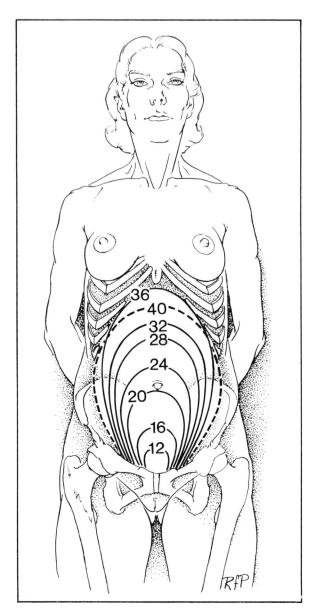

FIGURE 16.2
Height of fundus by week of gestation.

tion. Although the mucus may be thicker than non-pregnant vaginal discharge, there should be no unusual odor, color or consistency. If any of these symptoms exist, a vaginal infection should be considered.

Vaginal Changes. Like the cervix, the vagina also takes on a blue-like color at about 6 to 8 weeks after conception (*Chadwick's sign*). The physiologic reason is the same as for the cervical changes—increasing vascularity and edema. The vaginal walls change in the introitus and vaginal area to prepare for labor. There is an increase in the thickness of the vaginal mucosa, a loosening of the connective tissue and hypertrophy of the smooth muscle (Pritchard, et al., 1985).

The vaginal secretions also thicken and may have a white rather than clear appearance. The pH is more acidic due to increased lactic acid production. The acid nature of the vagina may help prevent bacterial production.

Ovarian Changes. The ovulatory function of the ovaries ceases when pregnancy occurs. The corpus luteum still functions and stimulates progesterone production during the first 4 weeks of pregnancy. Thereafter, the function of the corpus luteum also ceases.

Breast Changes. The breasts change significantly throughout pregnancy. Many of the early changes reported by the mother are subjective. Often this history helps the health care provider diagnose the pregnancy. Most significantly, in the first trimester, the breasts will feel tender and tingly to the mother. They might also be increasing in size. The examiner may notice this increase as well.

Metabolic Changes. Maternal weight gain is one of the most obvious changes that takes place. Most of the weight gain is due to the contents of the pregnancy (the fetus, placenta, amniotic fluid, etc.). The weight gain during the first trimester averages 2 to 4 pounds. The bulk of the weight gain should occur in the last 2 trimesters. The average total weight gain should be about 27 pounds (Naeye, 1979) with a range of 22 to 32 pounds considered acceptable.

Hematologic Changes. For some women, their blood volume can increase up to 45 percent during pregnancy (Pritchard , et al., 1985). The degree of increase varies greatly among women. The blood volume increases to meet additional vascular needs of the enlarged uterus; to nourish the mother from untoward effects of disrupted venous return in the supine and erect positions, and to compensate for the blood loss during the birthing process.

Cardiac output also increases markedly during pregnancy. It begins during the first trimester and stays elevated throughout the pregnancy.

Nasopharyngeal Changes. The oral and nasal mucosa can become hyperemic, edematous and boggy. The physiological response of the nasal mucosa may cause nasal stuffiness throughout the entire pregnancy. Although this symptom is not common, it can be very irritating to the patient. In addition, spontaneous bleeding of the gums occurs more easily in pregnancy.

Gastrointestinal Changes. Nausea and vomiting are most common in early pregnancy. There is no clear explanation regarding the etiology of this problem. One belief is that it is caused by increased human chorionic gonadotropin (HCG). This hormone is highest in the first trimester when nausea and vomiting are most frequently experienced. As the HCG decreases, so does the nausea and vomiting.

Interesting to note are the responses of the liver and gallbladder to pregnancy. There is some supposition, but not widely proven or experienced, that pregnancy predisposes a woman to gallstone formation. The only concrete evidence is that at the time of cesarean-section, the gallbladder is distended, and aspirated bile is thickened (Potter & Nestel, 1979). Liver function, on the other hand, remains essentially unchanged during pregnancy (Combes & Adams, 1971).

Skin Changes. The skin may change in pregnancy for two reasons—hormones and vascularity. Because of the many hormonal changes at the onset of pregnancy, many women report an increase in the incidence of acne. For other women, however, all acne clears up while they are pregnant. Some women also report an increase in generalized pruritis in early pregnancy. This is attributed to the increased estrogen in the body. Increasing vascular response can also occur in the skin. Excess heat is dissipated, and there can be an increase in perspiration and hot flashes.

Urinary Tract Changes. The urinary tract undergoes many changes throughout pregnancy. An early symptom of pregnancy is often urinary frequency. This is primarily due to the enlarging uterus which applies pressure on the bladder. Another belief about urinary frequency during the first trimester relates to hormonal changes affecting the smooth muscle of the bladder. The result is decreased bladder tone causing increased urination. This symptom usually disappears in the second trimester when the uterus moves out of the pelvis. Urinary frequency reappears in the final weeks of pregnancy.

SECOND TRIMESTER

The Uterus. Between the 12th and 16th weeks, the uterus becomes too large for the pelvic area and begins to grow into the abdominal cavity. As a result, the intestines are displaced laterally and superiorly. The uterus ascends toward the liver, causing a mild dextrorotation of the uterus. By the 16th week of gestation, the top of the fundus is halfway between the symphysis pubis and the umbilicus. By the 20th to 22nd week, the top of the uterus is at the level of the umbilicus (Fig. 16.2). It has been demonstrated that the fundal height in centimeters corresponds to the gestational age between the 18th and 30th weeks of gestation. (The method used to measure can be found on page 461.)

Cervical Changes. Many of the cervical changes discussed in the first trimester continue on through the second trimester. The physiological changes of the cervix are continuing toward one goal: sufficient cervical effacement and dilatation to allow for a spontaneous vaginal birth. The remarkable elastic structure of the connective tissue is what readies the cervix for dilatation. Connective tissue changes are ongoing throughout pregnancy but are more active in the second trimester than the first.

Vaginal Changes. During the second trimester, the increased vascularity continues in the vaginal vault. As a result of this, women may report a heightened sexual response.

The thick, white vaginal discharge present during the first trimester may either increase or decrease during this trimester. The pH continues to be acidic due to the increased amount of lactic acid from the glycogen in vaginal tissue.

Breasts. Breast size continues to increase throughout pregnancy. Venous distension, that looks like superficial skin veins, appears on both breasts. The nipples increase in size and take on a nodular-like appearance. They also darken and become more erectile. During this trimester, many women notice that a thick, white-yellow fluid, called *colostrum*, can be expressed from the nipples.

The areola also enlarge and darken. Nodular-like glands called *Montgomery's glands* appear on the areola. These are hypertrophied sebaceous glands. *Striae* (stretch marks) may also appear on the breasts during this trimester. They will have a reddened appearance. The size of the women's breasts and the extent to which they grow will affect the degree of striae.

Metabolic Changes. The most notable metabolic change in a woman during the second trimester is weight gain. She should gain about 11 pounds during this period. Her shape will change significantly as the uterus begins to rise out of the pelvis. Chemical alterations occur with protein, fat, and carbohydrate metabolism. Water metabolism also creates changes in the patient's body. Water retention occurs characteristically in later pregnancy (mostly during the third trimester). Because this symptom is associated with one of the most common complications of pregnancy, preeclampsia, the degree of water retention is a concern. In severe cases, this symptom may appear as early as the end of the second trimester. Inappropriate water retention may also be reflected in rapid maternal weight gain (Pritchard, et al., 1985).

Hematologic Changes. The maternal blood volume increases most rapidly during the second trimester. This hypervolemia is a result of an increase in plasma, followed by an increase in erythrocytes. The erythrocytes do not live long, but an increase in their production contributes to the added volume.

Although erythropoiesis (formation of red blood cells) increases throughout the pregnancy, the concentration of the hemoglobin and hematocrit decreases slightly in a normal pregnancy. The hemoglobin level of the nonpregnant woman is about 13.3 grams per deciliter. In a pregnant woman, the hemoglobin level is about 12.1 grams per deciliter at 32 to 34 weeks (Pritchard, et al., 1985). A hemoglobin level below 11.0 grams is indicative of an anemia, usually iron deficiency, not the physiological hypervolemic response.

Cardiovascular Changes. The pulse rate at rest increases about 10 to 15 beats per minute from the 14th week of gestation to term. The heart sounds may also change slightly, but these slight variations are distinctly within normal limits. An increased splitting may be heard in the first heart sound (S_1). There is no distinct change in S_2, but an S_3 can easily be heard. A systolic ejection murmur is a normal finding and may be heard in almost all pregnant women. In a small percent of pregnant women, a diastolic murmur can also be detected. The EKG should show no changes except for a slight axis deviation.

Blood pressure is monitored very carefully during pregnancy. During the second trimester, a slight decrease in arterial blood pressure is likely to occur. It will increase in the third trimester, but should do so no more than 15 mm Hg systolically or 30 mm Hg diastolically (Pritchard, et al., 1985).

Respiratory Changes. The respiratory system does not alter appreciably during this trimester of pregnancy. There are some changes that take place as the pregnancy progresses, but most of those are dependent on the uterus enlarging and the diaphragm elevating. Oxygen consumption increases about 15 percent after the 16th week of gestation.

The respiratory rate does not vary much throughout pregnancy, even in the more advanced stages. Abdominal breathing, however, replaces thoracic breathing around the 24th week. This compensatory mechanism assures adequate ventilation to both mother and fetus.

Urinary Tract Changes. Urinary frequency in this trimester is unusual. It exists primarily during the first and third trimesters. There are other changes during these weeks that affect renal function. Glomerular filtration rate (GFR) and renal plasma flow (RPF) increase in the early stages of pregnancy. The GFR increases as much as 50 percent by the beginning of the second trimester. Because the GFR and RPF increase, there is a decrease in the following: Blood urea nitrogen (BUN), serum uric acid and serum creatinine (Pritchard, et al., 1985).

Some women have *orthostatic proteinuria* (proteinuria only when standing). In the absence of hypertension, edema, renal infection or renovascular disease, mild proteinuria is not considered a problem.

Gastrointestinal Changes. Throughout the second trimester, the abdominal organs are beginning to be displaced. This leads to a variety of changes within the gastrointestinal system. Organs are not located exactly where they are normally located, and this can result in some discomfort common to a progressing pregnancy. The abdominal organs also respond to the hormonal changes of pregnancy.

One common gastrointestinal symptom of pregnancy is heartburn. This usually begins in the second trimester but may increase as the pregnancy progresses. There are two explanations offered for this problem. The most obvious reason for the heartburn is related to the displacement of abdominal organs. The position of the stomach probably facilitates acid secretion moving into the lower esophagus, causing esophageal reflux.

Hormonal influences that directly effect the gastrointestinal tract offer the second explanation. Hydrochloric acid secretion is decreased by the increased estrogen production, causing esophageal reflux. In addition, the increased progesterone, which prolongs gastric emptying time, sets up a reverse peristalisis, causing *pyrosis* (heartburn) (Bobak & Benson, 1984).

Another common discomfort during pregnancy is constipation. This is the result of an increased amount of progesterone, produced by the placenta, causing smooth muscle relaxation. The smooth muscle relaxation not only decreases gastric motility, but prolongs emptying and increases water absorption (Bobak & Benson, 1984). The degree of constipation varies depending on all these factors as well as diet, fluid intake and iron sources.

Skin Changes. Skin pigment is affected during pregnancy in a variety of ways. Most of the more obvious changes occur after the first trimester. A melanocyte stimulating hormone is known to be elevated during pregnancy. Although not much is known about the causes of the pigmentary changes, it is believed that the alterations in pigment are related to this increased hormone.

There are two common manifestations as

a result of the pigment changes in some pregnant women. The first is called *linea nigra* which is a thin, brown line that appears on the lower abdomen. It extends from the umbilicus to the symphysis pubis. As the abdomen enlarges, it may get darker but will fade after delivery.

The other manifestation is called *chloasma*, also known as the mask of pregnancy. This can best be described as brown patches that are visible on the face and neck. Chloasma may also occur in women taking oral contraceptives. As with the linea nigra, chloasma will resolve after giving birth (Pritchard, et al., 1985).

Another pigment change that will occur in almost all pregnant women is the deepening of color of the areola and nipples.

Musculoskeletal Changes. Lordosis (an increase in the concavity of the lumbar spine) will occur in all pregnant women as their pregnancy progresses. The more the abdomen protrudes, the more pronounced the lordosis will be. This is a compensatory mechanism which acts to aid the mother's body in carrying the pregnancy in a comfortable and balanced fashion. For mechanical purposes, the center of gravity is shifted.

Another musculoskeletal change is the result of hormonal influence. There is an increased movement of the sacroiliac, sacrococcygeal and pubic joints. These changes begin during the second trimester, as the fetus grows and the uterus increases in size. Not until the third trimester does the woman notice back discomfort and decreased coordination.

Leg cramps can become a common problem. The exact etiology is not clearly understood, nor has it been carefully studied. There is some belief, however, that it is related to an increase serum phosphorus and insufficient calcium intake (Bobak & Benson, 1984).

THIRD TRIMESTER

Uterine Changes. The uterus undergoes by far the most dramatic change during pregnancy. The total volume of the uterus and its contents may exceed 5 liters. The uterus itself weighs 50 to 70 grams in its non-pregnant state and it weighs over 1,000 grams at term. The dimensions of the uterus change dramatically as

well. The uterus is 6 centimeters long before pregnancy occurs. At term it is 32 centimeters long. The depth of the uterus is 2 to 3 centimeters when non-pregnant and may be 22 centimeters or larger at the time of delivery. Remembering that the uterus grows up and out of the pelvic area, another important milestone is that the uterus often reaches the xiphoid process at about 36 weeks gestational age.

During that last 2 weeks of pregnancy, the uterus begins to move down into the pelvic cavity in preparation for delivery. The shape of the uterus changes, and the fundal height decreases slightly as the fetus descends into the pelvis. This is known as *lightening.* The mother often describes this as, "the baby is dropping." Others may remark that she looks "less pregnant." The mother may also describe the sensation of finding herself less short of breath, but with increased urinary frequency. This relieves the pressure on the diaphragm, so the shortness of breath decreases. As the baby's head drops, the pressure increases on the mother's bladder so that the urinary frequency increases. When the biparietal diameter of the fetal skull is below the pelvic inlet, the head is said to be engaged (Figs. 16.3, 16.4, 16.5). In the multipara this usually occurs dur-

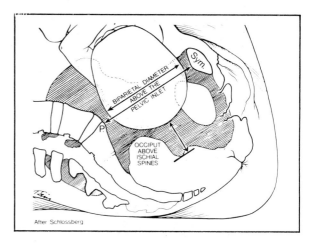

FIGURE 16.3
When the lowermost portion of the fetal head is above the ischial spines, the biparietal diameter of the head is not likely to have passed through the pelvic inlet and therefore is not engaged (P = sacral promontory; Sym = symphysis pubis). (From Pritchard, J. A., et al. Williams Obstetrics (17th ed.). Norwalk, Conn.: Appleton-Century-Crofts, 1985, p. 228.)

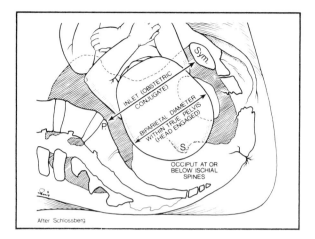

FIGURE 16.4
When the lowermost portion of the fetal head is at or below the ischial spines, it is usually engaged. Exceptions occur when there is considerable molding or caput formation, or both (P = sacral promontory; Sym = symphysis pubis; S = ischial spine). (From Pritchard, J. A., et al. Williams Obstetrics (17th ed.). Norwalk, Conn.: Appleton-Century-Crofts, 1985, p. 228.)

ing the early stages of labor. In the primipara this often takes place during the last weeks of pregnancy.

Throughout the entire pregnancy, the uterus has irregular contractions. There is no pattern of regularity to these movements. In fact, in the third trimester, one can lay a hand on the woman's abdomen to feel it tighten and loosen. These contractions are named for the man who described their occurrence and are known as *Braxton Hicks* contractions. During the last weeks of pregnancy, they increase in

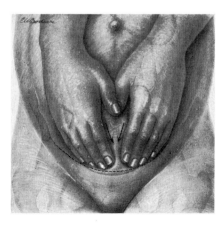

FIGURE 16.5
If the fingers converge when palpating the lateral aspects of the fetal head, it is not engaged. (From Pritchard, J. A., et al. Williams Obstetrics (16th ed.). Norwalk, Conn.: Appleton-Century-Crofts, 1980, p. 283.)

frequency and intensity to some degree. Braxton Hicks contractions may be mistaken for labor.

Cervical Changes. There are few changes in the cervix during this trimester until term. As the baby moves into the pelvis, a woman may have some irregular contractions causing the cervix to begin to dilate. This is especially true in multiparous women (Figs. 16.6, 16.7, 16.8, 16.9). As stated earlier, the mucus plug, formed in the cervix during the first trimester, is expelled just prior to or at the onset of labor. This plug is often referred to as bloody show, because it is blood tinged. As active labor begins, the cervix changes dramatically. The cervix effaces and dilates, so the baby's head can pass through the pelvis (Fig. 16.10).

The Vagina. Most of the changes that take place in the vagina during the third trimester are to prepare for the birth of the baby. With the remarkable expansive ability of the vaginal walls, certain structural changes occur. The walls are constantly increasing in length, while the mucosa thickens significantly. The connective tissue loosens and the smooth muscle hypertrophies. Although these are gradual changes, most take place as term approaches.

Breast Changes. Breast changes continue as in the second trimester. The yellow fluid, colostrum, is still able to be expressed. Lactation does not begin until after delivery. In fact, the fluid the baby nurses from the mother for the first 2 to 3 days of life is colostrum. It is considered healthy for the baby to nurse colostrum, due to immunologic benefits, until the mother's milk supply is established.

Abdomen. As the uterus enlarges, the abdomen gets bigger and changes shape. The ascension of the uterus into the abdomen causes more and more displacement of the other organs.

Stretch marks, or *striae*, often appear on the abdomen during this trimester. As in the breast, the striae will have a reddened appearance. They are likely to be at the lower abdomen, but may appear anywhere on the abdomen. Striae may also be found on the hips and thighs. There is little to do to prevent or get rid of these marks. However, after the baby is born and the mother's abdomen decreases

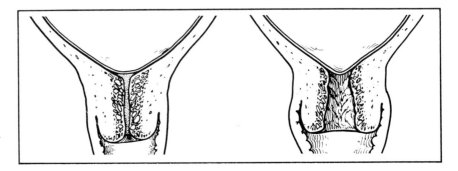

FIGURE 16.6
Cervix near the end of pregnancy but before labor. Left: Primigravida; Right: Multipara. (From Pritchard, J. A., et al. Williams Obstetrics (17th ed.). Norwalk, Conn.: Appleton-Century-Crofts, 1985, p. 312.)

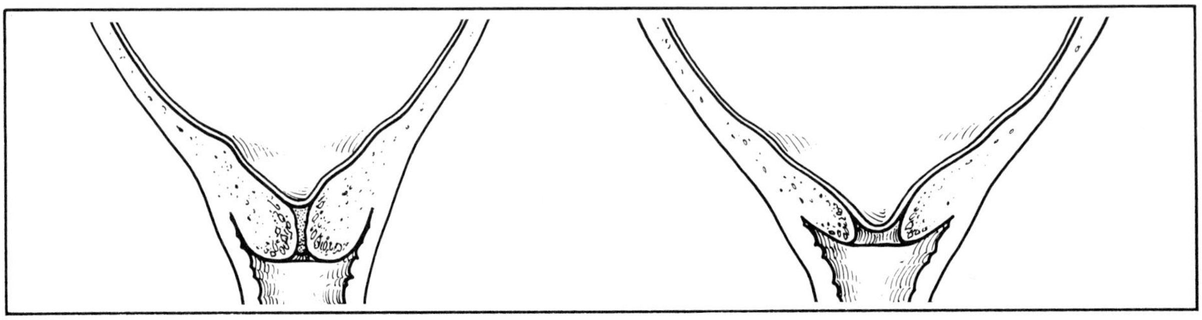

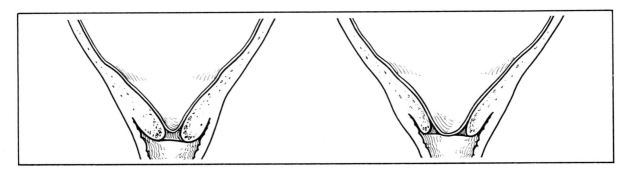

FIGURE 16.7
Beginning effacement of cervix. Note dilatation of internal os and funnel-shaped cervical canal. Left: Primigravida; Right: Multipara. (From Pritchard, J. A., et al. Williams Obstetrics (17th ed.). Norwalk, Conn.: Appleton-Century-Crofts, 1985, p. 312.)

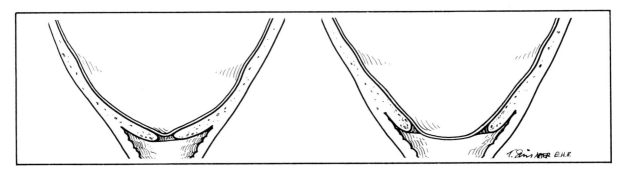

FIGURE 16.8
Further effacement of cervix. Left: Primigravida; Right: Multipara. (From Pritchard, J. A., et al. Williams Obstetrics (17th ed.). Norwalk, Conn.: Appleton-Century-Crofts, 1985, p. 312.)

FIGURE 16.9
Cervical canal obliterated, i.e., the cervix is completely effaced. Left: Primigravida; Right: Multigravida. (From Pritchard, J. A., et al. Williams Obstetrics (17th ed.). Norwalk, Conn.: Appleton-Century-Crofts, 1985, p. 312.)

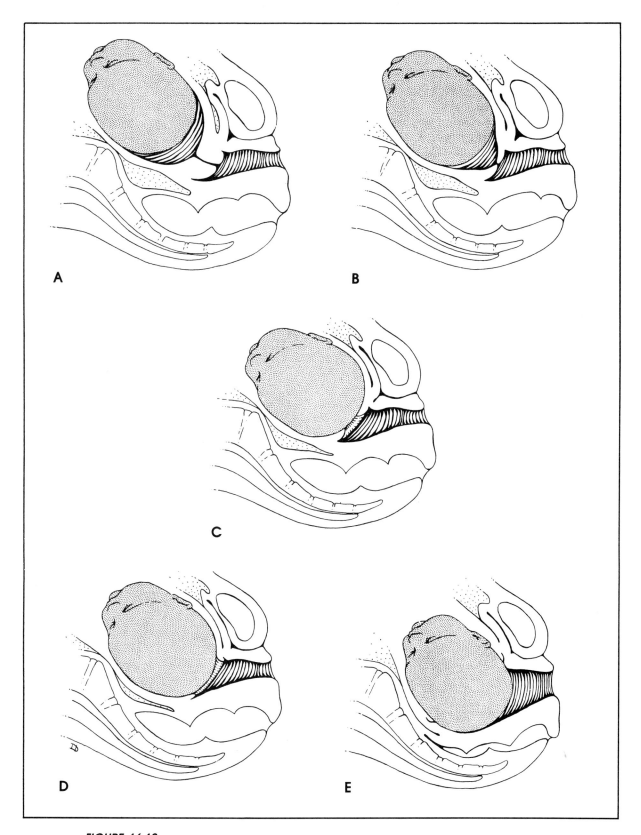

FIGURE 16.10

Dilatation of the cervix. **A.** *Cervix thick and closed.* **B.** *Cervix effaced.* **C.** *Cervix effaced and dilated 2 to 3 cm.* **D.** *Cervix half open.* **E.** *Cervix fully dilated and retracted.* *(From Oxorn, H. Human Labor and Birth (5th ed.). Norwalk, Conn.: Appleton-Century-Crofts, 1986.)*

in size, they will have more of a silver color and fade to some degree.

There is a rather fun feature relating to observing the abdomen during this trimester. If one watches the abdomen, when the mother feels movement, there is likely to be visible movement in the abdomen. A kick is a quick common movement to observe.

Metabolic Changes. During this trimester, the mother should gain about 10 pounds. This may average out to 1 pound a week, especially toward the latter part of the trimester. Many women stop gaining a couple of weeks prior to term. Some may even lose a small amount of weight as they approach their 40th week.

If a weight gain of 24 pounds is broken down into the products of the pregnancy, the contents are: blood volume, 3½ pounds; breasts, 2 pounds; amniotic fluid, 2 pounds; the uterus, 2½ pounds; and the fetus, 7½ pounds. The remaining pounds are probably due to fluid retention and some fat deposits (Pritchard, et al., 1985).

A large portion of the retained fluid is water. The water content of the fetus, placenta, and amniotic fluid as extracellular fluid are the main contributors of excess fluid. An accumulation of up to 6 liters can cause an edematous response in the woman, most frequently seen in the ankles and lower legs. This fluid increase in lower extremities may also be due to an increase in venous pressure below the level of the uterus. The fluid is often absorbed when the mother lies down. The venous pressure will decrease when she is in a lateral position.

Hematologic Changes. Some of the clotting mechanisms increase during pregnancy. This is another compensatory mechanism to protect the mother during the birthing process. There are increases in Factor I (plasma fibrinogen), Factors VII (proconvertin), VIII (antihemophiliac globulin), IX (plasma thromboplastin component) and X (fibrin-stabilizing factor) (Pritchard, et al., 1985).

Clotting times do not vary much in the pregnant woman. The platelet count also remains relatively stable throughout pregnancy. What does change, however, is the sedimentation rate. This is partially due to the increased fibrinogen. For this reason, it is important to note that a sedimentation rate cannot be used during pregnancy for diagnostic purposes.

Cardiovascular Changes. After many years of research, some conclusions about the cardiovascular response to late pregnancy have been reached. It is now believed that the cardiac output increases during the first trimester and remains elevated throughout the duration of pregnancy as stated earlier (Pritchard, et al., 1985). Late in pregnancy, however, the cardiac output increases even more when the woman lies in a lateral recumbent position (as opposed to a supine position). When lying in a supine position, the enlarged uterus causes slowing of the venous return to the heart.

The heart, like other organs in the abdominal and thoracic cavity, is displaced up and to the left. As the pregnancy progresses into the third trimester, this becomes even more true. Systolic murmurs, which are normal in pregnancy, may be exacerbated with increasing displacement.

The blood pressure rises slightly from the second to the third trimester. As during the second trimester, any sustained rise of more than 30 mm Hg systolic or 15 mm Hg diastolic is considered problematic.

Respiratory Changes. During the third trimester, as the uterus approaches the xiphoid process, the diaphragm is pushed up. Slight dyspnea may occur. With this displacement, there is an increase in the respiratory rate and the tidal volume. The vital capacity and the breathing capacity, however, remain unchanged. The residual volume and functional residual capacity decrease. All of these changes are a result of the elevation of the diaphragm.

Urinary Tract Changes. The kidney continues to change throughout pregnancy. The GFR (glomerular filtration rate) and RPF (renal plasma flow) have been increasing throughout the pregnancy. In the third trimester, the GFR remains elevated, but the RPF decreases to almost a prepregnant level. The exact reason for this is not clearly understood.

As the uterus enlarges, the bladder continues to be pushed out of the pelvis. Eventually, frequency of urination is again a complaint. This is due to the head of the fetus (or the presenting part) putting pressure on the bladder as it begins to descend into the pelvis.

Gastrointestinal Changes. The stomach is displaced upwards as a result of the growing uterus causing a widening of the diaphragm, making room for a herniation in some women. A hiatal hernia is a protrusion of the stomach through the esophageal hiatus of the diaphragm.

If a woman has *hemorrhoids* during pregnancy, they are likely to be caused by either constipation or an increase in venous pressure in the veins below the level of the uterus. Women who have problems with constipation are good candidates for hemorrhoids in pregnancy. The increased venous pressure on the veins below the level of the uterus is most likely to occur in the last trimester. If the venous pressure increases as pregnancy approaches term, the hemorrhoids can be proportionately worse. Some women have vulvar varicosities rather than hemorrhoids as a response to the increased venous pressure.

Skin Changes. For women whose acne has been increased in the first two trimesters, there is likely to be an improvement in the third trimester. Other skin conditions like seborrhea or psoriasis have not shown any dramatic improvement during pregnancy.

As the pregnancy approaches term, striae are likely to be much more evident. As stated earlier, there is no treatment for these. Reassuring the patient that they will improve and become less prominent after delivery, is the most honest information the provider can give.

In addition to the occurrence of *spider angiomas* and *telangiectasis,* (see Chapter 3, Chart 3.7) another benign skin condition may occur called *palmar erythema* (reddening of the palms). It is of no significance and resolves shortly after delivery. Telangiectasis and palmar erythema may occur together; both are probably due to the increased estrogen during pregnancy.

Musculoskeletal Changes. In the latter stages of pregnancy, the joint mobility and lordosis (see Chapter 14, page 357) that began in the second trimester are increased. This may result in low back discomfort which is aggra- vated if accompanied by nerve compression. The sensations are particularly common beneath the inguinal ligament, causing the discomfort in the groin and thigh areas.

PSYCHOLOGICAL CHANGES OF PREGNANCY

Changes in the Mother

Just as pregnancy involves dynamic physiological changes, it also mandates a significant developmental adjustment. The childbearing experience involves the incorporation of a new aspect of personality for the woman. The woman incorporates a maternal identity gradually and systematically in the process of being pregnant. In the early stages of pregnancy, concerns and preparations for the birth of the child are of minimal priority. Rather, these early stages find the pregnant woman focusing on confirming the pregnancy and adapting to changes in herself that are both psychological and physical in nature.

The childbearing experience results in an inevitable disequilibrium. Relationships with one's family members, their work and their social environment must be altered in order to make a place for this child. The pregnant woman has two major tasks to complete. They are 1) to keep herself and family intact as an ongoing system and 2) to facilitate the assimilation of this child into the existing system (Rubin, 1984). These two major tasks can be further delineated into the following:

1. To seek safe passage of the child;
2. To seek acceptance by the significant members of the family;
3. To seek total acceptance of oneself as the mother of this child; and
4. To give meaning to the giving of oneself.

In the first trimester, the pregnant woman is likely to focus on her own "safe passage." It is usually toward the end of the second trimester that one can ascertain that the woman is aware of the child within her and attaches considerable value to the child. By the third trimester, the concerns of the woman are for both self and baby. She recognizes that what endangers one will endanger the other.

Seeking safe passage is evidenced by the woman's decision to seek prenatal care and her interest in gaining a knowledge base for the childbearing experience. She may do this by attending childbirth preparation classes, reading relevant literature, or by searching out women who have had this experience.

Nursing assessment needs to include the evaluation of how well the pregnant woman deals with this task. For example, a young teenager may have great difficulty accomplishing this task as a result of her developmental status. Typically, teens have a limited concept of future time and are struggling with other personal identity issues including those related to body image. This can conflict with her need to care for herself as a pregnant woman who even now plays a role in the care of this child whom she does not yet know.

Coping with the dangers and threats to herself and the child continue throughout the pregnancy. The woman must constantly regulate these sources of anxiety in order to cope effectively. The health care provider is usually viewed as the major resource for this task. Therefore, assurance as to the normalcy of various symptoms and accurate information that assists the woman to sort out the myths versus the realities of childbearing are integral components of prenatal health care.

In the process of gaining acceptance of the child by others, stress is experienced incrementally throughout the pregnancy. During the first trimester, even the prospect of the loss of part of the woman's world is cause for distress. It is important that the family nurture this new child, but this acceptance by the family is contingent upon their ability to take in another member and to make the necessary adjustments. This may be a particularly difficult task to accomplish for a single or divorced woman whose sexual partner may reject her or the child, or even for the married couple who did not expect to further enlarge their family with yet another child. The 14-year-old pregnant girl usually finds herself ill-equipped to orchestrate the necessary changes needed and finds it difficult to gain acceptance of her pregnancy from her family and many societal groups.

It is important to regularly assess the degree to which the pregnant client has achieved this task. One cannot assume that the marital status of the client dictates the ease with which the woman can gain the necessary acceptance of the pregnancy and addition of a child to the family system.

Acceptance of oneself as a mother to this child is a third important task. In the first trimester, it is not unusual to find a lack of acceptance even in the woman who was hoping for a pregnancy at this point in her life. She may be consumed by the dramatic changes she observes including the nausea, fatigue, and changes in physical appearance. During the first trimester, most women seek out acceptance of pregnancy by others as a means to her own acceptance. As fetal movement is progressively experienced by the woman in the second trimester, a maternal protectiveness toward this child develops. There is usually an increased sense of well-being and more energy available to the pregnant woman at this time which allows her to "bind in" to her unborn child. The latter part of the third trimester finds most women growing impatient with the length of the pregnancy and vascillating between holding on to the unborn child and yet wanting to "let go" of the pregnancy. Assessing the woman's feelings toward the pregnancy, explaining the normalcy of the stages of acceptance of this child to the woman, and supporting the transitions between stages are important aspects of the nurse's role.

The fourth task, that of giving of oneself and finding meaning in that, is the most complex of the tasks of childbearing. During the first trimester, women typically view the demands of pregnancy as being high and the benefits as minimal. As the other tasks are achieved, the woman has the motivation and energy to deal with the meaning of this experience. She gives a child to her partner, a sibling to her other children, a grandchild to her parents and her partner's parents, and society gains a new member. The woman also receives this child. During the third trimester, most women are highly responsive to receiving from others. Her interpersonal reserves are somewhat depleted at this time and she is particularly delighted to have others giving to her in the form of personal attention, companionship, nurturance, and even gifts. The deprivations caused by pregnancy must be offset by the narcissistic pleasures. Eventually, there is an acceptance of the ongoing sacrifices and life adjustments one makes in order to experience motherhood.

Time and space are altered as the pregnant woman seeks to achieve her maternal tasks. Depending upon when the woman is aware of her pregnancy, there is usually not more than 7 to 8 months during which to adjust psychologically to the obvious changes. In the first trimester, the end point of the pregnancy and the birth of the child seem very distant into the future. The second trimester finds the woman "turning inward" to her pregnancy and the child. She often prefers more space in her outer world. As the second trimester ends, most women experience a growing sense of their vulnerability. Her inner space is stretched to accommodate this child resulting in some need for restriction of her physical movement. Home is usually perceived as a safe refuge, and she is not as anxious to travel. The third trimester finds many women feeling that this pregnancy has gone on long enough; yet there is a sense that time is running out. This can be a very lonely experience for the pregnant woman.

Changes in the Father

FIRST TRIMESTER

When a man is made aware of the fact that he has helped create a new life, many feelings are aroused in him. Many men report a sense of pride that their genes will be reproduced and that they have helped create this baby. Because we live in a patriarchal society, many men have pleasure in knowing that the family name will be carried on.

Men are also likely to experience some of the same ambivalent feelings that a newly pregnant woman does. The change in responsibility, the expectations of fatherhood, the economic burdens of parenthood quickly become a reality. This is as stressful for the father as the mother.

The father does not have the physical symptoms or changes that the woman experiences. Feelings of helplessness, empathy, and frustration exist if the woman is having a significant number of first trimester discomforts. Trying to adjust to the mood swings and fatigue that the newly pregnant woman often

has can be taxing and frustrating for him, too. It is fair to say, in the final analysis, that the first trimester evokes many new and exciting, yet anxious and ambivalent feelings for both the mother and father.

SECOND TRIMESTER

As the woman feels better in the second trimester, the father usually does too. Some of the worries about her health are now gone. Since she is probably more like herself again, their relationship is more like itself again.

Many men find the second trimester physical changes in a woman very exciting. The fact that her sexual desire and response may be heightened may be exciting for him, too. It is important to reassure the father that he cannot hurt the baby during intercourse, except under certain circumstances when problems exist. Once he has an understanding of this information, he should no longer hesitate to enjoy a warm satisfying sexual relationship with his partner.

Another very exciting time for the parents during this trimester is when they first hear the baby's heartbeat. If the father attends the prenatal visits with the mother, he will be able to hear the baby's heartbeat as early as she does. If he in unable to come along, the provider should try to schedule a time when he can come so that he can hear the heartbeat, too. The pregnancy becomes much more of a reality if the couple can share this excitement.

As the trimester progresses, he should eventually be able to feel the baby move. When both parents can put their hands on the abdomen and feel a thump, even more reality sets in. Many pregnant couples find watching and feeling the mother's abdomen for fetal movements a very special and intimate time together.

THIRD TRIMESTER

For the father there are probably anxious and exciting feelings similar to those of the mother during this trimester. He is both apprehensive and enthusiastic about the impending changes. For different reasons than those of the mother, the father is nervous about the birth itself. Although he may not experience the actual physical discomforts, he is very concerned about how he can help her, what his role will be, and how he will do in this very important supporting role. There is usually a concern about something terrible happening to his partner or to the baby. This may be a conscious or unconscious fear. On the other hand, the enthusiasm about this new role as father and the many fulfilling thoughts that the role brings with it are very exciting.

During this trimester, the father may feel more helpful and useful. If the parents are participating in childbirth classes, he can begin to see what his role will be during labor and delivery. Many of the childbirth classes encourage certain breathing and relaxation exercises be practiced at home. This gives the couple the opportunity to work at something to make the birth easier for both.

The physical preparation of the home to accommodate the new baby is a large part of the father's role, too. Again, this gives the couple something to work on together. It provides an opportunity for each member to feel productive and mutually helpful.

THE DIAGNOSIS OF PREGNANCY

Diagnosing pregnancy is not a clear and simple process. There are several diagnostic processes used to help confirm the suspicions. Many laboratory tests are available including tests of the blood and urine. Some of these tests can detect pregnancy as early as 7 days after conception and others require 42 days to pass following the first day of the last menstrual period. With technology advancing as quickly as it is, each year new tests are developed that have greater accuracy in confirming pregnancy at an earlier stage. None of these tests, however, can be utilized alone to diagnose pregnancy. There are many conditions that can result in a false positive or a false negative pregnancy test. Therefore, laboratory results must be supported with data obtained from an accurate history and physical examination.

The diagnosis of pregnancy is divided up into *presumptive symptoms and signs*, *probable signs*, and *positive signs of pregnancy* (Chart 16.2). The earlier the pregnancy, the more difficult it is to make an absolute diagnosis. It is important for health care providers to always consider the possibility of pregnancy in a woman during her menstruating years. What appears to be an isolated complaint of fatigue may indeed be a symptom of pregnancy.

Presumptive Symptoms and Signs

Many of the indicators of pregnancy in the early stages are based on a woman's subjective sensations and objective signs found on physical examination. The most commonly reported subjective symptoms are: a missed period(s), breast tenderness, nausea or vomiting, frequency of urination, questionable fetal movement, increased vaginal discharge, fatigue, weight gain, and constipation. These are referred to as the presumptive symptoms of pregnancy.

The most common objective signs in early pregnancy are: changes in vaginal mucosa and discharge, breast changes, pigment changes, acne and hirsutism, striae and telangiectasis, and bleeding gums. These are the presumptive signs of pregnancy.

Certainly, the greater the number of presumptive symptoms and signs a woman has, the stronger the likelihood of a pregnancy. Some women experience many changes and some very few.

PRESUMPTIVE SYMPTOMS

Cessation of Menses. This is often the first indication a woman has that she may be pregnant. The reliability of the cessation of menses is much greater after the second missed period. Some women have some vaginal bleeding around the time of their period when they are newly pregnant. The bleeding is usually less in quantity and lasts for a shorter period of time. This bleeding is more likely to occur in multiparas (Pritchard, et al., 1985). Therefore, it is very important when eliciting historical data from the patient to not only ask when the LMP was, but also to describe its length and the amount of bleeding. Asking the patient to compare the bleeding to other menstrual periods might provide a more accurate frame of reference for dating the pregnancy.

Other conditions cause a cessation of menses, too. Emotional disorders, chronic diseases, irregular ovulatory patterns, use of oral

CHART 16.2
PRESUMPTIVE, PROBABLE, AND POSITIVE SIGNS AND SYMPTOMS OF PREGNANCY

Presumptive Symptoms and Signs	Probable Signs	Positive Signs
Symptoms:		
Cessation of menses		
Breast tenderness		
Nausea and/or vomiting		
Frequency of urination		
Questionable fetal movement		
Increased vaginal discharge		
Fatigue		
Weight gain		
Constipation		
Signs:		
Altered vaginal mucosa and discharge	Increasing size of abdomen	Fetal heart heard by examiner
Pigment and breast changes	Ballottement of uterus	Fetal movement felt by examiner
Acne	Braxton Hicks contractions	X-Ray or ultrasound of uterus
Hirsutism	Cervical changes (Goodell's sign)	
Striae	Uterine changes (Hegar's sign)	
Telangiectasis	Ability to outline fetus	
Bleeding gums	Results of pregnancy tests	

contraceptives, long distance running, and stress are some things that can alter a woman's menstrual cycle. The nurse must be comprehensive in her history taking so that the right data is elicited.

Breast Tenderness. This symptom of early pregnancy often is confusing for the patient. Many women have breast tenderness prior to menses, too. A tingling sensation is often reported with the tenderness. Breast enlargement may start as early as the third week in pregnancy.

Nausea or Vomiting. The range of these symptoms varies greatly. Some women experience only the slightest nausea for a brief period of time during the day. Others are miserable with both nausea and frequent vomiting. The nausea and vomiting may occur as early as the sixth week of pregnancy and is usually resolved by the end of the 12th week. Nausea and vomiting that continues into the second trimester requires consultation. Distastes for certain foods or odors commonly occur along with this complaint.

Frequency of Urination. This symptom is very common in newly pregnant women. The common belief is that the frequency is caused by the growing uterus and its pressure on the bladder. As the uterus grows into the abdomen, the pressure decreases and the frequency subsides. Toward the end of pregnancy the frequency resumes when the baby's head begins its descent into the pelvis.

Questionable Fetal Movement. A later, but still presumptive symptom is fetal movement. Many women report a fluttering sensation and are unsure whether this is "feeling life" or "feeling gas." A multipara may notice this as early as the 16th to 20th weeks. A primigravidous woman is more likely to notice these sensations between the 18th to 20th weeks (Bobak & Benson, 1984). This feeling of life is called *quickening.* It is helpful in making the diagnosis of pregnancy, but once again it is not conclusive. When estimating the EDC, the date the woman notices quickening can be helpful for calculating purposes.

Increased Vaginal Discharge. Another early indicator of pregnancy is often an increased vaginal discharge. There should be no itching or burning accompanying the discharge. Some women report a musty, but unoffensive odor. This can be the presenting sympton for the woman who is concerned she has a vaginal infection. Further history taking may reveal other presumptive symptoms. When the history reveals information like an odorous, burning, oddly colored discharge, then infection must be ruled out.

Fatigue. This very common symptom may start shortly after conception. The reason for this is not clearly understood, but the symptom often remains prevalent through the first trimester.

Weight Gain. This should not be a dominant symptom of early pregnancy, since only a 3- to 4-pound weight gain is expected in the first trimester. Other causes of weight gain should be considered.

Constipation. The physiological response to the hormonal influence may affect some women. It may appear early and remain throughout the pregnancy.

PRESUMPTIVE SIGNS

Altered Vaginal Mucosa and Discharge. In the early weeks of pregnancy, the vaginal mucosa often pales or has the bluing (Chadwick's sign) referred to earlier. This color change is not exclusive to pregnancy. Any situation that causes congestion in the pelvic organs may discolor the vaginal mucosa (Pritchard, et al., 1985).

When doing the pelvic exam, the examiner may notice a significant amount of clear-to-cloudy vaginal discharge. A microscopic evaluation of this discharge should not show any pathological organisms such as hyphae, spores, clue cells or trichomonads.

Pigment Changes and Breast Changes. There are some pigment changes common in pregnancy. Again, these are only indicators and are not reliable enough to confirm the diagnosis of pregnancy.

Chloasma and linea nigra usually occur during the second trimester. They are more common in dark-complected women. The nipples, areola, and vulva may also darken. These hyperpigmented areas usually resolve after delivery.

There are other causes of these pigment changes. A woman taking oral contraceptives or a woman with Addison's disease may have similar skin responses.

Acne and Hirsutism. In some women, these conditions become more of a problem during pregnancy and, in other women, less. There is no way to predict which women will have which changes. In either case, a change in either direction may be an indicator of pregnancy.

Striae and Telangiectasis. Striae are more likely to develop as the pregnancy advances. The abdomen and breasts are the most common locations, but they may also appear on the hips and thighs.

Telangiectasis appear in some women. Their appearance may go unnoticed by the woman. They are most likely to occur on the face, chest, neck, and arms.

Bleeding Gums. This is not a frequent sign, but it does happen to some women. The exact cause is unknown, but it may be due to the increased estrogen.

PROBABLE SIGNS

The probable signs of pregnancy are additional objective data obtained on physical examination or through laboratory procedures. They include: *increasing size of the abdomen; ballottement in the uterus; Braxton Hicks contractions; cervical changes* (e.g., consistency and color); *uterine changes* (e.g., size, shape and consistency); ability to *outline the fetus,* and *results of pregnancy tests.*

Abdominal Changes. The uterus begins to rise out of the pelvis and grow into the abdominal cavity at about 12 weeks (Fig. 16.2). The uterus at 12 weeks is palpable just above the symphysis pubis. As the uterus grows up into the abdominal cavity, the abdomen takes on a protruding appearance. This protrusion continues to increase throughout the pregnancy.

Ballottement. About halfway through the pregnancy, the fetus can be ballotted within the amniotic fluid. When the examiner pushes on the uterus, the small fetus will sink in the amniotic fluid momentarily and then return to its original position. The examiner will feel the fetus rebound against her hand as it returns to its original location. Ballottement may also be used later in the pregnancy to determine the position of the baby's head.

Braxton Hicks Contractions. From the early stages of pregnancy, the uterus undergoes irregular, painless contractions. These may be brought on by massaging the uterus. There are pathological conditions of the uterus that may bring on similar contractions. Physiologically, movements within the abdomen like peristalsis may be mistaken for Braxton Hicks contractions.

Cervical Changes. Cervical changes are significant in early pregnancy. The softening (Goodell's sign) of the cervix gives positive clues to help diagnose the pregnancy. The examiner must always take an accurate history because the woman taking oral contraceptives may also have a softened cervix.

Uterine Changes. It is often difficult to diagnose pregnancy by a bimanual exam in the very early stages of pregnancy. As the pregnancy progresses, this exam becomes more valuable. During the 6th to 8th week, the softening of the isthmus of the uterus (Hegar's sign) can be felt. This also helps to confirm one's suspicion. The uterus itself, at this point, is taking on a more round shape. By 12 weeks' gestation, the diameter of the uterus is up to 8 centimeters.

Chemical Pregnancy Tests. The chief substance looked for in many pregnancy tests is HCG. HCG exists in maternal plasma and urine, and when identified is considered a probable sign of pregnancy. Although this is what most pregnancy tests are based on, the data is not 100 percent reliable. Certain situations give a false positive or a false negative result. One reason for this is that the amount of HCG in the body during pregnancy varies. The quantity is very small during the first few days and may not be detected in less sensitive methods of testing. Furthermore, the HCG also decreases after the 4th month. A further reason for inaccuracy occurs if proteinuria exists. The test will also provide a false negative result. The most accurate and earliest diagnostic test is a *serum pregnancy*. This test detects the presence of HCG in the blood serum. The results can be positive before the first missed period. A woman can have this test done one week after her believed date of conception. The test is expensive and is usually reserved for the woman, who for either health or personal reasons, needs to know very early whether or not she is pregnant.

Outline of the Fetus. In the last half of pregnancy, the body parts of the fetus may be palpated through the mother's abdomen. (See description of Leopold maneuvers, page 467.) The closer to term, the easier it is to locate the body parts. Some tumors can mimic the small body parts palpable through the abdomen. For this reason, this data is only probable, not a positive sign of pregnancy.

Positive Signs of Pregnancy

The three positive signs of pregnancy are:

1. The *fetal heart* (heard by the examiner),
2. The *fetal movement* felt by the examiner; and
3. An *x-ray* or *ultrasound* of the fetus.

FETAL HEART TONE

A normal *fetal heart rate* ranges from about 120 to 160 beats per minute. The instruments used to detect the fetal heart are the doppler (Fig. 16.11, left), the fetoscope (Fig. 16.11, right), and the stethoscope. The doppler allows one to hear the baby's heart beat earlier in the pregnancy than the other two instruments. Through the use of ultrasonic waves, this instrument can pick up the fetal heart by the 14th or 15th week of gestation. Sometimes the heart can be heard as early as the 12th week of gestation. The sound is very easy to hear. Another very nice feature of the doppler is that the provider can share this sound with the parents at the same time. With the fetoscope, the fetal heart can be heard around the 17th to 18th week. This method requires more time and practice. All practitioners are encouraged to become skilled with this method. The stethoscope is the hardest way to find the fetal heart tones. Although it is still used on occasion, the other two methods are much more efficient.

The maternal pulse can also be detected. This is relatively easy to differentiate from the fetal heart by counting the different rates. Also helpful is palpating the mother's radial pulse

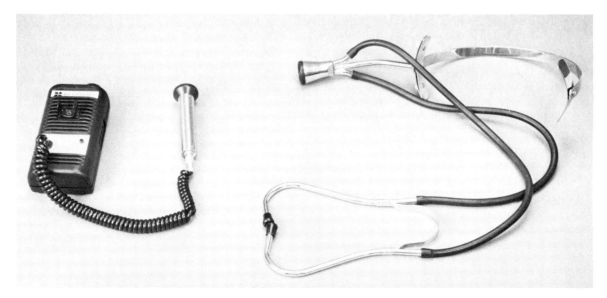

FIGURE 16.11
Equipment used to listen for fetal heart sounds. **Left.** *The Doppler.* **Right.** *The fetoscope.*

while counting the audible rhythmic sound. The rate heard should *not* be synchronous with the palpated radial rate. If it is, the examiner can then assume that she is hearing maternal pulse.

The uterine *souffle* is a blowing sound that is synchronous with the maternal pulse. The uterine souffle represents blood passing through the uterine vessels. Large tumors of the ovarian or uterine area may also cause this sound.

The *funic or umbilical cord souffle* is a sharp whistling noise heard simultaneously with the fetal heart. The sound is the result of blood flowing through the umbilical arteries. It is not constantly heard throughout pregnancy. The sound occurs in less than one quarter of all pregnant women (Pritchard, et al., 1985).

FETAL MOVEMENT FELT BY THE EXAMINER

Sometimes the movement of the fetus can be palpated by the examiner shortly after the 20th week. However, the further into the pregnancy the woman is, the easier it is to palpate the fetal movements. The first movements the examiner may feel are light, non-descript sensations. The more advanced the pregnancy becomes, the more likely a kick or thud-like sensation is to occur. When the movement is strong, it is likely to be seen as well.

X-RAY OR ULTRASOUND OF THE FETUS

An x-ray of the abdomen to detect the presence of a fetus is not commonly used anymore because of the obvious genetic hazard of roentgen rays. However, it does produce a positive diagnosis of pregnancy after about the 16th week of gestation. The fetal skeleton is visualized in the film. The first viable signs are the points of ossification (Pritchard, et al., 1985).

Ultrasound has been proven to be much safer. It also gives more detailed and accurate information than an x-ray. This painless test can detect a small white gestational ring as early as 6 weeks after the last menstrual period. The length of the embryo gives a general estimate of fetal age. Certain congenital problems can be visualized as well at this time. If there are suspicions of fetal death, this can be detected by ultrasound as early as 6 weeks.

As the pregnancy progresses, the age of the fetus can be accurately ascertained by use of the ultrasound. This is done by measuring the bipolar diameter of the baby's head using ultrasound waves. With some newer equipment, the baby's genitalia can be visualized. Ultrasound is also used to detect fetal position. If a breech position is suspected, ultrasound helps to confirm that by presenting a picture of the fetal lie in the uterus. Ultrasound is not routinely used in the assessment of the prenatal patient.

PRENATAL ASSESSMENT

Prenatal care has been revolutionized within the last century. Statistics have proven the worth of comprehensive prenatal care. The morbidity and mortality rates for both the mother and baby have dropped dramatically in the last 50 years. In the United States, in 1935, there were 12,544 reported maternal deaths, whereas in 1982 there were 330 (Chart 16.3). Although that figure represents 330 deaths too many, the decrease is striking. Many government dollars are spent today on federally funded programs that continue to provide and improve maternal–child health care.

There are many important aspects of quality prenatal care. It begins with a complete and accurate assessment of the prenatal patient. The nurse must place as much emphasis on the history as she does on the physical. It is fairly simple to conclude that a strong fetal heart rate of 120 to 160 is within normal limits. However, if the patient is not asked about swelling of her ankles and fingers, detrimental changes can be overlooked. The historical and physical data lay the foundation for patient teaching which is a critical aspect of prenatal care.

The frequency of prenatal visits will depend on the philosophy and expectations of the clinic or office. Usual scheduling for non-high risk patients might include visits monthly for the first 6 or 7 months, then bi-monthly until the 9th month and weekly after that. It is essential to remind the patient regularly that this type of schedule is a guideline only, and if there are problems, the patient should never hesitate to call and make an appointment.

The patient should be seen immediately if she presents or calls with any of the following danger signals: *vaginal bleeding, swelling of the face or fingers, severe or continuous headache, dimness or blurring of vision, abdominal pain, persistent vomiting, chills or fever, dysuria* or *escape of fluid from the vagina* (Pritchard, et al., 1985) (Chart 16.4).

Certain portions of the routine prenatal history and physical are common to each visit throughout the pregnancy. There are other parts of the prenatal visit that are not relevant or appropriate at certain times during the pregnancy.

CHART 16.3
MATERNAL MORTALITY IN THE UNITED STATES 1935–1982

	Maternal Deaths		Rate Per 100,000 Live Births		
Year	Number	Total	White	Other	
1935	12,544	582.1	530.6	945.7	
1940	8,876	376.0	319.8	773.5	
1945	5,668	107.2	172.1	454.8	
1950	2,960	83.3	61.1	221.6	
1955	1,901	47.0	32.8	130.3	
1960	1,579	37.1	26.0	97.9	
1965	1,189	31.6	21.0	83.7	
1970	803	21.5	14.4	55.9	
1975	403	12.8	9.1	29.0	
1980	334	9.2	6.7	19.8	
1982[a]	330	8.9	—	—	

[a] Provisional.
(From Pritchard, J. A., et al. Williams Obstetrics (17th ed.). Norwalk, Conn.: Appleton-Century-Crofts, 1985, p. 3.)

History

All the principles of history taking apply in the assessment of the prenatal patient, as well as any other patient. Listening, questioning, observing, and integrating are always critical elements of eliciting a thorough history.

THE INITIAL PRENATAL HISTORY

The areas of primary importance on which the nurse should focus, when pregnancy is suspected are: *demographic data, menstrual history, presumptive symptoms, past obstetric history, current health problems, occupational hazards, present medication usage, feelings about pregnancy, support systems, family history,* and *past medical history* (Chart 16.5).

Demographics. The patient's age, occupation, marital status, religion, and even her address may have implications for her pregnancy. If

CHART 16.4
DANGER SIGNALS OF PREGNANCY

Vaginal bleeding
Swelling of face or fingers
Severe or continuous headache
Dimness or blurring of vision
Abdominal pain
Persistent vomiting
Chills or fever
Dysuria
Escape of fluid from the vagina

CHART 16.5
INITIAL PRENATAL HISTORY

Demographic data
Menstrual history
Presumptive symptoms
Past obstetric history
Current health problems
Occupational hazards
Present medication usage
Feelings about pregnancy
Support system
Family history
Past medical history

she is under 18 or over 35, there is an increased risk for some congenital anomalies like Mongolism. If the patient lives in an area where there are potentially harmful substances (i.e., radiation, water spoilage, etc.), this may also put her in a high-risk category. The important issue is that the health care provider must be looking thoroughly at the history and results of the physical for red flag signals that might indicate potential danger for the mother and the child.

Menstrual History. Eliciting a complete menstrual history is essential. A history that is incomplete may result in misleading information. Questioning must go beyond the date of the last menstrual period. A woman who reports missing two periods offers a stronger likelihood of pregnancy than the woman who has only missed one period. If a woman has an irregular menstrual cycle, the dates of the last or last two menstrual periods is usually not the most accurate source of information for diagnostic or calculating purposes.

Presumptive Symptoms. Inquiring about whether or not any presumptive symptoms exist is important for the data base. Other than amenorrhea, the more common presumptive symptoms to ask about are: nausea or vomiting, urinary frequency, fatigue, increased vaginal discharge, breast tenderness, mood swings, skin changes, weight gain, abdominal enlargement, constipation, and questionable fetal movement.

Obstetric History. A complete and detailed history should be obtained. The most important areas of concern are: total number of pregnan-

cies, outcomes of each, dates of births, weights of babies, types of deliveries, lengths of gestations, lengths of labors, complications during prenatal or postpartum periods, types of feeding for babies, current health of children, and use of RhoGAM if indicated.

Current Health Problems or Concerns. The nurse should take this opportunity to investigate any current health problems or concerns, from irregular bowel habits to joint aches and pains. A thorough investigation of a problem, not previously evaluated, is necessary.

Occupational Hazards. A history of present and past employment situations should be elicited. Any exposure to toxins should be explored.

Present Medications. A precise, accurate history regarding medications is crucial. It is important to find out not only the types of medications, but also length of usage, frequency and dose of each prescription. Over-the-counter drug usage should be explored.

Any recent, but not present, use of medications should be inquired about. A woman may not have been on anything for a month or two, but she may be three months pregnant when she first seeks prenatal care. A thorough history regarding oral contraceptive usage anytime in the past should be taken.

Feelings About the Pregnancy. A woman's positiveness, reluctance, fears or anxieties should be carefully explored and assessed. Addressing the issue of whether it is a planned or unplanned pregnancy is necessary very early in the prenatal visits. A woman's feelings about being pregnant can be a tremendous support or drain to her throughout the nine months. Most women have concerns about the physical, emotional, and role changes to be encountered. Appropriate patient education and counseling can help to relieve much of the anxiety. For the woman who does not want to be pregnant, but chooses to remain so, there are very different counseling needs. For this difficult situation, the involvement of a nurse with the proper skills and empathy is necessary.

Support System. A brief inquiry regarding the patient's support systems is very worthwhile. If there is a husband or significant other who is involved as a main support, the nurse should inquire about the extent to which the patient wants this other person's participation. If the patient states she wants this other person to be actively involved, then the nurse should make it clear that he or she is also welcome to the prenatal visits and prenatal classes, etc. In a case where there are no support systems available or involved, the nurse faces further investigation and counseling.

Family History. A quick overview of the family history is important in the early visits. Exploring the health status of grandparents, parents, siblings of both the mother and father, and other children, is necessary. Finally, an inquiry about any family members on either side with: diabetes, cancer, cardiovascular disease, renal disease, mental illness, seizure disorders, mental retardation, tuberculosis, neuromuscular disease, unusual causes of death, multiple pregnancies or complications with pregnancies should be permanent data on the patient's chart.

Past Medical History. Any significant illnesses or hospitalizations should be recorded. Included in this should be a brief description of the course of the illness or hospitalization, any complications and the outcome. The most up-to-date information about allergies, childhood illnesses, and immunizations should also be elicited.

FIRST TRIMESTER PRENATAL REVISIT HISTORY
The approach to prenatal care during the first trimester has a theme. The nurse must determine the patient's feelings about being pregnant, identify her level of discomfort with early pregnancy symptoms, assess her nutritional practices, and identify her ideas about work or daily activities during pregnancy.

The subjective areas to be explored at each first trimester visit are:

1. Questions, complaints, or concerns?
2. Changes noted in body since last visit or since first pregnant?
3. Presence or update of first trimester discomforts? (i.e., fatigue, nausea, etc.)

4. Presence of danger signals?
5. Appetite, nutritional practices, typical 24-hour diet?
6. Vaginal discharge?
7. Maintenance or interference with daily activities, work, exercise, etc.?
8. Sexual concerns?
9. Use of medications (other than vitamins) and reasons?
10. Feelings about pregnancy—partner's feelings, etc.?
11. Reading about pregnancy—what type, need for suggestions?

SECOND TRIMESTER PRENATAL REVISIT HISTORY
Many of the first trimester discomforts are either resolving or have been resolved by the beginning of this trimester. Therefore, the focus of the visits change. The mother's abdomen is enlarging as the baby grows during this trimester. About the 20th week, the fetal heart tones are audible and she begins to feel life. For her, all these signs confirm the reality of the pregnancy. Because she is feeling better, it is now appropriate for the nurse to concentrate on the woman's personal experiences or adjustments. The following history is important to elicit during the next 13 weeks.

The subjective areas to be explored at each second trimester visit are:

1. Questions, complaints or concerns (new since the last visit)?
2. Changes noted in body since last visit (i.e., feeling life)?
3. Presence or update of first trimester symptoms or new discomforts (hemorrhoids, constipation, heartburn, etc.)?
4. Presence of danger signals?
5. Feeling signs of life, flutters, kicks?
6. Appetite—24-hour diet history?
7. Vaginal discharge?
8. Maintenance or interference with daily activities or work?
9. Sexual concerns or difficulties?
10. Use of medications since last visit?
11. New feelings about pregnancy? Mother's and father's adjustment?
12. Thoughts about feeding the baby by breast or bottle?
13. Interest in further reading?

THIRD TRIMESTER PRENATAL REVISIT HISTORY
During this time, the frequency of prenatal visits will increase. The baby's growth and development and mother's overall health status may change more dramatically from week to week. The thrust of the history takes a somewhat different approach, but basically the same history is taken with some additions.

The subjective areas to be explored at each third trimester visit are:

1. Questions, complaints, or concerns (new or since last visit)?
2. Changes noted in body since last visit, (i.e., urinating more frequently)?
3. Presence or update of second trimester symptoms or new discomforts (difficulty sleeping, back pain, etc.)?
4. Presence of danger signals?
5. Feeling life? Where being kicked? Can visualize abdomen move?
6. Appetite—24-hour diet?
7. Vaginal discharge?
8. Maintenance or interference with daily activities? Able to keep working? When does she plan to stop?
9. Sexual concerns—issues concerning intercourse? Difficulty finding comfortable positions?
10. Preparation for baby—nursery, help at home, etc.
11. Understanding when to contact physician or nurse when labor begins?
12. Updated plans for feeding baby—breast or bottle?
13. Anxieties about birth and new parenting role?
14. Attendance of prenatal classes? Practicing exercises? Plan to be supported by whom during labor and delivery?
15. Readings? Further interest?

Physical Assessment

Ideally at the time of the initial visit, a complete physical examination, including a pelvic, is performed. The following objective data is obtained at every revisit: *weight, blood pressure, fundal height, fetal heart rate* and *location, CVA tenderness, presence of varicosities* and *edema, Homans' sign, patellar deep tendon reflexes* (some health care providers do this

for baseline information in case *hyperreflexia* occurs), and *urine* for protein and sugar (Chart 16.6). Additional data to be obtained varies with the week of gestation.

THE INITIAL PRENATAL EXAMINATION
The areas of the initial complete physical examination that are of primary importance in assessing the pregnant patient include: general assessment; height and weight; pulse and blood pressure; skin; eyes, ears, nose, throat exam; thyroid and lymph nodes of the neck; breast exam; examination of the lungs and heart; abdominal exam; a pelvic exam including a speculum exam, bimanual and clinical pelvimetry; extremities; musculoskeletal, neurological, and specific laboratory studies.

1. *General.* The woman's emotional status, appearance and affect are assessed.
2. *Height and weight.* The patient's height and weight are necessary for baseline purposes. It is also helpful to look back through the patient's previous record for general weights and heights during past pregnancies. These numbers will directly influence the nutritional counseling done during the pregnancy.
3. *Blood pressure.* This is a critical measurement to monitor throughout the pregnancy. Any change from the baseline should be carefully noted. A blood pressure of 140/90 mm Hg is considered a sign of preeclampsia, as is any rise of 30 mm Hg systolic or 15 mm Hg diastolic from the baseline pressure. (Pritchard, et al., 1985)

CHART 16.6
OBJECTIVE DATA OBTAINED AT EVERY PRENATAL VISIT[a]

Weight
Blood pressure
Fundal height
Fetal heart rate
CVA tenderness
Presence of varicosities
Presence of edema
Homans' sign
Urine for protein sugar

[a] Additional data may be indicated depending on the week of gestation or if a problem exists.

4. *Skin.* Examination includes inspection for lesions and moles, scars, striae, linea nigra, and chloasma.
5. *Eyes.* Visual acuity is assessed. The external eye examination includes the conjunctiva, sclera, and pupillary reaction to light and accommodation. A complete funduscopic examination should be performed.
6. *Ears.* The auricle is inspected and an otoscopic examination is done.
7. *Nose and throat.* The nasal passages are inspected and checked for patency. The anterior and posterior pharynx are examined. Close attention is paid to the condition of the teeth and gums.
8. *Neck.* The anterior and posterior cervical nodes are palpated. The thyroid is palpated for enlargement and irregularities.
9. *Breasts.* The breasts are inspected for symmetry, venous pattern, changes in areola color, swelling, and dimpling. They are palpated for tenderness, consistency, masses, and nipple discharge. A woman is likely to notice breast enlargement within the first trimester. On exam, more nodular tissue may be felt due to the hypertrophy of the areola. Toward the end of the first trimester, the superficial veins in the breasts will become more visible beneath the skin's surface. The nipples will become larger and more deeply pigmented, as well.
10. *Lungs.* Examination of the lung includes respiratory rate and auscultation of the lung fields.
11. *Heart.* The heart is palpated for heaves and thrills and for the point of maximum impulse. The heart is auscultated in the sitting and lying positions. Murmurs and extra sounds are noted.
12. *Abdominal examination.* The value of the abdominal exam will depend on the length of gestation. If the gestational age is more than 12 weeks, the examiner will be able to palpate the uterus in the abdominal cavity with deep palpation. The kidneys, spleen and liver are palpated (when possible). Last, CVA tenderness is assessed.
13. *Speculum examination.* Changes visualized in the introitus, vagina, and cervix will also be affected by the gestational age. Early signs will be the bluing or cyanotic appearance of the vaginal organs (Chadwick's sign). A moderate amount of clear to cloudy discharge will be visible during the speculum exam. The discharge should not be gray, yellow, green, frothy, or have a thick white cottage cheese-like texture. There should be no foul odor. If there is any doubt in the examiner's mind, a microscopic evaluation should be done. A Pap smear is usually taken at this time, too. The results of the Pap smear may help identify a vaginal infection. Further speculum examinations are usually not performed again during the pregnancy unless a problem arises.
14. *Bimanual examination.* The outcome of this exam will depend strictly on gestational age. The further along the pregnancy is, the easier it is to determine gestational age. In the very early weeks of pregnancy, the softening of the cervix (Goodell's sign) is usually fairly evident. The isthmus between the cervix and uterus will also soften (Hegar's sign) considerably. Uterine enlargement prior to 12 weeks of gestation is often hard to determine.
15. *Clinical pelvimetry.* Clinical pelvimetry is the measurement of the diameters of the boney pelvis. It is an assessment of the adequacy of the pelvis for delivery. The examination is somewhat uncomfortable for the patient so it is done after the internal examination of the soft pelvic organs. This evaluation is included as part of the initial examination and may be repeated again late in the 3rd trimester (Varner, et al., 1980).

    Prior to performing clinical pelvimetry, it is important that the nurse take two measurements of her hands because they will be used as the measurement instruments. First, the distance between the tip of the middle or longest finger to the juncture of the first finger with the thumb is measured. Second, the fist is measured across the knuckles.

    It is important to establish an organized procedure for performing the examination of the bony pelvis. This avoids missing important aspects of the examination and contributes to the pa-

tient's comfort. The following bony pelvis landmarks are assessed:
a. Subpubic arch
b. Pelvic side walls
c. Ischial spines
d. Interspinous diameter
e. Sacrosciatic notch
f. Sacrum
g. Coccyx
h. Diagonal conjugate
i. Intertuberous diameter

The *subpubic arch* is at the inferior margin of the symphysis pubis (Fig. 16.12). The angle of the subpubic arch is palpated by inserting two fingers horizontally into the vagina just beneath the

arch (Fig. 16.13). If two fingers fit in this location the arch is probably at least a 90-degree angle which is optimal. Next, each *pelvic side wall* is palpated to determine if it is straight, convergent, or divergent. To examine the side walls, the vaginal fingers sweep down the lateral walls of the pelvis to the ischial spines at the point of the widest transverse diameter of the pelvic outlet. On examination, the side walls normally feel fairly straight.

The *ischial spines* are palpated bilaterally (Fig. 16.12). Each spine is assessed as being blunt (or flat), prominent (or sharp), or encroaching. The

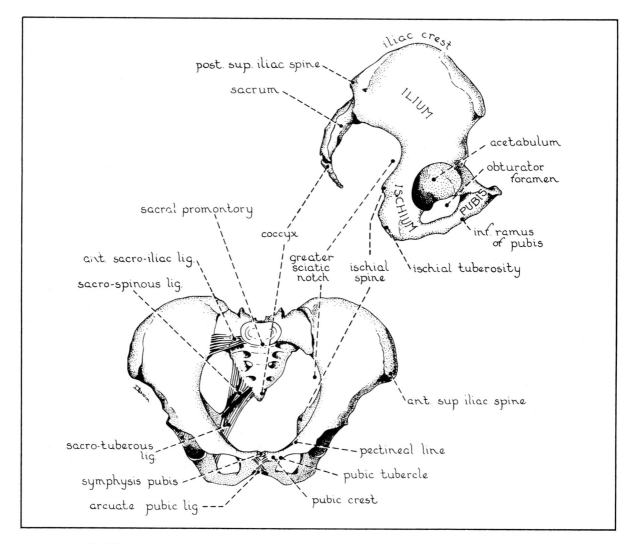

FIGURE 16.12
Bones and joints of the pelvis. (From Oxorn, H. Human Labor and Birth (5th ed.). Norwalk, Conn.: Appleton-Century-Crofts, 1986.)

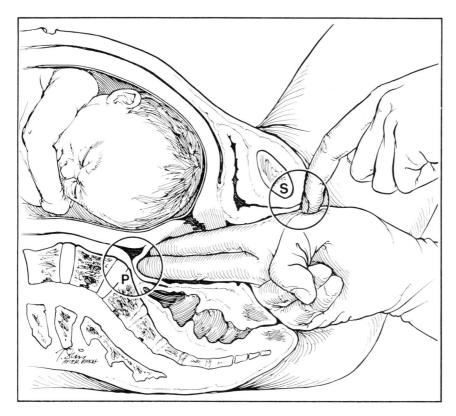

FIGURE 16.13
*Vaginal examination to deter-
mine the diagonal conjugate (P
= sacral promontory, S = symphysis pubis). (From Pritchard,
J. A., et al. Williams Obstetrics
(17th ed.). Norwalk, Conn.:
Appleton-Century-Crofts, 1985,
p. 227.)*

distance between the two spines (interspinous diameter) is measured by placing one examining finger on one spine
and spreading the examining fingers to
reach the other spine. Many individuals'
fingers do not spread to the normal measurement of 11.5 centimeters.

The shape and height at the sacrosciatic notch is assessed. The length
of *sacrospinous ligament* (Fig. 16.12) extending from the ischial spine to the sacrum is determined. This measurement,
which is the same as the width of the
sacrosciatic notch, is normally 2 to 3
fingerbreadths.

The examining fingers are moved
down the sacrum to the coccyx. First
the shape of the *sacrum* is determined.
It may be hollow, flat, or curved. The
sacrum is generally hollow. Next, by applying firm pressure on the coccyx it is
described as movable or fixed.

The measurement of the *diagonal
conjugate* (Fig. 16.13) is the last of the
internal measurements because it can
be very uncomfortable. This is the measurement of the distance between the

sacral promontory and the lower border
of the symphysis pubis. Two fingers are
placed in the posterior fornix of the vagina, and juncture of the finger and
thumb is located just to the side of the
urethra to avoid trauma. The vaginal
fingers are gently moved backward up
the sacrum until the middle finger
presses against the *sacral promontory*
(Fig. 16.13). By exerting pressure on the
juncture of the first finger and thumb
the examiner can extend her reach.
Once the sacral promontory is reached
with the middle finger, the free hand
is used to mark the point on the examining hand which is touching the symphysis pubis. The vaginal hand is removed
and the distance from the tip of the middle finger to the mark on the finger
which was at the symphysis pubis is
measured. If this measurement is 11.5
centimeters or greater, the inlet is usually assumed to be adequate. If the examiner is unable to reach the sacral promontory she knows that the diagonal
conjugate is longer than her examining
fingers which were measured earlier.

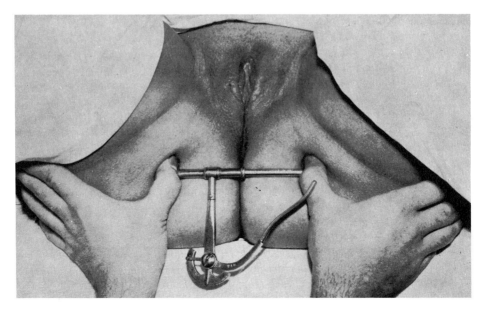

FIGURE 16.14
Mensuration of transverse diameter of outlet with Thoms' pelvimeter. Using the examiner's pre-measured fist will work also. (From Pritchard, J. A., et al. Williams Obstetrics (16th ed.). Norwalk, Conn.: Appleton-Century-Crofts, 1980, p. 284.)

Finally, the distance between the ischial tuberosities (*intertuberous diameter* or the *transverse diameter of the outlet*) (Fig. 16.14) is measured. This can be determined by placing the premeasured fist between the tuberosities. It is usually 7 to 8 centimeters in length.

16. *Extremities.* The legs are inspected for varicosities. Homans' sign is performed. The feet, legs, and hands are checked for edema.
17. *Musculoskeletal.* The patient is screened for orthopedic problems, mobility and shape of her spine.
18. *Neurologic.* Deep tendon reflexes, upper, and lower motor coordination are assessed.
19. *Laboratory studies.* Baseline laboratory information varies from clinic to clinic. The most common tests include: (1) hematocrit or hemoglobin, (2) serology, (3) blood type, (4) RH factor, (5) rubella titre, (6) Pap smear, (7) GC culture, and (8) urinalysis for protein and glucose with a microscope examination for bacteria or an alternative screening for bacteria. All black patients and those of Mediterranean origin should be tested for sickle-cell trait or disease. Some clinics require a broad spectrum of blood

tests such as those found in an SMA-6, SMA-12, or complete blood count (CBC).

THE FIRST TRIMESTER PRENATAL REVISIT PHYSICAL EXAMINATION

The objective foci for prenatal visits during the first trimester include:

1. *Weight.* An expected 2 to 4 pounds should be gained during these 13 weeks. The weight should be measured at each visit.
2. *Blood pressure.* No change is expected. Compare each prenatal visit's blood pressure to baseline information. The blood pressure should be taken at each visit.
3. *Abdomen.* There are probably not many changes in the abdomen during this trimester. The fundus is only palpable just above the symphysis pubis at 12 weeks. Thus, most of the abdominal changes are more evident in the last two trimesters. CVA tenderness is assessed.
4. *Extremities.* The legs are inspected for varicosities. Homans' sign is performed. The feet, legs and hands are checked for edema.
5. *Neurologic.* The patellar deep tendon reflexes are assessed if the patient is hypertensive, or preeclampsia is suspected. The patient may be hyperreflexive if pre-

eclamptic. Other reflexes are tested if indicated.

6. *Laboratory procedures.* At every prenatal visit, the urine is tested for glucose and protein. Spillage of glucose in the urine may be a sign of gestational diabetes. Therefore, any presence of glucose in the urine should be investigated further. Trace protein is not usually considered abnormal. One plus or greater protein in the urine may also be indicative of a problem. Along with edema and elevated blood pressure, proteinuria is a key feature of preeclampsia. Most commonly, this condition does not appear until the third trimester. As with glycosuria, proteinuria should be investigated.

THE SECOND TRIMESTER PRENATAL REVISIT PHYSICAL EXAMINATION

Because the mother usually feels well and this trimester does not harbor a great deal of risk, there is no need to increase the frequency of the visits. If problems begin to emerge, then this approach, of course, will change. The objective concerns are:

1. *Weight.* If the patient gained only the expected 2 to 4 pounds during the first trimester, then it is reasonable for her to gain a total of 12 to 14 pounds during this trimester. This usually averages out to about 1 pound per week.
2. *Blood pressure.* No change is expected.
3. *Skin.* The skin should be inspected for spider nevi, telangiectasia and presence of acne. Spider nevi and telangiectasia may emerge during the second and third trimesters. They commonly appear on the neck, thorax, face, and arms.

   The response to acne is individual. It may be more or less, but significant changes should be recorded.
4. *Breasts.* The breasts continue to grow in size. Other breast changes that took place in the first trimester might be enhanced. Toward the end of this trimester, the patient may notice that she can express colostrum from the nipples. No further examination, other than the initial evaluation, is necessary unless a problem arises.
5. *Abdomen.* Significant changes take place in the abdominal cavity during this trimester. The uterus should be palpated abdominally at each prenatal visit to measure the fundal height and to help confirm the existence of a fetus. Fetal movement can be felt and seen by the examiner later in this trimester.

As the pregnancy advances, palpating the fundus of the uterus becomes easier. There are three methods used to measure the height of the fundus. The first two methods give a gross calculation. They give the examiner a general idea of where the uterus is, compared to where it is expected to be.

For the first two methods, the patient is in a supine position with her abdomen exposed. The examiner places the ulnar sides of her hand on the abdomen, a few fingerbreadths above where she expects to find the top of the fundus. She then moves her hand down towards the uterus, palpating deeply about a fingerbreadth between each palpation. Eventually, the soft subcutaneous tissue of the abdomen will disappear and she will feel a rounded, solid, firm edge. This is the top of the uterus or fundus. The distance from the symphysis to the umbilicus or umbilicus to the xiphoid process is estimated and recorded (i.e., halfway between the umbilicus and xiphoid). According to the second method the examiner counts the number of fingerbreadths the fundus is below the xiphoid or umbilicus (i.e., the fundus is 2 fingerbreadths below the xiphoid).

The third method uses a more precise estimate. Between the 18th and 36th week, this method can be used. Again, the patient is in the supine position with her abdomen exposed. A cloth or paper tape measure with centimeters is needed. The tape measure is placed and held down with one finger at the symphysis pubis (Fig. 16.15). Then holding the tape between the examiner's straightened index and middle fingers of the opposite hand the tape is extended over the uterus to the top of the fundus. Between the 18th and 36th week, the uterus grows 1 centimeter per week. The measurement in centimeters should equal the gestational age until about the 36th week when the fundus is at the level of the xiphoid process.

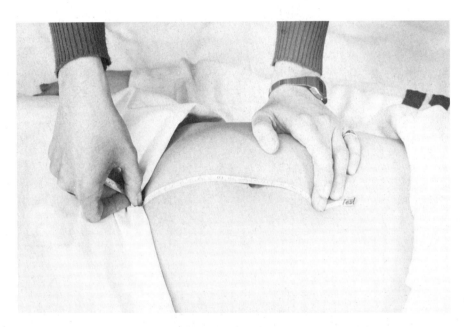

FIGURE 16.15
Measuring fundal height.

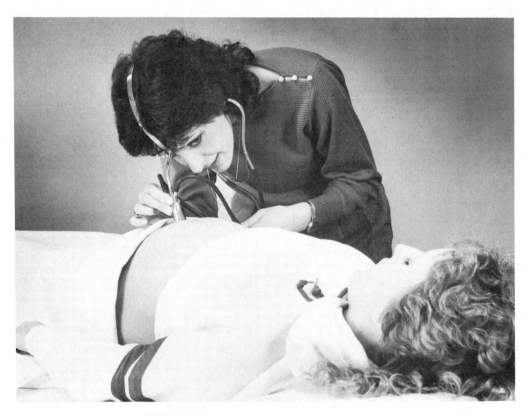

FIGURE 16.16
Listening for a fetal heart sound with a fetoscope.

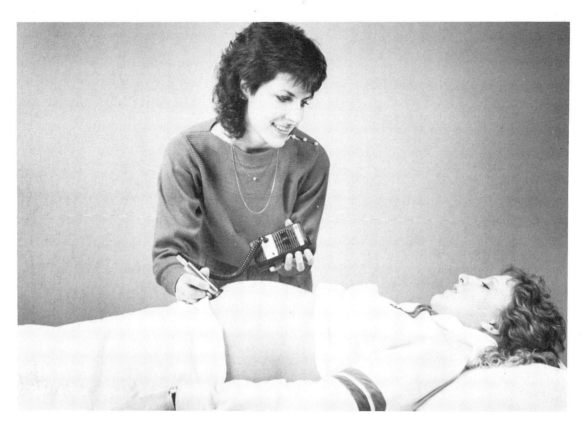

FIGURE 16.17
Listening for a fetal heart sound with a Doppler.

Around the 20th week, the fetus can be palpated. The examiner pushes down firmly on the uterus and then releases her hand. As she is easing up on the applied pressure, the fetus will ballott against her hand. A firm sensation will hit her hand momentarily as she is releasing her hand. This is a probable sign of pregnancy.

Another occurrence in this trimester is that the patient reports feeling life. The sensation goes from flutters to kicks. If the examiner can feel or see the fetus move, a positive sign of pregnancy can be recorded.

More likely, however, the first positive sign will be hearing a fetal heart (Figs. 16.16 and 16.17). The type of equipment and the parity of the mother will affect when the fetal heart rate can first be heard. In the early stages of listening for this, the sounds can be most clearly heard just above the symphysis pubis.

Later in the pregnancy, the location of the fetal heart will depend on the position of the fetus. It is usually heard most clearly through the back of the fetus.

Finally, CVA tenderness is assessed.

6. *Extremities.* The extremities should be inspected and palpated carefully at each visit. Mild bilateral ankle edema may appear as the pregnancy progresses through this trimester. This usually appears after the patient has been on her feet for an extended period of time. Mild ankle edema goes away after getting up in the morning or when a woman puts her feet up for awhile. If there are no other symptoms of preeclampsia (proteinuria and elevated blood pressure), then it is usually not worrisome. However, if facial edema or significant hand or facial swelling exists, further investigation is indicated.

Some leg varicosities may be visible in the latter part of this trimester. Their location, smoothness, and tenderness

464

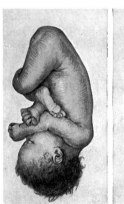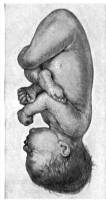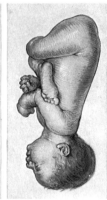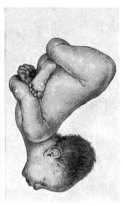

FIGURE 16.18
Differences in attitude of fetus in vertex, sinciput, brow, and face presentations. (From Pritchard, J. A., et al. Williams Obstetrics (17th ed.). Norwalk, Conn.: Appleton-Century-Crofts, 1985, p. 236.)

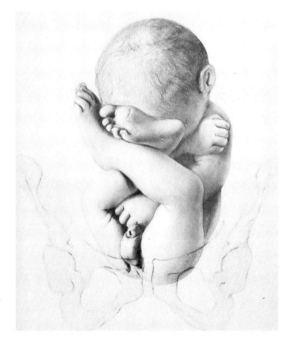

FIGURE 16.19
Frank breech presentation. (From Pritchard, J. A., et al. Williams Obstetrics (17th ed.). Norwalk, Conn.: Appleton-Century-Crofts, 1985, p. 236.)

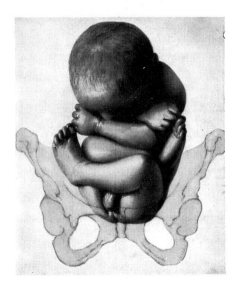

FIGURE 16.20
Complete breech presentation. (From Pritchard, J. A., et al. Williams Obstetrics (17th ed.). Norwalk, Conn.: Appleton-Century-Crofts, 1985, p. 236.)

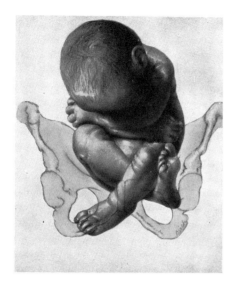

FIGURE 16.21
Incomplete breech presentation. (From Pritchard, J. A., et al. Williams Obstetrics (17th ed.). Norwalk, Conn.: Appleton-Century-Crofts, 1985, p. 236.)

should be recorded. If they are large, distended, tender to touch and tortuous, further evaluation is required.

Varicose veins can occur in the legs, vulva, or perineum (hemorrhoids). These may be very uncomfortable and may make an otherwise fairly uneventful pregnancy, very uncomfortable. As with severe leg varicosities, vulvar or perineal involvement should be recorded precisely. There are local, safe remedies that can be implemented to help relieve the discomfort.

7. *Neurologic.* The patellar deep tendon reflexes are assessed if indicated. (See "First Trimester Visit: Neurologic," page 460.)

8. *Laboratory procedures.* A urine glucose and protein is performed at each visit. Some providers like to have a one-hour obstetric glucose or a two-hour post prandial glucose tolerance screening test and a hematocrit (HCT) obtained between 26 and 30 weeks. An Rh titre is obtained if the woman is Rh negative.

THE THIRD TRIMESTER PRENATAL REVISIT PHYSICAL EXAMINATION

The objective information needed to be gathered during the last trimester includes the following:

1. *Weight.* Up to this point in the pregnancy, the patient should have gained about 18 pounds. An additional 8 to 10 pounds will be gained this trimester. Total weight gain should be about 24 to 30 pounds. A sudden and large weight gain (1 lb. in a week), especially in this trimester, may be an indicator of fluid retention and potential preeclampsia.

2. *Blood pressure.* If a problem is to arise regarding blood pressure, it is likely to be in the third trimester. An elevation over earlier stated figures (see p. 456) is a major criteria for preeclampsia. A second reading should always be taken to confirm the elevation.

3. *Breasts.* Breast changes continue through term. Unless a problem exists, examination is unnecessary.

4. *Abdomen.* Continued assessment of the abdomen is necessary at each prenatal visit. At this point in the pregnancy, the uterus is well above the umbilicus and by the 36th week, it is at the level of the xiphoid. The fundal height should be measured.

The other important portion of the abdominal exam during this trimester is *Leopold maneuvers.* These maneuvers are used to determine the *lie of the fetus and the presenting part.* The lie of the fetus is the relationship of the long axis of the fetus to the mother (Pritchard, et al., 1985). The lie can be transverse, longitudinal or oblique (Fig. 16.14). The presenting part refers to that part of the baby which is most prominently situated in the pelvis or birth canal. The presenting part can be the head (vertex) (Fig. 16.18), shoulder, brow, face, or breech (Figs. 16.19–16.21). In a longitudinal lie, the

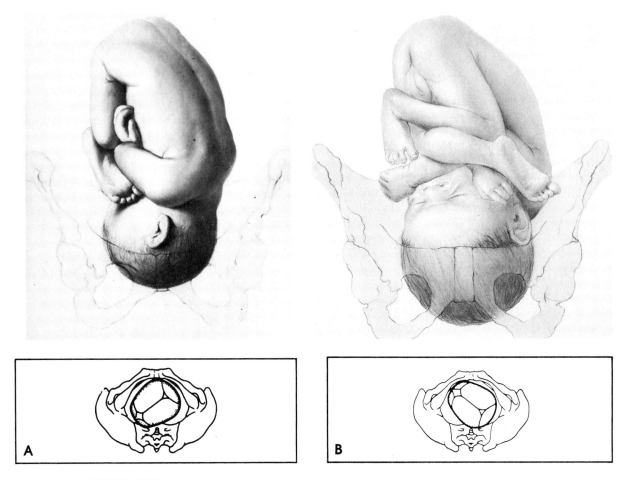

FIGURE 16.22
Vertex presentation: **A.** Left Occipito-Anterior. **B.** Left Occipito-Posterior. (From Pritchard, J. A.,
et al. Williams Obstetrics (17th ed.). Norwalk, Conn.: Appleton-Century-Crofts, 1985, p. 237.)

presentation is either vertex or breech. In a transverse presentation, the shoulder is the presenting part (Pritchard, et al., 1985).

For the most part, the shape of the fetus is in a *flexed* position. The fetus is usually bent upon itself with the chin often pointing down toward the chest, and the back is almost convex. The arms and legs are crossed over the thorax and abdomen. In some instances, the baby may be in a more extended position. This is most evident by the position of the head. When this occurs in a cephalic presentation, the presenting part will be the face.

The fetus can lie in one of two *positions* in relation to the mother's pelvis. The part of the baby's body that lies in the birth canal will face either right or

left. Therefore, with each presentation, there may be either a right or left position (Figs. 16.22–16.25).

The frequency of presentations at term approximates: 96 percent—vertex; 3.5 percent—breech; 0.3 percent—face; and 0.4 percent—shoulder (Pritchard, et al., 1985). Almost two-thirds of the vertex presentations are in the left position.

The terminology for presenting parts and position is based on the above information. The presentations are: *left or right occipital, left or right sacral, left or right mental (face)*. Remembering that the presenting position can be transverse (T), anterior (A), or posterior (P), one can include 6 varieties of these three presentations (Figs. 16.22–16.26). Because it is difficult to distinguish the position of the

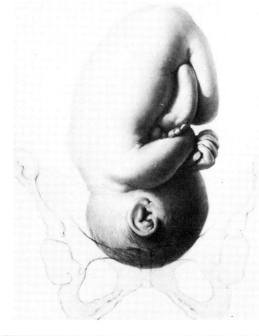
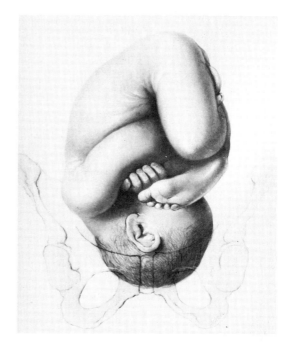
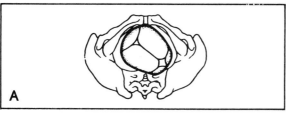
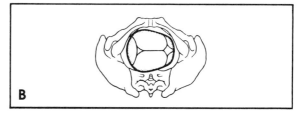

FIGURE 16.23
Vertex presentation: **A.** Right Occipito-Anterior. **B.** Right Occipito-Transverse. (From Pritchard, J. A., et al. Williams Obstetrics (17th ed.). Norwalk, Conn.: Appleton-Century-Crofts, 1985, p. 238.)

shoulder in relation to the pelvis, it is accepted that all transverse lies are referred to as shoulder presentations.

Knowing all this theoretical information about position, presentation and lie, it is possible for the examiner to use *Leopold's maneuvers* to determine how the baby is situated in utero.

There are four *Leopold maneuvers.* For each maneuver the mother should be lying flat on her back (although a pillow may be placed under her knees) and the abdomen exposed. For the first three maneuvers, the nurse stands at the patient's bedside (either side) and faces the patient. For the fourth maneuver she reverses her position and faces the patient's feet.

The first Leopold maneuver is used to determine the location of the baby's head. As described earlier, the head of the fetus will ballot when pushed on. The back and rump of the baby will *not* rebound to the examiners hand like the head does. If the head ballots in the pelvis, then a cephalic presentation seems likely. If in the lower abdomen, the examiner feels nodular-like bumps and the head ballots up toward the xiphoid, a breech presentation is more likely (Fig. 16.27).

The second Leopold maneuver helps to locate the baby's back. It is performed with the examiner's hands placed on either side of the patient's abdomen. Gentle, but firm pressure is applied on one side of the abdomen, and then the other; feeling for a long, smooth hard structure. This is the back. The limbs on the opposite side will feel like bumps. These are

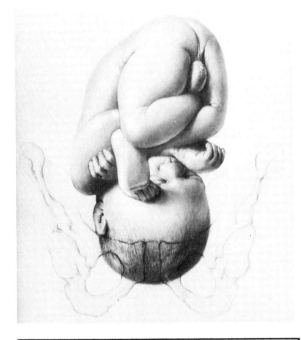

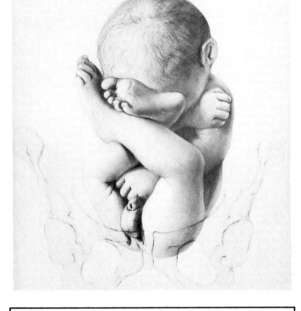

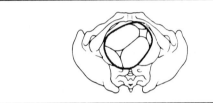

FIGURE 16.24
Vertex presentation: **C.** *Right Occipito-Posterior. (From Pritchard, J. A., et al. Williams Obstetrics (17th ed.). Norwalk, Conn.: Appleton-Century-Crofts, 1985, p. 239.)*

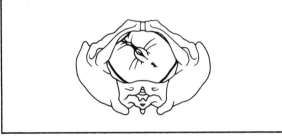

FIGURE 16.26
Breech presentation: Left sacrum posterior position. (From Pritchard, J. A., et al. Williams Obstetrics (17th ed.). Norwalk, Conn.: Appleton-Century-Crofts, 1985, p. 240.)

FIGURE 16.25
Face presentation: Right and left, anterior and posterior positions. (From Pritchard, J. A., et al. Williams Obstetrics (17th ed.). Norwalk, Conn.: Appleton-Century-Crofts, 1985, p. 239.)

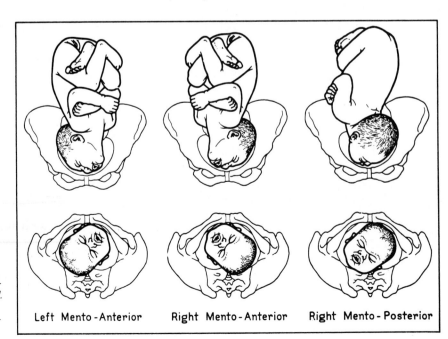

Left Mento-Anterior   Right Mento-Anterior   Right Mento-Posterior

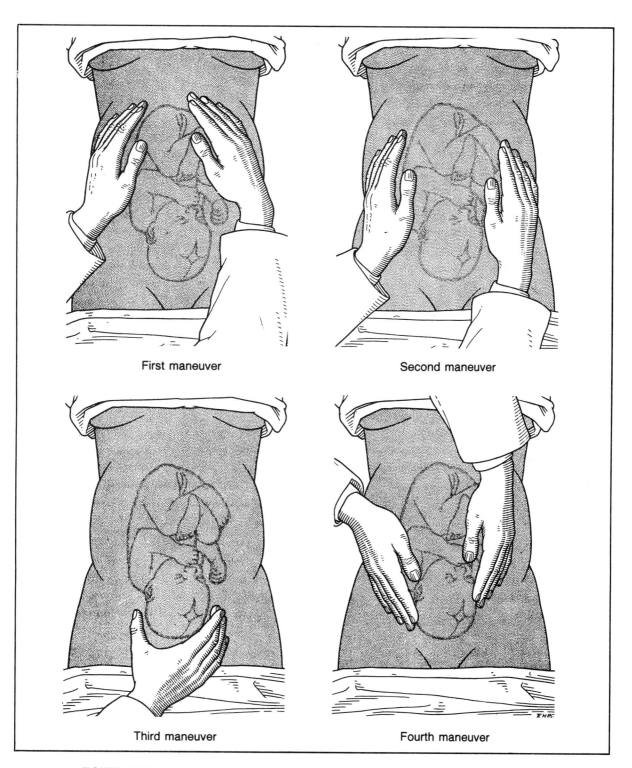

First maneuver

Second maneuver

Third maneuver

Fourth maneuver

FIGURE 16.27
Palpation in left occiput anterior position (maneuvers of Leopold). (From Pritchard, J. A., et al. Williams Obstetrics (17th ed.). Norwalk, Conn.: Appleton-Century-Crofts, 1985, p. 241.)

elbows, knees, feet, or hands (Fig. 16.27).

The third maneuver helps to determine if the head is engaged in the pelvis. For this maneuver, the examiner uses only one hand. If the right hand is used, she places it over the symphysis area (Fig. 16.27). She puts her right thumb on the mother's right side (right of umbilical line), and fingers on the left. The goal is to try to determine if the presenting part is engaged. Firm pressure is used. If the head moves back and forth easily, it is probably not engaged. If the head does not move, it may well be engaged.

The fourth maneuver is used to determine which side the cephalic prominence is on. In some women, this data may be very hard to obtain, especially if the patient is obese. The examiner changes her position for this. She stands facing the mother's feet (Fig. 16.27) with both hands applied on either side of the uterus. Firm pressure is applied around the area of the pelvis. If the musculature around the abdominal wall is tight, ask the patient to take a deep breath and let it out slowly. As she lets it out, the examiner applies pressure to gain some entry into the pelvic inlet. If the head is presenting, the rounded cephalic prominence will stop further access to the inlet. In a vertex presentation, the cephalic prominence is on the same side as the small nodular bumps of fetal extremities, felt earlier. In the fetus with a face presentation, the cephalic prominence will be on the same side as the back (Pritchard, et al., 1985). The level to which the fetus has descended into the pelvis is a direct reflection of the value of this test. Finally, CVA tenderness is assessed.

5. *Extremities.* Examining the extremities is very important during this trimester. The examination is the same as in the second trimester. It is likely that ankle edema will increase during these weeks. Whether or not it is relieved after the feet are elevated for a period of time should be explored. Many women are unable to wear rings on their fingers any longer. Finger edema and puffiness around the periorbital areas should be carefully evaluated. Recording precisely how much edema exists at each visit, will help to know if there is any change over certain periods of time.

6. *Neurologic.* The patellar deep tendon reflexes are assessed at each visit as indicated. (See "First Trimester Visit: Neurological," p. 460.)

7. *Laboratory procedures.* A urine glucose and protein is performed at every visit. At approximately 34 to 36 weeks, the hematocrit, VDRL, GC culture and urinalysis with a screening for bacteria may be repeated, if indicated. Blood glucose screening may be repeated at this time if the woman is at risk.

EXAMPLE OF A RECORDED HISTORY AND PHYSICAL

SUBJECTIVE:

Reason for Visit: "I'm 36 weeks pregnant and I'm here for my weekly visit."

Patient considers herself to be in "very good health," and states that pregnancy has been progressing without any problems. Patient reports feeling activity in uterus throughout day, but especially when first lying down at night. She and husband both see and feel movement.

Denies any bleeding or other vaginal discharge, swelling of face, feet or fingers (still able to wear and remove wedding ring), headache, change or problem with vision, abdominal pain, vomiting, chills or fever, or pain or burning with urination. Also states she has no constipation.

Eats 3 meals daily. Drinks 4 glasses of milk, watches snacking, avoids salt. Plans to breastfeed. She is no longer using soap on nipples. She and husband are finishing up birthing classes and practice breathing exercises at home. Patient also attends weekly exercise class at hospital for expectant mothers. Nursery is ready and suitcase is packed. Feels husband has been very supportive. They are both nervous about labor and delivery.

OBJECTIVE:

Gravida 1; Para 0; AB 0

Weight: 142 pounds (pre-pregnant weight 120 pounds)

B.P. 122/76 (pre-pregnant blood pressure 120/70)

Urine: Negative for protein and glucose

Abdomen: Head ballotts above symphysis pubis. Fetal heart heard in L side of abdomen at the level of umbilicus—Rate 146
FUNDAL HEIGHT: 36 cm.
Linea nigra present
No costovertebral angle tenderness

Extremities: No varicosities of legs. No edema of fingers, feet, or ankles

REFERENCES

Bobak, I., & Benson, R. (1984). Maternity Care: The Nurse and the Family (3rd ed.). St. Louis: C. V. Mosby.

Combes, B., & Adams, R. (1971). Pathophysiology of the liver in pregnancy. In N. S. Assali, (Ed.), Pathophysiology of Pregnancy, Vol. 1. New York: Academic Press.

Naeye, R. (1979). Weight gain and the outcome of pregnancy. American Journal of Obstetrics and Gynecology, 135:3.

Potter, J., & Nestel, P. (1979). The hyperlipidemia of pregnancy in normal and complicated pregnancies. American Journal of Obstetrics and Gynecology, 133:165.

Pritchard, J. A., McDonald, P. C., & Gant, N. F. (1985). Williams Obstetrics (17th ed.). Norwalk, Conn.: Appleton-Century-Crofts.

Rubin, R. (1984). Maternal Identity and the Maternal Experience. New York: Springer.

Varner, M. W., Cruikshank, D. P., & Laube, D. W. (1980). X-ray pelvimetry in clinical obstetrics. Obstetrics and Gynecology, 56:296.

Appendix A

WORKSHEET FOR PATIENT HISTORY

NAME _____

ADDRESS _____

AGE _____ SEX _____ MARITAL STATUS _____

RACE _____ RELIGION _____

OCCUPATION _____

USUAL SOURCE OF MEDICAL CARE _____

SOURCE AND RELIABILITY OF INFORMATION _____

CHIEF COMPLAINT/REASON FOR VISIT:

HISTORY OF PRESENT STATE OF HEALTH:

PAST HISTORY:

Childhood Illnesses:

Immunizations:

Allergies:

Hospitalizations and Serious Illnesses:

Accidents and Injuries:

Medications:

Habits:

Prenatal History: *

Labor and Delivery History: *

Neonatal History: *

FAMILY HISTORY:

REVIEW OF SYSTEMS:

General:

Skin and Mucous Membranes:

Hair:

Nails:

** Recorded for all children 5 years of age and under and older children with a congenital
or developmental problem.*

Head:

Eyes:

Ears:

Nose and Sinuses:

Mouth:

Throat:

Neck:

Nodes:

Breasts:

Respiratory:

Cardiovascular:

Gastrointestinal:

Genitourinary:

Back:

Extremities:

Neurologic:

Hematopoietic:

Endocrine:

NUTRITIONAL HISTORY:

SOCIAL DATA:

Family Relationships and Friendships:

Ethnic Affiliation:

Occupational History:

Educational History:

Economic Status:

Daily Profile:

Living Circumstances:

Pattern of Health Care:

DEVELOPMENTAL HISTORY:

SEXUAL HISTORY:

EXERCISE AND ACTIVITY PATTERNS:

STRESS PATTERNS:

Appendix B

EXAMPLE OF A RECORDED PHYSICAL EXAMINATION

NAME: L.R.   **Age:** 19   **Sex:** Female

HEIGHT: 5'5"   **WEIGHT:** 125 lbs.

VITAL SIGNS: T. 98.2° F. orally   P. 60 radial   R.15

B.P.: *Arm*   **Standing:**   *Right* 98/68/64   *Left* 98/68/62

Sitting: 102/72/68   106/70/66

Supine: 108/70/66   106/68/64

Leg   120/80/74

GENERAL:

Well-developed, well-nourished, young-looking adult. Articulate and pleasant. Ambulates without difficulty and is in no distress.

SKIN:

Uniformly pinkish white in color, soft, warm, moist, elastic. No edema, masses, or lesions. Occasional lentigos over anterior and posterior trunk. Hair is thick, brown, straight, and shoulder-length. Nails are firm. No clubbing, biting, or discolorations.

HEAD:

Cranium is normocephalic, with no tenderness. Scalp shows no lesions, lumps, scaling, or parasites. Face is symmetrical at rest and without edema. Alert and expressive.

EYES:

Visual Acuity: Snellen (no corrective lenses) R:20/20, L:20/25

Alignment: Corneal light reflex symmetrical; no strabismus.

Visual Fields: Full fields.

Extraocular Movements: Intact. No nystagmus.

Lids: No lid lag, edema, or crusting.

Lacrimal Apparatus: No tenderness, masses, or discharge.

Conjunctiva: Clear.

Cornea: No abrasions.

Sclera: White and without redness.

Anterior Chamber: No narrowing.

Irises: Uniformly blue.

Pupils: Equal and round. React to light and accommodation.

Lenses: No opacities.

Funduscopic: Red reflex elicited bilaterally. Disc margins sharp. A–V ratio 3:4. No A–V nicking, hemorrhages, exudate, or papilledema noted. Maculas unremarkable.

EARS:

Hearing: Hears whispered voice at 2 feet bilaterally. Weber—does not lateralize. Rinné—AC > BC bilaterally.

External Ear: No lesions, scaling, or tenderness bilaterally.

Otoscopic: Canals clear. Tympanic membranes—pearly gray; shiny light reflex; no redness, bulging, or retraction. Landmarks visible.

NOSE AND SINUSES:

Nasal septum midline. No tenderness with palpation. Mucosa moist, red, and without inflammation or lesions. Turbinates visualized. No polyps. Frontal and maxillary sinuses are without tenderness.

ORAL CAVITY:

No mouth odor. No lesions or bleeding of lips, gums, or tongue. Mucous membranes pink and moist. Teeth well aligned. No plaque or obvious decay. Tongue movement symmetrical. No swelling or lesions. Pharynx pink and without exudate. Tonsils present, without enlargement.

NECK:

No edema, masses, or tenderness. Trachea midline. Thyroid non-tender and not palpable. No lymphadenopathy.

CHEST:

Abdominal breathing. Respirations regular. No signs of labored breathing. Excursion symmetrical. A–P diameter within normal limits. Tactile fremitus equal bilaterally. No masses or tenderness. Lung fields resonant. Diaphragmatic excursion 3 cm. right side, 2 cm. left. Posterior thorax—vesicular breath sounds throughout. Anterior thorax—bronchovesicular breath sounds over bronchial tree, otherwise vesicular. No adventitious breath sounds.

CARDIAC AND PERIPHERAL VASCULAR:

Pulses: +3 and equal; elastic; regular rate and rhythm; of normal contour (see stick figure illustration).

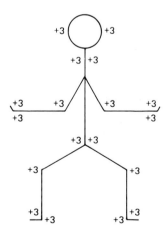

Cardiac: Apical pulse 60 and of regular rate and rhythm. No visible or palpable masses, abnormal pulsations, lifts, or heaves. No palpable pulsations in the epigastric area. PMI 2 cm. wide, palpable in the fifth ICS in the MCL and is a short sound synchronous with S_1. Percussion not done. S_1 is a single sound and is loudest at the apex; S_2 is loudest at the base and is split slightly with inspiration. No S_3, S_4, rubs, murmurs, or extra sounds heard.

Carotid Artery: No bruits auscultated.

Jugular Veins: External and internal jugular veins are elevated 2 cm. above the sternal angle with the head of the bed elevated 45°. The *a* wave is synchronous with S_1, as the *v* wave is with S_2.

BREASTS:

Symetrical, small. No scars, lesions, dimpling, masses, or tenderness bilaterally. Nipples everted. No discharge or crusting.

ABDOMEN:

Symmetrical. No protruberance. Strong muscle tone. No scars or striae. Bowel sounds audible in all four quadrants. No bruits over aorta or renal arteries. No masses or tenderness. Liver edge palpable, nontender. Span of 7 cm. at MCL. Spleen nontender or palpable. Kidneys not palpable, no CVA tenderness. Bladder not distended or tender. No inguinal, femoral, or umbilical hernias. Inguinal and femoral lymph nodes not palpable or tender.

GENITALIA:

External: Female hair distribution, no lesions. Introitus pink. Bartholin's and Skene's glands not palpable; no discharge from urethra.

Vagina: Mucosa pink, without lesions. Well rugated. No discharge. No cystocele or rectocele. Strong muscle tone.

Cervix: Pink, nulliparous os. Anterior, firm, mobile. No erosions, cysts, or lesions.

Uterus: Small, pear-shaped, firm. Anteflexed. No mases or tenderness.

Adnexae: Ovaries and tubes not palpable or tender.

Rectum: No lesions, rashes, hemorrhoids. Strong sphincter tone. No masses.

MUSCULOSKETAL:

Neck: Full range of motion without pain. Temporomandibular joint—no slipping or crepitation.

Back: Sits without slouching. No tenderness of vertebral column or paravertebral muscles. No deformity or curvature. Full extension, lateral bending, and rotation. Heights of shoulders and scapulae equal. No pain or discomfort with full ROM.

Extremities: Arms and legs symmetrical. Full ROM of all joints without pain, tenderness, or crepitation. No redness, swelling varicosities, or edema. Epitrochlear nodes not palpable. No muscle atrophy.

NEUROLOGIC:

Mental Status: Alert and oriented to time, person, and place. Can recall recent and past events. Able to name nationally elected officials. Able to interpret abstract thought—i.e., "Don't change horses in the middle of the stream."

Motor Function: Even, regular gait. Able to perform heel to toe walking. No ataxia. Finger grip strong bilaterally. Romberg—able to stand with eyes closed without falling. Able to hop, skip, and do deep-knee bends. Rapid alternating movements of finger to nose and heel sliding down shin done without difficulty. No tremor, tic, or fasciculations.

Sensory: Able to distinguish sharp from dull on face and extremities. Position—able to distinguish up and down movements of toes and fingers bilaterally.

Deep Tendon Reflexes: All intact, +2, symmetrical (see stick figure illustration).

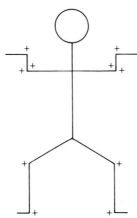

Cranial Nerves:
    I: Not done.
    II, III, IV, and VI: See *Eye.*
    V: Jaws strong, lateral movement intact. Sensation of face intact. See *Sensory.*
    VII: Smiles, wrinkles forehead, puffs cheeks, whistles. Symmetrical facial movements.
    VIII: See *Ear.*
    IX, X: Gag reflex present. Symmetrical rise of uvula and palate. Uvula midline.
    XI: Shoulders rise symmetrically in shrug of shoulders and able to resist push.
    XII: No asymmetry, fasciculations, or tremor of the tongue.

Index

Italicized page numbers refer to charts and figures.